SEQUOIA & KINGS CANYON

NATIONAL PARKS

YOUR COMPLETE HIKING GUIDE

Including Surrounding Lands in Golden Trout,
Jennie Lakes, John Muir, and Monarch Wildernesses
and Giant Sequoia National Monument

MIKE WHITE

 WILDERNESS PRESS ... *on the trail since 1967*

Sequoia and Kings Canyon National Parks: Your Complete Hiking Guide

1st EDITION 2012
   2nd printing 2017
This new edition is a compilation of Kings Canyon National Park *and* Sequoia National Park, *both published in 2004.*

Copyright © 2012 by Mike White

Front cover photos copyright © 2012 by Mike White
Interior photos, except where noted, by the author
Maps: Mike White and Scott McGrew
Cover design: Scott McGrew
Interior design and layout: Larry B. Van Dyke
Editor: Laura Shauger

ISBN 978-0-89997-672-3

Manufactured in the United States of America

Published by: **Wilderness Press**
　　　　　　　An imprint of AdventureKEEN
　　　　　　　2204 First Avenue South, Suite 102
　　　　　　　Birmingham, AL 35233
　　　　　　　(800) 443-7227
　　　　　　　info@wildernesspress.com
　　　　　　　www.wildernesspress.com

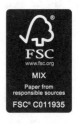

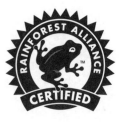

Visit our website for a complete listing of our books and for ordering information.

Distributed by Publishers Group West

Cover photos: Main: Hell-for-Sure Lake in John Muir Wilderness (Trips 86 and 87)
　　　　　　Top (inset): Redwood on Wolverton Cutoff Trail in the Giant Forest (Trip 30)

SAFETY NOTICE: Although Wilderness Press and the author have made every attempt to ensure that the information in this book is accurate at press time, they are not responsible for any loss, damage, injury, or inconvenience that may occur to anyone while using this book. You are responsible for your own safety and health while in the wilderness. The fact that a trail is described in this book does not mean that it will be safe for you. Be aware that trail conditions can change from day to day. Always check local conditions, know your own limitations, and consult a map.

Dedication

True friendship is a priceless treasure. For many, many years my wife and I have been abundantly blessed with the tremendously good fortune of knowing our dearest friends, Tic and Terrie Long. Together the four of us have shared dreams and heartaches, laughs and tears, adventures and mishaps, and triumphs and struggles. May God in his grace fill the rest of our days with many more moments together resulting in an even deeper friendship.

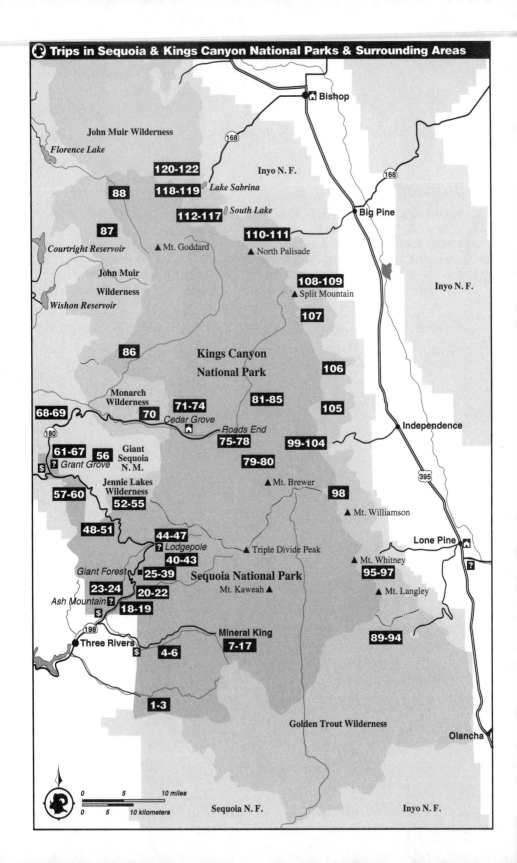

Contents

East Side Trips 305

BACKPACK TRIP FEATURES

Note: Time of year headings represent the average time in the season when trails become snow free. Times may vary from year to year depending on variables such as the amount of snowfall during the winter and the rate of snowmelt in the spring.

The scenery and solitude ratings listed for each trip are on a scale of 1 to 10, with 1 representing the most visited and least scenic.

WEST SIDE							
Trip Number and Name	Route	Scenery	Solitude	Difficulty	Days	Length (round-trip)	Elevation Gain/Loss
MARCH							
24. Colony Mill Road	↗	6	10	Ⓜ	2	16	+5,170'/-1,085'
LATE APRIL							
59. Redwood Mountain: Hart Trail	↻	8	7	Ⓜ	2	7.25	+2,065'/-2,065'
60. Redwood Mountain: Sugar Bowl	↻	8	7	Ⓜ	2	6.6	+2,130'/-2,130'
LATE MAY							
3. Garfield-Hockett Trail	↗	7	9	Ⓜ	2–4	20	+5,880'/-935'
31. Bearpaw Meadow	↗	7	5	Ⓜ	2–3	21	+4,085'/-3,155'
JUNE							
5. Atwell-Hockett Trail	↗	7	9	Ⓜ	2–4	20	+3,690'/-1,785'
MID-JUNE							
52. Stony Creek Trail	↗	7	8	Ⓢ	2	11.5	+2,875'/-405'
53. Jennie Lakes Loop	↻	7	7	Ⓜ	2–4	17.8	+4,135'/-4,135'
78. Sphinx Creek	↗	7	6	ⓂⓈ	2	12.4	+3,745'/-215'
LATE JUNE							
45. Twin Lakes	↗	7	5	Ⓜ	2–3	13.5	+3,030'/-285'
EARLY JULY							
8. Mosquito Lakes	↗	8	7	Ⓜ	2–3	6.5	+2,135'/-375'
9. Eagle Lake	↗	8	5	Ⓜ	2	6.5	+2,285'/-55'
10. White Chief Canyon	↗	8	6	Ⓢ	2–3	8	+2,360'/-150'
12. Franklin Lakes	↗	8	3	Ⓜ	2–3	11	+2,910'/-465'
17. Great Western Divide Loop	↻	7	8	Ⓜ	4–6	37.7	+13,175'/-13,175'

Trip Number and Name	Route	Scenery	Solitude	Difficulty	Days	Length (round-trip)	Elevation Gain/Loss
40. Mehrten and Alta Meadows	↗	8	5	M	2–3	11.8	+2,600'/-570'
54. Seville Lake	↗	7	9	M	2	13.2	+1,455'/-955'
71. East Kennedy Lake	↗	8	6	S	2–3	22	+7,280'/-1,690'
80. East Lake and Lake Reflection	↗	9	8	M	2–4	27	+5,420'/-410'
84. Copper Creek Trail to Granite Basin	↗	8	7	S	2–3	19	+5,735'/-685'
87. Red Mountain Basin	↗	9	8	M	3–5	30.5	+4,035'/-1,375'
MID-JULY							
13. Franklin Pass and Sawtooth Pass Loop	↻	9	5	S	3–5	27.5	+9,250'/-9,250'
14. Crystal Lake	↗	8	7	MS	2–3	7.5	+3,675'/-500'
16. Little Five and Big Five Lakes Loop	↻	9	8	M	3–5	26.5	+9,930'/-9,930'
31. Nine Lakes Basin	↗	10	7	M	3–5	42	+7,270'/-3,390'
32. High Sierra Trail: Crescent Meadow to Whitney Portal	╱	10	8	MS	8–14	62	+18,475'/-16,835'
41. Alta Peak	↗	10	6	S	2–3	13.4	+4,265'/-330'
43. Lakes Trail	↻	9	4	M	2–3	11.5	+2,795'/-535'
46. Kings-Kaweah Divide	↻	9	9	M	5–9	52	+14,100'/-14,100'
79. Circle of Solitude	↻	10	9	MS	5–10	68	+18,700'/-18,700'
81. Charlotte Lake	↗	8	5	M	2–3	29	+5,890'/-535'
83. Rae Lakes Loop	↻	10	2	MS	3–5	39	+7,500'/-7,500'
85. State and Horseshoe Lakes	↗	7	6	S	3–4	36	+7,735'/-2,275'
86. Middle Fork Kings River	╱	10	10	S	7–11	82.6	+15,950'/-14,025'
88. Martha Lake	↗	10	9	M	4–6	46	+4,830'/-1,175'

EAST SIDE

Trip Number and Name	Route	Scenery	Solitude	Difficulty	Days	Length (round-trip)	Elevation Gain/Loss
LATE JUNE							
108. Red Lake	↗	8	10	S	2–3	9	+4,200'/-1,065'
109. Birch Lake	↗	8	10	S	2–3	11	+4,615'/-300'
MID-JULY							
89. Chicken Spring Lake	↗	8	5	M	2	8.2	+1,400'/-90'
90. Cottonwood Pass and New Army Pass Loop	↻	8	7	M	2–4	19	+4,115'/-4,115'
91. New Army Pass Trail	↗	8	5	E	2–3	13	+1,650'/-215'
92. Cottonwood Lakes	↗	7	3	E	2–3	11.8	+1,450'/-300'
93. Soldier Lakes and Rock Creek	↗	8	8	M	2–4	29.2	+2,555'/-445'
94. Cottonwood Lakes to Whitney Portal	↗	10	5	MS	3–5	35	+8,070'/-9,805'
95. Mount Whitney	↗	10	1	S	2–3	21.4	+7,830'/-1,875'
96. Meysan Trail	↗	7	8	MS	2	10.2	+3,860'/-310'
97. John Muir Trail: Whitney Portal to Onion Valley	↗	10	2	MS	4–7	44.5	+15,250'/-13,250'
98. Shepherd Pass Trail	↗	7	9	S	3–5	25	+6,785'/-2,205'
99. Robinson Lake	↗	6	7	M	2	3	+1,340'/negligible
100. Kearsarge and Bullfrog Lakes	↙	8	4	M	2–3	14.4	+2,685'/-1,415'
101. Charlotte Lake and Rae Lakes Basin	↙	10	3	M	3–5	28.6	+4,050'/-2,685'
102. Trans-Sierra Trek: Onion Valley to Cedar Grove	↗	8	4	M	2–3	22.3	+2,845'/-4,140'
103. John Muir Trail: Onion Valley to South Lake	↗	10	4	MS	5–8	61.2	+17,260'/-14,535'
104. Golden Trout Lakes	↗	7	7	M	2	5	+2,295'/-80'
105. Baxter Pass Trail	↗	6	10	S	2–3	22	+6,650'/2,430'
106. Sawmill Pass Trail	↗	6	10	S	2–3	25	+7,325'/1,550'
107. Taboose Pass Trail	↗	8	10	S	2–4	23.5	+6,205'/1,065'
110. Brainerd and Finger Lakes	↗	10	6	S	2–3	10	+3,740'/-700'

Trip Number and Name	Route	Scenery	Solitude	Difficulty	Days	Length (round-trip)	Elevation Gain/Loss
111. Big Pine Lakes	↻	10	4	M	2–4	12.5	+3,170'/-3,170'
112. Long, Saddlerock, and Bishop Lakes	↗	8	3	M	2–3	8.4	+1,740'/-260'
113. Dusy Basin and Le Conte Canyon	↗	10	4	M	3–5	26	+2,585'/-3,680'
114. John Muir Trail: South Lake to North Lake	↗	10	7	MS	5–8	55.1	+10,580'/-11,150'
115. Chocolate Lakes Loop	↻	7	6	M	2–3	7.2	+1,690'/-1,690'
116. Treasure Lakes	↗	6	7	M	2	8	+1,765'/-450'
117. Tyee Lakes	↗	5	7	M	2	8	+2,560'/-25'
118. Sabrina Basin	↗	9	4	M	2–4	14	+2,860'/-680'
119. George Lake	↗	4	8	M	2	6.6	+2,025'/-170'
120. Lamarck Lakes	↗	8	6	M	2–3	6	+1,700'/-50'
121. Evolution Basin via Lamarck Col	↗	10	6	M	3–5	21	+4,510'/1,600'
122. Piute Pass Trail to Humphreys Basin and Piute Canyon	↗	9	5	MS	3–5	34	+2,600'/-3,800'

DAYHIKE TRIP FEATURES

Note: Time of year headings represent the average point in the season when trails become snow free. Times may vary from year to year depending on variables such as the amount of snowfall during the winter and the rate of snowmelt in the spring.

The scenery and solitude ratings listed for each trip are on a scale of 1 to 10, with 1 representing the most visited and least scenic.

WEST SIDE							
Trip Number and Name	Route	Scenery	Solitude	Difficulty	Length (round-trip)	Elevation Gain/Loss	
ALL YEAR							
1. Putnam and Snowslide Canyons	↗	6	9	M	6.8	+2,690'/-460'	
2. Ladybug Camp and Cedar Creek	↗	5	9	M	5.6	+1,880'/-325'	
18. Potwisha Pictographs Loop	↺	5	6	E	0.5	+205'/-205'	
19. Marble Falls	↗	6	6	M	6.6	+1,750'/-295'	
20. Middle Fork Kaweah River: Hospital Rock to Potwisha	↗	6	8	E	2.4	+345'/-935'	
21. Paradise Creek Trail	↗	6	8	M	4.6	+975'/-280'	
22. Middle Fork Kaweah River: Hospital Rock to Panther Creek	↙	6	8	M	5.5	+1,325'/-935'	
23. North Fork Trail	↗	5	9	M	8.4	+1,415'/-555'	
MARCH							
24. Colony Mill Road: North Fork to Colony Mill Ranger Station	↗	6	10	M	16	+5,170'/-1,085'	
EARLY APRIL							
44. Tokopah Falls	↗	8	3	E	3.8	+700'/-40'	
LATE APRIL							
29. High Sierra Trail: Crescent Meadow to Panther Creek	↗	7	5	M	5.4	+850'/-800'	
EARLY MAY TO MID-MAY							
25. Colony Mill Road: Crystal Cave Road to Colony Mill Ranger Station	↙	6	10	M	4	+865'/-245'	
27. Bobcat Point Loop	↺	7	8	E	1.25	+255'/-255'	
30. Giant Forest East Loop	↺	8	7	M	8.5	+2,370'/-2,370'	
34. Sunset Rock	↗	6	3	E	1.6	+215'/-115'	

Trip Number and Name	Route	Scenery	Solitude	Difficulty	Length (round-trip)	Elevation Gain/Loss
35. Big Trees Trail	↻	7	1	E	1	Negligible
36. Hazelwood Nature Trail	↻	7	2	E	0.5	Negligible
37. Trail of the Sequoias	↻	8	6	M	6.1	+1,325'/-1,325'
38. Circle Meadow Loop	↻	8	6	E	3.8	+675'/-675'
39. Congress Trail	↻	8	1	E	3.1	+550'/-550'
50. Lost Grove to Dorst Campground	↗	6	6	E	2.3	+555'/-545'
51. Cabin Creek Trail	↗	5	8	E	0.8	+165'/-120'
59. Redwood Mountain Grove: Hart Trail Loop	↻	7	7	M	7.25	+2,065'/-2,065'
60. Redwood Mountain Grove: Sugar Bowl Loop	↻	7	7	M	6.6	+2,130'/-2,130'
66. General Grant Tree Trail	↻	8	1	E	0.5	+100'/-100'
70. Deer Cove Trail	↗	5	9	M	6.8	+2,720'/-620'
73. Cedar Grove Overlook	↗	6	6	MS	4.8	+1,525'/-115'
74. Hotel and Lewis Creeks Loop	↻	7	7	MS	6.4	1,970'/-2,090'
75. Zumwalt Meadow Nature Trail	↻	6	2	E	1.5	Negligible
76. River Trail	↗	5	3	E	2.5	+35'/-225'
77. Kanawyer Loop Trail	↻	6	3	E	4.7	+265'/-265'
82. Mist Falls	↗	7	4	M	7.8	+765'/negligible
LATE MAY						
3. Garfield-Hockett Trail to Garfield Creek	↗	5	10	M	10	+4,150'/-200'
4. East Fork Grove	↗	5	9	M	5	+525'/-820'
7. Cold Springs Trail	↗	6	6	E	1.2	+350'/-20'
33. Moro Rock Loop	↻	8	5	M	4.4	+1,475'/-1,475'
58. Buena Vista Peak	↗	7	4	E	2	+975'/-445'
61. Big Stump Grove	↻	6	5	E	2	+325'/-325'

Trip Number and Name	Route	Scenery	Solitude	Difficulty	Length (round-trip)	Elevation Gain/Loss
62. Hitchcock Meadow	↗	5	7	E	1.2	+20'/-290'
63. Sunset Loop	↻	6	6	M	5.75	+1,885'/-1,885'
65. North Grove Loop	↻	6	7	E	1.5	+355'/-355'
67. Park Ridge Lookout	↻	8	5	E	5.6	+1,430'/-1,430'
68. Chicago Stump	↗	7	9	E	0.6	Negligible
69. Boole Tree	↻	7	9	E	2.25	+740'/-740'
EARLY JUNE						
26. Huckleberry Meadow Loop	↻	6	6	E	3.75	+840'/-840'
28. Crescent and Log Meadows Loop	↻	7	5	E	2.2	+435'/-435'
48. Little Baldy	↗	7	4	M	3.5	+735'/-85'
49. Muir Grove	↗	8	7	M	4.2	+530'/-515'
56. Evans Grove	↗	6	10	M	4	+595'/-920'
57. Big Baldy	↗	7	6	M	4.4	+975'/-445'
72. Don Cecil Trail to Lookout Peak	↗	8	7	MS	10	+4,000'/-225'
MID-JUNE						
6. Paradise Peak	↗	7	9	M	10	+2,990'/-185'
52. Stony Creek Trail to Jennie Lake	↗	7	8	S	11.5	+2,875'/-405'
64. Azalea and Manzanita Trails Loop	↻	6	6	M	4.6	+1,200'/-1,200'
78. Sphinx Creek	↗	7	6	MS	12.4	+3,745'/-215'
LATE JUNE						
45. Twin Lakes	↗	7	5	M	13.5	+3,030'/285'
47. Wuksachi Trail	↗	5	8	M	3	+220'/-430'
EARLY JULY						
8. Mosquito Lakes	↗	8	7	M	6.5	+2,135'/-375'
9. Eagle Lake	↗	8	5	M	6.5	+2,285'/-55'
10. White Chief Canyon	↗	8	7	M	7.5	+2,360'/-150'

Trip Number and Name	Route	Scenery	Solitude	Difficulty	Length (round-trip)	Elevation Gain/Loss
12. Franklin Lakes	↗	8	3	MS	11	+2,910'/-465'
40. Mehrten and Alta Meadows	↗	8	5	M	11.8	+2,600'/-570'
41. Alta Peak	↗	10	6	S	13.4	+4,265'/-330'
42. Panther Gap Loop	↻	8	5	M	7	+1,720'/-1,720'
54. Seville Lake	↗	7	9	M	13.2	+1,455'/-955'
55. Mitchell Peak	↗	8	9	M	6.5	+2,090'/-365'
MID-JULY						
11. Farewell Gap	↗	8	7	M	11	+3,320'/-455'
14. Crystal Lake	↗	8	7	MS	7.5	+3,675'/-500'
15. Monarch Lakes	↗	7	5	M	6.5	+2,740'/-200'
43. Lakes Trail	↻	9	4	M	11.5	+2,795'/-535'

EAST SIDE

Trip Number and Name	Route	Scenery	Solitude	Difficulty	Length (round-trip)	Elevation Gain/Loss
LATE JUNE						
108. Red Lake	↗	8	10	S	9	+4,200'/-1,065'
109. Birch Lake	↗	8	10	S	11	+4,615'/-300'
EARLY JULY						
115. Chocolate Lakes Loop	↻	7	6	M	7.2	+1,690'/-1,690'
116. Treasure Lakes	↗	6	7	M	8	+1,765'/-450'
MID-JULY						
89. Chicken Spring Lake	↗	8	5	M	8.2	+1,400'/-90'
91. New Army Pass Trail	↗	8	5	E	13	+1,650'/-215'
92. Cottonwood Lakes	↗	7	3	E	11.8	+1,450'/-295'
95. Mount Whitney	↗	10	1	S	21.4	+7,830'/-1,875'
96. Meysan Trail	↗	7	8	MS	10.2	+3,860'/-310'
99. Robinson Lake	↗	7	7	M	3	+1,330'/negligible
100. Kearsarge and Bullfrog Lakes	↗	8	5	M	14.4	+2,685'/-1,415'
102. Trans-Sierra Trek: Onion Valley to Cedar Grove	↗	8	5	MS	22.3	+2,845'/-4,140'
104. Golden Trout Lakes	↗	7	7	M	5	+2,295'/-80'
110. Brainerd and Finger Lakes	↗	10	6	S	10	+3,740'/-700'
111. Big Pine Lakes	↻	10	4	M	12.5	+3,170'/-3,170'
112. Long, Saddlerock, and Bishop Lakes	↗	8	2	M	8.4	+1,740'/-260'
117. Tyee Lakes	↗	5	7	M	8	+2,520'/negligible
118. Sabrina Basin	↗	9	4	M	14	+2,860'/-680'
119. George Lake	↗	4	8	M	6.6	+2,025'/-170'
120. Lamarck Lakes	↗	8	6	M	6	+1,700'/-50'
122. Piute Pass Trail to Humphreys Basin	↗	9	5	M	14	+2,175'/-450'
LATE JULY						
121. Evolution Basin via Lamarck Col	↗	10	6	M	21	+4,510'/-1,600'

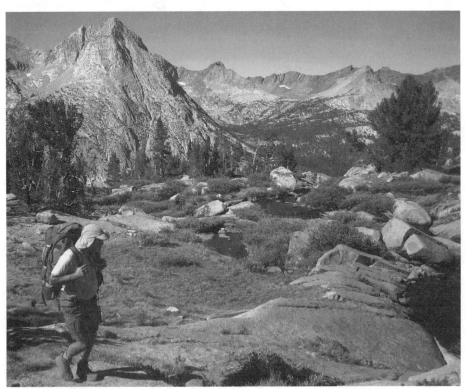

Darwin Creek (Trip 121)

Preface

The first editions of this guide were published as two books in 2004, one for each of the two parks. For this edition, we have combined the two books into one, primarily because the two parks, even though they have two names and encompass two geographic areas, are managed as one unit. Publishing one guide produces a fairly hefty, but more seamless treatise on the heart of the High Sierra. Besides, most backpackers do not carry an entire guidebook in their packs anyway, since they can photocopy the sections specific to a particular trip.

The near-record winter of 2010–2011 and subsequent late-arriving summer drastically shortened the 2011 backpacking season. Consequently, I was unable to complete as much fieldwork as I would have preferred, although I have made every attempt to ensure that all the information in the second edition is as up to date as possible. If you discover errors, please bring them to the attention of Wilderness Press.

The greater Sequoia-Kings Canyon region remains one of my most favorite destinations for dayhiking, backpacking, and climbing. May this guide help you to discover the incomparable riches of the Range of Light.

Thanks to the Creator for the majesty of creation and specifically for the wonder and beauty of the High Sierra. My gratitude also goes to my wife, Robin, without whom none of my projects would gain any traction. Having solo hiked much of the Sequoia and Kings Canyon backcountry, I have been fortunate to have company on many trips and would like to thank fellow travelers Stephen White, Carmel Bang, Tic Long, Andy Montessoro, Bob Redding, Chris Taylor, Dal and Candy Hunter, Lisa Kafchinsky, Art Barkely, Joe Tavares, Kim Small, Darrin Munson, Keith Catlin, and Jerry Hapgood.

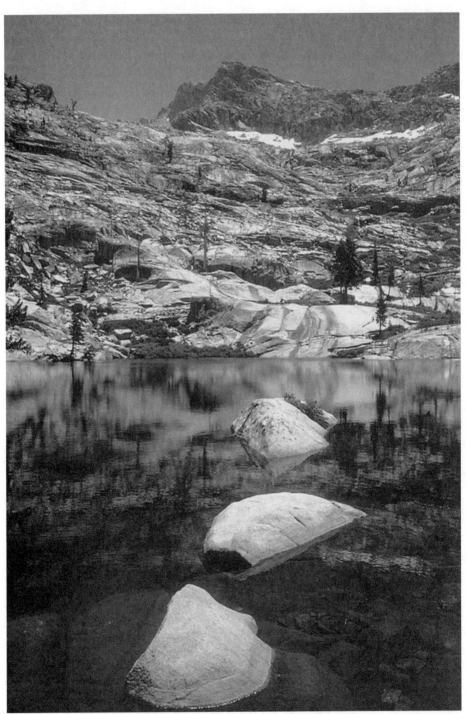

Emerald Lake on the Lakes Trail (Trip 43)

Introduction

To stand atop a craggy peak and gaze through the clear blue skies of the High Sierra across the sparkling granite landscape of the Sequoia and Kings Canyon backcountry is a truly rapturous and transcendent experience. A similar stirring is found at the base of a cinnamon-colored giant sequoia, one's face warmed while gazing skyward by the few rays of dappled sunlight that reach the forest floor through a towering canopy of massive limbs holding feathery green foliage. Gaze upon the rushing and turbulent waters of a wild river coursing through a canyon of vertical rock rising thousands of feet above and you're likely to experience the same emotions that swept over John Muir when he first saw Kings Canyon and later declared this chasm to be "a rival to Yosemite."

Human History

People have been interacting with the greater Sequoia and Kings Canyon area for centuries. Their influence on the land has been an important element of the evolution of the parks, the surrounding wilderness, and the frontcountry.

Native Americans and Early Settlement

The Native Americans who resided in the Sequoia and Kings Canyon region have been divided into four separate tribes—the Monache, Tubatulabal, Owens Valley Paiute, and Yokut. These four groups traveled extensively within the region, hunting, trading, and establishing summer camps. Several sites within the parks provide evidence of some of these settlements, with Hospital Rock in Sequoia perhaps the most visited by modern-day tourists.

Early European-American explorers, such as Jedediah Smith and John C. Frémont, tended to avoid the rugged, high mountains of the High Sierra in favor of more easily negotiated terrain to the north and south. Dissuaded by the difficult topog-

raphy, early explorers knew little about the area until settlers in the San Joaquin Valley began venturing into the mountains in the mid-1850s.

Hale D. Tharp, a rancher from the Three Rivers area, was perhaps the first Caucasian to see the sequoias in the Giant Forest. At the invitation of some friendly Potwisha in 1856, Tharp headed east toward the mountains to see the rumored Big Trees and to scout a summer range for his livestock. He followed the Middle Fork Kaweah River upstream to Moro Rock and then climbed up to Log Meadow. A couple of years later, he retraced his route to the Giant Forest, continued north into the Kings River drainage, and then returned to his ranch by way of the East and South Forks of the Kaweah. Subsequently, Tharp grazed his cattle each summer in Log Meadow, using a fallen and burned out sequoia as a makeshift cabin.

Increasing settlement in the San Joaquin Valley ultimately spelled doom for the Native Americans, as exposure to various diseases decimated their populations. Surviving members of the four tribes either traversed the Sierra to the less desirable high desert on the east side of the range or remained on the west side and attempted to adapt to the white man's culture. Additional pressure was placed on the Native American population when an even greater number of Euro-Americans settled in the area, lured by the prospects of gold, lumber, and fertile ranchland.

Exploitation of Resources

Much to the disappointment of the hordes of miners seeking their fortune, the southern Sierra proved to be a major bust in the search for precious metals. Mineral King, perhaps the preeminent site in the region, was imagined to be the area's equivalent to Sutter's Mill in the northern Sierra. However, the site never produced a commercially viable quantity of either gold or silver.

Lumbermen turned out to be as equally disillusioned as their mining counterparts. The discovery of the giant sequoia wetted the appetites of entrepreneurs who anticipated enormous profits from milling lumber from such gigantic trees. Unfortunately for the lumbermen, the sequoia wood proved to be too brittle for most construction purposes. Fortunately for the species, the labor-intensive effort required to fell the big trees turned out to be a commercially unviable enterprise. The mills never made much of a profit—some even lost money—and most of the sequoia wood was used for fence posts or shakes. Sadly, many lumber companies failed to realize the relatively poor quality of sequoia lumber until after entire groves were destroyed. Converse Basin, one of the finest stands of big trees, witnessed the destruction of every significant sequoia save one—the Boole Tree, which turned out to be the eighth-largest sequoia in the world.

Unlike mining and lumbering, cattle and sheep grazing in the San Joaquin Valley was fairly profitable, which ultimately produced a growing competition among ranchers for rangeland. In order to feed their herds and flocks properly, ranchers and sheepherders searched farther and farther afield for green pastures, inflicting extensive environmental damage on the meadows on the west side of the southern Sierra. Fires, set by the ranch-

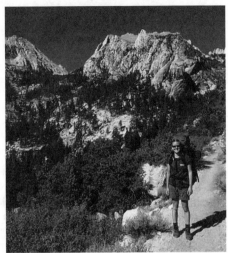

Hiker on the Mt. Whitney Trail (Trip 95)

ers and sheepherders to clear pastures and create passage, ran unchecked throughout the range. Thousands of hooves trampled sensitive meadows each season. The resulting erosion produced by the combination of spreading fires and trampling stock created inevitable watershed degradation.

California Geographical Survey

While the ranchers and loggers were investigating the natural resources of the area, the California Geographical Survey, under the leadership of Josiah D. Whitney, began exploring the High Sierra. The survey's charge was to ascend the high peaks to obtain precise measurements that would enable accurate mapping of this previously uncharted region. As part of the 1864 survey, William H. Brewer led Clarence King, Richard D. Cotter, James T. Gardiner, and Charles F. Hoffman from Visalia to a base camp at Big Meadow. Proceeding east into the high mountains, the party climbed and named Mt. Silliman along Silliman Crest and Mt. Brewer on the Great Western Divide.

From a campsite near Mt. Brewer, King and Cotter left the others behind to make a multiday attempt on Mt. Whitney. Although failing to reach the range's highest summit, the pair did scale 14,048-foot Mt. Tyndall, a mere six miles northwest. Following the climb, the party regrouped near Mt. Brewer and returned to Big Meadow.

Undeterred by the failed attempt on Mt. Whitney, King tried again, leading a small party from Three Rivers up the recently constructed Hockett Trail to Kern River. After following the river north for several miles, they veered away toward the big peak. Ultimately, their summit bid fell short by 300 to 400 vertical feet.

Following the second failed attempt, King join the resupplied and expanded survey party at Big Meadow in order to explore the Kings River area, which they would compare favorably to Yosemite Valley. After exploring the South and Middle Forks, and the Monarch Divide separating the two gorges, the party traveled upstream along Bubbs Creek and over the Sierra Crest at Kearsarge Pass, before descending to Fort Independence in Owens Valley.

From Independence, the group journeyed north through Owens Valley, eventually crossing back over the Sierra Crest at Mono Pass before establishing a base camp at Vermillion Valley (currently under the waters of Lake Edison). Although the exact route is undetermined, the survey headed south toward Le Conte Divide, from where Cotter, and a soldier named Spratt, made a 36-hour assault on Mt. Goddard, turning back about 300 feet below the summit. Returning to Vermillion Valley after yet another failed summit bid, the party headed north to Wawona, concluding the survey for the year. The California Geographical Survey made a more limited expedition along the east side of the range in 1870, before disbanding in 1874.

Despite failing to reach the summits of Mt. Whitney and Mt. Goddard, the Brewer Party was the first group of explorers to develop a significant understanding of the topography, botany, and geology of the High Sierra. In addition to scientific findings, the survey named several significant features, including Mt. Whitney, the highest summit in the continental United States.

Seeds of Preservation

Over his lifetime, John Muir made nine separate excursions into the backcountry of Sequoia and Kings Canyon, ultimately increasing public awareness of the beauty and majesty of the region as a whole and of the giant sequoias in particular. Over time, an increasing number of concerned citizens joined Muir to champion the cause of protecting the unique character of the region. These citizens included George W. Stewart, the youthful city editor of one of Visalia's newspapers. Eventually, national and international figures lent their voices to the idea of setting aside this area as parkland.

As ranching and farming increased in the San Joaquin Valley, so rose the demand for water for irrigation. Watershed degradation from mining, logging, and grazing in the southern Sierra conflicted with the agricultural needs of the ranchers and farmers downstream. Concern over water issues, combined with a growing preservationist ethic, created increased opposition to the unmitigated consumption of the area's natural resources and the environmental destruction of the landscape.

The first official step toward the establishment of a national park in the region occurred in 1880, when Theodore Wagner,

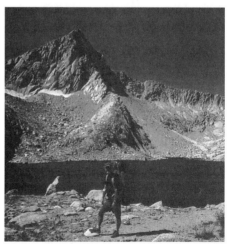

Backpacker near Columbine Lake, Sawtooth Pass Trail (Trip 13)

US Surveyor General for California, suspended four square miles of Grant Grove, prohibiting anyone from filing a land claim. Unfortunately, a 160-acre claim had already been filed adjacent to the area (Wilsonia remains in private hands to the present day). Although little progress toward preservation was made in subsequent years, the seeds of a grand idea had been planted.

The Kaweah Colony

A group of socialist utopians from San Francisco created one of the more colorful chapters in the history of the region. Armed with a big dream, a heady dose of gumption, and a limited supply of capital, thirty-some members of the Cooperative Land and Colonization Association filed claims on nearly 6,000 acres of prime timberland within the Giant Forest. As a means of funding their utopian society, the colonists planned to build a road from Three Rivers to a proposed mill near their timber claims to harvest timber and mill it for sale.

Controversy swirled around the legality of the colonists' land claims, which became an ongoing dilemma. Despite the brewing controversy, nearly 160 colonists were camped along the North Kaweah River in 1886, ready to begin construction on their wagon road. Idealism and optimism reigned within the colony, as they successfully built the road over the following four years. Despite using only hand tools, the quality of construction and the grade of the road were remarkable. Coaxing a steam tractor named Ajax to a saddle at the end of the road, the colonists erected a portable sawmill. However, a variety of complications prohibited them from fully realizing their dream, including inexperience, internal squabbles, insufficient funds, and an inability to secure full title to their land claims. By 1892 the dream ended and the remaining trustees officially dissolved the colony.

Although the utopian dream of the Kaweah Colony was short-lived, their road had a much longer life. Eventually extended from Colony Mill to the Giant Forest by

the US Army, the road was opened to one-way traffic in 1903, serving as the principal access to Sequoia for the next few decades.

Creation of Sequoia and General Grant National Parks

While the Kaweah colonists were busy with the construction of their road, political winds had shifted unfavorably in Washington, DC, as a more development-friendly Department of Interior assumed power. In 1889, the General Land Office reopened for private sale several townships west of Mineral King, which alarmed George W. Stewart and others sympathetic toward preserving this area. The tract offered for sale included Garfield Grove, one of the finest giant sequoia groves in the southern Sierra, along with expansive Hockett Meadows. In response to this threat, Stewart vigorously courted public opinion and successfully maneuvered through political channels to pass a bill on September 25, 1890, setting aside 76 square miles of Sierra forest as a public park.

Mystery shrouds the next step in the process of setting aside Sequoia and Kings Canyon National Parks. Unbeknownst to Stewart and his associates, another bill came before Congress a mere six days after passage of the bill for Sequoia, establishing Yosemite as a national park. Attached to the Yosemite measure was the addition of five townships to Sequoia, including the area around the Giant Forest and four sections surrounding Grant Grove. No one knows for certain who was behind the bill's additions, or how the size increased by more than five hundred percent from the original proposal. However, on October 1, 1890, Yosemite and General Grant National Parks were born and Sequoia National Park was greatly enlarged. Speculation points toward Daniel K. Zumwalt, a Southern Pacific Railroad agent, as the man behind the bill, but his motivation remains unclear.

Management of the new parks became problematic quite quickly. By the following spring, Captain Joseph H. Dorst and the Fourth Cavalry had the unenviable task of protection, although the mission for the new national parks was ill defined. They spent most of that first summer dealing with the Kaweah colonists, who had rather unjustly been denied their claims in the Giant Forest. A small contingent of the colonists resurfaced near Mineral King to log sequoias for the leased Atwell Mill. The government initially took issue with the project, harassing the colonists for much of the summer, but eventually acquiescing after determining the mill was located on private land and was a perfectly legal operation. However, the colonists proved to be inexperienced and failed to turn a profit. By the time the lease came up for renewal the following year, the colony had disbanded. During the remainder of the summer and into autumn, Dorst and his men explored the parks, dealing with problems of logging, grazing, and squatting.

Stewart, Muir, and others continued their push to place more lands under federal protection. As a result, in 1893, President William Henry Harrison signed a presidential proclamation creating the Sierra Forest Reserve, which removed most of the central and southern Sierra from private sale. The preserve was reclassified as Sequoia

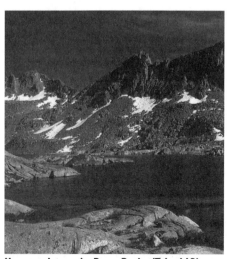

Unnamed tarn in Dusy Basin (Trip 113)

National Forest in 1905, placing the area under the jurisdiction of the Department of Agriculture, which was more concerned with resource management than preservation. During the first part of the 20th century, the idea of a large national park for the southern Sierra still had life, but very little progress was made toward that goal.

The military continued their minimally successful attempt at protecting the parks until 1914, when Walter Fry became the first civilian superintendent of General Grant and Sequoia National Parks. By then the Colony Mill Road had been extended into the Giant Forest. Also, the Mt. Whitney Power Company had constructed several hydroelectric power plants on branches of the Kaweah River. Aside from these improvements, most of the area was still virtually untouched by any form of development. Ongoing cattle grazing, private inholdings, lack of access, and poor facilities plagued Fry's administration.

The Reign of the National Park Service

In 1916 Congress created the National Park Service, with Californian Stephen T. Mather appointed as the first director. Mather was quite familiar with the Sequoia region, having organized an expedition of notable persons to traverse the range in 1915. Armed with firsthand knowledge, along with a Park Service mandate for conservation and enjoyment of the parks, Mather ushered in a new era of park management.

Mather was given two mandates for Sequoia—acquisition of private lands inside the park and expansion of the park's boundary to include the High Sierra and Kings Canyon. Acquiring private inholdings was a fairly easy proposition compared to park enlargement, which drew staunch opposition from nearly every quarter, including ranchers, hunters, and Mineral King property owners. Additional opponents included the Los Angeles Bureau of Power and Light and San Joaquin Light and Power Company, which hoped to build hydroelectric dams at

Cedar Grove and Tehipite Valley. Even the Forest Service joined the opposition, reluctant to give up lands currently under its control with mineral, timber, and grazing potential. A scaled-down proposal to expand the park was passed in 1926, incorporating lands east over the Sierra Crest, but omitting Mineral King and Kings Canyon.

The Generals Highway, from Ash Mountain to the Giant Forest, opened in 1926, replacing the old Colony Mill Road. Nine years later the road was extended to Grant Grove. Easier access, combined with America's growing fascination with the private automobile, led to a dramatic rise in park visitation, which in turn sparked a need for new and expanded facilities. In addition to improving roads and utilities, an extensive network of trails was built (including sections of the John Muir and High Sierra Trails), campgrounds were improved, a number of government and public structures were erected, and a concession monopoly was granted. Completion of a road from Grant Grove to Kings Canyon accelerated development of campgrounds along the South Fork Kings River, but more significant projects were put on hold until the question of hydroelectric dams was settled.

Initially, the park improvements seemed to be a good and necessary way to accommodate the growing number of visitors. However, as both visitation and development continued to increase, ills such as traffic jams, congestion, and overcrowding began to characterize the Giant Forest and, to a slightly lesser extent, Grant Grove. Environmental concerns created by a meteoric rise in tourists and rampant development provided a real threat to the long-term health of the park, particularly the sequoia groves.

Additional management concerns surfaced with threats to vegetation and wildlife. Fire suppression was the rule of the day, allowing a dangerous buildup of fuels that could produce potentially disastrous forest fires. The previous ban on stock grazing was lifted, throwing open the door to severe environmental damage to meadows and

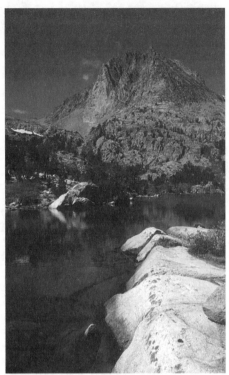

Two Eagle Peak and Fifth Lake, Big Pine Lakes (Trip 111)

other vegetation. Wildlife management suffered similar setbacks. The last grizzly bear in California was shot during the 1920s near Horse Corral Meadow. Increased conflicts between humans and black bears put "problem" bears at risk. The evening garbage feast at Bear Hill (Sequoia's garbage dump), where marauding bears put on a show for tourists, was emblematic of the times.

A philosophical shift occurred when Colonel John R. White became park superintendent from 1920 to 1938 and 1941 to 1947. He made visible efforts to reduce the effects of excessive visitation at the Giant Forest, placing limits on future development and moving many of the government facilities to other areas of the park. Unfortunately, he had little impact on limiting the number of concessionaires. Perhaps his greatest accomplishment was in defeating several proposed roads into the Sequoia backcountry, including two trans-Sierra links, one from Cedar Grove to Independence, and another between Porterville and Lone Pine. Colonel White also squelched the notion of the Sierra Way, a mountain highway that would have connected Yosemite and Sequoia, with a link between the Giant Forest and Mineral King through Redwood Meadow.

The Creation of Kings Canyon National Park

While management confronted issues of overcrowding at the Giant Forest, the fight to preserve Kings Canyon escalated. In 1935, Interior Secretary Harold Ickes proposed the creation of Kings Canyon National Park, most of which should be managed as wilderness. Opposition came from four distinct groups. San Joaquin Valley business professionals saw extensive commercial potential in Kings Canyon. The Forest Service favored a multiuse approach and was once again reluctant to relinquish authority over currently held lands. Central Valley ranchers were concerned about possible reductions in irrigation water. Power companies maintained their interest in building hydroelectric dams on both the South and Middle Forks of the Kings River.

Compromises were eventually made to secure passage of a national park bill for Kings Canyon, most notably the exclusion of Cedar Grove and Tehipite Valley, which pacified the commercial and power interests. Ranchers were assuaged by a promise to build a dam for irrigation storage at Pine Flat Reservoir. After some political intrigue between two local congressional representatives, President Franklin D. Roosevelt signed the bill establishing Kings Canyon National Park on March 4, 1940. Along with a vast area of wilderness, the new park included the old General Grant National Park and Redwood Mountain. Kings Canyon and Tehipite Valley were added to the park in 1965, eliminating the possibility of dams on the South Fork and Middle Fork Kings River.

The Battle for Mineral King

Following the establishment of Kings Canyon National Park, controversy over Mineral King began to swirl. Responding to the demands from the public for more recreational facilities, in 1949 the multiuse-oriented Forest Service sought proposals from private developers for a ski resort at Mineral King. No suitable developer with the necessary capital was found until the Walt Disney Company was awarded a temporary permit in 1966. Disney's proposal included a large-scale Swiss village, with two hotels, 14 ski lifts, and parking for 3,600 vehicles. The Sierra Club deemed the small subalpine valley unsuitable for such a large-scale development, initiating a series of legal battles to thwart the project and obtaining a restraining order in 1969.

The Sierra Club tied up Disney in the courts long enough for public opinion to turn against the proposed resort. Another strike against Disney occurred when California withdrew its proposal to construct a new state highway from Three Rivers to Mineral King, requiring potential developers to come up with several million more dollars for construction, as well as having the responsibility of acquiring all the necessary permits for a route crossing both state and federal lands. As the public's awareness of environmental concerns grew, Disney began to lose the public relations battle, putting the proposed development in serious jeopardy. On November 10, 1978, President Jimmy Carter signed into law the Omnibus Parks Bill, which, in part, added Mineral King to Sequoia National Park, permanently ending the notion of a ski area in the lovely valley.

Recent History

The post–World War II era was characterized by increased visitation, improvements to infrastructure, and the advancement of scientific research for the purposes of determining park policy. The Park Service instituted steps to protect the sequoias in the Giant Forest by reducing development. By

1972, campsites, picnic areas, and most structures were removed and relocated to less sensitive areas. The visitor center was moved to Lodgepole, and the gas station and maintenance facilities were moved to Red Fir.

Nearly twenty-five more years would be necessary before the Park Service finally resolved the problem of commercialism at the Giant Forest. Following the 1996 season, the historic Giant Forest Lodge was permanently closed, replaced by a new lodge at Wuksachi. Two years later, the commercial buildings had been removed, with four exceptions. The old market was renovated and remodeled into the Giant Forest Museum, which opened in 2001. Additional improvements at the Giant Forest included trails, interpretive displays, and new parking areas. A free shuttle bus system was instituted in 2004 in an attempt to reduce traffic on the nearby roads.

Cedar Grove eventually saw limited commercial development in 1978, when a lodge with 18 motel rooms, a snack bar, and general store was built—a small-scale fulfillment of the vision once held by the San Joaquin Valley's business professionals from so many years before. Construction of the John Muir Lodge has increased the number of overnight accommodations at Grant Grove, which never really suffered the extent of problems of overdevelopment experienced at the Giant Forest.

Wilderness and Backcountry Issues

Since 1984, nearly 90 percent of Sequoia and Kings Canyon has been managed as wilderness. Combined with the adjacent Forest Service wildernesses, a vast stretch of the southern Sierra remains wild. After decades of some neglect, the Park Service developed backcountry regulations and policies to prevent severe overuse and restore environmental health. By 1972, backcountry permits and quotas were in place to forestall the crush of backpackers in the more popular areas of the parks and surrounding wilderness areas. They put camping bans and stay limits in place for areas of severe overuse and banned campfires above certain elevations. In addition, rangers from both the Park Service and Forest Service began a campaign to educate visitors about wilderness ethics. More recently, both services began requiring the use of bear lockers and canisters in heavily used areas and strongly suggesting their use in others.

Sequoia and Kings Canyon have faced many challenges and undoubtedly await more trials in the future. Although visitation is below the peak levels experienced during the late '80s and early '90s, managing hundreds of thousands of visitors per year can be a daunting task. Even more difficult is dealing with consequences produced beyond the park's borders, such as air pollution from heavily populated urban areas of western California, which creeps into the Sierra and threatens animal and plant life (including giant sequoia seedlings), reduces visibility, and produces acid rain. Illegal marijuana cultivation plagues remote areas in the western foothills and promises to be an ongoing dilemma because of a lack of personnel and proper funding to deal with the situation. Fortunately, backpackers will experience few, if any, of these problems while on the trail, with perhaps the notable exception of securing a wilderness permit.

Flora and Fauna

Encompassing the change in elevation from near the floor of the San Joaquin Valley to Mt. Whitney, the Sequoia and Kings Canyon region of the southern Sierra supports a diverse cross section of plant and animal life within several distinct communities. The following general divisions should not be viewed as definitive descriptions. Consult the bibliography for additional resources on plants and animals in the Sierra Nevada.

The Foothills

Plant Life: The western fringe of Sequoia National Park includes the Sierra foothills, a low-elevation zone extending from the edge of the San Joaquin Valley east to elevations between 4,500 and 5,000 feet. The foothills plant community is characterized by a Mediterranean climate, with mild temperatures, winter rain, and dry summers. Average rainfall varies from as little as 10 inches per year in the lowlands to as much as 40 inches per year in the upper elevations. Much of the vegetation may appear parched and dry throughout much of the year, but following the rainy season, the hills come alive with a vibrant carpet of green, sprinkled with a brilliant display of wildflowers.

Grasslands cover the lower slopes of the foothills, as they rise from the broad plain of the Central Valley. Nonnative grasses have mostly overtaken the native species. Periods of drought, coupled with severe overgrazing in previous centuries, have favored the invasive European annual grasses over the native species.

Diverse woodlands alternate with chaparral on the higher slopes east of the grasslands. Generally, woodland occupies shady slopes where the soil is damp, while chaparral flourishes on dry and sunny slopes. Foothills woodland is characterized by savannalike growth of trees and grasses, including oaks (blue, live, valley, and canyon), California buckeye, laurel, and redbud.

Dry, rocky slopes in the foothills are typically carpeted with chaparral, a tangle of shrubs that includes chamise (greasewood), manzanita, ceanothus, buckeye, flowering ash, mountain mahogany, and California coffeeberry. Fire plays an important role in the chaparral community, regularly burning areas every 10 to 40 years.

Although the foothills zone is generally considered to be a dry environment, rivers, streams, and creeks flow through the area, transporting meltwater from the High Sierra toward the thirsty valley below. A varied plant community thrives along these watercourses, well-watered by the plentiful moisture. Cottonwood, willow, alder, oak,

POISON OAK

Poison oak is found in both the foothills woodland and chaparral communities. As the saying goes, "leaves of three, let it be." Poison oak leaves typically grow in groups of three; they are bronze and shiny in spring, green in summer, and scarlet in fall. The leaves usually fall off the plant prior to winter. Poison oak may grow as a creeping plant, erect shrub, or even a small tree under the right conditions. All parts of the poison oak plant, including branches, stems, leaves, and even roots, contain the oil urushiol, which is the causal agent for the rash that may develop after contact. Even a microscopic drop of urushiol is enough to trigger a reaction in people sensitive to the oil. The toxin may penetrate the skin within less than 10 minutes after being exposed to it.

Upon contact, immediately wash your skin or attempt to absorb the oil with dirt. Touching clothing that has come in contact with the plant is oftentimes just as potent as direct contact. Wash contaminated clothing in soap and hot water as soon as possible. If a rash develops, treat the affected area with hydrocortisone cream. For severe reactions, consult a physician.

laurel, and sycamore are common streamside associates.

Animal Life: The mild, Mediterranean climate of the foothills region is hospitable to a wide variety of creatures. Common woodland amphibians include three varieties of salamander and the California newt. Several varieties of lizards can often be seen scurrying across the trail. Snakes are quite common in this zone as well, with the western rattlesnake receiving the most attention from humans.

Several varieties of rodents find a home in the foothills, including gray squirrel, dusky-footed wood rat, and deer mouse. Rabbit species include the brush rabbit, black-tailed jackrabbit, and Audubon's cottontail. Bats can often be seen around dusk, as they flit through the sky searching for insects. Medium-size mammals, such as the raccoon, ringtail, gray fox, skunk, and coyote are familiar residents. Larger mammals in the foothills include mule deer and two reclusive cats, the bobcat and mountain lion.

Numerous birds can be found in the foothills—far too many for a casual list of even the common species. Familiar raptors include the red-tailed hawk, golden eagle, American kestrel, and great horned owl. The California quail is the most common game bird. The turkey vulture, the ubiquitous buzzard of the California sky, is also common.

Montane Forest

Plant Life: Above the foothills region, a zone of mixed coniferous forest, composed of conifers and deciduous trees, extends across the west slope of the southern Sierra roughly between 4,500 and 7,500 feet. The two most dominant conifers are the three-needled ponderosa pine *(Pinus ponderosa)* and the white fir *(Abies concolor)*. Generally, ponderosas are found in relatively dry areas, while white firs occupy soils with more moisture. Mature ponderosas can obtain heights between 60 and 130 feet.

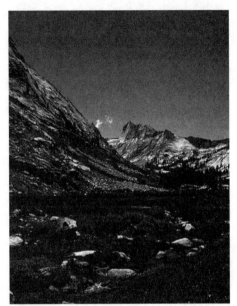

Ranger Meadow, Deadman Canyon Trail (Trip 46)

At higher elevations in the zone, Jeffrey pines replaces ponderosa pines. Closely related to the ponderosa pine, Jeffrey pines are more adaptable to the colder temperatures and increased snowfall of the upper limits of the montane forest. A host of other evergreens may intermix with these conifers, most commonly incense cedar and sugar pine. Some of the more common deciduous trees include dogwood and black oak.

On the east side of the range, in the rain shadow below the Sierra Crest, the montane forest is found between elevations of 7,000 and 9,000 feet. Stands are typically less dense and less diverse than in their western counterpart. The forest is composed primarily of Jeffrey pine and white fir.

As expected, streamside environments within the montane forest harbor many more species of trees, shrubs, and plants. On the west side, quaking aspen, black cottonwood, bigleaf maple, nutmeg, laurel, Oregon ash, and numerous varieties of willow line the banks of rivers and streams. Riparian zones on the eastside are home to quaking aspen, Fremont cottonwood, black cottonwood, and water birch.

Animal Life: The esantina salamander, western toad, and Pacific tree frog are the three most commonly seen amphibians in the montane zone. Reptiles include a wide variety of lizards and snakes, including the western rattlesnake, which is common up to around 6,000 feet. A wide variety of birds, including songbirds, woodpeckers, and raptors live in this zone.

Similar to the foothills, the montane forest is home to many rodents, including the broad-handed mole, Trowbridge shrew, deer mouse, pocket gopher, northern flying squirrel, chipmunk, and dusky-footed wood rat. Bats also frequent the evening sky above the montane forest. In addition to the medium and large mammals of the foothills zone, the porcupine and long-tailed weasel and black bear also reside in the montane forest.

Weighing up to 300 pounds, the black bear *(Ursus americanus)* is the largest mammal in the Sierra and ranges from cinnamon to black in color. A female typically gives birth to two cubs every other winter. She cares for her offspring through the summer and following winter, before forcing them to fend for themselves the following spring. Male bears do not participate in raising the cubs, and would possibly kill and eat them if the mother did not fiercely protect them.

Giant Sequoia Groves

Plant Life: The giant sequoia *(Sequoiadendron gigantean)* sets the Sierra Nevada apart from all other forests in the world. When Europeans first reported trees of such stature, their claims were largely discounted by virtually all who had not seen them firsthand. A few of these "Big Trees" were chopped down, cut into pieces, and sent to expositions, where they were carefully reassembled, only to be viewed as hoaxes by an unbelieving public. Few could comprehend that a living tree could attain such enormous size. Unfortunately, when lumbermen caught wind of the Big Trees, they turned a lustful gaze toward the stately monarchs. Only after hundreds of sequoias were felled, did the lumbermen realize the brittle wood had little commercial value, good for nothing more than fence posts and shakes (shingles). Only after conservationists waged an arduous battle lasting many decades did the giant sequoias receive the appropriate protection. Today, the Big Trees are safe and secure in three national parks, a national monument, and a handful of state parks.

Not only is the giant sequoia the largest species of tree by volume on the planet, the statuesque conifer lives within only 75 groves on the west side of the Sierra Nevada. All but eight of these groves are found within the greater Sequoia and Kings Canyon ecosystem. The largest groves are Redwood Mountain in Kings Canyon National Park and the Giant Forest in Sequoia National Park. Most of the largest individual specimens are also found within this area, with the General Sherman Tree receiving top honors, followed by Washington, General Grant, President, and Lincoln—all five within the park boundaries.

Giant sequoias may reach heights between 150 and 300 feet, with widths between 5 and 30 feet. The trees have cinnamon-colored bark with deep furrows. For such a huge tree, the oblong cones are rather small at 2 to 3 inches. Limbs on mature trees are oftentimes as big as the trunks of other conifers, bearing branches of lacy, flat, blue-green foliage.

Rather than pure stands, the giant sequoia grows in a mixed coniferous forest made up of white fir, sugar pine, incense cedar, and dogwood. Somewhat less drought tolerant than other Sierra conifers, the Big Trees are found only in areas of moist soil at elevations between 4,500 and 8,400 feet. Average yearly precipitation in sequoia groves varies between 45 and 60 inches, but the soil's ability to hold moisture throughout the typically dry summers is perhaps more important to the sequoia's long-term survival.

Although the sequoia has an extensive root system, the roots are generally shallow in relation to their immense size. Most mature trees meet their ultimate demise, not

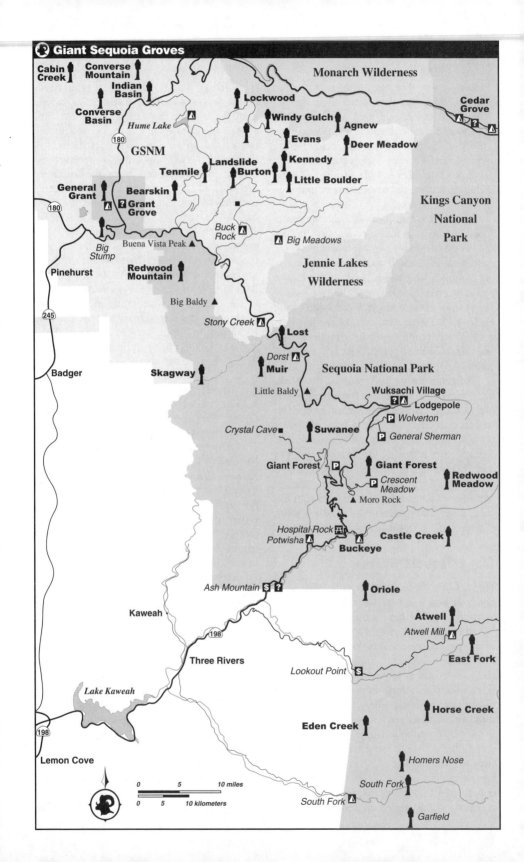

from the more common maladies of forest fire, disease, or insect infestation but from simply toppling over.

Thick bark makes the sequoia highly resistant to both insects and fire. Typically, the only insult a forest fire leaves on a giant sequoia is a black scar on the lower trunk. Forest fires help giant sequoias propagate. Their small cones require extreme heat in order to open and release their oatmeal-size seeds. Fire also clears the forest floor, making way for the tiny sequoia seedlings and minimizing competition with other plants for moisture and light. Although fire suppression was the rule of the past for park and forest management, modern-day foresters use controlled burns in sequoia groves and elsewhere in the forest to restore this natural process and reduce the accumulation of fuels that could produce unnaturally intense wildfires.

Animal Life: The animals in giant sequoia groves are similar to those found in the montane forest.

Red Fir Forest

Plant Life: Unlike the mixture of trees in the montane forest, the stately red fir is often the sole species in the climax forest on the west slope of the Sierra. Growing to heights between 60 and 130 feet, red fir is quite susceptible to lightning strikes. Mature specimens are between 2 and 4 feet wide, with maroon-brown bark with red furrows. Their branches sweep down and curve up at the end, bearing short, blue-green needles and 5- to 8-inch long cones.

The tall trees often form such dense cover that competitors and understory plants cannot survive—any plant that does grow in the red-fir zone must be shade tolerant. Where red-fir stands are less dense, associates may include lodgepole pine, western white pine, Jeffrey pine, western juniper, and quaking aspen (one small stand of mountain hemlock occurs in this zone in Sequoia National Park). White fir oftentimes intermingles with red fir along the lower end of this zone.

IDENTIFYING RED AND WHITE FIRS

The easiest way to differentiate a white fir from a red fir, which are similar in appearance, is by examining a tree's bark. The bark on a mature red fir is maroon-brown, while white fir has grayish bark. Also, the slightly longer needles of the white fir are twisted at the base and have white lines; the shorter red fir needles are four-sided and not twisted.

Red fir prefers deep, well-drained soil and is found in the southern Sierra roughly between 7,000 and 9,000 feet, from Kern County northward. The species thrives in areas receiving the greatest amount or precipitation, usually in the form of winter snowfall.

Animal Life: Inhabitants of the higher elevations of the upper forest zones must adapt to more severe weather conditions and periodically scarce food supplies. Common amphibians in the red fir forest are limited to two varieties each of salamanders, frogs, and toads. Reptiles include the garter snake and three types of lizard.

Ordinary small mammals you might encounter in this zone include the deer mouse, pocket gopher, vole, shrew, broadhanded mole, pika, chipmunk, chickaree, Belding ground squirrel, golden-mantled ground squirrel, northern flying squirrel, beaver, white-tailed jackrabbit, and yellow-bellied marmot. Bats are commonly seen around lakes and meadows in the evening. Medium-size animals include the red fox, porcupine, coyote, long-tailed weasel, fisher, ermine, wolverine, badger, and pine marten. The Sierra bighorn sheep lives in this zone but is very reclusive. Black bear and mule deer are the most common large mammals.

Mule deer *(Odocoileus hemionus)* are quite numerous in the southern Sierra, since their main predators, the grizzly bear and the wolf, are now extinct in California.

Mountain lions are their most common predators today. Starvation and disease are the most common causes of death for mule deer. Mature males may exceed 200 pounds. Each March, males shed their antlers and start to regrow them again in April.

Although not as numerous as in the lower zones, a vast number of birds find a home in the upper forest belt. Among some of the more interesting species are the blue grouse, dipper, and mountain bluebird. The most common (and occasionally obnoxious) bird known to backpackers is the Steller's jay, whose bold exploits to snatch human food has earned it the nickname "camp robber."

Lodgepole Pine Forest

Plant Life: Perhaps no tree is more closely associated with the High Sierra than the lodgepole pine. Found between 8,000 and 11,000 feet in the southern Sierra, this versatile conifer with pale gray bark flourishes in soils where red fir struggles because the soil is either too wet or too dry. In stark contrast to the red fir, which is almost exclusively found in California, the two-needled lodgepole pine is one of the most widespread trees in the American West. Typically tall and thin, they reach heights of 50 to 100 feet, and their cones are 1 to 2 inches long.

Although commonly found in exclusive stands, the lodgepole also intermingles with western white pine and whitebark pine in the higher elevations and red fir in the lower elevations. Quaking aspen and lodgepole oftentimes grow together in areas that have plentiful groundwater. On the east side of the range, lodgepole pines are common between 9,000 and 11,000 feet, where the western white pine is the most common associate.

Animal Life: Animals found in the lodgepole pine forest are similar to those found in the red fir forest.

Subalpine Zone

Plant Life: Roughly occurring between 9,500 and 12,000 feet, the subalpine zone straddles the Sierra Crest and bridges the gap between the mighty forest of the lower elevations and the austere realm above timberline.

The most common conifer in this zone is the interesting foxtail pine, with its characteristic pendulous branches. This five-needled pine is similar in appearance to the bristlecone pine. The foxtail pine grows only in Inyo and Tulare Counties in the southern Sierra and in the Klamath Mountains of northern California. Mature specimens reach heights between 20 and 45 feet, and they bear purplish, prickly cones 2 to 5 inches long. Foxtail pines occasionally can be found in pure stands along the eastern fringe of Sequoia National Park and along the Kern River. The most common associate is the majestic whitebark pine, an oftentimes multitrunked tree that survives the harsh conditions just below timberline, sometimes in the form of a windblown shrub. Less common associates include western white, lodgepole, and limber pines.

Forests are but one part of the diverse subalpine zone. Mountain lakes, craggy peaks, and granite-covered slopes are common features of the subalpine landscape,

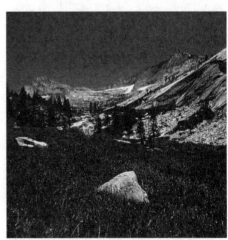

Meadow on the Lone Pine Creek Trail (Trip 14)

as are numerous grass-and-sedge-covered meadows harboring a vast array of midsummer wildflowers.

Animal Life: Animals found in the subalpine zone are similar to those found in the red fir forest.

Alpine Zone

Plant Life: The alpine zone occurs at the highest elevations in the Sierra, where the growing season is measured in weeks rather than months. Harsh conditions characterize this zone, with lower temperatures and cloudier skies allowing snow to linger longer than in other zones, despite the fact that the alpine zone receives less snowfall. At elevations above 12,000 feet, frost can occur at any time during the summer, and cool temperatures, nearly constant winds, and a significant lack of precipitation produce desertlike conditions. Generally poor, granitic soils further limit the number of species able to adapt to this harsh climate.

Most alpine plants have successfully adapted to their environment by developing a low-growing, compact, and drought-tolerant form, which allows them to avoid the full brunt of the wind, grow closer to the warmth of the soil, and survive on low amounts of moisture. Most alpine plants are perennial, using less energy than annuals, which must produce an entirely new plant each season. Vegetation in the alpine zone can be divided into two classifications: alpine meadow and alpine rock.

Alpine meadows are common in the upper realm of the Sierra where a sufficient layer of moist soil is present. Meadows are generally composed of grasses and sedges, with alpine sedge and common sedge the most common. A wide array of wildflowers put on a showy, colorful display over the course of an abbreviated summer, capitalizing on the greater amount of available moisture. Among them is Sierra primrose, an alpine wildflower preferring moist, rocky soils with reddish blossoms on a 1- to 4-inch stem. There are a limited variety of shrubs,

including alpine willow, snow willow, laurel, and heather, in small groupings.

Vegetation grows in small patches in the alpine rock community, unlike the large swaths of foliage in alpine meadows. Open gravel flats and scree areas produce a smattering of alpine plants. The protected microclimates found in boulder fields are oftentimes more suited to the survival of a diverse group of plants; wildflowers are most common, but a few shrubs grow here as well.

Animal Life: Aside from insects and invertebrates, few animals find a permanent home in the rarified alpine zone, where both food and shelter are in short supply. The only common residents are the heather vole, marmot, and pika. Yellow-bellied marmots often sunbathe on the tops of boulders. These usually chubby beasts have brown backs, dull yellow undersides, with white around their eyes and a dark band above their nose. They utter a sharp whistle when alarmed, which accounts for the common name of "whistle pig."

Sierra bighorn sheep may venture into these heights during the summer, but they generally prefer areas at or below timberline. Similarly, black bears make occasional appearances in the alpine zone but are much more common in the lower elevations. Although many different species of birds frequent the alpine zone, only the rosy finch is as common here as it is in the upper forest zones.

Pinyon-Juniper Woodland

Plant Life: On the east side of the range and in the rain shadow of the Sierra Nevada, between roughly 6,000 and 9,000 feet, is the pinyon-juniper woodland. Typically, this zone receives a mere 5 to 15 inches of precipitation per year, most of which falls as winter snow, with the rest coming from random summer thunderstorms. This zone is composed primarily of widely scattered singleleaf pinyon pine (*Pinus monophylla*), with Sierra juniper and curl-leaf mountain mahogany as its two most common

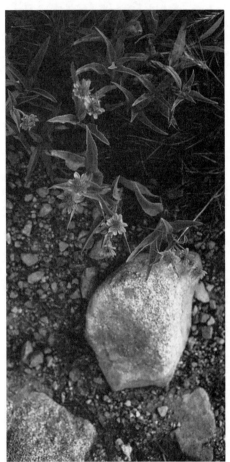

Wildflowers near Golden Trout Lake (Trip 104)

to the area immediately outside the riparian zone. Quaking aspen, cottonwood, willow, oak, birch, and ash are common streamside trees, which may intermix with conifers from the forest zones above. Currant, wild rose, and a variety of willows are typical riparian shrubs.

Animal Life: A wide variety of amphibians, reptiles, birds such as the sage grouse and red-tailed hawk, and insects find a home in the pinyon-juniper woodland, as do an assortment of mammals. Small mammals, including several species of mice, squirrel, vole, rabbit, shrew, and chipmunk are quite common. Larger mammals, such as the coyote, skunk, badger, and mule deer, are familiar residents as well. Coyotes *(Canas latrans)* subsist as omnivores on a wide-ranging diet. Their whelps and howls are commonly heard after sundown.

Sagebrush Scrub

Plant Life: Fortunately, only a few east side trails pass through the extremely hot and dry conditions found in the sagebrush scrub zone. This zone receives less than 12 inches of precipitation per year, most of which falls during the winter months. Occasionally, a welcome thunderstorm waters the parched ground and produces the characteristically pungent aroma of wet sagebrush.

At first glance, the gray-green sagebrush creates a seemingly unbroken band of vegetation across the lower foothills above Owens Valley. However, closer inspection reveals a diverse flora, including a mixture of bitterbrush, rabbitbrush, desert peach, and spiny hopsage interspersed within the sagebrush. Before native perennial grasses were overgrazed and replaced by invasive annuals, a healthy mixture of bunchgrasses filled the sagebrush scrub zone. After uncommonly wet winters and springs, the high desert produces a vivid display of wildflowers from late spring into early summer.

Animal Life: Animals found in the sagebrush scrub zone are similar to those found in the pinyon-juniper woodland zone.

associates. Trees in this zone often grow in the form of large shrubs, although the pinyon can reach between 20 and 25 feet in height with spherical cones 1.5 to 2 inches long. Something of a gourmet item today, the seeds were a staple of the Paiute tribe's diet. Sagebrush, rabbitbrush, and bitterbrush commonly make up this zone's understory.

Spring and early summer may bring a colorful display of wildflowers, including drought-tolerant species like paintbrush, lupine, and mules ears, to the woodland.

Along the banks of eastern Sierra streams in this zone, a dense display of wildflowers, shrubs, and trees flourish in stark contrast

Geology

Although the origins of the Sequoia and Kings Canyon regions are somewhat speculative, geologists have determined the composition of the rock forming the area's soaring peaks and deep canyons. Even a cursory examination by the untrained eye reveals granite to be the overwhelming rock type in the High Sierra. These light-colored, salt-and-pepper speckled, coarse-grained rocks include granite, granodiorite, and tonalite (formerly referred to as quartz diorite). These rocks also contain varying amounts of minerals such as quartz, feldspar, biotite, and hornblende.

The Sierra Nevada Batholith, a term geologists use to describe the massive pluton of rock forming the range stretching 300 miles in length and 50 miles in width, was formerly a band of molten magma below the earth's surface. The magma eventually cooled and crystallized, and was subsequently uplifted and exposed to form the Sierra Nevada as we know them today.

A much smaller percentage of rock in the Sierra is metamorphic. Typically dark in color and variegated in appearance, metamorphic rocks are considered older than the much more common granitic rocks. Remnants of these rocks are scattered across the Sequoia and Kings Canyon region, and four distinct metamorphic terranes have been identified. A number of caves, including Crystal Cave near the Giant Forest and Boyden Cave near Kings Canyon, were discovered in concentrations of marble, a type of metamorphic rock.

An even smaller percentage of the region's geologic composition includes volcanic rock. Within park boundaries, this rock type is nearly nonexistent, the lone exception being a very old volcanic intrusion near Windy Peak along the Middle Fork Kings River. Smatterings of other volcanic activity are evident in small pockets west of Kings Canyon and southeast of Sequoia near Golden Trout Creek. The most noticeable evidence of volcanism in the area occurs east of Kings Canyon National Park in the Big Pine Volcanic Field, where passing motorists on US Highway 395 can easily see cinder cones and lava flows.

The Sequoia and Kings Canyon area is home to some of North America's most impressive canyons. Modern geologists recognize the importance of both erosion and glaciation in the formation of these canyons. In the lower elevations, the erosive power of water is clearly evident, resulting in V-shaped canyons, such as the lower South Fork and Middle Fork Kings River. The characteristic U-shaped canyons cut by former glaciers are found in the higher elevations.

Speculation on the role of glaciers in the sculpting of the upper canyons of the Sierra Nevada is as old as John Muir himself, who proposed the notion back in the late 1800s. Whatever the extent of their importance in the past, today's glaciers occupy a very small percentage of territory in the

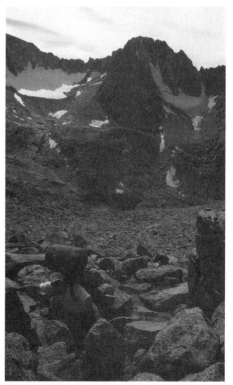

Negotiating talus on the Lamarck Col cross-country route (Trip 121)

uppermost realm of the High Sierra (usually above 12,000 feet on the north and east faces of the highest peaks). Despite their lack of size, these remaining glaciers add a touch of alpine beauty to these otherwise rocky mountains, The largest glacier in the Sierra is Palisade Glacier, a pocket of ice less than one square mile in size.

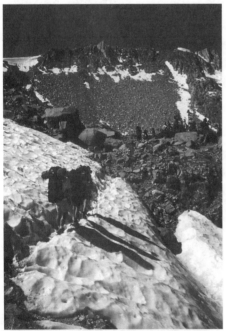

Backpackers negotiate the snow-covered trail on the way to Bishop Pass (Trip 103)

Climate

The Sierra Nevada experiences a wide range of weather within the four seasons, which greatly affects the recreational opportunities for exploring this majestic landscape.

Summer

Most visitors to Sequoia and Kings Canyon National Parks and surrounding wilderness areas come to the region during the summer months. Compared to many other North American mountain ranges, the Sierra Nevada is typically blessed with an abundance of mild, dry, and sunny weather. Summers are particularly fine, as 95 percent of the annual precipitation falls between November and March. Occasional summer thunderstorms account for the remainder, but they occur with much less regularity than in the Rocky Mountains, for instance. Summer temperatures are generally mild. However, they vary considerably from the foothills to the alpine heights.

When the snow has mostly melted in the highest parts of the Sierra, backpacking season begins in earnest. Warm weather usually persists in the High Sierra from mid-July into September. Although summers in the Sierra usually bring dry, sunny days, thunderstorms are not uncommon, particularly in the month of July, requiring backpackers to be prepared for fickle weather conditions. Usually thunderstorms resolve fairly quickly, but infrequent monsoonal storms lasting two to three days or longer are not completely out of the question. Afternoon highs during summer often creep up into the high 60s and low 70s in the high country, although the temperature may actually feel much warmer due to the increased solar radiation prevalent at higher altitudes. July is also when the mosquito population explodes, with a peak usually lasting over a two-week period. If you plan a trip for July, be sure to pack plenty of repellent and bring a tent.

Early to mid-August is the prime time for backpacking because thunderstorms are less common, a major frontal system is unlikely to affect the area, and the mosquito population has abated to a more manageable level. Lakes in the High Sierra, although rarely warm, are not as cold as earlier in the summer, offering refreshing opportunities for an enjoyable swim. Late August into early September brings less daylight, pleasant but slightly cooler temperatures, and far fewer mosquitoes. By then, the wildflower season has passed its peak and the meadows have started to dry out, but fewer people are on the trails.

Autumn

Pleasant Indian summer conditions generally continue for another month or so beyond the middle of September, but the reliably good weather usually comes to an end, at least in the upper elevations, by late October. Days are considerably shorter and temperatures noticeably cooler, especially at night. Backpackers should carry plenty of warm clothing and bring a multiseason tent instead of a lightweight one. By sometime in November of most years, the Sierra has experienced its first significant snowfall of the season, prompting most recreationists to think about winter pursuits. Autumn can be a fine time to enjoy the lower elevation trails and footpaths on the west side of the range. Fall is a pleasant season for hiking in the foothills, after the extreme summer heat has abated and the autumn foliage is at peak color.

Winter

The mountains of the Sierra Nevada usually receive a significant amount of precipitation during the winter. Except for the foothills, most of that precipitation falls in the form of snow, when cold Pacific storms may dump substantial amounts of the white stuff during the height of winter. However, significant winter snowfall is not always guaranteed in the southern Sierra since the

region experiences periods of drought from time to time. Nevertheless, below freezing temperatures, high winds, and a lack of daylight even in dry years tend to discourage all but the intrepid few from backcountry pursuits during the winter months.

Most winter visitors to the park stay overnight at Grant Grove or Wuksachi Village and then cross-country ski or snowshoe during the day. Even fewer ski or snowshoe from Wolverton to stay overnight at the Pear Lake Ski Hut. For diehard hikers, winter can be a good time to visit the foothills because the trails usually stay snow-free throughout the year.

Spring

Late March and April may see extremely variable weather conditions: fair and mild in some years or an extension of winter in others. During periods of stable weather and with slightly longer days, the High Sierra is a perennial favorite among backcountry skiers, many of whom attempt multiday, trans-Sierra treks.

During the spring, the low elevations found in the foothills produce conditions quite favorable to off-season hiking. Although fall is a good time for hiking in the foothills, spring is perhaps the best time because the High Sierra is still cloaked in winter's mantle, the foothills are green from winter rains, the wildflowers are in bloom, and the deciduous trees are leafing out.

Above the foothills, snow-free hiking isn't available typically until later in May, after the highway into Kings Canyon has been opened and the trails in the Giant Forest and Grant Grove are no longer covered with snow. Once the spring thaw is underway, the snow line marches steadily up the mountainsides, opening more and more trails along the way. By June, most west-side paths are accessible into the Sequoia and Kings Canyon frontcountry, but the High Sierra usually remains snowbound until early to mid-July.

Average Precipitation and Temperatures in the Foothills

MONTH	PRECIPITATION (inches [cm])	MAXIMUM (°F [°C])	MINIMUM (°F [°C])
January	4.7 (11.9)	57 (14)	36 (2)
February	4.3 (10.9)	61 (16)	39 (4)
March	4.8 (12.2)	64 (18)	41 (5)
April	1.8 (4.6)	70 (21)	46 (8)
May	0.8 (2.0)	79 (26)	52 (11)
June	0.3 (0.8)	89 (32)	61 (16)
July	0.1 (0.3)	97 (36)	68 (20)
August	0.06 (0.2)	96 (36)	67 (20)
September	0.1 (0.3)	91 (33)	52 (11)
October	1.2 (3.0)	80 (27)	43 (6)
November	2.7 (6.9)	67 (19)	37 (3)
December	3.0 (7.6)	62 (28)	36 (2)

Average Precipitation and Temperatures in the Giant Forest

MONTH	PRECIPITATION (inches [cm])	MAXIMUM (°F [°C])	MINIMUM (°F [°C])
January	7.32 (18.6)	41.2 (5.1)	23.2 (-4.9)
February	8.02 (20.4)	43.5 (6.4)	23.8 (-4.6)
March	6.63 (16.8)	47.6 (8.7)	25.6 (-3.6)
April	4.75 (12.1)	52.8 (11.6)	30.1 (-1.1)
May	1.78 (4.5)	59.0 (15)	35.9 (2.2)
June	0.42 (1.1)	67.5 (19.7)	43.6 (6.4)
July	0.11 (0.3)	77.2 (25.1)	51.3 (10.7)
August	0.17 (0.4)	76.8 (24.9)	49.9 (9.9)
September	0.44 (1.1)	72.4 (22.4)	45.2 (7.3)
October	1.54 (3.9)	61.7 (16.5)	38.1 (3.4)
November	4.11 (10.4)	49.9 (9.9)	30.4 (-0.9)
December	8.0 (20.3)	42.8 (6.0)	26.1 (-3.3)

Traveling in the Backcountry

Recreating in the greater Sequoia and Kings Canyon region may present some significant challenges. The following information will help make your journey a pleasant one.

Fees

Entrance fees are collected at the Ash Mountain Entrance Station (where Highway 198 becomes the Generals Highway), the Lookout Point Entrance Station on Mineral King Road, and the Big Stump Entrance Station on Highway 180. If you enter the parks at an unmanned station, be prepared to pay the appropriate fee upon exiting.

TYPE OF PASS	FEE	DURATION	TERMS
Weekly Pass	$20 per vehicle	7 days	Access to Sequoia and Kings Canyon
Annual Pass	$30 per vehicle	1 year	Access to Sequoia and Kings Canyon
America the Beautiful (interagency pass)	$80	1 year	Access to all federal recreation sites, including national parks, national forests, and FWS, BLM, and Bureau of Reclamation lands
Senior America the Beautiful	$10 (62 or over)	Lifetime	Access to all federal recreation sites, including national parks, national forests, and FWS, BLM, and Bureau of Reclamation lands

About the Parks and Surrounding Forest Service Lands

Tourist-related facilities in Sequoia and Kings Canyon are not as developed or concentrated as those in the more popular Yosemite Valley to the north. However, visitors should find an adequate range of services.

Information

Sequoia and Kings Canyon National Parks
47050 Generals Highway
Three Rivers, CA 93271
559-565-3341
www.nps.gov/seki

Inyo National Forest
351 Pacu Lane, Suite 200
Bishop, CA 93514
760-873-2400
www.fs.usda.gov/inyo

Sequoia National Forest
1839 South Newcomb Street
Porterville, CA 93257
559-781-4744
www.fs.usda.gov/sequoia

Sierra National Forest
1600 Tollhouse Road
Clovis, CA 93611
559-297-0706
www.fs.usda.gov/sierra

Park Service Ranger Stations and Visitor Centers

Mineral King Ranger Station
Open daily 7 a.m.–4 p.m.,
June to mid-September.
Books, maps, first-aid supplies, and wilderness permits.

Ash Mountain Visitor Center
559-565-4212
Open daily 8 a.m.–6 p.m. through
early September, then 8 a.m.–4:30 p.m.
Exhibits, books, maps, bear canisters,
first-aid supplies, wilderness permits,
and a pay phone.

Giant Forest Museum
559-565-4480
Open daily 9 a.m.–7 p.m.
Exhibits, books, maps, and first-aid
supplies.

Lodgepole Visitor Center
559-565-4436
Open daily 7 a.m.–5 p.m.
Movies, exhibits, books, maps, first-
aid supplies, wilderness permits, a pay
phone, and Crystal Cave tickets.

Kings Canyon Visitor Center
(Grant Grove)
559-565-4307
Open daily 8 a.m.–6 p.m. through early
September, then 8 a.m.–5 p.m.
Movie, exhibits, books, maps, first-aid
supplies, bear canisters, wilderness permits, and a pay phone.

Cedar Grove Visitor Center
559-565-3793
Open daily 9 a.m.–5 p.m.,
May through early September.
Books, maps, first-aid supplies, bear
canisters, and a pay phone.

Roads End Wilderness Permit Station
Open daily 7 a.m.–3 p.m.,
May through late September.
Maps, bear canisters, and wilderness
permits.

West Side Forest Service
District Ranger Stations

Sierra National Forest
High Sierra Ranger District
29688 Auberry Road
P.O. Box 559
Prather, CA 93651
559-855-5355

Sequoia National Forest
Hume Lake Ranger District
35860 East Kings Canyon Road
Dunlap, CA 93621
559-338-2251

Inyo National Forest
Eastern Sierra Interagency
Visitor Center
Junction of US Highway 395
and State Route 136
Lone Pine, CA 93545
760-876-6222;

White Mountain Ranger District
798 North Main Street
Bishop, CA 93514
760-873-2500

Lodging

A variety of overnight accommodations are
available inside the parks, although reservations are highly recommended during peak
summer season. Some of the parks' facilities remain open year-round. Communities
surrounding the parks, including Fresno,
Visalia, and Three Rivers on the west side
and Lone Pine, Independence, Big Pine, and
Bishop on the east side, offer additional
lodging options.

Mineral King (Silver City)

Silver City Resort
Open late May to November.
559-561-3223 (summer)
559-734-4109 (winter)
reservations@silvercityresort.com
www.silvercityresort.com

Lodgepole Area

Wuksachi Village
(Delaware North Companies)
Open all year.
www.visitsequoia.com

Bearpaw Meadow High Sierra Camp
(Delaware North Companies)
Open mid-June to mid-September.
www.visitsequoia.com

**Pear Lake Ski Hut
(Sequoia Natural History Association)**
Open December through April.
559-565-3759
www.sequoiahistory.org

Giant Sequoia National Monument

Montecito Sequoia Lodge
Open all year.
800-227-9900
www.montecitosequoia.com

Stony Creek Lodge
Open May through early October.
866-522-6966
www.sequoia-kingscanyon.com

Grant Grove

Grant Grove Cabins
Open all year.
866-522-6966
www.sequoia-kingscanyon.com

John Muir Lodge
Open all year.
866-522-6966
www.sequoia-kingscanyon.com

Kings Canyon Lodge
Open April to November.
559-335-2405
www.thekingscanyonlodge.com

Campgrounds

Both Sequoia and Kings Canyon offer an extensive array of improved campgrounds. The surrounding national forests also offer numerous camping options.

For reservations, call 877-444-6777 or visit www.recreation.gov.

On the west side, for Sequoia and Kings Canyon National Parks, here are the campgrounds by area:

- **Mineral King:** Atwell Mill and Cold Spring
- **Foothills:** Potwisha, Buckeye Flat, and South Fork
- **Lodgepole:** Lodgepole and Dorst

- **Grant Grove:** Azalea, Crystal Springs, and Sunset
- **Cedar Grove:** Sentinel, Sheep Creek, Canyon View, and Moraine

For Giant Sequoia National Monument, campgrounds by area include:

- **Hume Lake Area:** Princess, Hume Lake, Tenmile, and Landslide
- **Big Meadows Road and Stony Creek Area:** Stony Creek, Upper Stony, Horse Camp, Buck Rock, and Big Meadows

On the east side, there are numerous campgrounds in two separate US Forest Service ranger districts:

- **Mt. Whitney Ranger District:** Cottonwood Pass, Golden Trout, Lone Pine, Whitney Portal, Whitney Trailhead, Upper Grays Meadow, Lower Grays Meadow, and Onion Valley
- **White Mountain Ranger District:** Sage Flat, Upper Sage Flat, Big Pine Creek, Palisade Glacier, Clyde Glacier, Big Trees, Four Jeffrey, Intake 2, Bishop Park, Sabrina, Willow, and North Lake

Pack Trips

A number of private individuals and companies offer pack service for trips into the parks and surrounding forest lands. Each outfitter operates under a permit issued by the governing agency. Check with either the Park Service or Forest Service about current status, as the pack services that hold permits may change from year to year.

West side park services include:

**Big Meadow Corral
(Delaware North Park Services)**
559-564-3404 (summer)
559-564-6429 (winter)
www.visitsequoia.com

**Cedar Grove Pack Station
(Delaware North Park Services)**
559-565-3464
www.visitsequoia.com

**Grant Grove Stables
(Delaware North Park Services)**
559-335-9292 (summer)
559-337-1273 (winter)
www.visitsequoia.com

Horse Corral Pack Station
559-565-3404 (summer)
209-742-6400 (winter)
www.highsierrapackers.org

East side pack services include:

Bishop Pack Outfitters
760-873-4785
www.bishoppackoutfitters.com

Cottonwood Pack Station
760-878-2015

Glacier Pack Train
760-938-2538

Mt. Whitney Pack Trains
760-873-8331
www.rockcreekpackstation.com

Pine Creek Pack Station
760-387-2797 (summer)
760-387-2627 (winter)

Rainbow Pack Outfitters
760-873-8877
www.rainbowpackoutfit.com

Rock Creek Pack Station
760-935-4493
www.rockcreekpackstation.com

Sequoia Kings Pack Train
800-962-0775 (summer)
760-387-2627 (winter)
www.sequoiakingspacktrain.com

Additional Park Facilities

To reduce environmental concerns, gasoline is not available within park boundaries, except for in emergencies. Motorists approaching the parks from the west will find the least expensive fuel in Visalia or Fresno. Closer to the parks, prices tend to rise. Gas is available in Three Rivers, Hume

Lake, Clingan's Junction, and at Kings Canyon Lodge.

East side travelers won't find any bargain prices in the towns along US 395, but Bishop is the least expensive.

Here are a few other key park facilities on the west side:

- **Post offices:** Lodgepole and Grant Grove
- **Showers and laundry:** Lodgepole, Grant Grove, and Cedar Grove
- **Groceries and supplies:** Lodgepole, Grant Grove, and Cedar Grove
- **Snack bar and deli:** Lodgepole, Grant Grove, and Cedar Grove
- **Restaurants:** Wuksachi Village and Grant Grove

Nonprofit Organization

Sequoia Natural History Association (SNHA) is a nonprofit organization dedicated to supporting education, interpretation, research, and the natural and historic preservation of Sequoia and Kings Canyon National Parks, Devils Postpile National Monument, and Lake Kaweah. SNHA is committed to enriching the experiences of visitors and promoting public awareness of the significance of public lands through educational programs, publications, and financial support.

The SNHA participates in the following activities:

- Operation of visitor center bookstores
- Operation of the Sequoia Field Institute and Beetle Rock Education Center
- Publication of the Sequoia and Kings Canyon National Parks newsletter
- Free and low-cost school programs
- Tours of Crystal Cave
- Operation of the Pear Lake Ski Hut
- Purchasing supplies for ranger programs
- Financing active protection of black bears
- Field seminar courses

- Funding visitor center and trail exhibits
- Providing information staff at visitor centers
- Publishing books and maps of the parks
- Funding scientific research within the parks

Membership categories include: park partner for $25 per year, green partner for $40 per year, supporter for $65 per year, business sponsor for $150 per year, and park guardian for $300 per year. Membership benefits include the following: a 15-percent discount on visitor center and online purchases, discounts at Pear Lake Ski Hut and on all Sequoia Field Institute seminars and naturalist services, copies of the biannual *Seedlings* and *Nature Connections* newsletters, a monthly email newsletter, a 10- to 20-percent discount at most other national park visitor center bookstores, connection coupons, volunteer opportunities, and discounts on local lodging. For more information, contact them at: 47050 Generals Highway #10, Three Rivers, CA 93721, 559-565-3759, 559-565-3728 (fax). Email them at snha@sequoiahistory.org or learn more at **www.sequoiahistory.org.**

Wilderness Ethics and Trail Courtesy

The American wilderness evokes notions of wild and undeveloped places, where humans are simply visitors who leave no trace of their presence. The "leave only footprints, take only photographs" motto popularized during the back-to-earth movement of the 1970s embodies just such a principle. The goal of all visitors, hikers, backpackers, and equestrians should be to leave a wilderness area as they found it, if not better.

The following backcountry guidelines should keep the wild in wilderness. When camping:

- Camp a minimum of 100 feet from any water source.
- Choose a campsite away from trails.
- Never build improvements (fireplaces, rock walls, drainage swales, etc.).
- Camp on exposed dirt or rock surfaces not on vegetation.
- Use only downed wood for campfires; never cut trees (dead or alive).
- Use only existing fire rings.
- Never leave a campfire unattended.
- Fully extinguish all campfires by thoroughly soaking them with water.

To keep yourself healthy and the wilderness pristine, please:

- Bury waste in soil six inches deep, a minimum of 100 feet from trails, and at least 500 feet from water sources.
- Pack out toilet paper in heavily used areas.
- Cook only the amount of food you can eat to avoid having to dispose of leftovers.
- Wash and rinse dishes, clothes, and yourself a minimum of 100 feet from water sources; never wash in lakes or streams.
- Pack out all trash—do not attempt to burn plastic or foil packaging.
- Filter, boil, or treat all drinking water.

On the trail, always:

- Stay on the trail; do not cut switchbacks.
- Preserve the serenity of the backcountry; avoid making loud noises.
- Yield the right-of-way to uphill hikers.
- Yield the right-of-way to equestrians; step well off the trail on the downhill side.
- Avoid traveling in large groups.
- Because trail conditions can change, either from natural or human causes, hikers should check with ranger stations for updates before starting a hike.

Sequoia and Kings Canyon National Parks have some park-specific regulations:

- Group size is limited to 15 (8 for parties traveling off of developed trails).

- Pets, weapons, wheeled vehicles, hunting, and motorized equipment are prohibited.

- Campfires are prohibited above 10,400 feet in Sequoia National Park, above 9000 feet in the Kaweah River drainage, and above 10,000 feet in Kings Canyon National Park. Campfires are also prohibited at Mineral King Valley, Nine Lakes Basin, Hamilton Lakes, Upper Big Arroyo, Pinto Lake, Lower Crabtree Meadow, Granite Basin, and Redwood Canyon.

- Food must be stored so that it is completely inaccessible to bears. Food must be stored in bear canisters or food lockers on the Rae Lakes Loop, in Dusy Basin and Palisade Basin, and along Rock Creek.

- Do not camp within 100 feet of lakes and streams.

- Camping is limited to 25 people per night at Pear and Emerald Lakes at designated sites only. Advanced reservations are not available for these sites. Permits are issued by the Lodgepole trailhead office.

- Stock users should consult the park website for current grazing regulations.

Inyo National Forest has its own regulations:

- Group size is limited to 15.

- Bear canisters are required for the Cottonwood Lakes, Mt. Whitney, Kearsarge Pass, and Bishop Pass areas.

- Campfires are prohibited in Meysan Creek, North Fork Lone Pine Creek, Anvil Camp (Shepherd Creek), Onion Valley, Taboose Creek, and South Fork and North Fork Big Pine Creek.

Stock users are responsible for following no-trace practices within the parks and surrounding wilderness areas. A downloadable PDF is available on the Sequoia and Kings Canyon National Parks website detailing the specific regulations pertaining to stock use (**www.nps.gov/seki/planyourvisit/stock-reg.htm**).

The Bear Facts and Other Animal (and Insect) Concerns

Bears

The range of the grizzly bear used to include the Sierra Nevada, but the last grizzly in California was shot near Horse Corral Meadows in the early 1900s. Since then, the common American black bear has been the only ursine species in the range. Despite their name, black bears vary in color from jet black to cinnamon. Quick, agile, and oftentimes quite large, mature males can weigh around 300 pounds. Active both day and night, black bears have a highly developed sense of smell. More common on the west slope, they usually stay between 5,000 and 8,000 feet, occasionally traveling through higher elevations. As omnivores, black bears subsist mainly on vegetation and are typically not aggressive toward humans. Bears unfamiliar with human food sources tend to be quite shy and retiring, avoiding human contact at virtually any cost. However, black bears that have grown accustomed to human food and garbage through our carelessness can become destructive and potentially threatening.

Once bears discover food in coolers, cars, or backpacks or garbage from unsecured trash bins, reconditioning them away from these food sources is extremely difficult. Bears frequenting developed campgrounds in search of food tend to be the boldest and potentially most dangerous culprits. Relocating such animals has not proven to be 100 percent effective, since they generally find a way back to habited areas in search of food. "Problem" bears then face death at the hands of wildlife officials.

Despite a reputation for being dumb animals, bears have figured out how to thwart previous attempts to hang food in the backcountry. Nowadays, when attempts are made to counterbalance stuff sacks full of food from a tree limb, a bear might simply climb the tree and either sever the cord or break off the branch. Mother bears often send cubs up the tree to knock the bags to the ground. The counterbalance method was never foolproof for backpackers camping at or above timberline, where trees were either too low to the ground or absent altogether.

Several years ago, park and forest service officials in the Sierra implemented a plan to help minimize bear-human conflicts in the backcountry. They outfitted popular backcountry campsites in bear-prone areas with metal bear lockers, started requiring bear canisters in high-traffic areas, and encouraged hikers to use them elsewhere. This plan has been in effect for many years and, for the most part, has successfully broken the bear's association between backpackers and food. Requiring the full cooperation of all recreationists along the urban fringe, the plan has been less effective near developed campgrounds. When visiting the parks, everyone is responsible for storing food-related items away from the bears so that they do not become accustomed to seeking human food or garbage as a food source.

Bearproof canisters may add a few pounds to your backpack, but this burden should be offset with the knowledge that the life of a bear may be spared. Plus, having food safely secured in a canister should help hikers sleep more soundly. Despite the emphasis on protecting food from bears, recreationists should not be discouraged from hiking or backpacking in the High Sierra, as actual bear sightings are benign and fairly rare.

The following guidelines will enhance your experience while helping to protect the bears:

At campgrounds:

- Leave extra or unnecessary food and scented items at home.
- Store all food, food containers, and scented items in securely latched bear lockers.
- Dispose of all trash in bearproof garbage cans or dumpsters.
- Never leave food out at an unattended campsite.

In the backcountry:

- Don't leave backpacks unattended in plain sight while on the trail.
- At camp, empty backpacks and open all flaps and pockets.
- Keep all food, trash, and scented items in a bearproof locker or canister.
- Pack out all trash.

Everywhere:

- Don't allow bears to approach food— make noise, wave your arms, and throw rocks. Be bold, but keep a safe distance between you and the bear. Use good judgment.
- If a bear gets into your food, you are responsible for cleaning up the mess.
- Never attempt to retrieve food from a bear.
- Never approach a bear, especially a cub.
- Report any incidents or injuries to the appropriate agency.

Within Sequoia and Kings Canyon National Parks, hikers must use bear canisters in the following places: within the wilderness area bordered by Sawmill Pass and the Woods Creek drainage on the north, Forester Pass and the Kings-Kern Divide on the south, the Sierra Crest on the east, and Cedar Grove, South Fork of the Kings River, and Sphinx Crest on the west (including all trail corridors and cross-country routes within the area); within the Dusy Basin wilderness areas including all camp areas from Bishop Pass to the junction with the John Muir Trail in Le Conte Canyon and all cross-country areas in Dusy Basin and Palisades Basin; and within the Rock Creek Wilderness area of Sequoia National Park including all camp areas in the Rock Creek drainage, including Miter Basin, Soldier Lake, Siberian Outpost, and Rock Creek proper. (Specifically, the area is defined as areas [including cross-country routes] in the Rock Creek drainage west of Cottonwood and New Army Passes, south of Crabtree Pass, south of Guyot Pass, and north-northwest of the Sequoia National Park boundary and Siberian Pass.)

Within Inyo National Forest, hikers must use bear canisters in the following areas: Bishop Pass, Cottonwood Lakes, Cottonwood Pass, Kearsarge Pass, and the Mt. Whitney Zone.

Bear lockers are installed in many backcountry locations. In Sequoia National Park, there are bear lockers at Hockett Plateau, including Hockett Meadow, South Fork Meadow/Rock Camp, and Upper Camp/South Fork Pasture; Mineral King, including Franklin Lake and Lower Monarch Lake; Kern Canyon, including Lower Funston Meadow, Upper Funston Meadow, Kern Hot Springs, and Junction Meadow; Little Five Lakes, Cliff Creek, and Chagoopa Plateau, including Moraine Lake, Big Arroyo Crossing, Lost Canyon, Big Five Lakes, Little Five Lakes, Pinto Lake, and Cliff Creek and Timber Gap Junction; Rock Creek, including Lower Soldier Lake, Lower Rock Creek Lake, and Lower Rock Creek crossing (PCT); Lodgepole, including Mehrten Creek Crossing (on the High Sierra Trail, or HST), 9 Mile Creek Crossing (HST), Buck Creek Crossing (HST), Bearpaw, Upper Hamilton Lake, Emerald Lake, Pear Lake, Clover Creek South Crossing (Twin Lakes Trail), J O Pass Trail and Twin Lakes Trail Junction, and Twin Lakes; Tyndall and Crabtree, including Lower Crabtree Meadow, Crabtree Ranger Station, Wallace Creek (on the JMT), Tyndall Creek Frog Ponds, and Tyndall Creek (JMT).

In Kings Canyon National Park, there are bear lockers at Sugarloaf Valley and Roaring River, including Ranger Lake, Lost Lake, Seville Lake, Comanche Meadow, Sugarloaf Meadow, and Roaring River Ranger Station; Kings Canyon, including Lower Tent Meadow (Copper Creek Trail) and Frypan Meadow (Lewis Creek Trail); Bubbs Creek (canisters required, lockers are reserved for JMT and PCT thru-hikers), including Sphinx Creek, Charlotte Creek, Lower Junction Meadow, Junction Meadow and East Creek, East Lake, at 9,900 feet in elevation (JMT), Vidette Meadows, and at the junction of the Center Basin Trail and JMT; Woods Creek (canisters required, lockers reserved for JMT and PCT thru-hikers), including Lower Paradise Valley, Middle Paradise Valley, Upper Paradise Valley, Woods Creek crossing (JMT), Arrowhead Lake, and Middle Rae Lake; Kearsarge area, including Kearsarge Lakes and Charlotte Lake.

Cougars (Mountain Lions)

The chances of seeing a big cat in the backcountry are extremely small since they are typically shy, avoiding human contact at nearly all costs. They are much more likely to see you, especially while you are hiking in the western foothills area. Unlike omnivorous black bears, cougars are strictly carnivorous, with mule deer as the main staple of their diet. When hunting for deer is poor, they supplement with smaller animals. A typical mountain lion is estimated to kill 36 deer per year, and the overall health of the deer herd is directly linked to the predatory nature of the cats, since the cats cull the weaker members. Experts recommend you do the following to avoid running into a cougar or react to an encounter with one:

- Don't hike alone, especially in the foothills zone.
- Don't leave small children unattended; pick them up if a cat approaches.
- Don't run since flight indicates you are prey.
- Make yourself appear as large as possible—don't crouch or try to hide.
- Hold your ground, or back away slowly while facing the cat.
- If the cat is aggressive, make noise, wave your arms, and throw rocks.
- If the animal attacks, fight back.
- Report any encounters or injuries to the appropriate agency.

Marmots

The largest member of the squirrel family, chirping marmots hardly seem threatening to humans. However, these herbivores have been known to wreak havoc on radiator hoses and wiring in cars parked at Mineral King trailheads, especially in spring (this hankering seems to taper off by midsummer). Many a vehicle has been disabled by their rare proclivity for dining on automobile parts, leaving drivers stranded until they can arrange for repair services. Unsuspecting drivers have transported these furry creatures to other parts of the park and as far away as Southern California! Check with the rangers at the Mineral King Ranger Station for the current conditions. Some backpackers surround their vehicles with wire to keep them safe.

Marmots in other parts of the High Sierra, particularly near popular campsites, have been known to chew through backpack straps, hiking boots, and rubber grips on trekking poles. Once they associate humans with food, they will often tear through backpacks in search of treats. In marmot-infested areas, store your food in canisters or bear lockers, or hang it from a tree.

Rattlesnakes

Although rattlesnakes are common to the foothills community on the west side of the Sierra and the pinyon-sagebrush zone on the east side, human encounters with them are relatively rare. Actual bites are even less frequent, and fatalities are almost nonexistent in adults. While rattlers live in a wide range of environments, pay close attention when hiking near creeks below 6,000 feet in elevation. These reptiles seek sun when temperatures are cool and retreat into the shade when temperatures are warm. During the summer months, they are often nocturnal.

Rattlesnakes are not aggressive and will seek escape unless cornered. Never provoke a rattlesnake. If you happen to encounter one, back away quickly. On the rare occasion you or someone in your party is bitten, seek medical attention immediately.

Ticks

Very uncommon in the High Sierra, ticks are most prevalent in the foothills zone, especially in spring following particularly wet winters. These blood-sucking pests would be a mere nuisance if they weren't also carriers of debilitating diseases, such as Lyme disease or Rocky Mountain spotted fever. Although rare in the southern Sierra, these tick-borne conditions can be serious if left untreated. If you are bitten by a tick, especially one that may have been attached for 24 hours or more, watch for a bull's-eye rash, flulike symptoms, headache, rash, fever, or joint pain. Consult a physician if any of these symptoms persist.

Myths, old wives tales, and urban legends abound regarding the removal of a tick from human flesh. The medically accepted method advises the use of a pair of tweezers to gain a solid hold and the application of gentle traction to back the tick out. After you have removed it, thoroughly wash the area with antibacterial soap, completely dry the skin, and then apply an antibiotic ointment. Monitor your health for the next several days. Prevention is the best medicine; observe the following guidelines when traveling in tick country:

- Apply an effective repellent on skin and clothing, and reapply often.
- Wear long-sleeved shirts and long pants, and tuck your pant legs into the top of your socks.
- Inspect your entire body regularly (at least a couple times a day). Check your clothing thoroughly.

Mosquitoes

While they are not a major health concern, nothing can ruin a backcountry trip faster than a horde of pesky mosquitoes. Fortunately, the mosquito cycle in the Sierra Nevada builds for a short time in early summer, peaks for about two weeks, and then steadily diminishes; the peak of mosquito season varies from year to year, but unfortunately climaxes during the height of wildflower season.

Mosquitoes seem to prefer some people to others. For those who are so cursed, supposed deterrents seem to be the modern era's equivalent of snake oil, including sleeping under a pyramid, ingesting a boatload of vitamin B, bathing yourself in a vat of hand lotion, or using some high-frequency device to drive the bugs away. Although the only surefire method of avoiding these ubiquitous pests is to stay away, most outdoor recreationists find this alternative justifiably unacceptable. The following guidelines may help to minimize the aggravation of mosquito season:

- Use an effective repellent containing a high concentration of DEET. Lemoneucalyptus oil may also work, but it never hurts to bring a repellent with DEET just in case.
- Wear long-sleeved shirts, long pants, and a head net when necessary.
- Select wind-prone campsites, bring a tent, and avoid camping near marshy areas.

Maps

Hikers and backpackers can choose from a number of recreational maps for the popular Sequoia and Kings Canyon region, including the maps provided in this guide.

USGS Topographic Maps

The 7.5-minute quadrangles, published by the US Geological Survey, are the most accurate and detailed maps available. You can purchase the USGS maps ($8 per sheet in 2012) directly from the USGS website

(**www.store.usgs.gov**) and at Park Service or Forest Service visitor centers. Some outdoor retailers offer customers the ability to customize and print maps using the 7.5-minute maps as a base. Long-distance backpackers may favor maps at a smaller scale since the 1:24,000 scale of the 7.5-minute quads may require them to carry numerous maps.

USGS Map Name	Trip Numbers
1. Dennison Peak	1–3
2. Moses Mountain	1–3
3. Silver City	4–6
4. Mineral King	7–17
5. Chagoopa Falls	13, 32
6. Johnson Peak	90, 93, 94
7. Cirque Peak	89–94
8. Shadequarter Mountain	23, 24
9. Giant Forest	18–22, 24–30, 33–39, 48
10. Lodgepole	17, 26–32, 37–47
11. Triple Divide Peak	17, 31, 32, 46, 79
12. Mt. Kaweah	32, 79, 97
13. Mount Whitney	32, 90, 93–95, 97
14. Mt. Langley	32, 92, 94, 96
15. General Grant Grove	56–67
16. Muir Grove	49–54
17. Mt. Silliman	45, 46, 53–55
18. Sphinx Lakes	46, 79
19. Mt. Brewer	79, 80, 97, 98
20. Mt. Williamson	79, 97, 98
21. Hume	68, 69
22. Wren Peak	56
23. Cedar Grove	70–74
24. The Sphinx	75–85, 102
25. Mt. Clarence King	79–81, 83, 97, 100–103, 105
26. Kearsarge Peak	97, 99–105
27. Rough Spur	86
28. Tehipite Dome	86
29. Slide Bluffs	71, 86
30. Marion Peak	85, 86
31. Mt. Pinchot	103, 106, 107
32. Aberdeen	106, 107
33. Courtright Reservoir	86, 87
34. Blackcap Mountain	86–88
35. Mt. Goddard	86, 88, 114
36. North Palisade	86, 103, 111–114
37. Split Mountain	103, 108–111
38. Fish Springs	107–109
39. Ward Mountain	86–88
40. Mt. Henry	86–88, 114, 122
41. Mt. Darwin	86, 114, 118, 120–122
42. Mt. Thompson	103, 111–119
43. Coyote Flat	110, 111
44. Florence Lake	88
45. Mt. Hilgard	114, 122
46. Mt. Tom	114, 122

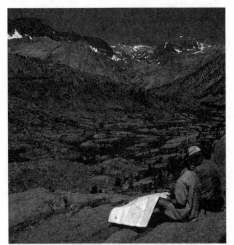

Hikers study the map above Palisade Basin (Trip 113).

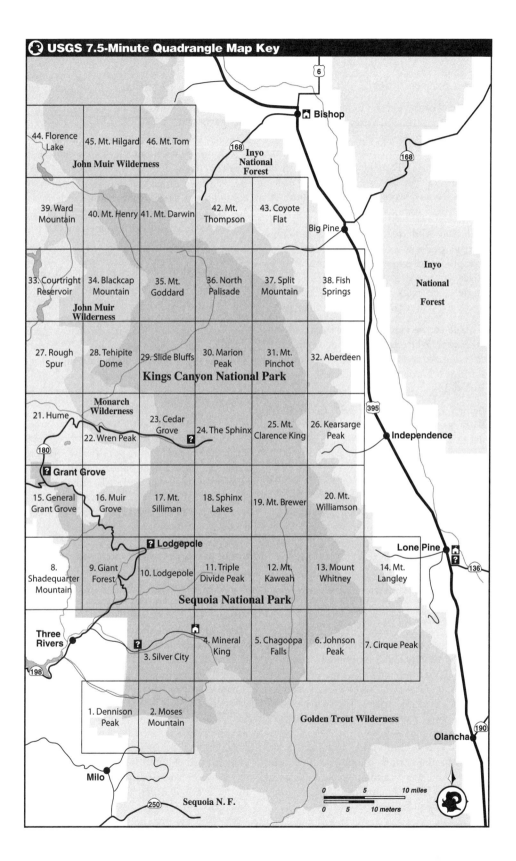

USGS 7.5-Minute Quadrangle Map Key

Forest Service Maps

The US Forest Service publishes a variety of maps covering the greater Sequoia and Kings Canyon region. National Forest maps are suitable for trip planning and driving to trailheads. USFS wilderness maps can be used on the trail. Maps can be purchased online (**www.nationalforeststore.com**) or from ranger stations and visitor centers.

John Muir Wilderness and Sequoia and Kings Canyon Wilderness: A three-sheet set of topographic maps suitable for backcountry use, covering nearly every trip described in this guide (exceptions include Grant Grove and Redwood Mountain, 1 inch = 1 mile, $12).

A Guide to the Monarch Wilderness and Jennie Lakes Wilderness: A topographic map covering the two wilderness areas along the southwest border of Kings Canyon National Parks (2 inches = 1 mile, $8).

Golden Trout Wilderness and South Sierra Wilderness: A topographic map of the wilderness areas south of Sequoia National Park (1 inch = 1 mile, $8).

Inyo National Forest: Covers the entire Inyo National Forest (0.5 inch = 1 mile, $12).

Sequoia National Forest: Covers the entire Sequoia National Forest (0.5 inch = 1 mile, $9).

Sierra National Forest: Covers the entire Sierra National Forest (0.5 inch = 1 mile, $9).

Other Maps

The SNHA publishes a set of four, foldout maps with concise descriptions of popular dayhikes in the Cedar Grove, Giant Forest, Grant Grove, Lodgepole, and Mineral King areas of the parks. You can purchase these maps online (**www.sequoiahistory. org**) or at park visitor centers and stores ($3.50 each). Both Tom Harrison Maps (**www.tomharrisonmaps.com**) and National Geographic (**www.nationalgeographic.com**) publish additional maps for the Sequoia and Kings Canyon region.

Wilderness Permits

With the exception of entering the Whitney Zone via the Mt. Whitney Trail from Whitney Portal, dayhikers do not need a permit for the national parks or national forests. Hikers who plan on traveling into the Whitney Zone, a roughly 5-mile by 2.5-mile area of the John Muir Wilderness that borders Sequoia National Park along the Sierra Crest, will need to procure one of the 100 day-use permits that Inyo National Forest issues each day. Day-use permits can be reserved through a lottery held each year in February, subject to a $15 per person fee. The Eastern Sierra Interagency Visitor Center at the junction of US 395 and Highway 136 south of Lone Pine issues any unused permits free. Consult the Inyo National Forest website (**www.fs.usda.gov/inyo**) for further information.

Overnight Trips

All overnight users entering the backcountry in Sequoia and Kings Canyon National Parks must get a valid wilderness permit from the ranger station or visitor center closest to the trailhead. The main park wilderness office is at 47050 Generals Highway #60, Three Rivers, CA 93271, 559-565-4239 (fax).

Approximately 75 percent of the daily trailhead quota, which is in effect from late May through September, is set aside for reserved permits. Beginning March 1, permits can be reserved up to two weeks in advance of departure. Permit forms can be downloaded from the park website (**www. nps.gov/seki**) and either faxed or mailed when completed to the wilderness office (the NPS plans to set up an online reservation system by 2012). A $15 per person fee must accompany your application (VISA, MC, check, or money order). Reserved permits can be picked up from the issuing station after 1 p.m. the day before departure and will be held until 9 a.m. the morning of the trip. You must notify the ranger station if you are will be picking up your permit past this time since reserved permits are released to first-come, first-served back-packers at that time.

The remaining 25 percent of the daily trailhead quota and any cancelled reservations are available for free walk-in permits, beginning after 1 p.m. the day before departure. Unclaimed reservations may become available after 9 a.m. the morning of a trip.

Wilderness permits are required year-round for all overnight visits, and all trails entering wilderness areas in Inyo National Forest have quotas in effect. The quota period for overnight stays in John Muir Wilderness is between May 1 and September 15. The quota period for overnight stays in Golden Trout Wilderness is between the last Friday in June through September 15. Outside of the quota period, backpackers can self-issue permits from Forest Service ranger stations and visitor centers. Up to 60 percent of the quota can be reserved up to six months in advance for $5 per person (Inyo National Forest plans to have an online reservation system in place by 2012). The remaining 40 percent is available as free walk-in permits, available from any USFS ranger station or visitor center, one day ahead of the departure date. Contact the Wilderness Permit Office (760-873-2483) for more information.

Day hiking and backpacking permits for entry into the Mt. Whitney Zone are issued through a lottery system (see Trip 95).

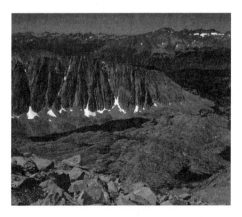

Westward view from Mt. Whitney (Trip 95)

Winter in the Sequoia and Kings Canyon Area

While most recreationists visit the Sequoia and Kings Canyon area in the summer and some during the shoulder seasons of spring and fall, winter can be a magical time to enjoy a wide range of activities.

Hiking and Backpacking

Although the greater Sequoia and Kings Canyon region doesn't provide an abundance of off-season hiking and backpacking opportunities, a few possibilities do exist. A handful of trails in the foothills region of Sequoia National Park offer some year-round, snow-free hiking (see Trips 1, 18–22, and the initial segments of 23–24). At least one of the nearby campgrounds remains open all year, and lodging is available both inside the park and in the nearby town of Three Rivers.

Snowshoeing and Cross-Country Skiing

During winters of average snowfall, recreationists can enjoy snowshoeing and cross-country skiing opportunities in both parks. Marked trails in the Giant Forest and Lodgepole areas of Sequoia National Park lure snow lovers each winter, as do similar winter trails in Grant Grove in Kings Canyon National Park. More adventurous winter enthusiasts with the requisite winter skills will have a huge area of backcountry mostly to themselves, where an unlimited number of multiday excursions are possible. Late winter and early spring, with increasing daylight and more stable weather, can make the snow-covered High Sierra a fine place for backcountry pursuits. Anyone desiring to stay overnight in the parks backcountry or surrounding wilderness areas must secure a self-issue wilderness permit from a visitor center or ranger station. Be sure to check with rangers about restrictions and current conditions before embarking into the backcountry.

On the west side of Sequoia National Park, the Generals Highway is kept open

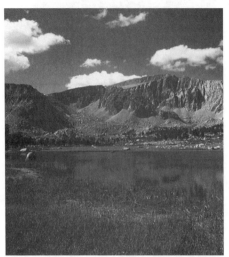

Lake 3 in Cottonwood Lakes Basin (Trip 92)

during the winter months from Three Rivers to Wuksachi Village. The foothills area offers year-round hiking, information, and exhibits at the Ash Mountain Visitor Center, camping at Potwisha Campground, and picnicking at Hospital Rock. Farther up the road in the Giant Forest, the museum is open all year, and marked trails lead past giant sequoias, including the largest of all, General Sherman. Wolverton has a snowplay area, snack bar, and rentals. The Lodgepole Campground is open all year for those not adverse to snow camping. Wuksachi Village provides lodging throughout the year, with a restaurant, small gift shop, and cross-country ski and snowshoe rentals; ranger-led snowshoe walks are held on some weekends and holidays.

Wolverton is also the trailhead for the strenuous 6-mile route to Pear Lake Ski Hut. Equipped with a pellet stove, lanterns, propane stove, cooking utensils, and indoor toilet, the lodge sleeps ten cross-country skiers or snowshoers. Private individuals may rent the hut from the middle of December through the end of April. Reservations made through a lottery process are required. Downloadable registration forms are available through the Sequoia Natural History Association website (**www.sequoiahistory. org**). Using the Pear Lake Ski Hut as a base

camp, winter recreationists can make forays into the dramatic scenery of the nearby Tableland area.

Access to the west side of Kings Canyon National Park is via Highway 180. The road is kept open in winter from the park entrance through Grant Grove Village to the junction with the Hume Lake Road near Princess Meadow. From there, the road is plowed to Hume Lake, where Hume Lake Christian Camps operates a general store (that sells gasoline), gift shop, post office, and snack bar during limited hours. Snow play areas near Grant Grove include Big Stump and Columbine. Facilities in Grant Grove that remain open all year include the visitor center, market (cross-country ski and snowshoe rentals), restaurant, gift shop, and post office. Lodging is available during winter at John Muir Lodge and Grant Grove Cabins. Marked trails through Grant Grove lead past giant sequoias; ranger-led snowshoe walks are held on some weekends and holidays.

Motorists entering the parks from the west are required to carry chains at all times, even if their vehicles are equipped with four-wheel-drive. The road from the Y-junction between the Kings Canyon Highway (Highway 180) and Wuksachi Village is usually closed during winter storms (sometimes for days), reopening after snowplows have safely cleared the snow. During snowy periods, the road may be open only to guests staying at Montecito Sequoia Lodge, who are allowed to travel the road only in caravans at three scheduled times during the day.

As well as lodging and dining, Montecito Sequoia Lodge offers 30 to 50 kilometers of groomed trails for cross-country and skate skiing. Other winter activities at the lodge include snowshoeing, snowboarding, tubing, sledding, sleigh rides, snow biking, ice skating, and snow play. Rentals and lessons are also available. Check out their website, **www.montecitosequoia.com**, for rates and more information.

Long and sometimes difficult access, combined with reduced commercial activity, ensures that the east side of the High Sierra sees few winter visitors. Away from the hubs of Mammoth Village and June Lake ski areas, the range can seem totally deserted from December to April. Consequently, winter recreationists have the opportunity to enjoy the dramatic scenery of high peaks, steep-walled canyons, and frozen lakes in solitude. Getting to snow that is deep enough for skiing or snowshoeing is oftentimes the most challenging aspect of an eastside trip. Few roads other than the major north-south thoroughfare of US 395 are plowed during the winter. The only SnoPark on this side of the range is Rock Creek, located west of Toms Place, well north of the Sequoia-Kings Canyon region. For those willing to endure such obstacles, the High Sierra backcountry abounds with possibilities during the winter. Within the greater Sequoia-Kings Canyon region, the town of Bishop offers the widest range of services for winter travelers on the east side of the Sierra.

About This Guide

This guide is designed primarily for hikers in search of dayhiking opportunities in and around Sequoia and Kings Canyon National Parks and for backpackers looking to explore the area's majesty on anything from short weekend trips to multi-week excursions. Some aspects of the evaluations of the trails in this guide are subjective, but every effort has been made to ensure that the descriptions are meaningful to the average trail user.

The 122 trips described in this guide are divided into two main sections: west side trips include 88 hikes or backpacks in 11 subregions. East side trips cover 34 excursions in 2 subregions. A brief introduction to each subregion precedes the trip descriptions, which will familiarize hikers with the area. Information regarding access, services, campground locations and facilities, and nearest ranger stations follows, along with helpful tips specific to the area.

Symbols

Each description begins with a display of symbols, denoting the following characteristics of each trip.

Trip Difficulty

E = Easy

M = Moderate

MS = Moderately strenuous

S = Strenuous

Type of Trip

↗ = Out-and-back

/ = Point-to-point (shuttle required)

↻ = Loop

↺ = Semiloop

Duration

DH = Dayhike (single-day outing)

BP = Backpack

BPx= Extended backpack (overnight trip with three or more nights in the backcountry)

  X = Cross-country route (backpack requiring some cross-country travel)

Trip Information

Each trip description includes the following information:

Distance

Distances are listed in miles. The mileage value for each trip is the total round-trip mileage.

Elevation

Elevation figures listed are in feet. The first set of numbers represents the starting elevation, followed by all the significant high and low points. The second set of numbers represents the elevation gain, elevation loss, and the total combined elevation gain and loss. (To convert feet to meters, multiply by 0.3048).

Season

This entry lists the general period for when the trail should be open and mostly free of snow. However, these conditions vary considerably from year to year, depending on a particular winter's snowpack and severity.

Use

This entry gives you a general idea of the trail's popularity (light, moderate, heavy, and extremely heavy) and an idea of how many other people to expect along the way. Packed trails are tourist destinations, which may have hundreds of people during the most popular season. On heavy and packed backpack trails, campsites may be in short supply on weekends though probably not on weekdays. Some of this book's hikes have sections that vary significantly in usage.

Map

USGS 7.5-minute topographical maps covering the area are listed in this category. Occasionally, supplemental maps are also recommended.

Trail Log

Many of the longer trips have a trail log that lists the trail's highlights, such as trail junctions, stream crossings, lakes, summits, and campsites, along with their corresponding mileage. Shorter trips with only a single destination as a point of interest do not have a trail log.

Trip Description

The main body of the description includes an introduction of the route, directions to the trailhead, and a fairly detailed guide to the trail. In the margins beside the main trip description, quick-reference icons indicate various features found along the route, such as:

🏕 = Campgrounds and campsites

〜 = Swimming areas

◉ = Noteworthy views

✿ = Seasonal wildflowers

◇ = History

🌲 = Giant sequoia groves

Options and Regulatory Information

Options, indicated by ◻️O, allow you to extend your trip with side trips, alternate routes, additional cross-country routes, and peaks that you may want to climb in the vicinity.

Regulatory information, indicated by ◻️R, lists details about permits, quotas, and any specific restrictions for a given trip.

Map Legend

This map legend identifies the symbols and styles used on the maps.

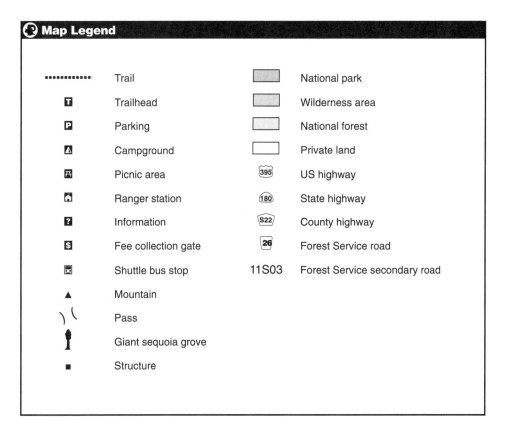

▪▪▪▪▪▪▪▪▪▪▪▪	Trail	�	National park
T	Trailhead		Wilderness area
P	Parking		National forest
⛺	Campground		Private land
🏕	Picnic area	(395)	US highway
🏠	Ranger station	(180)	State highway
❓	Information	(S22)	County highway
$	Fee collection gate	26	Forest Service road
🚌	Shuttle bus stop	11S03	Forest Service secondary road
▲	Mountain		
) (	Pass		
🌲	Giant sequoia grove		
▪	Structure		

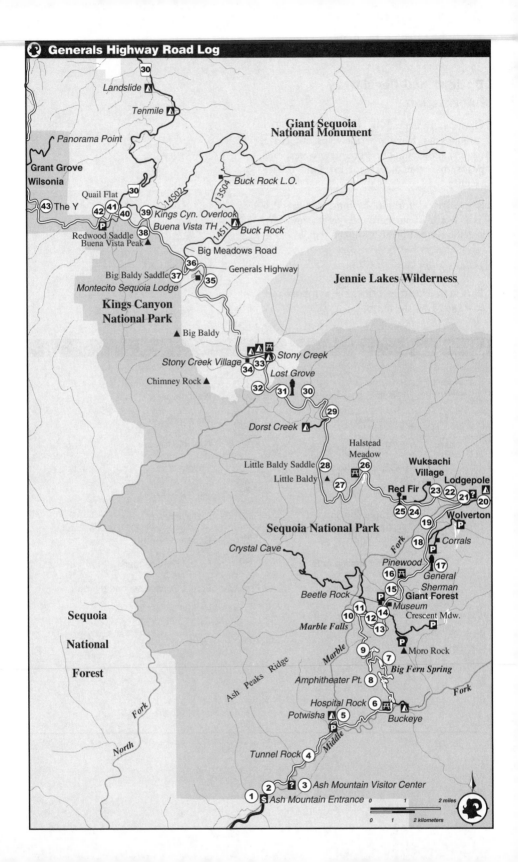

Giant Sequoia
National Monument

Landslide

Tenmile

Panorama Point

Grant Grove
Wilsonia

Quail Flat

Buck Rock L.O.

The Y

Kings Cyn. Overlook
Buena Vista TH

Buck Rock

Redwood Saddle
Buena Vista Peak

Big Meadows Road

Generals Highway

Jennie Lakes Wilderness

Big Baldy Saddle
Montecito Sequoia Lodge

Kings Canyon
National Park

Big Baldy

Stony Creek Village
Stony Creek

Lost Grove

Chimney Rock

Dorst Creek

Halstead
Meadow

Little Baldy Saddle

Little Baldy

Wuksachi
Village

Lodgepole

Red Fir

Wolverton

Sequoia National Park

Crystal Cave

Corrals

Pinewood

General
Sherman

Beetle Rock

Giant Forest
Museum

Crescent Mdw.

Sequoia

National

Forest

Marble Falls

Moro Rock

Big Fern Spring

Amphitheater Pt.

Ash Peaks Ridge

Hospital Rock

Potwisha

Buckeye

Tunnel Rock

Ash Mountain Visitor Center

Ash Mountain Entrance

North

Fork

Middle

Fork

0   1   2 miles

0   1   2 kilometers

Generals Highway Road Log

The Generals Highway connects the two prominent generals of Sequoia and Kings Canyon National Parks, the General Sherman and General Grant giant sequoia trees. The highway begins at the Ash Mountain Entrance in Sequoia at the park boundary with the community of Three Rivers, after State Highway 198 has passed through the town of Visalia and by Lake Kaweah. The highway technically ends at the General Grant Tree Road junction in Kings Canyon. Completed in 1926, the Generals Highway replaced the Colony Mill Road as the principal access for motorists to the Giant Forest in Sequoia National Park. In modern times, the road is open from the Ash Mountain Entrance to Grant Grove, with periodic closures during winter storms beyond the Wuksachi junction.

① **0.0 mile**

Ash Mountain Entrance: The Ash Mountain Entrance heralds the visitor's arrival to the west boundary of Sequoia National Park. The journey into the park begins in the foothills plant community, a typically hot and arid environment during the summer. Initially, the road follows Middle Fork Kaweah River upstream through a chaparral-covered canyon.

② **0.2 mile**

Entrance Sign: Shortly beyond the Ash Mountain Entrance, a pullout on the right-hand shoulder lets visitors stop and admire the newly restored welcome sign. Created in the 1930s by a member of the Civilian Conservation Corps, the sign was patterned after an Indian head (or buffalo) nickel, commemorating the link between Chief Sequoyah of the Cherokee and the naming of the parks' most compelling feature, *Sequoiadendron giganteum,* the giant sequoia. Be on the alert for pedestrians; many visitors stop for the customary photograph in front of the old sign.

③ **0.7 mile**

Ash Mountain Visitor Center: Open daily, the Ash Mountain Visitor Center offers visitors an excellent opportunity to acquaint themselves with the park, with a modest selection of interpretive exhibits, as well as an assortment of books, maps, and gifts. Rangers on staff are available to answer questions, write wilderness permits, and rent bear canisters. The visitor center has restrooms, a pay phone, and a small picnic area across the highway.

④ **2.3 miles**

Tunnel Rock: When the Generals Highway was originally built during the 1920s, the road passed beneath this massive boulder.

⑤ **3.8 miles**

Potwisha Campground: Potwisha, named for a band of Monache Indians, is an all-year campground, with running water, flush toilets, picnic tables, and a pay phone. At this campground at 2,100 feet, summer temperatures can be quite hot—the more temperate conditions during spring and fall offer more pleasant camping. The campground also provides a trailhead for the 3-plus-mile hike up a stretch of Marble Fork Kaweah River to Marble Falls (see Trip 19, page 107).

Directly across the highway from the entrance is a broad flat containing the campground dump station and parking for the short Potwisha Pictographs Loop (see Trip 18, page 105). The Middle Fork Trail to Hospital Rock can also be accessed from here (see Trip 20, page 109).

⑥ 6.1 miles

Hospital Rock: The highway continues upstream through Middle Fork Kaweah River canyon until bending north at a fair-size flat known as Hospital Rock. Humans have frequented this hospitable area for hundreds of years, with Native Americans establishing residence as early as the mid-1300s. During the late 1850s, when Hale Tharp passed through on his way to the

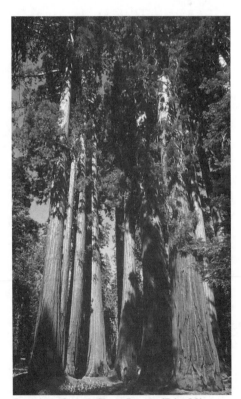

Founders Group, Giant Forest (Trip 30)

Giant Forest, hundreds of Monache were residing here and at Potwisha until introduced diseases devastated their population. After most of the Native Americans were gone, the area continued to provide a convenient camp for ranchers, settlers, and explorers. In 1873, James Everton accidentally shot himself in the leg and convalesced at this site, which became known as Hospital Rock.

Nowadays, Hospital Rock is a picnic area with running water, restrooms, and oak-shaded tables. Interpretive signs provide information about the former residents, and visitors may find pictographs on some of the nearby rocks. The Middle Fork Trail to Potwisha begins on the uphill side of the picnic area (see Trip 20, page 109).

Across the highway from the entrance to the picnic area, is a paved road to **Buckeye Campground,** open mid-May to mid-October. Inside the campground is the trailhead for the Paradise Creek Trail, but hikers will have to walk the 0.6-mile road from Hospital Rock because only campground guests may park at the trailhead (see Trip 21, page 110). A dirt road beyond the campground access road leads another 1.3 miles to a trailhead for the upper section of the Middle Fork Trail (see Trip 22, page 111).

⑦ 9.5 miles

Big Fern Spring: Beyond Hospital Rock, the Generals Highway begins a steep and winding climb up the south wall of the Giant Forest Plateau toward the Giant Forest. Built in the 1920s and 1930s, this highway is something of an engineering marvel. On the way to Big Fern Spring, the vegetation transitions from the drought-tolerant vegetation of the foothills zone to broadleaf evergreens, such as live oaks and laurels, with an occasional incense cedar serving as a harbinger of the coniferous forest above. The spring is named for the giant chain fern, largest of the native Californian ferns.

⑧ 11 miles

Amphitheater Point: The broad turnout here offers a wide-ranging panorama encompassing the full breadth of Sierra Nevada life zones. The precipitous slopes below are cloaked with the classic oak forest and chaparral of the foothills zone. Directly above lies the distinctive exfoliated granite dome of Moro Rock, bordered by the coniferous forest carpeting the Giant Forest Plateau. In the distance are some of the airy summits of the Great Western Divide, offering the first images of the mighty High Sierra.

⑨ 12.6 miles

Deer Ridge: From Amphitheater Point to Deer Ridge, the Generals Highway offers glimpses of two distinct rock types—the classic salt-and-pepper-colored granites typically associated with the Sierra and much older metamorphic rocks. Most of the metamorphic rocks are red, but patches of white rocks can be seen scattered across the terrain as well. The white cliffs seen from the vicinity of Deer Ridge are usually made of marble. Since marble is water-soluble over the course of geologic time, natural caverns often form in this rock, with Crystal Cave being the most famous of these caverns in Sequoia and Kings Canyon National Parks.

⑩ 13.5 miles

Eleven Range Point: This point is named for its expansive vista, encompassing up to eleven mountain ridges, depending upon the air quality. Unfortunately, the ubiquitous haze coating the atmosphere above the San Joaquin Valley usually clouds the view. Air pollution from Southern California and the Central Valley poses the most significant risk to humans and the natural environment in the parks. Oftentimes, Sequoia and Kings Canyon suffer some of the worst air quality in the national park system.

⑪ 14.5 miles

Giant Forest: The steep and winding climb eventually leads to the Giant Forest, where a roadside sign heralds your arrival. Gone are the oaks and laurels of the upper foothills zone, replaced by varieties of tall, slender, and straight-trunked trees with short branches, which can tolerate the snowy winters common to the mid-elevation forests. The Giant Forest is the home of the world's largest living organism, the giant sequoia. Common conifer associates of the Big Trees include incense cedars, sugar pines, and white firs. Deciduous dogwoods are also prevalent, offering beautiful accents of showy white flowers in spring and colorful foliage in autumn.

⑫ 14.6 miles

Commissary Curve: Crystal Cave Road branches away from the Generals Highway at a sharp bend named for the supply station that served men of the US Cavalry, who protected the park in the early 1900s before the creation of the NPS. Crystal Cave Road follows the upper course of the old Colony Mill Road for 6.4 miles to a parking lot for Sequoia's only visitor-accessible cave tour. Tickets for the daily tours may be acquired at either the Foothills or Lodgepole Visitor Centers. The road to the cave is open only from mid-May to late October and is *not* recommended for vehicles longer than 22 feet.

⑬ 15.1 miles

The Four Guardsmen: Here the highway divides briefly to pass among four stately giant sequoias, which are each estimated to be more than 1,000 years old.

⑭ 16.7 miles

Giant Forest Village: The several-mile ascent from Middle Fork Kaweah River culminates in your arrival at Giant Forest Village, the center of human activity on the plateau. To the left is a short stretch of road to the visitor parking lot, a bus stop for the Moro Rock-Crescent Meadow shuttle, and access to the **Beetle Rock Education Center.** The center, operated by the Sequoia Natural History Association, is a hub for naturalist activities,

NPS-sponsored meetings, outreach events, and the Family Nature Center.

On the right is the Moro Rock-Crescent Meadow Road, which leads to the namesake features plus several trailheads (see Trips 26–32, page 123). Although visitors may drive a private vehicle to either **Moro Rock** or **Crescent Meadow**, traffic jams on the narrow roads and crammed parking lots are persistent problems. Therefore, riding the free shuttle bus to these destinations is highly recommended.

Proceeding ahead on the Generals Highway, the **Giant Forest Museum** is the structure on the right, housed in the renovated old market building, originally designed by renowned architect Gilbert Stanley Underwood. The museum has interpretive exhibits and informational displays about the human and natural history of the Giant Forest. The museum also serves as a hub for several connecting trails of varying lengths leading into the heart of the forest (see Trips 33–39, page 145).

⑮ 17.1 miles

Round Meadow: The half-mile-long Big Trees Trail encircles Round Meadow, offering a short and leisurely hike past some prime examples of mature sequoias on a circuit around a flower-covered meadow. Interpretive signs and benches along the way offer an opportunity for a leisurely stroll. A small lot allows handicapped parking for the wheelchair-accessible trail. Everyone else must begin at the museum (see Trip 35, page 149).

⑯ 18 miles

Pinewood Picnic Area: As part of the Giant Forest's restoration, this former employee-housing site was converted to a picnic area in 2000. The area is complete with picnic tables, grills, and restrooms. Group and handicapped-accessible sites are also available.

⑰ 19.2 miles

General Sherman: Handicapped parking and a shuttle stop occupy the former parking area for access to the General Sherman Tree, at more than 52,000 cubic feet, the world's largest living organism. Giant sequoias grow only in areas with very specific soil, water, and climate conditions, and the Sherman Tree is located near the northern boundary of the Giant Forest. To visit the tree, either ride the free shuttle bus system, or continue driving on the Generals Highway to the Wolverton junction and then follow signs to the General Sherman Tree parking lot.

⑱ 19.8 miles

Wolverton Junction: Here Wolverton Road branches away from the Generals Highway and heads eastward. At 0.5 mile from the highway, a right turn eventually leads to the expansive **General Sherman** parking area (restrooms and shuttle bus stop). From there, a 0.4-mile paved path descends to the largest of the giant sequoias. Along the way, the path is imprinted with a cross section of the base of the Sherman Tree, which allows visitors to gain some understanding of the tree's massive size. A gap in the forest here also allows photographers an unobstructed view of the tree. The popular Congress Trail continues beyond General Sherman (see Trip 39, page 156).

Continuing ahead from the General Sherman junction, Wolverton Road travels another mile to a large parking area near Wolverton Meadow, which serves as the trailhead for the Lakes and Panther Gap Trails (see Trips 42 and 43, page 164) and a connection to the Alta Trail (see Trips 40 and 41, page 160). During the winter, Wolverton is a center for winter recreation.

⑲ 20.2 miles

Wolverton Creek: A short distance beyond Wolverton Junction, the Generals Highway crosses Wolverton Creek, one of the tributaries of Marble Fork Kaweah River.

⑳ 21.2 miles

Lodgepole: Similar to the Giant Forest in elevation, the Lodgepole area maintains an entirely different feel, situated in a deep, glacier-carved canyon near the banks of Marble Fork Kaweah River. Although not usually common at elevations below 7,500 feet, lodgepole pines grace the forest in this relatively cool canyon and give the area its name. As the commercial and administrative center of Sequoia, Lodgepole boasts a visitor center, wilderness permit office, market, gift shop, snack bar, deli, laundry, shower facility, post office, picnic area, year-round campground, and the Walter Fry Nature Center. It is the trailhead for the Twin Lakes Trail and the popular 2-mile dayhike to Tokopah Falls (see Trips 44 and 45, page 170).

㉑ 21.3 miles

Marble Fork Bridge: Just past the Lodgepole junction, the Generals Highway crosses a bridge over Marble Fork Kaweah River and passes a service road to employee housing on the right and the serene Lodgepole Picnic Area on the left.

㉒ 21.5 miles

Silliman Creek: Another tributary of Marble Fork Kaweah River, Silliman Creek drains Silliman Lake near the south base of Silliman Peak.

㉓ 22.1 miles

Clover Creek: The highway crosses Clover Creek over a handsome arched bridge of hand-hewn stone. A small pullout on the left, upper side of the creek could be used for parking for further exploration of the bridge and creek.

㉔ 22.8 miles

Wuksachi Junction: As part of the restoration of the Giant Forest, all lodging was moved away from the environmentally sensitive giant sequoia grove to Wuksachi Village in 1999. Along with 102 rooms, the village

has a dining room, gift shop, and conference facilities, as well as a trailhead for the Wuksachi Trail (see Trip 47, page 182).

㉕ 23.2 miles

Red Fir Junction: During the Giant Forest's restoration, maintenance facilities were also relocated to Red Fir. A short distance past the junction is a gate, where the NPS will periodically close the Generals Highway during winter storms. Beyond this gate you'll see little development for the next several miles, as a relatively quiet section of road weaves through mid-elevation forests composed mainly of firs and pines.

㉖ 24.9 miles

Halstead Meadow and Picnic Area: The highway passes a picturesque meadow bisected by Halstead Creek. Just past the creek on the left is the Halstead Picnic Area, with picnic tables, grills, and vault toilets but no running water.

㉗ 26.2 miles

Suwanee Creek: The highway inauspiciously crosses Suwanee Creek, which appears to the casual observer to be little more than a pleasant stream. Hidden from view a mile to the south is Suwanee Grove, a somewhat inaccessible 100-acre pocket of forest harboring nearly 300 giant sequoias, one of the many lesser-known giant sequoia groves in Sequoia and Kings Canyon.

㉘ 27.8 miles

Little Baldy Saddle: After climbing for several miles, the Generals Highway tops out at Little Baldy Saddle, which sits on the divide between the Marble Fork and North Fork of the Kaweah River. The right-hand shoulder allows vehicle parking for hikers bound for the top of Little Baldy, one of several granite domes poking above the surrounding forest on the west side of the parks. The 1.75-mile hike to the site of a former fire lookout leads to a fine view of the surrounding parklands (see Trip 48, page 184).

㉙ 29.4 miles

Dorst Creek Campground: An access road on the left-hand side of the highway leads down to the fir-shaded campground, open from late June through early September. Although popular, Dorst emits an ambiance of being one of the quieter campgrounds in the parks. Several trails emanate from the campground, including the 2-mile hike to Muir Grove, where hikers can commune with the giant sequoias without the hubbub usually found in the more popular groves (see Trip 49, page 185).

㉚ 30.4 miles

Cabin Creek: Immediately past the highway bridge over Cabin Creek is a small pullout, from where a little-used trail follows the west bank of the creek toward a junction of a trail heading west to Lost Grove (see Trip 50, page 187) and then continuing south to Dorst Campground (see Trip 51, page 188).

㉛ 31.3 miles

Lost Grove: Despite its location next to the Generals Highway, Lost Grove is one of the more serene giant sequoia groves in the parks accessible by automobile. The grove is sheltered in a narrow ravine, well-watered by a tributary of Dorst Creek, which produces conditions compatible for growth of the Big Trees. Containing nearly 200 specimens in 50 acres, the upper part of Lost Grove on the north side of the highway has a short nature trail. A longer trail on the south side heads south and then east to Dorst Campground (see Trip 50, page 187). This grove is certainly not "lost" nowadays, but the origin of its name remains unclear.

㉜ 31.9 miles

Sequoia National Park boundary: A historic sign marks your departure from national parklands at the entrance to Giant Sequoia National Monument. Formerly, these lands were simply part of Sequoia National Forest until President Bill Clinton designated the monument in 2000. While the National Park Service is responsible for the parks, the US Forest Service retains oversight of the monument, which includes 33 giant sequoia groves on the west flank of the Sierra.

㉝ 34 miles

Stony Creek Campgrounds and Day Use Area: Two Forest Service campgrounds, three group campgrounds farther up the highway, and a picnic area provide recreational opportunities near Stony Creek, a tributary of North Fork Kaweah River. The upper campground also has a small parking area at the trailhead for the Stony Creek Trail (see Trip 52, page 191).

㉞ 34.4 miles

Stony Creek Village: On the left side of the highway is a seasonally open lodge with motel-style accommodations, a general store, restaurant, showers, and gas station.

㉟ 38.2 miles

Montecito Sequoia Lodge: Also on the left side of the highway, Montecito Sequoia is an all-season, all-inclusive resort near a private lake. Lodging is available in hotel-style rooms, suites, or cabins.

㊱ 38.7 miles

Big Meadow Road Junction: The Big Meadow Road provides access to Horse Camp, Buck Rock, and Big Meadows Campgrounds and Buck Rock Lookout, as well as trailheads for trips into Jennie Lake Wilderness (see Trips 53–56, page 193).

㊲ 39.3 miles

Big Baldy Saddle: The highest point on the Generals Highway is reached at Big Baldy Saddle (approximately 7,600 feet), which also coincides with the Kings Canyon National Park's east boundary. For the next few miles, the highway follows the boundary between the park on the left and national forest land to the right. A broad shoulder at the saddle provides parking for the Big Baldy Trail, which travels 2-plus-miles to the top of a granite dome with a fine 360-degree view (see Trip 57, page 202).

38 41.3 miles

Buena Vista Trailhead: A small parking area on the left-hand side of the highway provides limited parking for the 1-mile hike to the top of Buena Vista Peak and a view of the Redwood Mountain area (see Trip 58, page 204).

39 41.4 miles

Kings Canyon Overlook: On the right-hand side of the Generals Highway is a parking for an overlook of the deep clefts of the South Fork and Middle Fork Kings River canyons, some of the deepest canyons in North America. Interpretive signs help to identify the distant snow-clad peaks rising above these deep holes, which provide the headwaters for these two forks of the Kings River. Closer at hand to the northeast is Buck Rock Lookout.

40 42.4 miles

Quail Flat Junction: The major junction at Quail Flat provides access to a variety of destinations. The narrow, dirt road on the left leads 1.7 miles to Redwood Saddle, where trails access Redwood Mountain Grove, the largest giant sequoia grove on the planet, where thousands of giant sequoias thrive in the drainages and hillsides of aptly named Redwood Mountain (see Trips 59–60, page 205).

Paved Tenmile Road to the right leads to Tenmile and Landslide Campgrounds, and Logger Flat and Aspen Hollow Group Campgrounds, on the way to Hume Lake. The lake offers swimming at Sandy Cove, picnicking at Powder Can, and camping at Hume Lake Campground. Hume Lake

Christian Camps above the southwest shore has a general store with gas pumps, a snack shop, gift shop, and boat rentals available to the general public.

From Quail Flat, FS Road 14S02 leads to remote giant sequoia groves, including the Kennedy Meadows Trailhead and Evans Grove (see Trip 56, page 199).

41 43.1 miles

Redwood Canyon Overlook: A pullout on the left-hand side of the highway offers a wide-ranging view of the Redwood Mountain Grove. Careful observation soon reveals the characteristically round crown of giant sequoias, which differs from the tops of its usual associates—white firs, incense cedars, and sugar pines. More than 15,000 specimens of giant sequoia larger than one foot in diameter, along with tens of thousand younger sequoias, call the grove home.

42 43.4 miles

Kings Canyon National Park boundary: At 0.3 mile from the overlook, the Generals Highway forsakes the national forest land present on the right-hand side for the last few miles and now travels wholly within Kings Canyon National Park.

43 46.1 miles

Y-junction with Kings Canyon Highway: Although the Generals Highway technically continues another 2.8 miles to the General Grant Tree, for our purposes the road log for the Generals Highway ends at the Y-junction with Kings Canyon Highway. A left turn at the junction will lead shortly out of the park beyond the Big Stump Entrance and toward Fresno. A right turn will continue through Grant Grove and ultimately into Kings Canyon proper.

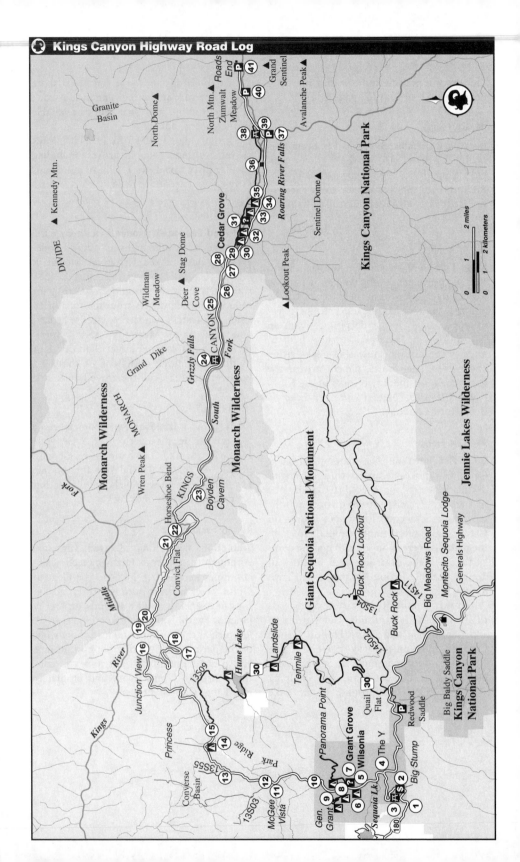

Kings Canyon Highway Road Log

Kings Canyon Highway provides the lone vehicular access into its namesake canyon, dead-ending at aptly named Roads End. State Highway 198 proceeds eastbound from Fresno across the broad plain of the San Joaquin Valley before climbing through the foothills zone and into the mid-elevation forests to the Big Stump Entrance into Kings Canyon National Park. The 40-mile journey from the Big Stump Entrance to Roads End requires a minimum of an hour to complete without stops along the way, as the curvy road winds down into the canyon. Kings Canyon Highway is usually open beyond the Hume junction from late April to mid-November.

Since most motorists approach Kings Canyon from the Fresno area via Highway 180, this road log begins at the west boundary of Kings Canyon National Park.

① 0.0 mile

Kings Canyon National Park boundary: Highway 180 climbs out of the San Joaquin Valley up the west slope of the Sierra and enters national parkland.

② 0.8 mile

Big Stump Entrance Station: The old entrance station was removed in 2005 due to the high probability of an old sequoia tree toppling onto the site and was temporarily relocated to the Big Stump Picnic Area parking lot.

③ 1.4 miles

Big Stump Picnic Area: Hopefully, this picnic area, which served as the temporary entrance station, will be refurbished when the new entrance station opens, with restrooms and picnic tables available to the public. In winter, Big Stump has been also used as a snow play area. A short nature trail loop through Big Stump Grove attracts tourists, while a longer 2-mile loop and a trail to Hitchcock Meadow offer a bit more solitude (see Trips 61–62, page 212).

④ 2.4 miles

Y-junction with Generals Highway: Here the Generals Highway heads south through the western finger of Kings Canyon National Park and across Giant Sequoia National Monument to the north part of Sequoia National Park. Kings Canyon Highway continues ahead toward Grant Grove.

⑤ 3.5 miles

Wilsonia: On the right-hand side of the highway, a road heads into a private inholding within Kings Canyon National Park, filled mainly with rustic cabins. The first official step toward the establishment of a national park occurred in 1880, when Theodore Wagner, US Surveyor General for California, suspended four square miles of Grant Grove, prohibiting any interested parties from filing a land claim. Unfortunately, a 160-acre claim had already been filed adjacent to the area. Subsequent efforts to buy the land were unsuccessful, leading to the privately owned Wilsonia area you see today.

⑥ 3.6 miles

Sunset Campground: Sunset Campground on the left is the first of the campgrounds in the Grant Grove area. It is open from late May to September.

⑦ 3.8 miles

Grant Grove Village: Grant Grove is the main hub of services within Kings Canyon National Park. Facilities include a visitor center, restrooms, lodging, restaurant, general store, gift shop, post office, and public showers. A number of hiking trails emanate from the area as well (see Trips 63–67, page 215).

⑧ 4 miles

Grant Tree Road and Crystal Springs Road: A mere 0.2 mile from the entrance to Grant Grove Village is an intersection with the Grant Tree Road on the left and the Crystal Springs Road on the right. The Grant Tree Road travels 0.75 mile to a large parking lot (restrooms) near the start of the nature trail loop around the General Grant Tree (see Trip 66, page 220). This road also accesses the Azalea and Swale Campgrounds and the trailhead for the North Grove (see Trip 65, page 219).

The Crystal Springs Road leads to Crystal Springs Campground and John Muir Lodge in the Grant Grove area before continuing roughly northeast to the parking lot for the short walk to Panorama Point (see Trip 67, page 222).

⑨ 4.2 miles

Stables: Horseback rides are available from the Grant Grove Stables during the summer months.

⑩ 5.2 miles

Kings Canyon National Park boundary: Just before the boundary between the park and Giant Sequoia National Monument, the highway crosses the North Boundary Trail. Beyond the boundary, the highway enters

lands administered by Sequoia National Forest.

⑪ 6.6 miles

McGee Vista Point: From a pullout on the left-hand side, you have a sweeping view of the western Sierra. An interpretive sign offers information about the McGee Burn forest fire of 1955.

⑫ 6.9 miles

Cherry Gap: Here the Kings Canyon Highway reaches its high point (approximately 6,800 feet). On the left, FS 13S03 heads into Converse Basin, where thousands of giant sequoias were sacrificed to the lumberman's axe in the late 1800s and early 1900s. Only a small percentage remains, including the Boole Tree, eighth largest (see Trip 69, page 225), of what was once the largest grove of giant sequoias in the world.

⑬ 8.2 miles

FS Road 13S55: On the left, another dirt Forest Service road heads into Converse Basin.

⑭ 9.8 miles

Princess Meadow: Near lovely Princess Meadow is the right-hand turn into Princess Campground. Look for deer and other wildlife in the meadow right after dawn or before sunset.

⑮ 10 miles

Hume junction: The Hume Road on the right leaves Kings Canyon Highway and makes a steep, winding descent on narrow road to Hume Lake. Along the way are some airy views. The lake, which is a reservoir created by a dam, offers swimming at Sandy Cove, picnicking at Powder Can, and camping at Hume Lake Campground. Hume Lake Christian Camps above the southwest shore has a general store with gas pumps, a snack shop, gift shop, and boat rentals available to the general public. In winter, the Kings Canyon Highway is closed past this junction.

⑯ 14.6 miles

Junction View: For about the previous 3 miles, you've had limited views of the deep hole created by the Kings River. At this pullout is a staggering view straight down to where Middle and South Forks converge thousands of feet below. Near this confluence, the two canyons reach their greatest depths. When measured from the top of Spanish Mountain, the South Fork Canyon at 7,800 feet is one of the deepest gorges in North America, more than 2,500 feet deeper than the Grand Canyon. While the Middle Fork is wild and virtually inaccessible except by hardy hikers, the highway continues upstream along the South Fork into the heart of Kings Canyon.

⑰ 16.8 miles

Ten Mile Creek: The highway crosses a bridge over Ten Mile Creek, which carries water released from Hume Lake dam down to the Kings River. Between here and Yucca Point, the road closely follows the creek

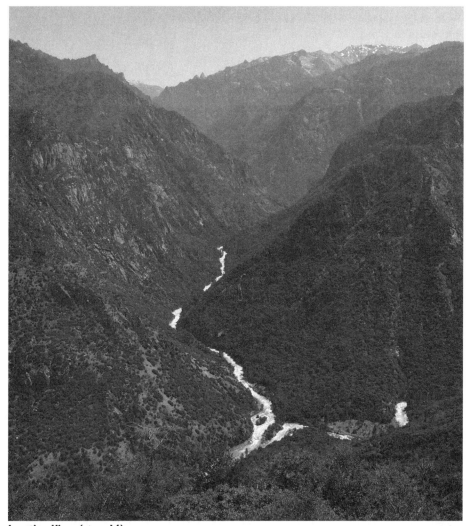

Junction View (stop 16)

downstream, providing a definite contrast between the riparian foliage alongside the creek and the chaparral-covered hillsides away from the water.

⑱ 17 miles

Kings Canyon Lodge: This rustic resort has been in operation since the late 1930s, offering cabin-style lodging, a restaurant, ice cream bar, and gasoline from the oldest double-gravity gas pumps in the country.

⑲ 18.1 miles

Yucca Point Trailhead: The highway drops into the inner gorge of Kings Canyon near Yucca Point, a point on a knife-edge ridge 200 feet above the road, which also serves as the westernmost boundary of Monarch Wilderness. Watch for the namesake plant through this section, especially in late spring and early summer, when the upper part of the plant is covered with white, bell-shaped flowers. A moderately steep, 2.5-mile trail descends more than 1,000 feet from the trailhead to the confluence of the Middle and South Forks of the Kings River. Anglers accessing the South and Middle Forks of the Kings River are this trail's primary users.

⑳ 18.6 miles

Lockwood Creek Vista: A half mile from Yucca Point is a broad, paved turnout on the left with an interpretive sign about birds commonly seen soaring above the canyon. The visual highlight of a stop here is in the opposite direction, especially when a year with abundant water enhances a beautiful display of cascades and falls on Lockwood Creek, which tumbles down a narrow, steep, and rocky side canyon. Shortly beyond the turnout, the highway crosses over the creek and continues down toward the river amid the towering metamorphic rock walls of the canyon.

㉑ 19.5 miles

Convict Flat Picnic Area: Construction of the Kings Canyon Highway began in 1929 and took ten years to complete. Much of the

work was done by convicts. The picnic area resides on the former site of the prisoner camps.

㉒ 22.3 miles

Horseshoe Bend Vista: The pullout at Horseshoe Bend offers a dramatic view of the canyon, where high, unbroken cliffs composed of hard metamorphosed rock forced the South Fork to take a winding detour.

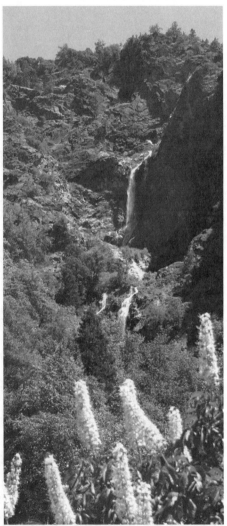

Waterfall in Lockwood Creek Canyon (stop 20)

㉓ 23.5 miles

Boyden Cavern: On the right-hand side of the highway, just prior to a bridge over the South Fork, is the turnoff for Boyden Cavern. The west side of the Sierra has considerable deposits of marble. Caves are formed when underground channels of water erode away some of the minerals in such marble over time. A private concessionaire, under supervision of the Forest Service, offers 45-minute tours of Boyden Cavern from April through November. The tour visits many extraordinary features, including various stalagmites, stalactites, draperies, and columns.

Beyond the first bridge over South Fork Kings River, the highway closely follows the river upstream, which can become quite a torrent during spring snowmelt.

㉔ 28.7 miles

Grizzly Falls Picnic Area: A small picnic area (restrooms) on the left side of the highway under the shade of mixed forest provides a pleasant rest stop. Just 50 yards above the picnic area is Grizzly Falls, which drops 80 feet over a ledge of granite. The falls can be quite robust in spring and early summer, when melting snow on the south side of the Monarch Divide high above fills Grizzly Creek and its tributaries.

㉕ 30.4 miles

Deer Cove Trailhead: A small parking area on the left-hand side of the highway marks the beginning of the Deer Cove Trail, an infrequently used, dead-end trail that climbs into the Monarch Wilderness (see Trip 70, page 229).

㉖ 30.8 miles

Turnout: This unmarked turnout offers another chance to stop and view the South Fork.

㉗ 31.5 miles

Kings Canyon National Park boundary: After the long, winding descent across Forest Service lands, you once again enter the national park, at the geological gate of the more famous section of Kings Canyon. Below here, the canyon has a V-shaped aspect, formed by the erosional forces of the South Fork Kings River. Above, the canyon adopts more of a U-shape, with a broader valley floor and steeper canyon walls composed of the characteristic Sierra granite, which has led geologists to the conclusion that glaciers were primarily responsible for the formation of the upper part of Kings Canyon.

㉘ 31.4 miles

Lewis Creek Trailhead: Shortly past the park boundary, the highway spans Lewis Creek and continues 0.2 mile to the trailhead on the left shoulder (see Trips 73 and 74, page 236). The creek is one of the many watercourses born high up in the mountains that tumble down the steep wall of the canyon toward a union with the South Fork. Similarly, since the only way out of the canyon is up, most of the trails starting in the bottom of the canyon climb steeply.

㉙ 32.1 miles

South Fork Bridge: Thinking back to the first bridged crossing of the South Fork, the river was a boulder-strewn torrent racing toward the San Joaquin Valley below. Here, the broad and shallow river has adopted a more placid course because it's flowing through the flatter and wider valley created by the glaciers.

Just prior to the bridge, a paved road branches off to the left, which is the back way into the Cedar Grove complex and the most direct route from here to the pack station and Hotel Creek Trailhead (see Trips 73 and 74, page 236).

㉚ 32.6 miles

Sheep Creek Campground: Kings Canyon is blessed with many fine campgrounds, Sheep Creek being the first you'll encounter on your way upstream. Open from May to mid-November, the 111-site campground is run on a first-come, first-served basis. Ranger programs run during July and August.

③ 33.1 miles

Cedar Grove: The broad, forested flat of Cedar Grove has long been the center of human activity in Kings Canyon. Bedrock mortars on the opposite side of the river testify to the presence of Native Americans before the arrival of European settlers. In 1897 the area's first hotel was constructed on this site, and the park service eventually established their headquarters here in the 1930s. Today, Cedar Grove Village offers motel-style lodging at Cedar Grove Lodge, which also has a snack bar and small store, with public showers and a laundromat nearby. A small visitor center provides exhibits, books, and maps and rents bear canisters. Cedar Grove also has a picnic area with restrooms. The stables offer horseback rides and pack trips.

Although hard to imagine today, a dam at the lower end of the valley was once slated to inundate this area with a reservoir. Thanks to rigorous conservation efforts, a dam was eventually built farther downstream at Pine Flat instead, sparing Kings Canyon from a fate similar to the one that befell Hetch Hetchy in Yosemite.

③ 33.3 miles

Don Cecil Trailhead: Barely noticeable on the right-hand shoulder is the trailhead for the 5-mile trail to a viewpoint atop Lookout Peak (see Trip 72, page 234). A fair number of hikers use this trail, but most of them go no farther than a mile to a refreshing grotto at a crossing of Sheep Creek.

③ 33.5 miles

Canyon View Campground: Canyon View is the next campground you pass in Kings Canyon, with 23 sites and 5 group sites open on a first-come, first-served basis, from May to October as needed.

③ 33.8 miles

Moraine Campground: Moraine is the next campground you pass in Kings Canyon, with 120 sites open on a first-come, first-served basis, from May to October as needed.

③ 34 miles

Canyon View Vista Point: On the left-hand shoulder, just past the entrance to Moraine Campground, the vegetation parts enough to allow one of the few unimpeded views of U-shaped Kings Canyon along the highway.

③ 35.2 miles

Knapps Cabin: During the Roaring Twenties, a wealthy Santa Barbara businessman named George Knapp organized lavish fishing trips to Kings Canyon. A small cabin at this site was used to store his extravagant fishing gear.

③ 36.1 miles

Roaring River Falls: The highway once again crosses the South Fork on a bridge and soon comes to the parking area for Roaring River Falls. A short, paved path climbs to the base of the falls, where water that flows from below the divide separating Kings Canyon and Sequoia parks spills dramatically into a deep green pool. A gently graded footpath follows the South Fork upstream from the parking area to Zumwalt Meadow and Roads End.

③ 36.3 miles

Pullout: On the left-hand side of the highway is an informal picnic area.

③ 36.5 miles

Upper Kings River Bridge: Keen eyes will notice the diminished flow of the river above the confluence with Roaring River, which carries nearly as much water as the main South Fork.

⑩ 37.6 miles

Zumwalt Meadow: After crossing Granite Creek, the highway comes to a parking area near Zumwalt Meadow, where a 1.5-mile long nature trail (see Trip 75, page 239) crosses a bridge over the South Fork and then circles the fringe of Zumwalt Meadow. For a small fee, you can pick up a brochure at the start of the trail containing information pertaining to the natural history of the area and corresponding to the numbered posts positioned along the way. From the meadow are fine views of two of the upper canyon's most imposing features, the granite hulks of North Dome and Grand Sentinel.

㊶ 38.4 miles

Roads End Loop: Less than a mile from Zumwalt Meadow, where Copper Creek meets the South Fork, the highway reaches a conclusion at aptly named Roads End, where a 0.3-mile loop provides access to day-use and overnight parking lots. Other than the wilderness permit cabin near the Roads End Trailhead, restrooms and a couple of picnic tables are the last signs of civilization at the western edge of the Kings Canyon wilderness. From here, hiking trails provide the only means of access to the lands beyond (see Trips 76–85, page 241).

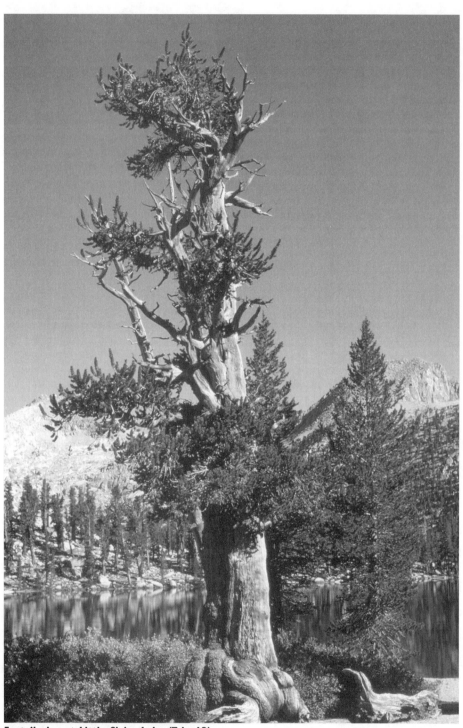

Foxtail pine at Little Claire Lake (Trip 13)

West Side Trips

The west side of the Sierra Nevada rises steadily from the broad plain of the San Joaquin Valley toward the protected lands of Sequoia and Kings Canyon National Parks. Heading east, the verdant agricultural land of the San Joaquin Valley gives way to the grasslands and chaparral of the foothills zone, which in turn give way to the dense timber of the mid-elevation forests. A few roads penetrate the heart of these areas of towering conifers and scattered groves of giant sequoias, but auto-bound visitors to the parks must stop well below the granite cirques and serrated peaks of the High Sierra. Steadily rising, roadless terrain continues through the red fir and lodgepole pine forests into the subalpine and alpine zones, which eventually culminates at the apex of the Sierra Crest forming the eastern boundary of both parks.

Recreationists entering Sequoia and Kings Canyon National Parks from the west will experience a wide range of topography, flora, and fauna. The foothills region of Sequoia offers year-round hiking opportunities in the drainages of the South Fork and Middle Fork Kaweah Rivers. In the spring, once Mineral King Road reopens and the Giant Forest is snow free, fortunate hikers are blessed with splendid opportunities to stand beneath a massive sequoia, stroll along a tumbling stream, or gaze across a verdant, wildflower-covered meadow. Midsummer, the height of the outdoor season, lures backpackers with the siren call of the magnificent backcountry within the parks and surrounding wilderness areas.

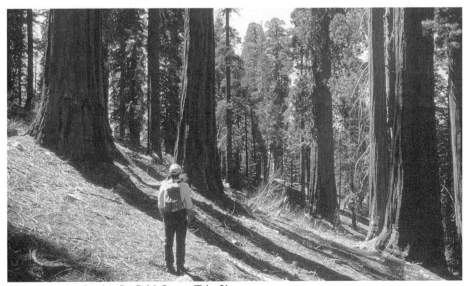

Giant sequoias in the Garfield Grove (Trip 2)

Introduction to South Fork Kaweah River

Situated in the extreme southwest corner of Sequoia National Park, the South Fork Kaweah River Trailhead provides access to some of the lowland trails of the foothills zone, a plant community composed primarily of oak woodland and chaparral. As opposed to the classic Sierra granite of the higher elevations, much of the foothills zone is covered with crumbling metamorphic rock, primarily marble, schist, and slate. Steep-walled, brush-filled canyons cut by turbulent rivers and streams characterize the topography in this area.

Due to the milder climate at these altitudes, recreationists have opportunities for off-season hiking on trails that typically see little use. Fall, winter, and spring can be ideal times for trips to the South Fork, although summer visitors can beat the heat by hiking earlier or later in the day. During the summer season, backpackers use the Garfield-Hockett Trail as a gateway into the mid-elevation forests and meadows of the Hockett Plateau and backcountry beyond.

In the past, a more extensive network of trails crisscrossed the southwest corner of

Campground							
Campground	Fee	Elevation	Season	Restrooms	Water	Bear Boxes	Phone
South Fork (12 miles from Hwy. 198)	No	3,600 feet	All year	Vault	No	Yes	No

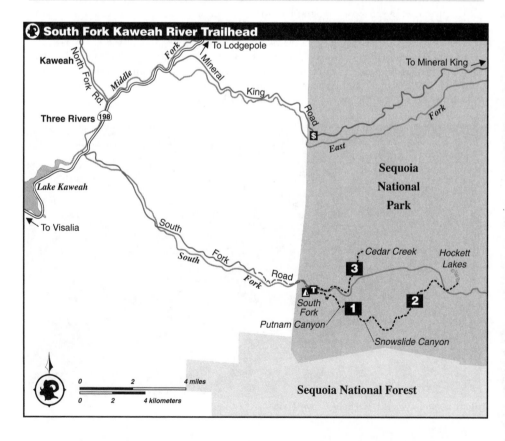

the park, but many of these paths are now overgrown. Unmaintained trails that still appear on some maps should be considered difficult bushwhacks. The Ladybug Trail follows a section of the historic Hockett Trail, constructed during the Civil War for travel through the Sierra between Visalia and the silver mines east of Owens Valley. Illegal marijuana cultivation has occurred in the lower elevations of the park and adjoining national forests—check with the proper authorities for updates.

ACCESS: This area is open all year. South Fork Road branches away from Highway 198 near the fire station in the town of Three Rivers. The road dead-ends at the South Fork Campground after 12 miles.

AMENITIES: Three Rivers is a small, tourist-driven town near the west boundary of Sequoia National Park, 37 miles east of Visalia. A wide range of services includes motels, restaurants, gas stations, and general stores. No services exist along the South Fork Road beyond Three Rivers.

RANGER STATION: The nearest ranger station is the Foothills Visitor Center inside the park. Wilderness permits may be available from the campground host at South Fork Campground in the summer or by self-registration at the trailhead the rest of the year. The South Fork Ranger Station has not been staffed for several years.

GOOD TO KNOW BEFORE YOU GO: At these low elevations, hikers should be on the lookout for ticks, rattlesnakes, and poison oak. Mountain lions live in the foothills zone, although they have presented few, if any, problems in the past. However, *don't leave small children unattended.* The Park Service recommends against hiking alone in mountain lion country.

SOUTH FORK KAWEAH RIVER TRAILHEAD

TRIP 1

Putnam and Snowslide Canyons

Ⓜ ↗ DH

DISTANCE: 4.2 miles, out-and-back to Putnam Canyon

6.8 miles, out-and-back to Snowslide Canyon

ELEVATION: 3,620'/5,125', +1,830'/-230'/±4,120' to Putnam Canyon

3,620'/5,800', +2,690'/-460'/±6,300' to Snowslide Canyon

SEASON: All year to Putnam Canyon

March to December to Snowslide Canyon

USE: Light

MAPS: *Dennison Peak* and *Moses Mountain*

INTRODUCTION: While most Sierra hikers sit at home and eagerly await the snow-free months of summer, a few resourceful souls enjoy the year-round pleasures of the foothills zone in the southwest corner of Sequoia National Park. The 2-mile hike to Putnam Canyon and 3.25-mile hike to Snowslide Canyon on the Garfield-Hockett Trail provide fine opportunities for early and late season forays into the frontcountry, when the majority of higher trails are buried in snow. This trip passes through foothills woodland to Putnam Canyon and then continues through mixed coniferous forest with a smattering of giant sequoias. Fine views of Homers Nose and Dennison Peak provide visual delights along the way.

DIRECTIONS TO TRAILHEAD: Follow State Highway 198 to Three Rivers and turn east onto South Fork Road, approximately 7 miles southwest of the Ash Mountain

Entrance to Sequoia National Park. Follow South Fork Road 9 miles to the end of the pavement, and continue another 3 miles on a narrow, dirt road to free South Fork Campground (vault toilets). Proceed through the campground to a small, oak-shaded hikers' parking area.

DESCRIPTION: The signed Garfield-Hockett Trail begins from the edge of the campground access road a short way before the parking area. Proceed up the trail on a moderate, winding climb across an oak-studded hillside. Lush trailside vegetation includes a healthy population of poison oak and colorful spring wildflowers. Enter a side canyon, about a mile from the trailhead, and step across the first of many small streams you encounter on the way across the slopes below Dennison Peak. The moisture in these diminutive nooks creates a dramatic change in vegetation, and ferns, thimble-

berry, maples, nutmegs, alders, dogwoods, and cedar line the shady stream banks.

Continue climbing steadily through oak woodland to Putnam Canyon. Just below the trail, the sound of rushing water from Big Spring courses down the canyon, but chances are the creek will be dry after snowmelt where the trail crosses the streambed. Steep and narrow, Putnam Canyon is filled with boulders and low shrubs, creating an opening through which you have a fine view across South Fork Canyon of the bulbous granite dome of Homers Nose protruding from the opposite ridge.

Beyond Putnam Canyon, the steady climb continues, as a smattering of ponderosa pines, white firs, and incense cedars start to intermix with the deciduous trees of the oak woodland. Fortunately, the arrival of conifers coincides with the departure of the poison oak, although the lovely flowers

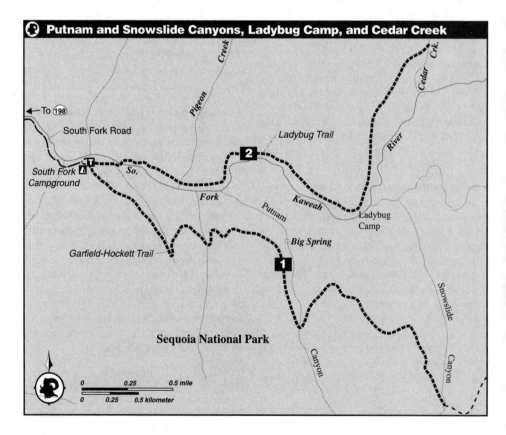

Putnam and Snowslide Canyons, Ladybug Camp, and Cedar Creek

and plants seen previously start to disappear as well. A mile from Putnam Canyon, you bid a final farewell to the oak woodland, as the trail bends southeast into a canyon near the western fringe of Garfield Grove. Farther on, a dozen or so giant sequoias dwarf the smaller conifers on the way to the crossing of the usually vigorous creek coursing down Snowslide Canyon.

For dayhikers, Snowslide Canyon is a fine early season goal because the winter snowpack generally covers the path beyond here until late spring.

TRIP 2

Ladybug Camp and Cedar Creek

M **DH** or **BP**

DISTANCE: 3.5 miles, out-and-back to Ladybug Camp

5.6 miles, out-and-back to Cedar Creek

ELEVATION: 3,620'/4,300', +960'/-180'/±2,280' to Ladybug Camp

3,620'/5,800', +1,880'/-325'/±4,410' to Cedar Creek

SEASON: All year to Ladybug Camp

March to December to Cedar Creek

USE: Light

MAPS: *Dennison Peak* and *Moses Mountain*

see map on p.58

TRAIL LOG

1.75 Ladybug Camp
2.75 Cedar Creek

INTRODUCTION: The Ladybug Trail offers a fine opportunity for off-season hiking. During March and April, blooming wildflowers complement the green grasslands, both of which are replenished by the winter rains. Also in spring, deciduous trees of the oak woodland leaf out, returning signs of life to their previously bare branches. South Fork Kaweah River is at full force at this time, cascading and churning through the foothills, before ultimately realizing a much tamer fate in the San Joaquin Valley. Fall adds a touch of crispness to the air and a splash of autumn color to the deciduous forest. Toss in the chance for an up-close experience with the giant sequoias at Cedar Creek, and you have the makings for a splendid outing. As with all foothills trips, watch for ticks, rattlesnakes, and poison oak.

DIRECTIONS TO TRAILHEAD: Follow State Highway 198 to Three Rivers and turn east onto South Fork Road, approximately 7 miles southwest of the Ash Mountain Entrance to Sequoia National Park. Follow South Fork Road 9 miles to the end of the pavement, and continue another 3 miles on narrow, dirt road to free South Fork Campground (vault toilets). Proceed through the campground to a small, oak-shaded hikers' parking area.

DESCRIPTION: From the parking area, head east upstream on a wide trail to the wood bridge spanning the South Fork Kaweah River and cross to the far side. Begin a moderate ascent through oak woodland and scattered boulders high above the river. Just before crossing the usually dry streambed of Pigeon Creek, you may notice the remnants of an old, now abandoned path that once led hikers steeply uphill to Homers Nose. Beyond Pigeon Creek, the trail ultimately emerges out of the forest to a fine view of the river below and also ahead to Putnam

Canyon and its cascading creek. A gentle climb then leads back into the trees and on to a log-and-boulder crossing of Squaw Creek 0.9 mile from the trailhead.

A moderate, 0.75-mile climb takes you away from the creek and back into the main canyon. Continue upstream, alternating between the filtered shade of oak woodland and the sun-drenched sky above patches of chaparral. A gentle descent heralds your arrival at the flat of Ladybug Camp alongside the swirling South Fork, where oaks, incense cedars, and a few ponderosa pines shade pleasant campsites. The area received its name from a wintering population of ladybugs.

Beyond Ladybug Camp, the trail continues upstream a short distance to an unofficial junction with a use trail heading straight ahead to an open area of rock slabs on a narrow bench. From this spot, directly above the river and across from the confluence of Garfield Creek, a breathtaking view unfolds when the tumbling river is flush with snowmelt, churning and plunging down the canyon.

THE BRIDGE THAT ISN'T

You may notice some reinforcing steel protruding out of rock on either side of the river just above the confluence with Garfield Creek, remnants of an old bridge that once spanned the South Fork. A trail that formerly led from the bridge up a ridge to connect with the Garfield-Hockett Trail was abandoned after the bridge collapsed from heavy snows in 1969.

From the Ladybug Camp junction, the main trail bends away from the river and climbs moderately up a grassy hillside dotted with oaks and cedars. Through gaps in the trees you have fine views of Homers Nose 4,000 feet above, a granite dome dubiously named by a surveyor for its resem-

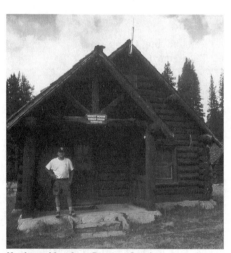

Hockett Meadow Ranger Station

blance to the nose of his guide, John Homer. Keen eyes will notice a smattering of giant sequoias across the canyon, their characteristic rounded tops thrusting skyward. These specimens of Garfield Grove represent the lowest-elevation sequoias in the Sierra. The views eventually disappear in a thickening forest of oaks and cedars on the approach to Cedar Creek. Along the banks, a number of sequoias tower over their neighboring conifers, with several younger sequoias sprinkled throughout the drainage.

□ A variety of options once existed for travel further into the Sequoia frontcountry beyond where maintained trail dead-ends at Cedar Creek. Hikers can still follow remnants of the old trail beyond the creek to a Y-junction, where a metal sign with punched-out letters gives directions to Cahoon Meadow and South Fork. Since the 1970s, neither trail has been maintained, and both are currently overgrown with brush and blocked by deadfalls and washouts. The South Fork branch descends to a grove of sequoias in the South Fork Canyon and an old campsite at Whiskey Log Camp, about 2 miles from Cedar Creek. However, the hiking is difficult and tedious; attempt it only if you have experience bushwhacking and hiking off-trail.

R Wilderness permits are required for overnight stays. Campfires are permitted.

SOUTH FORK KAWEAH RIVER TRAILHEAD

TRIP 3

Garfield-Hockett Trail to Garfield Grove and Hockett Lakes

Ⓜ ↗ DH or BP

DISTANCE: 10 miles, out-and-back to Garfield Creek

20 miles, out-and-back to Hockett Lakes

ELEVATION: 3,620'/7,700', +4,150'/-200'/±8,700' to Garfield Creek

3,620'/8,585', +5,880'/-935'/±13,630' to Hockett Lakes

SEASON: Late May to mid-October

USE: Light

MAPS: *Dennison Peak* and *Moses Mountain*

TRAIL LOG

3.25 Snowslide Canyon
5.0   Garfield Creek
9.25 South Fork crossing
10.0 Hockett Lakes

INTRODUCTION: Tucked quietly away in the southwest corner of Sequoia, Garfield Grove (named after a former president) and the contiguous Dillonwood Grove, compose one of the largest clusters of giant sequoias in the world. While hordes of tourists crane their necks to see the Big Trees in more popular areas such as the Giant Forest, Garfield Grove is cloaked in relative obscurity, awaiting discovery by the small number of devotees willing to hike 5 miles to the heart of the grove.

Beginning in foothills woodland, the trail climbs moderately through diverse plant communities, including riparian zones and mixed coniferous forest. Along with

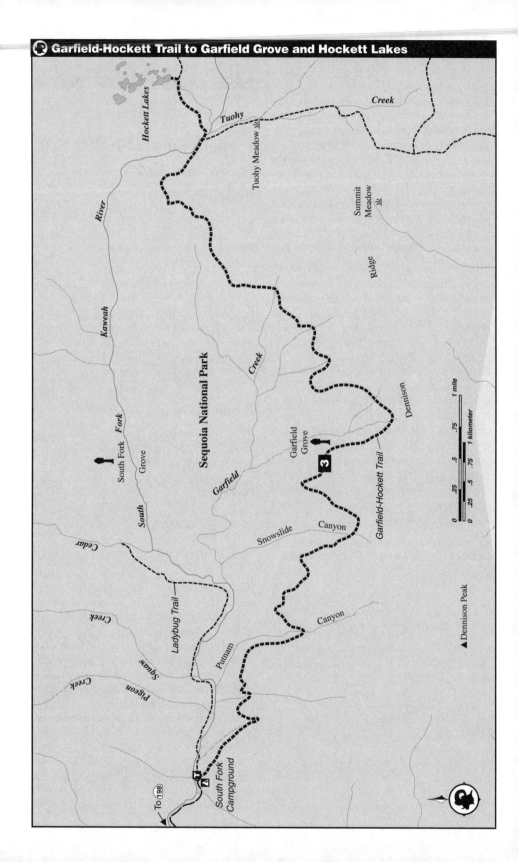

such diversity, the route offers refreshing streams and fine views on the way to Garfield Grove. After a 10-mile, 5,000-foot climb, backpackers reach first-rate camping and swimming at the serene Hockett Lakes.

While the low-elevation start offers off-season hiking opportunities (see Trip 1, page 57), backpackers bound for the high country beyond should get an early start to beat the summer heat. The typically high daily temperatures deter many recreationists, but the Garfield-Hockett Trail is the shortest route to Hockett Lakes. Perhaps the best bet for avoiding the stiff ascent during the heat of the day is to stay at the free South Fork Campground the night before and start hiking at the crack of dawn. Watch for poison oak, ticks, and rattlesnakes for the first 3 miles or so.

DIRECTIONS TO TRAILHEAD: Follow State Highway 198 to Three Rivers and turn east onto South Fork Road, approximately 7 miles southwest of the Ash Mountain Entrance to Sequoia National Park. Follow South Fork Road 9 miles to the end of the pavement, and continue another 3 miles on narrow, dirt road to free South Fork Campground (vault toilets). Proceed through the campground to a small, oak-shaded hikers' parking area.

DESCRIPTION: The signed Garfield-Hockett Trail begins from the edge of the campground access road a short way before the parking area. Proceed up the trail on a moderate, winding climb across an oak-studded hillside. Lush trailside vegetation includes a healthy population of poison oak and colorful spring wildflowers. Enter a side canyon, about a mile from the trailhead, and step across the first of many small streams you encounter on the way across the slopes below Dennison Peak. The moisture in these diminutive nooks creates a dramatic change in vegetation, and ferns, thimbleberry, maples, nutmegs, alders, dogwoods, and cedar line the shady stream banks.

Continue climbing steadily through oak woodland to Putnam Canyon. Just below

the trail, the sound of rushing water from Big Spring courses down the canyon, but chances are the creek will be dry after snowmelt where the trail crosses the streambed. Steep and narrow, Putnam Canyon is filled with boulders and low shrubs, creating an opening through which you have a fine view across South Fork Canyon of the bulbous granite dome of Homers Nose protruding from the opposite ridge.

Beyond Putnam Canyon, the steady climb continues, as a smattering of ponderosa pines, white firs, and incense cedars start to intermix with the deciduous trees of the oak woodland. Fortunately, the arrival of conifers coincides with the departure of the poison oak, although the lovely flowers and plants seen previously start to disappear as well. A mile from Putnam Canyon, you bid a final farewell to the oak woodland, as the trail bends southeast into a canyon near the western fringe of Garfield Grove. Farther on, a dozen or so giant sequoias dwarf the smaller conifers on the way to the crossing of the usually vigorous creek coursing down Snowslide Canyon.

Beyond the canyon, the trail returns to mixed forest on a steady, moderate ascent through the heart of Garfield Grove. The stately sequoias become more numerous after you reach the crest of a forested ridge, where the trail passes right by some of the larger specimens in the grove. At the 5-mile mark, step across the first of five branches of Garfield Creek—the luxuriant flora and delightful cascade in each of these five shady nooks offer inviting rest stops. Beyond the first branch of the creek, 3 miles of gently ascending tread lead to the far end of the grove.

Leaving the Big Trees behind, a steep climb leads to the crest of a red fir–forested ridge, followed by a brief descent to a broad ford of South Fork Kaweah River, 9.25 miles from the trailhead, where several shady campsites line the far bank. From the ford, follow the river upstream to a signed junction with the little-used Tuohy Creek Trail, which fords the South Fork and continues south beyond the park boundary to a trailhead at Shake Creek Campground.

From the junction, a winding, moderate climb heads away from the river and up a lodgepole-pine-covered hillside to gentler slopes above. Just past the crossing of the outlet, a short lateral branches to the southernmost Hockett Lake, 10 miles from the trailhead.

Hockett Lakes are a collection of shallow, grassy-banked bodies of water surrounded by a light forest of lodgepole pines. A pair of primitive campsites near the southernmost lake testify to the relative lack of overnight visitors and the strong possibility for solitude. The 5- to 8-foot deep lakes make fine swimming holes.

Beyond the junction of the lateral, the Garfield-Hockett Trail continues approximately 300 yards to a junction with a connector heading across Sand Meadows and a junction with the Atwell-Hockett Trail a mile farther.

O Although not as extensive as in former days, a fine network of connecting trails crisscross the Hockett Plateau. Along with the route described in Trip 5 (page 69), seldom-used trails lead south and east to a variety of obscure destinations.

R Wilderness permits are required for overnight stays. Campfires are permitted.

Introduction to Atwell Mill and Mineral King

One glimpse of the glacier-carved East Fork Kaweah River Canyon, with its alpine slopes rimmed by striking peaks, will convince onlookers of Mineral King's picturesque riches. Ironically, these scenic virtues had less to do with the area's eventual inclusion into Sequoia National Park than did its lack of mineral resources.

Prompted by the well-publicized mining booms in other areas of California and Nevada, hopeful miners poured into Mineral King (originally named Buelah) in the late 1880s, searching for the next mother lode. Miners extracted just enough ore to keep hopes alive, but it was never enough to make such a remote location profitable. The southern Sierra never yielded a significant strike of either gold or silver and was determined to be a bust by the turn of the century. The powerful San Francisco earthquake of 1906 triggered massive avalanches that leveled structures in Mineral King, serving as an exclamation point to the region's commercial woes.

The lumber to rebuild Mineral King after the avalanches had to come from somewhere, and so a sawmill was erected in 1879 at nearby Atwell Mill. A flume was also constructed between Oak Grove and Hammond to produce hydroelectricity. Unfortunately, a number of mighty sequoias were felled in the process, stumps of which are still visible in the vicinity of the mill. The mill ultimately suffered the same fate as the mines, as the cost of transporting lumber to viable markets in the San Joaquin Valley proved to be too expensive.

Another commercial interest invaded Mineral King in the early 1900s, when the Mt. Whitney Power Company built four rock-and-mortar dams at Crystal, Eagle, and Monarch Lakes. The dams were erected to regulate the flow of water into the aforementioned flume to maximize power generation at the company's hydroelectric plant in Hammond. Unlike the mines and mill, the dams and power plant remain in operation, currently owned by Southern California Edison.

Once mining and timber went by the wayside, the remaining inhabitants of Mineral King turned to the prospect of a resort community to maintain an existence in their beloved mountains. Unfortunately for the residents, the area failed to achieve much fame as a resort community, turning into a sleepy little burg after World War II.

The area's customarily mild winters and long-lasting snowpack prompted the Tulare County Board of Supervisors to sponsor a snow survey in 1947, which recommended that the board develop Mineral King as a winter sports destination. In 1949, the board solicited proposals from potential developers, but progress stalled until 1965, when they selected Disney Enterprises of Burbank as the contractor. Disney had ambitions to turn Mineral King into the foremost ski destination in the world, with a resort and amenities catering to more than 10,000 skiers per day. With eager cooperation from the Forest Service, Disney proceeded with their ambitious plans.

Plans for the megaresort ran headlong into the budding environmental movement of the 1970s. Protracted legal battles, negative public opinion, the excessive costs of constructing an all-weather road, and increased awareness of the area's avalanche potential combined to create forces too extreme for Disney to overcome. In 1978, President Jimmy Carter signed a bill incorporating the majestic Mineral King area into Sequoia National Park. Today, the park manages the area with the same sleepy atmosphere that prevailed much of the 20th century.

ACCESS: This area is open from late May until November 1. Between November and May, weather permitting, the road is open

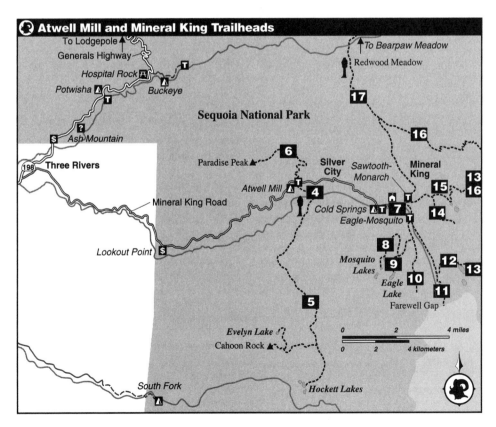

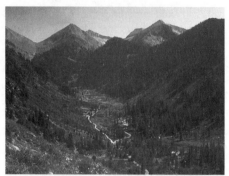

Mineral King as seen from the Sawtooth Pass Trail (Trip 13)

for the first 16.5 miles to a locked gate, 2.5 miles before Atwell Mill Campground. Access to Atwell Mill, Silver City, and Mineral King is via Mineral King Road, a sometimes steep, always narrow, often winding, partially dirt road that proceeds up the canyon of East Fork Kaweah River. Drivers must be constantly on alert for oncoming traffic, particularly during weekends. Plan to drive about an hour and a quarter to cover the 25-mile, 6,700-foot climb from Three Rivers to trailheads in Mineral King. *Gas is not available beyond Three Rivers.*

AMENITIES: The tourist-based community of Three Rivers, 37 miles east of Visalia and immediately west of the park entrance, offers a modicum of services, including motels, restaurants, gas stations, and stores.

The family-run Silver City Resort is usually open from late May into October, providing comfortable lodging in chalets and cabins, a limited selection of supplies (no ice or alcohol), dining, public showers, and ranger-led campfire talks on Thursday evenings. Many consider their fresh-baked pies to, be the resort's highlight. Call (559) 561-3223 in summer, or (805) 528-2730

off-season for more information, or visit their website at **www.silvercityresort.com.**

RANGER STATION: The rustic Mineral King Ranger Station, usually staffed from late May to late September, is located 22 miles from the junction of Highway 198 in Three Rivers. Backpackers can get wilderness permits during normal business hours (with reduced hours after Labor Day weekend). A limited selection of books and maps are available for purchase, and bear canisters can be rented. Call (559) 565-3768 for more information.

GOOD TO KNOW BEFORE YOU GO: Backpackers leaving vehicles overnight at trailheads in Mineral King should place all food and scented items in the storage shed directly opposite the ranger station because bear boxes are not available at the Tar Gap, Eagle-Mosquito, or Sawtooth-Monarch Trailheads.

Some of the plentiful marmots in Mineral King have developed a peculiar hankering for munching on car parts, such as radiator hoses, fan belts, and brake lines. Fortunately, this proclivity seems to be limited to early in the season (May and June), and by July these rodents turn to more nutritious fare. Check with rangers about current conditions. If your trip coincides with car-munching season, you may want to encircle your vehicle with chicken wire.

If you plan to camp at either Atwell Mill or Cold Springs Campgrounds, check the board at the Mineral King and Highway 198 junction in Three Rivers or at the Lookout Point Entrance Station for availability. Doing so could save you from a fruitless, time-consuming drive if the campgrounds are full.

Campgrounds

Campground	Fee	Elevation	Season	Restrooms	Water	Bear Boxes	Phone
Atwell Mill (18 miles from Hwy. 198)	$12	6,650 feet	Late May to November	Vault	Yes	Yes	No
Cold Springs (21.5 miles from Hwy. 198)	$12	7,500 feet	Late May to November	Vault	Yes	Yes	No

ATWELL MILL TRAILHEAD

TRIP 4

East Fork Grove

Ⓜ ↗ DH

DISTANCE: 5 miles, out-and-back

ELEVATION: 6,600'/6,240',
+525'/-820'/±2,690'

SEASON: Late May to November

USE: Light

MAP: *Silver City*

INTRODUCTION: Most hikers and backpackers who endure the rigors of the drive on Mineral King Road are bound for the high country above the valley, overlooking some of the lesser-known treasures along the way. Some of these neglected riches are found along the Atwell-Hockett Trail, which leads to a picturesque river canyon and a nearly forgotten grove of giant sequoias. On this 5-mile hike, visitors will enjoy the turbulent East Fork Kaweah River, which cascades through a narrow cleft of granite and a fine selection of Big Trees sans crowds.

DIRECTIONS TO TRAILHEAD: From the east end of Three Rivers, leave Highway 198 and turn onto Mineral King Road. Follow the road for 8 miles to the Atwell Mill Campground entrance and then continue another 0.2 mile to the signed trailhead parking area, which has a bear box, at the east end of the campground.

DESCRIPTION: Walk down a road toward the campground, which has water and vault toilets, for about 250 yards to the beginning of the signed Atwell-Hockett Trail. Follow a path past redwood stumps to a small meadow filled with relics from the long-abandoned Atwell Mill.

Through a mixed forest of black oaks, white firs, sugar pines, ponderosa pines, incense cedars, and sequoias, you veer away from the old mill site and descend around a hillside, soon dropping to diminutive

ATWELL MILL

In the 1870s, the Atwell Mill provided the town of Buelah (now Mineral King) with lumber for buildings and mines, also supplying a million board feet for a flume between Oak Grove and a hydroelectric plant in Hammond. The high cost of transporting lumber to the San Joaquin Valley eventually doomed the mill, but not before many stately giant sequoias near the mill succumbed to the logger's axe. Ironically, the brittle sequoia wood proved to be useful only for shakes and fence posts.

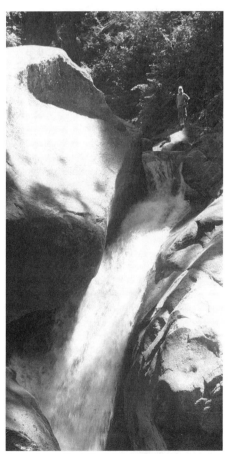

Cascade on East Fork Kaweah River

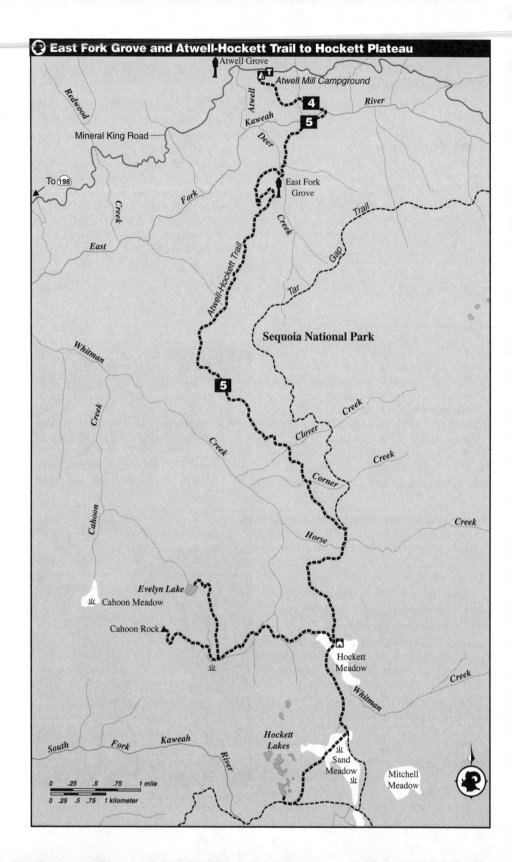

Deadwood Creek. The descent continues through forest another half mile to a stout steel-and-wood bridge spanning the granite cleft of East Fork Kaweah River, 1.25 miles from the parking area. The bridge offers a picture-postcard view of the cascading river plummeting over slabs and boulders down a narrow, sequoia-lined gorge.

Beyond the bridge, proceed through the East Fork Grove on a mild to moderate climb away from the river to Deer Creek, a good turnaround point for dayhikers. From the creek, the Atwell-Hockett Trail continues to the unceremonious southern end of the East Fork Grove.

ATWELL MILL TRAILHEAD

TRIP 5

Atwell-Hockett Trail to Hockett Plateau

Ⓜ ╱ BP

DISTANCE: 20 miles, out-and-back

ELEVATION: 6,600'/8,510', +3,690'/-1,785'/±10,950'

SEASON: June to late October

USE: Light

MAP: *Silver City*

TRAIL LOG

1.25	Cedar Creek
2.5	Deer Creek
7.25	Clover Creek
8.5	Tar Gap Trail junction
8.75	Horse Creek
10.0	Hockett Meadow

INTRODUCTION: Backpackers along the Atwell-Hockett Trail pass cascading streams and quiet forests with giant sequoias on the way to the Hockett Meadow, one of the largest and prettiest meadows in the park. The few backpackers and equestrians who visit the plateau usually access the area from Mineral King on the Tar Gap Trail, missing the scenic canyon of East Fork Kaweah River and the stately sequoias of the East Fork Grove.

After the first mile of descent to the East Fork, the remaining 9-mile trek along the Atwell-Hockett Trail is mostly a steady, pleasantly graded climb through mixed forest with occasional breaks in the trees allowing fine views of the surrounding terrain.

Once at pastoral Hockett Meadow, backpackers will find pleasant camping, stunning scenery, and unmatched serenity. A base camp here provides a fine outpost for additional hikes to attractive Evelyn Lake and tranquil Hockett Lakes, Cahoon Rock to enjoy its expansive views, or more remote destinations along the southern fringe of the park. Another highlight is the chance to see wildlife. Deer frequent Hockett Meadow, and hikers occasionally see bears along the trail.

DIRECTIONS TO TRAILHEAD: From the east end of Three Rivers, leave Highway 198 and turn onto Mineral King Road. Follow the road for 8 miles to the Atwell Mill Campground entrance and then continue another 0.2 mile to the signed trailhead parking area, which has a bear box, at the east end of the campground.

DESCRIPTION: Walk down a road toward the campground, which has water and vault toilets, for about 250 yards to the beginning of the signed Atwell-Hockett Trail. Follow a path past redwood stumps to a small meadow filled with relics from the long-abandoned Atwell Mill (see the sidebar in Trip 4, page 67, for historical information).

Through a mixed forest of black oaks, white firs, sugar pines, ponderosa pines, incense cedars, and sequoias, you veer away from the old mill site and descend around a hillside, soon dropping to diminutive Deadwood Creek. The descent continues through forest another half mile to a stout steel-and-wood bridge spanning the granite cleft of East Fork Kaweah River, 1.25 miles from the parking area. The bridge offers a picture-postcard view of the cascading river plummeting over slabs and boulders down a narrow, sequoia-lined gorge.

Beyond the bridge, proceed through the East Fork Grove on a mild to moderate climb away from the creek, passing a pair of rivulets on the way to Deer Creek. Leaving the creek, the trail climbs through a mixed forest of sugar and ponderosa pines, white firs, incense cedars, black oaks, and giant sequoias. The trail switchbacks and curves high above Deer Creek, leaving the Big Trees behind. Across a hillside above

the East Fork, the climb continues through mixed forest with an understory of chinquapin, mountain misery, thimbleberry, bracken fern, and hazel nut. Occasional breaks in the forest allow fine views down the East Fork and out to the San Joaquin Valley (haze permitting), including cars snaking along Mineral King Road.

Rounding a ridge, you find yourself above Horse Creek, with periodic views of Cahoon Rock and the backside of Homers Nose. After crossing a number of tiny brooks, the trail eventually reaches the densely vegetated banks of Clover Creek, 7.25 miles from the parking area. Above the near bank, a short use trail leads to a secluded campsite.

From Clover Creek, a steady half-mile ascent leads past a flower-filled, sloping meadow and continues to Corner Creek, where head-high wildflowers and plants carpet the drainage. Continue through fir forest and pockets of meadow for the next 0.75 mile to a signed Y-junction of the Tar Gap Trail from Mineral King, 8.5 miles from the parking area.

A few steps beyond the junction, you pass the indistinct junction with the abandoned Horse Creek Trail to Ansel Lake. The lake is very scenic, but the route

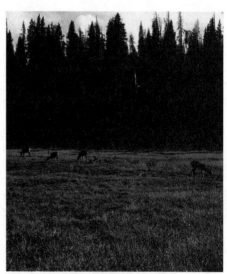

Deer at Hockett Meadow

is quite obscure and difficult to follow. A cross-country route from White Cloud Basin provides an easier way to Ansel Lake (see Trip 10, page 79). As you continue on the Atwell-Hockett Trail, a gentle descent leads to a series of spacious campsites along Horse Creek with a food storage cable nearby. Reach a ford of Horse Creek a short distance beyond the camp.

From the ford, cross a boggy area on a wood-plank bridge and begin a short climb around the nose of a red fir–forested ridge. A gentle descent through lodgepole pines follows, leading to the signed junction of the Evelyn Lake Trail near the north fringe of a large meadow. A short stroll beyond the junction brings you to the wide, open expanse of Hockett Meadow.

The signed trail toward Evelyn Lake and Cahoon Meadow leads to campsites not far from Whitman Creek, with a pit toilet and bear box. However, with a little effort, you can find better, more scenic sites around the fringe of Hockett Meadow.

SIDE TRIP TO EVELYN LAKE: From the junction with the Atwell-Hockett Trail, follow the Evelyn Lake Trail past campsites to the crossing of Whitman Creek and cross a meadow-lined smaller tributary 0.4 mile farther. A moderate ascent leads to a Y-junction, 1.7 miles from the Atwell-Hockett junction. Veer right at the junction and climb more steeply up a hillside of scattered trees and then along the crest of a view-packed ridge. A zigzagging descent from the end of the ridge leads through red firs to the shore of Evelyn Lake. The northeast shore offers campsites with a hitching post nearby, but more remote sites exist near the outlet. Most of the shoreline is covered with thick brush and a jumble of boulders, which makes getting around the lake a tad difficult. The lake is backdropped picturesquely by cliffs and offers good fishing and refreshing swimming. **END OF SIDE TRIP**

SIDE TRIP TO CAHOON ROCK: Follow the Evelyn Lake Trail to the Y-junction, 1.7 miles from the Atwell-Hockett junction. Veer left at the junction and follow a diminutive stream through moderate forest cover to a climb of a sandy slope below the summit of Cahoon Rock. Although the path becomes ill defined, the route to the top is obvious—make a short scramble over boulders to the summit, 1 mile from the junction.

The views are quite rewarding, especially if the usually hazy skies are clear from a recent shower or zephyr. The distant peaks of the Great Western Divide and the more immediate summits of Quinn Peak, Soda Butte, and Vandeveer Mountain fill the eastern skyline. Dennison Ridge is visible to the south; Homers Nose and the San Joaquin Valley beyond are the significant features in the west. **END OF SIDE TRIP**

SIDE TRIP TO HOCKETT LAKES: Continue on the Atwell-Hockett Trail, passing the ranger cabin and crossing a wood bridge over Whitman Creek. After a short climb up a hillside, parallel Hockett Meadow along the lodgepole-shaded fringe to a junction at the north end of Sand Meadow, 1.1 miles from the Evelyn Lake and Cahoon Rock junction.

Turn right at the junction and head across the northern fringe of Sand Meadow into lodgepole pine forest. After a mile, you reach the Garfield-Hockett Trail and head west for several hundred yards to the lateral leading to the southernmost lake. The Hockett Lakes are a collection of shallow, grass-lined lakes and ponds bordered by lodgepole pines, offering secluded camping and pleasant swimming. **END OF SIDE TRIP**

A base camp at either Hockett Meadow or Hockett Lakes allows for forays on isolated trails to a variety of destinations in the southern reaches of Sequoia National Park. With shuttle arrangements, you can combine this trip with the Garfield-Hockett Trail, reversing the description in Trip 3 and ending at the South Fork Trailhead.

Wilderness permits are required for overnight stays. Campfires are permitted.

ATWELL MILL TRAILHEAD

TRIP 6

Paradise Peak

Ⓜ ⟋ DH

DISTANCE: 10 miles, out-and-back

ELEVATION: 6,600'/9,362',
+2,990'/-185'/±6,350'

SEASON: Mid-June to late October

USE: Light

MAP: *Silver City*

INTRODUCTION: You won't have to fight the crowds here, as only a few hardy souls undertake the steep ascent to Paradise Peak. However, this climb up a south-facing slope to a superb view from the site of a former

lookout isn't as difficult as it seems. Giant sequoias in Atwell Grove, some of which are among the largest in existence, provide an added bonus.

DIRECTIONS TO TRAILHEAD: From the east end of Three Rivers, leave Highway 198 and turn onto Mineral King Road. Follow the road for 8 miles to the Atwell Mill Campground entrance and then continue another 0.2 mile to the signed trailhead parking area, which has a bear box, at the east end of the campground.

DESCRIPTION: From the parking area, head back down Mineral King Road for a quarter mile to the signed trailhead, where single-track tread begins a moderate climb through a mixed forest of white firs, ponderosa and sugar pines, incense cedars, and young sequoias with an understory of mountain misery and manzanita. Soon a series of switchbacks leads farther up

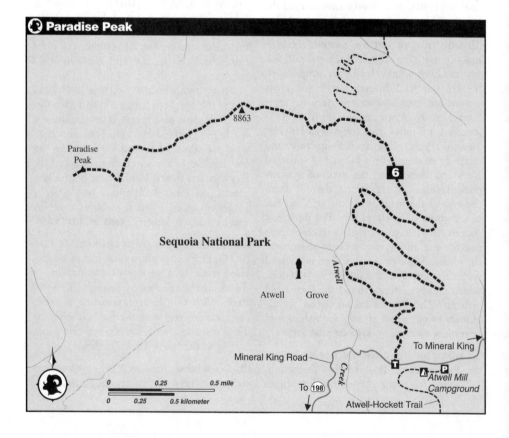

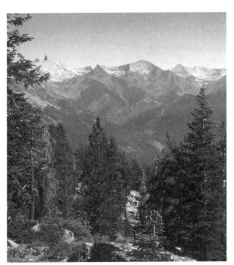

The Great Western Divide from Paradise Peak Trail

the slope. Medium-size sequoias begin to appear just past an opening in the forest and right before the crossing of a small fern- and alder-lined seasonal rivulet. Progressing up the hillside, you'll eventually see even larger sequoias, a few of which are some of the largest 20 to 30 specimens in the Sierra.

More zigzagging switchbacks lead up the hillside toward Atwell Creek—contrary to the trail route shown on the USGS map. If you need water, you'll have to thrash your way through thick brush to reach the creek, which is the only source along the entire route. Continue the switchbacking climb away from the creek to the crest of Paradise Ridge and a trail junction, 3.8 miles from the parking lot.

Amid a light forest of red firs and widely scattered patches of snowbush, chinquapin, and manzanita, the route to Paradise Peak turns west and follows gently graded tread along the ridge, a welcome change. After passing north of Peak 8863, watchful eyes may spot the crown of a sequoia growing at a higher elevation (8,800 feet) than any other, down-slope to the southeast. Continue along the ridge toward the summit over rocky terrain, where the tread falters a bit—watch for cairns or simply scramble over the rocks to the high point. The summit has a grand view to the east of the Great Western Divide and to the north of Castle Rocks and the granite domes of Big Baldy and Little Baldy.

To complete the experience, from the site of the old lookout, work your way through brush and around boulders to the base of the rock at the far end of the ridge, climb some rock steps, and then scramble up a short crack to the top. While trees block the view of the Great Western Divide, the vista to the west is quite impressive, including a glimpse straight down the canyon of Paradise Creek to Middle Fork Kaweah River. Additional points of interest include Moro Rock, Alta Peak, and the Generals Highway. You can see the Hockett Plateau clearly to the south.

TRIP 7

Cold Springs Trail

E / DH

DISTANCE: 1.2 miles, point-to-point

ELEVATION: 7,480'/7,810', +350'/-20'/±740'

SEASON: Late May through October

USE: Moderate

MAPS: USGS's *Mineral King* or
SNHA's *Mineral King*

INTRODUCTION: Most trails emanating from Mineral King climb steeply out of the valley. A rare exception, the Cold Springs Trail gently ascends along the East Fork Kaweah River between Cold Springs Campground and the Eagle-Mosquito Trailhead. Diehard backcountry types won't find the short trail very challenging, but the path is well suited for a family outing or an easy afternoon stroll. The scenery of Mineral King is always rewarding, and the short nature trail loop is an informative way to get acquainted with the ecology and history of the area.

DIRECTIONS TO TRAILHEAD:

START: From the east end of Three Rivers, leave Highway 198 and turn onto Mineral King Road. Follow the road for 22 miles to the Cold Springs Campground entrance, 2.5 miles past Silver City. Cross a bridge over East Fork Kaweah River and turn left at the first intersection. Travel 0.1 mile to the small parking area near Campsite 6.

END: Continue past the Cold Springs Campground entrance another 1.2 miles, passing the ranger station on the way, to the Eagle-Mosquito Trailhead parking area at the end of the road.

DESCRIPTION: From the trailhead, head upstream along the south bank of East Fork Kaweah River on gently graded tread, crossing a grassland dotted with aspens, cottonwoods, and a plethora of wildflowers in early summer. Reach a junction with the Cold Springs Nature Trail about 0.1 mile from the campground. The nature trail has interpretive signposts with pertinent information about the flora, geology, and mining history of Mineral King. The nature trail shortly loops back to the main trail.

The Cold Springs Trail continues upstream from the nature trail, passing delightful ponds and tumbling cascades well suited for wading and fishing. Farther on, switchbacks lead away from the river and into a stand of red firs. Beyond the trees, you emerge onto sagebrush-covered slopes, cross a number of side streams on wood bridges, and then descend rock steps to the final stretch of trail, passing several old cabins on the way to the Eagle-Mosquito Trailhead.

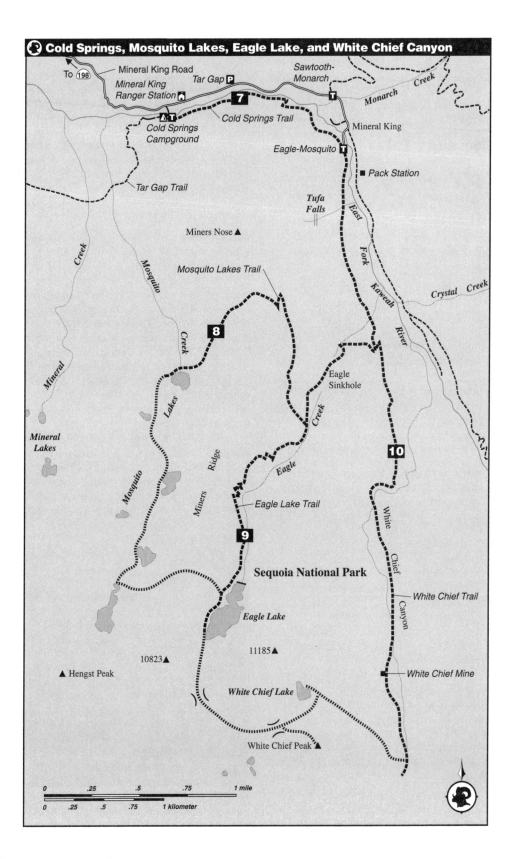

Cold Springs, Mosquito Lakes, Eagle Lake, and White Chief Canyon

To (198)
Mineral King Road
Mineral King Ranger Station
Tar Gap
Sawtooth-Monarch
Monarch Creek

7

Cold Springs Trail
Cold Springs Campground

Mineral King

Eagle-Mosquito

Tar Gap Trail

Pack Station

Tufa Falls

Miners Nose ▲

Mosquito Lakes Trail

East Fork Kaweah River

Crystal Creek

Creek

Mosquito

8

Eagle Sinkhole

Eagle Creek

Lakes

Creek

Mineral Lakes

Mineral

Miners Ridge

Eagle

Eagle Lake Trail

9

10

Sequoia National Park

White Chief Canyon

White Chief Trail

Eagle Lake

11185▲

10823▲

White Chief Mine

▲ Hengst Peak

White Chief Lake

White Chief Peak ▲

0   .25   .5   .75   1 mile
0   .25   .5   .75   1 kilometer

TRIP 8

Mosquito Lakes

Ⓜ ↗ **DH or BPx**

DISTANCE: 6.5 miles, out-and-back

ELEVATION: 7,815'/9,585',
+2,135'/-375'/±5,020'

SEASON: Early July to mid-October

USE: Moderate

MAPS: USGS's *Mineral King* or
SNHA's *Mineral King*

see
map on
p.75

TRAIL LOG

1.0 White Chief Canyon Trail junction
1.75 Eagle Lake Trail junction
3.25 Mosquito Lake #1

INTRODUCTION: The six enchanting Mosquito Lakes range from densely forest-rimmed to barren and rockbound. Formerly, the lakes were extremely popular destinations before the 1.5-mile trail from Cold Springs Campground was abandoned, camping at the Lake #1 was prohibited, and the trail beyond the first lake devolved into a cross-country route. Nowadays, a smattering of dayhikers trek up the newer trail to the first lake, but only a few of those travel farther off-trail to the upper lakes, offering a good chance of solitude for those who do make the journey.

At each of the lakes, the scenery is sublime, the swimming is refreshing, and the fishing for brook trout is reportedly good. Lake #3 has the best campsites for backpackers. Traces of the old trail still exist and cairns mark the way, which allows for straightforward route-finding. Be forewarned that these lakes received their name for a reason—be prepared for hordes of mosquitoes in early summer.

DIRECTIONS TO TRAILHEAD: From the east end of Three Rivers, leave Highway 198 and turn onto Mineral King Road. Follow the road past Atwell Mill Campground, Silver City, Cold Springs Campground, and Mineral King Ranger Station (which issues wilderness permits and has food storage areas) to the Eagle-Mosquito Trailhead parking area at the end of the road, 23.5 miles from Highway 198.

DESCRIPTION: Just south of the parking area, a dirt road heads past the Honeymoon Cabin and climbs gently up the East Fork Kaweah River Canyon through sagebrush scrub dotted with red firs, mountain maples, and a few western junipers. After a quarter mile, you cross Spring Creek on a removable wood bridge. Within earshot of the bridge but out of sight above the trail is Tufa Falls. The creek originates higher up the hillside and then follows a subterranean course through a band of marble before emerging a few hundred feet above the trail.

Just beyond Spring Creek, pass an unsigned lateral descending toward the river and proceed up the canyon, with good views of Crystal Creek cascading down the slope across the valley. Hop across willow-lined Eagle Creek and shortly arrive at the

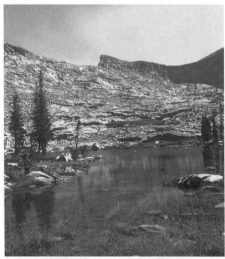

Lake #3 from Mosquito Lakes Trail

signed White Chief Canyon junction, 1 mile from the parking area.

Turn right at the junction and wrap around the hillside to a set of steep switchbacks that climb through pockets of meadow alternating with stands of red fir and lodgepole pine. The grade eases on the approach to Eagle Sinkhole, where Eagle Creek mysteriously disappears. Resume climbing, soon passing the Eagle Lake junction, 1.75 miles from the parking area.

From the junction, the trail ascends through red firs to the crest of Miners Ridge, from where a 0.75-mile switchbacking descent leads to Mosquito Lake #1, 3.25 miles from the trailhead. The oval-shaped lake is backed by a talus slope and encircled by lodgepole pines. Camping is banned here in an attempt to restore the native vegetation.

UNMAINTAINED TRAIL

Old signs near the outlet of Mosquito Lake #1 mark a junction with the unmaintained trail descending Mosquito Creek to a junction with the Tar Gap Trail, a half mile from Cold Springs Campground. This old trail was a shorter, but much steeper, route to the lakes.

A now unmaintained trail used to climb to the upper lakes, part of which is still evident as far up the canyon as Lake #3. From the outlet of Lake #1, follow distinct tread around the west shore and then head south up a steep hillside, where blazes and cairns will help guide you. To the east of Lake #2, another steep but short climb leads to Lake #3, where a pair of small islands and an amphitheater of towering white rock cliffs combine for some pretty scenery. Slabs on the south shore will entice sunbathers and swimmers, while anglers can ply the waters for brook trout. A sparse forest of lodgepole pines encircling the lake shade fine campsites.

Above Lake #3, signs of the old trail finally disappear for good. Cairns may be of assistance as you head cross-country up the next hillside to the right of a rocky slope. The route passes well to the east of Lake #4 and then proceeds toward irregularly shaped Lake #5, whose grassy shoreline is dotted with scattered lodgepoles, tucked against the cliffs of Miners Ridge.

The route to austere, treeless Mosquito Lake #6, the last lake in the chain, continues another quarter mile up the canyon.

O Off-trail enthusiasts can follow a short but challenging loop back to the trailhead by making an extremely steep ascent from the vicinity of Mosquito Lake #4 over Miners Ridge and down to Eagle Lake. From there, reverse the description in Trip 9 (page 78).

Mineral Lakes can be accessed via a straightforward route over a saddle directly west of Mosquito Lake #4.

R Wilderness permits are required for overnight stays. Campfires are prohibited. Camping is banned at Mosquito Lake #1.

see
map on
p.75

MINERAL KING TRAILHEAD

TRIP 9

Eagle Lake

Ⓜ ↗ **DH** or **BP**

DISTANCE: 6.5 miles, out-and-back

ELEVATION: 7,815'/10,045',
+2,285'/-55'/±4,680'

SEASON: Early July to mid-October

USE: Moderate

MAPS: USGS's *Mineral King* or
SNHA's *Mineral King* or Tom
Harrison Maps' *Mineral King*

TRAIL LOG

1.0   White Chief Canyon Trail junction
1.75   Eagle Lake Trail junction
3.25   Eagle Lake

INTRODUCTION: Crystalline Eagle Lake, reposing majestically in a deep glacial cirque, attracts flocks of anglers, photographers, dayhikers, and backpackers alike during the height of summer. The lake's popularity is well deserved due to the incredible scenery and is enhanced by the relatively short hiking distance of a little more than 3 miles. However, the rather stiff climb requires visitors to be in reasonable physical shape.

The Mt. Whitney Power and Electric Company dammed the lake in the early 1900s to regulate the flow of water at their generating plant downstream in Hammond. Southern California Edison regulates the water in the lake nowadays, and the level typically drops dramatically toward the end of the season, which somewhat diminishes the otherwise beautiful surroundings.

DIRECTIONS TO TRAILHEAD: From the east end of Three Rivers, leave Highway 198 and turn onto Mineral King Road. Follow the road past Atwell Mill Campground, Silver City, Cold Springs Campground, and Mineral King Ranger Station (which issues wilderness permits and has food storage areas) to the Eagle-Mosquito Trailhead parking area at the end of the road, 23.5 miles from Highway 198.

DESCRIPTION: Just south of the parking area, a dirt road heads past the Honeymoon Cabin and climbs gently up the East Fork Kaweah River Canyon through sagebrush scrub dotted with red firs, mountain maples, and a few western junipers. After a quarter mile, you cross Spring Creek on a removable wood bridge. Within earshot of the bridge but out of sight above the trail is Tufa Falls. The creek originates higher up the hillside and then follows a subterranean course through a band of marble before emerging a few hundred feet above the trail.

Just beyond Spring Creek, pass an unsigned lateral descending toward the river and proceed up the canyon, with good views of Crystal Creek cascading down the slope across the valley. Hop across willow-lined Eagle Creek and shortly arrive at the signed White Chief Canyon junction, 1 mile from the parking area.

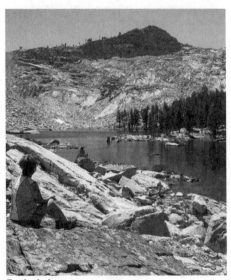

Eagle Lake

Turn right at the junction and wrap around the hillside to steep switchbacks that climb through pockets of meadow alternating with stands of red fir and lodgepole pine. The grade eases on the approach to Eagle Sinkhole, where Eagle Creek mysteriously disappears. Resume the climb, and soon reach the Eagle Lake junction, 1.75 miles from the parking area.

Climb mildly away from the junction alongside Eagle Creek to the far side of a meadow. From there, a steeper, switchbacking ascent of a hillside covered by red firs and lodgepole pines leads to an expansive talus slope. The trail makes a long ascending traverse across the talus slope toward the lip of Eagle Lake's basin. Along the way, the open topography allows for excellent views of Mineral and Sawtooth Peaks and the silver thread of cascading Crystal Creek across the canyon. The grade eventually eases beyond the talus, as you pass through pockets of grasses and shrubs, scattered boulders, and rock slabs amid a light forest of lodgepole pines. One final, steep pitch leads to the concrete dam and then along the west shore of Eagle Lake.

The stunning scenery of the steep-walled cirque is complemented by the soaring summit of Eagle Crest immediately south of the lake. Opposite, multicolored rock peaks rim the deep cleft of Mineral King Valley. Just past the dam, a use trail branches uphill to a primitive, screened pit toilet. Camping between the lake and the trail is banned; the best sites are about midway down the west shoreline. Anglers can fish for small to medium brook trout.

Cross-country enthusiasts can climb over Miners Ridge from the west shore of Eagle Lake to access the Mosquito Lakes Basin. The route is short, but quite steep, and is particularly rocky on the Mosquito Lakes side (see Trip 8, page 76).

Wilderness permits are required for overnight stays. Campfires are prohibited. Camping is banned between the shore of Eagle Lake and the trail.

MINERAL KING TRAILHEAD

TRIP 10

White Chief Canyon

M ↗ DH, BP, or **X**

DISTANCE: 7.5 miles, out-and-back

ELEVATION: 7,815'/10,030', +2,360'/-150'/±5,050'

SEASON: Early July to mid-October

USE: Moderate

MAPS: USGS's *Mineral King* or SNHA's *Mineral King* or Tom Harrison Maps' *Mineral King*

see map on p.75

TRAIL LOG

1.0 White Chief Canyon Trail junction
1.75 Eagle Lake Trail junction
3.75 Upper meadow

INTRODUCTION: All trails in the Mineral King area are blessed with fantastic scenery, and the White Chief Trail is no exception. Visitors will experience wonderful vistas, delightful meadows, and off-trail routes to exquisite lakes. To top it off, this trip offers caves, a rare feature in the area. Some of the caves are naturally occurring stone caverns, while others are mines—all are potentially dangerous. Hikers with caving or spelunking on their agenda should contact the rangers in Mineral King before embarking on an adventure into one of the caves. Additionally, some of the mines are private property, requiring the owner's permission for entrance.

DIRECTIONS TO TRAILHEAD: From the east end of Three Rivers, leave Highway 198 and turn onto Mineral King Road. Follow the road past Atwell Mill Campground, Silver City, Cold Springs Campground, and Mineral King Ranger Station (which issues wilderness permits and has food storage areas) to the Eagle-Mosquito Trailhead parking area at the end of the road, 23.5 miles from Highway 198.

DESCRIPTION: Just south of the parking area, a dirt road heads past the Honeymoon Cabin and climbs gently up the East Fork Kaweah River Canyon through sagebrush scrub dotted with red firs, mountain maples, and a few western junipers. After a quarter mile, you cross Spring Creek on a removable wood bridge. Within earshot of the bridge but out of sight above the trail is Tufa Falls. The creek originates higher up the hillside and then follows a subterranean course through a band of marble before emerging a few hundred feet above the trail.

Just beyond Spring Creek, pass an unsigned lateral descending toward the river and proceed up the canyon, with good views of Crystal Creek cascading down the slope across the valley. Hop across willow-lined Eagle Creek and shortly arrive at the signed White Chief Canyon junction, 1 mile from the parking area.

From the junction, head south on the White Chief Trail. If you thought the mile-long climb to the junction was tough, just wait; the next stretch of trail is as steep as any section of maintained trail in the parks.

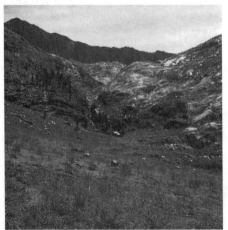

White Chief Meadow from the White Chief Canyon Trail

The excellent view of the canyon and the peaks above may temporarily distract you from the grueling ascent.

Eventually the grade moderates, as you head across sagebrush-covered slopes dotted with junipers and pass outcroppings of dark metamorphic rock. The grade eases even more on the approach to White Chief Meadow, 2 miles from the trailhead.

The ruins of Crabtree Cabin, on a low rise just west of the lower end of the meadow, is all that remains of a structure built by John Crabtree and used as a bunkhouse for miners working the nearby White Chief Mine. The trail soon crosses the creek and proceeds along the fringe of the flat. Over the years, numerous avalanches have swept the slopes above clean and littered the meadow with snags. The trail soon climbs a rib to a bench overlooking the meadow, where campsites nestle beneath red firs and lodgepole and foxtail pines. A resident deer herd can often be seen here around dusk.

Quickly leaving the trees behind, head across open, view-filled slopes, carpeted with wildflowers in season, including gentian, yarrow, and bluebell. The creek plays a game of cat and mouse in the canyon below, frequently disappearing and then reappearing; the seemingly erratic behavior is common for streams in areas of marble and limestone. At 2.75 miles, the trail crosses the main branch of the creek.

Ascend the far hillside beyond the creek and pass through tailings directly below the White Chief Mine, which was blasted out of a huge vein of marble. Do not explore the privately owned mine without permission from the owners.

Past the mine, ascend rocky slopes across the west wall of the canyon. The tread may be hard to follow here, but cairns should help to keep you on track. Continue up the canyon, passing numerous mine shafts, sinkholes, and caves to another creek crossing. Moving away from the creek on the east side of the drainage, you climb a grassy slope before returning to the creek and following it to a meadow-rimmed tarn at the head of the canyon. The upper canyon has

WHITE CHIEF MINE

John Crabtree and two companions claimed that a giant Indian spirit led them on an all-night vision quest to a natural marble cave with veins of pure gold. As ridiculous as the tale may seem now, their relation of their experience in San Joaquin Valley sparked the first wave of gold rush fever in Mineral King. Despite all the hoopla and the millions of dollars in investment capital, the mines never produced a single bar of either gold or silver.

ruins from old mining cabins and natural marble caverns.

[O] To reach lovely White Chief Lake from the upper meadow, strike out on a straight-forward cross-country route northwest 0.75 mile across the talus-filled slope beneath White Chief Peak. The remote lake has a few windswept campsites. Confident hikers can easily ascend White Chief Peak from the saddle directly northwest of it. A challenging off-trail route from the same saddle provides access to the broad pass (approximately 10,650 feet) 0.3 mile south of Eagle Lake, from where you could descend to the lake and then follow the Eagle Lake Trail back to the trailhead.

Beautiful, isolated Ansel Lake can be reached from either White Chief Lake or the upper meadow. Although many conclude the lake was named for famed photographer Ansel Adams, the name refers to Ansel Franklin Hall, a Sequoia Park ranger from 1916 to 1917.

[R] Wilderness permits are required for overnight stays. Campfires are prohibited.

MINERAL KING TRAILHEAD

TRIP 11

Farewell Gap

Ⓜ ↗ DH

DISTANCE: 11 miles, out-and-back

ELEVATION: 7,815'/10,680', +3,320'/-455'/±7,550'

SEASON: Mid-July to mid-October

USE: Light

MAPS: USGS's *Mineral King* or SNHA's *Mineral King* or Tom Harrison Maps' *Mineral King*

TRAIL LOG

3.25 Franklin Lakes Trail junction
5.5 Farewell Gap

INTRODUCTION: The Farewell Gap Trail was a popular route into the Kern River backcountry, at least until another trail was built over Franklin Pass. Nowadays, only the initial stretch of trail to the Franklin Lakes Trail junction is well traveled. However, hikers in good physical condition searching for excellent vistas will find the 5.5-mile climb to Farewell Gap quite rewarding, where the panorama of Mineral King and Little Kern River's upper basin create picture-postcard scenes.

DIRECTIONS TO TRAILHEAD: From the east end of Three Rivers, leave Highway 198 and turn onto Mineral King Road. Follow the road past the Atwell Mill Campground, Silver City, Cold Springs Campground, and Mineral King Ranger Station (which issues wilderness permits and has food storage areas) to the Eagle-Mosquito Trailhead parking area at the end of the road, 23.5 miles from Highway 198. If space is available in the small parking area near the bridge over East Fork Kaweah River, you could park there and shorten your hike a bit.

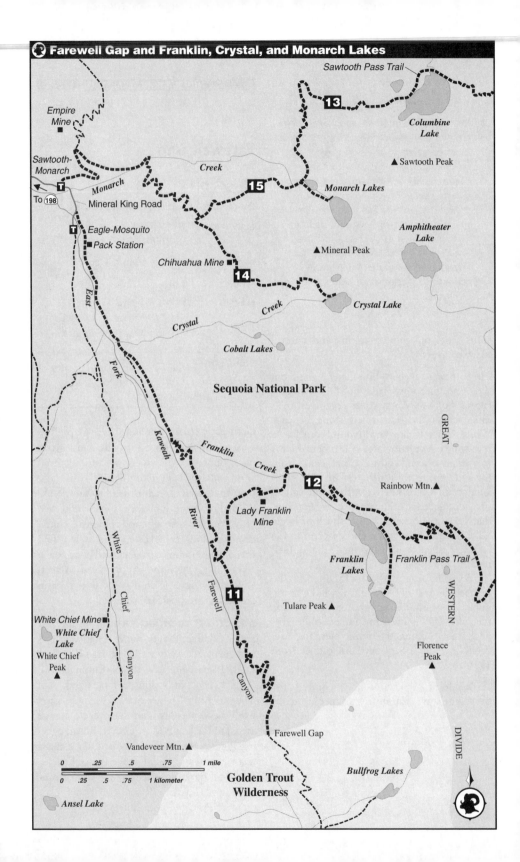

*Empire
Mine* ■

*Sawtooth-
Monarch* Ⓣ

To ⑲⑻

Creek

13

*Columbine
Lake*

▲ Sawtooth Peak

Monarch Mineral King Road

15

Monarch Lakes

*Amphitheater
Lake*

Ⓣ *Eagle-Mosquito*
■ *Pack Station*

Chihuahua Mine ■

14

▲ *Mineral Peak*

Crystal Lake

Crystal *Creek*

Cobalt Lakes

Sequoia National Park

East

Fork

Kaweah

Franklin *Creek*

12

Rainbow Mtn. ▲

GREAT

River

*Lady Franklin
Mine* ■

*Franklin
Lakes*

Franklin Pass Trail

Farewell

11

Tulare Peak ▲

WESTERN

White Chief Mine ■
*White Chief
Lake*

White Chief
Peak
▲

White

Chief

Canyon

Florence
Peak
▲

Canyon

Farewell Gap

DIVIDE

Vandeveer Mtn. ▲

Bullfrog Lakes

| 0 | .25 | .5 | .75 | 1 mile |
| 0 | .25 | .5 | .75 | 1 kilometer |

**Golden Trout
Wilderness**

Ansel Lake

DESCRIPTION: From the Eagle-Mosquito parking area, walk back down the road to the bridge over the river, and then follow single-track trail on a short climb to the Mineral King Pack Station access road. Follow the gently graded road through the open terrain of Mineral King Valley, passing the pack station's corrals along the way. Sagebrush, currant, and gooseberry grow alongside the road, while grasses and willows line the riverbanks. Farther upslope, a widely scattered forest gives the area an alpine character.

At 1.1 miles, you ford Crystal Creek and then veer left away from the road onto single-track trail at an unsigned junction; the road continues through Aspen Flat before ending at Soda Spring. A mild to moderate 0.75-mile climb from the junction leads to Franklin Creek and the start of a steep, switchbacking climb, interrupted near the midpoint by an ascending traverse. Fine views of the multihued peaks and valleys of the Mineral King area may distract you from the upward grind. Above the switchbacks, 3.25 miles from the parking area, reach a junction with the Franklin Lakes Trail.

Continue ahead on the Farewell Gap Trail, climbing high above the dwindling East Fork, soon reaching the first of twenty switchbacks that lead farther up into the canyon. The final leg of the climb is accomplished by a quarter-mile traverse culminating at the V-shaped notch of Farewell Gap, 2.25 miles from the Franklin Lakes junction.

The view from Farewell Gap is certainly awe-inspiring, with the entire Mineral King Valley spreading out before you, rimmed by vibrantly colored peaks. To the south, the equally colorful cleft of the Kern River creates a picture-postcard scene. If the oft-present winds fail to drive you from this picturesque aerie, the hours may drift by as you enjoy the breathtaking views.

The trail is infrequently used beyond Farewell Gap, especially after camping was banned at nearby Bullfrog Lakes. Adventurous souls in search of solitude have plenty of options within the Golden Trout Wilderness and Kern River backcountry. Vandeveer Mountain is a straightforward climb from Farewell Gap.

MINERAL KING TRAILHEAD

TRIP 12

Franklin Lakes

Ⓜ ↗ **DH** or **BP**

DISTANCE: 11 miles, out-and-back

ELEVATION: 7,815'/10,335',
+2,910'/-465'/±6,750'

SEASON: Early July to mid-October

USE: Heavy

MAPS: USGS's *Mineral King* or
SNHA's *Mineral King* or Tom
Harrison Maps' *Mineral King*

see
map on
p.82

TRAIL LOG

3.25 Franklin Lakes Trail junction
5.5 Lower Franklin Lake

INTRODUCTION: Scores of hikers and backpackers travel the popular Franklin Lakes Trail to access the picturesque lakes, cradled in a dramatic cirque beneath the Great Western Divide. As with most trails in the Mineral King area, this one climbs steadily out of the valley. Rainbow-colored metamorphic rock in Farewell and Franklin Canyons provides optical delights during the stiff ascent to the lakes.

DIRECTIONS TO TRAILHEAD: From the east end of Three Rivers, leave Highway 198 and turn onto Mineral King Road. Follow the road past Atwell Mill Campground, Silver City, Cold Springs Campground, and Mineral King Ranger Station (which issues wilderness permits and has food storage areas) to the Eagle-Mosquito Trailhead parking area at the end of the road, 23.5 miles from Highway 198. If space is available in the small parking area near the bridge over East Fork Kaweah River, you could park there and shorten your hike a bit.

DESCRIPTION: From the Eagle-Mosquito parking area, walk back down the road to the bridge over the river, and then follow single-track trail on a short climb to the Mineral King Pack Station access road. Follow the gently graded road through the open terrain of Mineral King Valley, passing the pack station's corrals along the way. Sagebrush, currant, and gooseberry grow alongside the road, while grasses and willows line the riverbanks. Farther upslope, a widely scattered forest gives the area an alpine character.

At 1.1 miles, you ford Crystal Creek and then veer left away from the road onto single-track trail at an unsigned junction; the road continues through Aspen Flat before ending at Soda Spring. A mild to moderate 0.75-mile climb from the junction leads to Franklin Creek and the start of a steep, switchbacking climb, interrupted near the midpoint by an ascending traverse. Fine views of the multihued peaks and valleys of the Mineral King area may distract you from the upward grind. Above the switchbacks, 3.25 miles from the parking area, reach a junction with the Franklin Lakes Trail.

Turn left at the junction and proceed up the Franklin Lakes Trail on a long ascending traverse across the slope below Tulare Peak, where views down to Mineral King Valley and up to red-and-orange-hued Franklin Canyon are quite striking. Sharp eyes may detect the tailings and shaft of the Lady Franklin Mine upslope above a pair of switchbacks. Reach a crossing of willow-lined Franklin Creek at 4.4 miles.

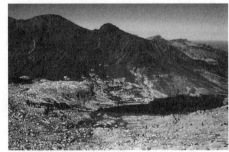

Franklin Lakes from trail

Continue the switchbacking climb above the creek. Soon the rock-and-mortar dam on the outlet of Franklin Lake springs into view, backdropped dramatically by the soaring peaks of the Great Western Divide, including aptly named Rainbow Mountain. Below the dam, a use trail heads shortly downhill to campsites along the creek. Continue climbing, as the trail leads high above the lower lake to a pair of side trails leading to hillside campsites.

Lower Franklin Lake is nestled in a picturesque basin below the multicolored peaks along the Great Western Divide. Campsites meeting the 100-foot regulation are in short supply, leaving only some semi-level sites above the north shore for the substantial number or backpackers who visit the area each summer day. Unfortunately, the lake's popularity coupled with a paucity of marginal campsites creates an ambiance more consistent with a trailer park than a backcountry haven.

Both designated camp areas (with bear boxes) on the north side of Lower Franklin Lake are partially shaded by a smattering of foxtail pines. A pit toilet is located down the southernmost access trail. Brook trout inhabit both lakes, but the crowd at the lower lake will probably prevent anglers from pulling out any trophy-size fish.

Backpackers who haven't expended all their energy getting to Lower Franklin Lake may be able to escape the crowds by continuing another half mile or so to campsites on the bench between the upper and lower lakes. The bench is treeless and exposed but sees far fewer visitors. A short romp over boulders from the bench leads to Upper Franklin Lake, directly below the steep cirque wall between Florence and Tulare Peaks.

From Franklin Pass, mountaineers can ascend Class 2 routes to the summits of either Rainbow Mountain or Florence Peak.

Wilderness permits are required for overnight stays. Campfires are prohibited.

MINERAL KING TRAILHEAD

TRIP 13

Franklin Pass and Sawtooth Pass Loop

S **𝒫** **BPx or X**

DISTANCE: 27.5 miles, loop

ELEVATION: 7,815'/11,760'/8,605'/11,710'/ 7,815', +9,250'/-9,250'/±18,500'

SEASON: Mid-July to mid-October

USE: Light

MAPS: USGS's *Mineral King* and *Chagoopa Falls* or Tom Harrison Maps' *Mineral King*

see map on p.82

TRAIL LOG

3.25	Franklin Lakes Trail junction
5.5	Lower Franklin Lake
7.4	Franklin Pass
10.0	Rattlesnake Creek and Soda Creek junction
10.5	Forester Lake
11.75	Little Claire Lake
16.4	Sawtooth Pass Trail junction
18.0	Big Five Lakes junction
21.5	Columbine Lake
22.3	Sawtooth Pass
24.0	Lower Monarch Lake
24.75	Crystal Lake Trail junction
26.9	Timber Gap Trail junction

INTRODUCTION: A bare minimum of three days provides an opportunity to experience one of Mineral King's classic loops, featuring alpine and subalpine lakes, deep forests, picturesque meadows, tumbling streams, and stunning views from two passes on the Great Western Divide. The red and orange hues of metamorphic rock surrounding Mineral King complement and contrast with the typical High Sierra granite. Crossing both Franklin and Sawtooth Passes, especially Sawtooth, which follows an unmaintained route on a difficult climb from Columbine Lake, followed by a tedious descent over loose soil to Monarch Lake, ensures backpackers will get a workout. Managing this demanding stretch requires more than rudimentary backpacking skills, which makes this loop one for experienced backpackers only.

Travelers with extra time will certainly want to take the short side trip to Big Five Lakes. The siren call of grand scenery and relative seclusion may lure backpackers off the main loop for an extended visit. Anglers should enjoy the temptations offered by prospects of landing some good-size brook trout.

DIRECTIONS TO TRAILHEAD: From the east end of Three Rivers, leave Highway 198 and turn onto Mineral King Road. Follow the road past Atwell Mill Campground, Silver City, Cold Springs Campground, and Mineral King Ranger Station (which issues wilderness permits and has food storage areas) to the Eagle-Mosquito Trailhead parking area at the end of the road, 23.5 miles from Highway 198. If space is available in the small parking area near the bridge over East Fork Kaweah River, you could park there and shorten your hike a bit.

DESCRIPTION: From the Eagle-Mosquito parking area, walk back down the road to the bridge over the river, and then follow single-track trail on a short climb to the Mineral King Pack Station access road. Follow the gently graded road through the open terrain of Mineral King Valley, passing the pack station's corrals along the way. Sagebrush, currant, and gooseberry grow alongside the road, while grasses and willows line the riverbanks. Farther upslope, a widely scattered forest gives the area an alpine character.

At 1.1 miles, you ford Crystal Creek and then veer left away from the road onto single-track trail at an unsigned junction; the road continues through Aspen Flat

before ending at Soda Spring. A mild to moderate 0.75-mile climb from the junction leads to Franklin Creek and the start of a steep, switchbacking climb, interrupted near the midpoint by an ascending traverse. Fine views of the multihued peaks and valleys of the Mineral King area may distract you from the upward grind. Above the switchbacks, 3.25 miles from the parking area, reach a junction with the Franklin Lakes Trail.

Turn left at the junction and proceed up the Franklin Lakes Trail on a long ascending traverse across the slope below Tulare Peak, where views down to Mineral King Valley and up to red-and-orange-hued Franklin Canyon are quite striking. Sharp eyes may detect the tailings and shaft of the Lady Franklin Mine upslope above a pair of switchbacks. Reach a crossing of willow-lined Franklin Creek at 4.4 miles.

Continue the switchbacking climb above the creek. Soon the rock-and-mortar dam on the outlet of Franklin Lake springs into view, backdropped dramatically by the soaring peaks of the Great Western Divide, including aptly named Rainbow Mountain. Below the dam, a use trail heads shortly downhill to campsites along the creek. Continue climbing, as the trail leads high

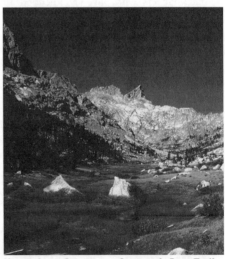

Upper Lost Canyon on Sawtooth Pass Trail

above the lower lake to a pair of side trails leading to hillside campsites.

Lower Franklin Lake is nestled in a picturesque basin below the multicolored peaks along the Great Western Divide. Campsites meeting the 100-foot regulation are in short supply, leaving only some semi-level sites above the north shore for the substantial number or backpackers who visit the area each summer day. Unfortunately, the lake's popularity coupled with a paucity of marginal campsites creates an ambiance more consistent with a trailer park than a backcountry haven.

Both designated camp areas (with bear boxes) on the north side of Lower Franklin Lake are partially shaded by a smattering of foxtail pines. A pit toilet is located down the southernmost access trail. Brook trout inhabit both lakes, but the crowd at the lower lake will probably prevent anglers from pulling out any trophy-size fish.

Backpackers who haven't expended all their energy getting to Lower Franklin Lake may be able to escape the crowds by continuing another half mile or so to campsites on the bench between the upper and lower lakes. The bench is treeless and exposed but sees far fewer visitors. A short romp over boulders from the bench leads to Upper Franklin Lake, directly below the steep cirque wall between Florence and Tulare Peaks.

From Lower Franklin Lake, the main trail heads southeast to a set of well-graded switchbacks. At the top of the switchbacks, a long ascending traverse leads to just below the crest of the ridge, from where a few short-legged switchbacks take you up to Franklin Pass (which is north of the low point), 7.4 miles from the parking area. Standing on this gap in the Great Western Divide, alpine scenery—including Mt. Whitney, 18 miles to the northeast above the deep cleft of Kern Canyon, and the Kaweah Peaks less than 10 miles to the north—spreads across the eastern horizon.

From the pass, wind down barren and sandy slopes. Eventually, very widely scattered, stunted, and contorted pines appear just before switchbacks lead down to a small meadow in the Rattlesnake Creek drainage. Pass a signed junction with the Shotgun Pass Trail on the right, and skirt the meadow, continuing down the canyon another half mile to a junction between the Rattlesnake Creek and Soda Creek Trails, 10 miles from the parking area.

Turn left onto the Soda Creek Trail, and proceed through light lodgepole pine forest on a mild, 0.5-mile ascent to Forester Lake. Grasses and pines rim the lake, which offers plenty of campsites spread around the shoreline. Anglers can fish for fair-size brook trout.

From the lake, a moderate climb, briefly interrupted by a short jaunt around a small meadow, leads to the top of a rise; after a moderate descent you reach Little Claire Lake, 11.75 miles from the parking area. Along the south shore, a large sandy slope dotted with foxtail pines makes for a fine camping area, with the bonus of an excellent view across the lake of 12,210-foot Needham Mountain. More mundane campsites can be found along the north shore near the outlet, close to the lip of the steep-walled canyon of Soda Creek. Anglers can ply the waters for good-size brook trout.

From Little Claire Lake, the trail drops 900 vertical feet over the course of a mile via switchbacks to a crossing of Soda Creek. For the next 3-plus miles, a mild, featureless descent along Soda Creek travels through lodgepole pine forest, with occasional clearings created by frequent avalanches sweeping down the sides of the canyon. Nearing the Lost Canyon junction, red firs, western white, and Jeffrey pines join the lodgepoles. At 16.4 miles is the signed Sawtooth Pass Trail junction.

Heading northeast from the junction, you climb to a crossing of Lost Canyon Creek, a pleasant oasis if the day is hot. Beyond the creek, the trail makes a zigzagging climb through light forest cover to a meadow with a lone campsite. A more moderately graded ascent continues up the canyon beyond the meadow to a junction of a trail to Big Five Lakes, 18 miles from the trailhead. A short distance from the junction up the Sawtooth Pass Trail, near the crossing of Lost Canyon Creek, are more campsites (with bear boxes).

SIDE TRIP TO BIG FIVE LAKES: From the junction, switchbacks climb up a hillside covered with chinquapin and lodgepole pines to a bench, where a tepid tarn offers the possibility of a fine swim and secluded camping above the heather-lined shore. Beyond the pond, the climb resumes around boulders and over slabs to the top of a ridge overlooking the deep cleft holding the Big Five Lakes. A steep, rocky descent from the ridge leads to the first lake, 2 miles from the Sawtooth Pass junction. There are good campsites near the outlet and along the north shore.

The main trail continues around the north side of the lake to an informal junction; take the right-hand fork and make a short, steep, zigzag up to a T-junction with the trail to Little Five Lakes.

From the T-junction, descend southwest to the north shore of the second lake, smallest in the chain. Backpackers will find excellent campsites around this lake. A short descent from the second lake leads to the third and largest of the Big Five Lakes and then along the north shore through a boggy meadow. An easy climb takes you to the fourth lake, where overnighters will find good campsites near the outlet. The trail becomes indistinct past the fourth lake, but the route to the uppermost lake is straightforward.

The Big Five Lakes have much to offer, not the least of which is that all five are strikingly beautiful. In addition, solitude is a reasonable expectation, due to the relatively long distances from trailheads and the steep passes on the Great Western Divide that must be crossed on the way. Anglers will appreciate the lack of pressure and the opportunity to land some good-size brookies. **END OF SIDE TRIP**

From the Big Five Lakes junction, continue upstream past campsites to cross Lost Canyon Creek. About 0.3 mile farther, you hop back over to the north side of the creek and proceed up the mostly forested canyon.

Eventually the trail breaks out of the forest into a boulder-strewn meadow providing good views of Needham Mountain, Sawtooth Peak, and the crest of the Great Western Divide. Scattered campsites offer the chance to linger in the upper basin.

The steep wall at the end of the canyon heralds the end of the mild climbing; the terrain forces the trail to climb more moderately toward Columbine Lake and Sawtooth Pass above. Switchbacks lead to the lip of the basin, where Columbine Lake immediately springs into view, 3.5 miles from the Big Five Lakes junction. A classic alpine lake, Columbine reposes in a deep, rocky bowl of granite slabs and boulders. The deep blue waters reflect the rust-colored, metamorphosed rock of the surrounding peaks. Cramped pockets of decomposed granite offer passable campsites just off the trail, but perhaps the best sites occur above the southwest shore.

Maintained trail ends at Columbine Lake and does not resume again until Monarch Lakes, well down the other side of Sawtooth Pass. Consequently, it may be challenging to determine the best route to the pass. A number of different paths offer variations on a theme. Fortunately, they all eventually converge on the sandy slope just below the pass. Some final switchbacks lead to stunning views from windswept Sawtooth Pass, 22.3 miles from the parking area. Empire Mountain and Sawtooth Peak grab your attention in the immediate foreground, while Mt. Whitney, Mt. Langley, and Cirque Peak rise above the east skyline. Perhaps the most impressive view is straight down the canyon of Monarch Creek to Mineral Creek below.

From the pass, a seemingly interminable, obnoxious descent zigzags across a shifting slope of loose dirt, gritty sand, and scree, where myriad paths crisscross the slope in haphazard fashion. Eventually reaching more stable ground below, you can finally take off your boots and dump out the accumulated debris. The only solace of this misadventure comes from knowing that at least you didn't have to climb up this insufferable slope.

After such a gruesome descent, you will appreciate the much more stable, though unmaintained trail to Monarch Lakes. Pass a bear box and fair campsites fashioned out of the rocky terrain on the way to Lower Monarch Lake, 1.7 miles from the pass. A path along the north shore provides a little-used route to the upper lake, where decent campsites are virtually nonexistent. Typically, the environs of the lower lake bustle with activity, with backpackers crowding into the limited campsites and dayhikers languishing around the shoreline.

Leaving Monarch Lakes, the trail crosses the outlet and begins a gently descending traverse below rust-colored cliffs and across a rocky slope devoid of plant life. After crossing a minor ridge, you leave the harsh surroundings behind, as the gentle descent continues through scattered pines and pockets of wildflowers, including lupine and paintbrush. Reach the Crystal Lake junction after a pair of switchbacks, 0.75 mile from Lower Monarch Lake.

From the junction, long-legged switchbacks continue the lengthy descent toward Mineral King Valley. Prior to the crossing of Crystal Creek, lush vegetation carpets the hillside. Beyond the creek, the trail descends along the edge of the canyon, where water gushes out of the opposite wall. Through open slopes of sagebrush, manzanita, chin-

quapin, and gooseberry, you continue down the canyon and then across the final slope above Mineral King, reaching a junction with the Timber Gap Trail at a switchback. After another 0.6 mile, you reach the Sawtooth-Monarch Trailhead, and then hike up the road to the Eagle-Mosquito Trailhead parking area.

[O] This area has many options for trip extensions, including forays deep into the heart of Sequoia's backcountry on the Rattlesnake, Big Arroyo, and Kern River Trails.

A pair of difficult cross-country routes leaves the Big Five Lakes area. The first climbs over Cyclamen Pass on the Great Western Divide and then drops to Cyclamen and Columbine Lakes. The second climbs over Bilko Pass and around the east side of the Great Western Divide to Columbine Lake.

Mountaineers can attempt a number of Class 2 routes: Florence Peak or Rainbow Mountain from Franklin Pass, Sawtooth Peak from Sawtooth Pass, Empire Mountain from Glacier Pass, or Mineral Peak from Monarch Lakes.

[R] Wilderness permits are required for overnight stays. Campfires are prohibited above 10,400 feet.

MINERAL KING TRAILHEAD

TRIP 14

Crystal Lake

Ⓜ ⤢ **DH or BP**

DISTANCE: 7.5 miles, out-and-back

ELEVATION: 7,820'/10,995',
+3,675'/-500'/±8,350'

SEASON: Mid-July to mid-October

USE: Light

MAPS: USGS's *Mineral King* or
SNHA's *Mineral King* or Tom
Harrison Maps' *Mineral King*

see
map on
p.82

INTRODUCTION: The Sawtooth Pass Trail is often crowded with hikers and backpackers bound for Monarch Lakes or Sawtooth Pass and other points east, but few veer away from the main trail toward Crystal Lake. Apparently, an extra half mile and 600 feet of elevation gain are enough to dissuade most travelers. Beyond the Sawtooth Pass and Crystal Lake junction, the tailings from and shaft of the Chihuahua Mine are vivid reminders of the high expectations miners and investors had for the Mineral King area—expectations that were never realized. The lake itself is quite picturesque and strikingly backdropped by steep, multicolored peaks; it makes a fine destination for either a dayhike or overnight backpack.

DIRECTIONS TO TRAILHEAD: From the east end of Three Rivers, leave Highway 198 and turn onto Mineral King Road. Follow the road past Atwell Mill Campground, Silver City, Cold Springs Campground, and Mineral King Ranger Station (which issues wilderness permits and has food storage areas) to the Sawtooth-Monarch Trailhead parking area, 0.8 mile from the ranger station and 23 miles from Highway 198.

DESCRIPTION: Climb steeply away from the Sawtooth-Monarch Trailhead up a hillside carpeted with sagebrush, manzanita, chinquapin, and gooseberry to a junction with the Timber Gap Trail at 0.6 mile. Turn right to continue on the Sawtooth Pass Trail, as the ascent assumes a more moderate grade on long-legged switchbacks. At 1.2 miles, you reach misnamed Groundhog Meadow, which should more appropriately refer to the resident yellow-bellied marmots inhabiting the rocky slopes of the Sierra. Cross Crystal Creek and follow a series of switchbacks in and out of shady red fir forest on the way to the Y-junction with the Crystal Lake Trail, 2.4 miles from the trailhead.

Veer left onto the lightly used Crystal Lake Trail and climb across the barren, avalanche-ridden slopes of Chihuahua Bowl, named for the nearby Chihuahua Mine, the ruins of which are visible from the trail on the southeast slope of the bowl. Beyond Chihuahua Bowl, the trail crests a ridge, from where you have good views amid 👁 scattered foxtail pines. A short descent off the ridge leads to an ascending traverse across the north side of upper Crystal Creek canyon, followed by a steep, switchbacking climb up to the narrow slot of Crystal Lake's outlet.

A lack of trees around the shoreline sends most overnighters to more sheltered campsites on a terrace just below the lake, ⌂ where gnarled foxtail pines offer a modicum of protection from the elements. The lake's brook trout will test the patience of anglers.

🔲 A faint path leaves the Crystal Lake Trail to descend along the outlet, from where a little-used, straightforward off-trail route heads to the dwarfish Cobalt Lakes.

Although maintained trail concludes at Crystal Lake, a short scramble over bluffs to the northeast leads to Little Crystal Lake, directly north of Crystal Lake and southeast of Crystal Peak. A direct off-trail route to the Monarch Lakes heads north from Little Crystal Lake, climbing 400 vertical feet to a saddle overlooking Upper Monarch Lake.

A steep but straightforward descent from there leads down a chute to the upper lake.

A short cross-country route connects Crystal Lake to Amphitheater Lake via Crystal Pass.

R Wilderness permits are required for overnight stays. Campfires are prohibited.

TRIP 15

Monarch Lakes

M ╱ DH

DISTANCE:	6.5 miles, out-and-back
ELEVATION:	7,820'/10,395', +2,740'/-200'/±5,880'
SEASON:	Mid-July to mid-October
USE:	Heavy
MAPS:	USGS's *Mineral King* or SNHA's *Mineral King* or Tom Harrison Maps' *Mineral King*

see map on p.82

INTRODUCTION: The reward for this hike's stiff climb is a pair of lovely subalpine lakes cradled in a picturesque cirque beneath multicolored, metamorphic rock peaks. Not only is the destination stunningly beautiful, but the views of Mineral King Valley during the ascent are equally impressive. Despite the climb—2,500 feet in 3-plus miles—this trip up the Sawtooth Pass Trail is fairly popular among backpackers and dayhikers alike. Since the overused campsites at the lake become extremely cramped during

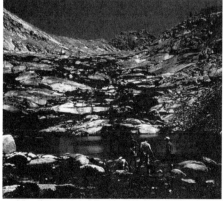

Hikers at Lower Monarch Lake

peak season, it is better to take this trip as a dayhike. If you insist on an overnight visit, *don't expect peace and quiet.* Experienced off-trail enthusiasts can enjoy more serene camping with the added bonus of a loop trip by camping at nearby Crystal Lake (see Trip 14, page 90) and then following a cross-country route over a saddle to Monarch Lakes (see this trip's options).

DIRECTIONS TO TRAILHEAD: From the east end of Three Rivers, leave Highway 198 and turn onto Mineral King Road. Follow 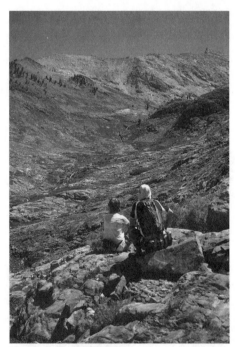 the road past Atwell Mill Campground, Silver City, Cold Springs Campground, and Mineral King Ranger Station (which issues wilderness permits and has food storage areas) to the Sawtooth-Monarch Trailhead parking area, 0.8 mile from the ranger station and 23 miles from Highway 198.

DESCRIPTION: Climb steeply away from the Sawtooth-Monarch Trailhead up a hillside carpeted with sagebrush, manzanita, chinquapin, and gooseberry to a junction with the Timber Gap Trail at 0.6 mile. Turn right to continue on the Sawtooth Pass Trail, as the ascent assumes a more moderate grade on long-legged switchbacks. At 1.2 miles, you reach misnamed Groundhog Meadow, which should more appropriately refer to the resident yellow-bellied marmots inhabiting the rocky slopes of the Sierra. Cross Crystal Creek and follow a series of switchbacks in and out of shady red fir forest on the way to the Y-junction with the Crystal Lake Trail, 2.4 miles from the trailhead.

From the junction, continue climbing up the Sawtooth Pass Trail. After a pair of switchbacks, cross a minor ridge at the edge of expansive and rock-strewn Chihuahua Bowl, and then follow a mildly rising traverse across a barren, austere slope well above the level of Monarch Creek, which courses through the deep canyon below. Eventually the trail curves toward more hospitable looking terrain once more, meeting the meadow-lined creek just below the outlet of Lower Monarch Lake. From there, a short climb leads to the west shore. Sandwiched between multihued Monarch

and Mineral Peaks on the Great Western Divide, the two Monarch Lakes nestle picturesquely in a scenic cirque. Scratched out of the rocky slopes to the west of the lower lake are exposed, overused campsites with bear boxes and a partially screened pit toilet nearby.

To reach the upper lake, find a use trail near the inlet amid a patch of willows, and follow it up a steep hillside to larger Upper Monarch Lake. Since most hikers go no farther than the lower lake, the upper lake should offer a reasonable dose of solitude away from the well-traveled Sawtooth Pass Trail.

[O] A steep but relatively straightforward cross-country route connects Monarch and Crystal Lakes. From Upper Monarch Lake, head south and ascend a steep chute to a saddle above. Descend toward the smallest lake below and then find a use trail leading to the shore of Lower Crystal Lake.

[R] Wilderness permits are required for overnight stays. Campfires are prohibited.

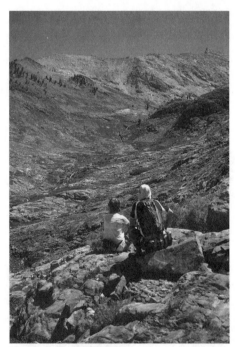

Monarch Creek Canyon

MINERAL KING TRAILHEAD

TRIP 16

Little Five and Big Five Lakes Loop

(M) (P) BPx

DISTANCE: 26.5 miles, loop

ELEVATION: 7,820'/9,511'/7,124'/
11,970'/9,580'/7,820',
+9,930'/-9,930'/±19,860'

SEASON: Mid-July to mid-October

USE: Moderate

MAPS: USGS's *Mineral King* or Tom
Harrison Maps' *Mineral King*

TRAIL LOG

2.25 Timber Gap
5.0 Black Rock Pass junction
7.5 Pinto Lake
10.7 Black Rock Pass
11.5 Little Five Lakes
12.5 Big Five Lakes Trail junction
14.1 Big Five Lakes
17.1 Sawtooth Pass Trail junction
20.5 Columbine Lake
21.25 Sawtooth Pass
23.0 Monarch Lakes

INTRODUCTION: This loop exposes backpackers to the best of what the Mineral King area has to offer. Both Little Five and Big Five Lakes basins contain picturesque lakes with excellent camping and fishing. Flower-carpeted meadows, rushing streams, and quiet forests, all in the shadow of the Great Western Divide, offer plenty of scenic delights along the way. Add alpine Columbine Lake and far-reaching views from nearby Sawtooth Pass, and you have nearly every component of a classic High Sierra trip. Mountaineers and cross-country enthusiasts have much to choose from as well.

Gaining such stunning attributes has a price—crossing three increasingly difficult passes with steep climbs. Reaching

Timber Gap is a relatively straightforward climb, gaining 1,700 feet in 2.25 miles, while getting to Black Rock Pass requires a 3-mile, 3,000-foot climb. The difficulty of Sawtooth Pass is not so much its distance or elevation, but the condition of the route, which isn't a trail at all but an unmaintained route; backpackers must pick one of many routes to scramble up on the east side of the pass and then endure a nasty descent down loose soils on the opposite side. The rigors of this loop require backpackers to be in excellent physical condition.

DIRECTIONS TO TRAILHEAD: From the east end of Three Rivers, leave Highway 198 and turn onto Mineral King Road. Follow the road past Atwell Mill Campground, Silver City, Cold Springs Campground, and Mineral King Ranger Station (which issues wilderness permits and has food storage areas) to the Sawtooth-Monarch Trailhead parking area, 0.8 mile from the ranger station and 23 miles from Highway 198.

DESCRIPTION: Climb steeply away from the Sawtooth-Monarch Trailhead up a hillside carpeted with sagebrush, manzanita, chinquapin, and gooseberry to a junction with the Timber Gap Trail at 0.6 mile. Turn left at the junction, climb less severely across open slopes, and then follow switchbacks through a copse of red firs providing pockets of welcome shade. Near 9,200 feet, leave the trees and make a long ascending traverse toward Timber Gap. Before reentering red fir forest just below the gap, take in one last view toward Mineral King. Reach the forested saddle of Timber Gap at 2.25 miles from the trailhead.

A forested, switchbacking descent leads away from the gap to a crossing of Timber Gap Creek, where a long swath of flower-bedecked meadow along the banks supplants a mixed forest. Continue down the verdant canyon, quickly crossing back over the main branch and then a number of lushly lined, spring-fed tributaries. Eventually the trail departs the Timber Gap Creek drainage and makes a short climb over the northeast lip of the canyon, before following

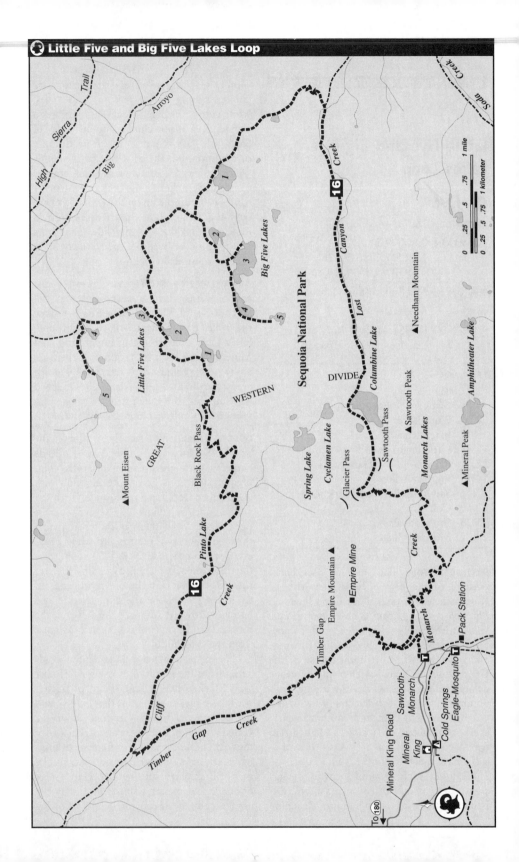

a switchbacking descent toward Cliff Creek below. At 5 miles, you boulder hop Cliff Creek and come to red fir–shaded campsites (which have a bear box) near a signed junction with the Black Rock Pass Trail.

From the junction, ascend southeast up the Black Rock Pass Trail through wildflowers, shrubs, and scattered firs, crossing a number of small rivulets lined with lush foliage. Farther up the canyon, you emerge from the forest to an extensive boulder field, where the creek adopts a temporarily subterranean course. The forward view includes a ribbonlike waterfall spilling down a rock wall on the south side of the canyon.

Switchbacks lead along the left-hand branch of the creek up the wall of the creek and on toward the meadows surrounding Pinto Lake. At 7.5 miles, you reach an unsigned junction with a use trail branching right toward campsites (which have a bear box). Nearby, diminutive Pinto Lake hides in a screen of willows. The lake offers surprisingly pleasant swimming.

Past a series of meadows, you climb through open terrain carpeted with sagebrush, chinquapin, and willow. The early summer flower display includes forget-me-nots, paintbrush, lupine, phlox, wallflower, yampa, larkspur, senecio, and Bigelow sneezeweed. Soon encounter the first of many switchbacks leading to the pass, 2,000 feet above. The interminable slog is made more tolerable by the incredible scenery along the way. First, Spring Lake comes into view, backdropped majestically by the sheer face of Peak 11480, followed by Cyclamen Lake, and then Columbine Lake. Finally, you can catch your breath at Black Rock Pass (approximately 11,670 feet), 10.7 miles from the trailhead. From the pass, Little Five and Big Five Lakes basins spill into the deep cleft of Big Arroyo, backdropped dramatically by the Kaweah Peaks. In the distance, Mt. Whitney and its surrounding summits pierce the eastern skyline.

A zigzagging descent from the pass leads to the first of the Little Five Lakes at 11.5 miles. Fine campsites above the north shore lure campers, while the prospect of catching the resident brook trout will tantalize anglers.

Reenter forest on the way toward the second highest lake, where more delightful campsites can be found above the north shore. Reach a junction with the Big Five Lakes Trail just after crossing the outlet. By continuing north for another mile on the Black Rock Pass Trail, you can access the remaining lakes in the Little Five Lakes chain via a use trail heading west, where solitude is almost guaranteed at the northern cluster of lakes.

From the Big Five Lakes junction, take the left-hand trail and head east across rolling terrain through lodgepole pine forest. Eventually, the trail bends south and contours around a ridge separating the Little Five and Big Five Lakes basins. Reach a junction with a trail accessing the four upper lakes at 14.1 miles.

To visit Big Five Lakes 2–5, descend southwest from the junction to the north shore of the second lake, smallest in the chain, where overnighters can locate excellent campsites. A short descent from there leads to the third and largest lake, where the trail proceeds through boggy meadows along the north shore. An easy climb beyond the third lake takes you to the fourth lake, which offers more good campsites near the outlet. The trail becomes faint beyond the fourth lake, but the route is clear to the uppermost lake. Good-size brook trout should provide anglers with plenty of challenges at all of the lakes.

From the Big Five Lakes junction, the Big Five Lakes Trail zigzags down a pine-covered hillside to an informal T-junction near the north shore of the first lake. Not surprisingly, the most accessible of the five lakes offers plenty of fine campsites spread around the shore. Remaining on the main trail, bear left (southeast) at the junction, and continue around the north shore of the lowest lake to the crossing of the outlet. A moderately steep climb leads away from the lake and up a rock-strewn hillside to the crest of a ridge above. After a short descent off the crest, the trail levels on a bench holding a tepid, heather-fringed pond, which

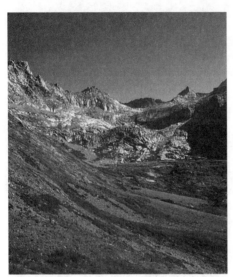

Upper Cliff Creek Basin on Black Rock Trail

〰 provides excellent swimming and secluded camping. Switchbacks below the pond lead down the hillside to a junction with the Sawtooth Pass Trail in Lost Canyon, 17.1 miles from the trailhead.

From the Big Five Lakes junction, continue upstream past campsites to a crossing of Lost Canyon Creek. A third of a mile farther, hop back over to the north side of the creek, and proceed up the mostly forested canyon. Eventually the trail breaks out of the forest into a boulder-strewn meadow providing good views of Needham Mountain, Sawtooth Peak, and the crest of the Great Western Divide. Scattered campsites offer you a chance to linger in the upper basin.

The steep wall at the end of the canyon heralds the end of the mild climbing, as the terrain forces the trail to climb more moderately toward Columbine Lake and Sawtooth Pass above. Switchbacks lead to the lip of the basin, where Columbine Lake immediately springs into view. A classic alpine lake, Columbine reposes in a deep, rocky bowl of granite slabs and boulders. The deep blue waters reflect the rust-colored, metamorphic rock of the surrounding peaks. Cramped pockets of decomposed granite offer passable campsites just off the

trail, but perhaps the best sites occur above the southwest shore.

Maintained trail ends at Columbine Lake and does not resume again until Monarch Lakes, well down the other side of Sawtooth Pass. Determining the best route to the pass may be a bit challenging because a number of different paths offer variations on a theme. Fortunately, no matter which route you choose, they all eventually converge on the sandy slope just below the pass. A final set of switchbacks leads to stunning views from windswept Sawtooth Pass. Empire Mountain and Sawtooth Peak grab your attention in the immediate foreground, while Mt. Whitney, Mt. Langley, and Cirque Peak rise above the east skyline. Perhaps the most impressive view is straight down the canyon of Monarch Creek to Mineral Creek below.

From the pass, a seemingly interminable, obnoxious descent zigzags across a shifting slope of loose dirt, gritty sand, and scree, where myriad paths crisscross the slope in haphazard fashion. Eventually reaching more stable ground below, you can finally take off your boots and dump out the accumulated debris. The only solace of this misadventure comes from knowing that at least you didn't have to climb up this insufferable slope.

After such a gruesome descent, hikers will greatly appreciate the much more stable trail to Monarch Lakes, despite the fact that this section is also unmaintained. Pass a bear box and fair campsites fashioned out of the rocky terrain on the way to Lower Monarch Lake. A path along the north shore provides a little-used route to the upper lake, where decent campsites are virtually nonexistent. Typically, the environs of the lower lake bustle with activity, with backpackers crowding into the limited campsites and dayhikers languishing around the shoreline.

Leaving Monarch Lakes, the trail crosses the outlet and begins a gently descending traverse below rust-colored cliffs and across a rocky slope devoid of plant life. After crossing a minor ridge, you leave behind the harsh surroundings, as the gentle descent continues through scattered pines and pockets of wildflowers, including lupine and paintbrush. Reach the Crystal Lake junction after a pair of switchbacks.

From the junction, long-legged switchbacks continue the lengthy descent toward Mineral King Valley. Prior to the crossing of Crystal Creek, lush vegetation carpets the hillside. Beyond the creek, the trail descends along the edge of the canyon, where water gushes out of the opposite wall. Through open slopes of sagebrush, manzanita, chinquapin, and gooseberry, you continue down the canyon and then across the final slope above Mineral King, reaching a junction with the Timber Gap Trail at a switchback. After another 0.6 mile, you reach the Sawtooth-Monarch Trailhead.

O Setting up a base camp at any of the lakes offers easy options for exploration of the Big Five Lakes and Little Five Lakes areas. Cross-country enthusiasts have many options along this loop. From Timber Gap, a 0.75-mile traverse southeast along the

EMPIRE CAMP AND MINE

The bunkhouse at Empire Camp was destroyed by an avalanche in 1880, while 20 miners slept inside. Four men were seriously injured, but fortunately no one was killed. The mine itself was not so lucky; work ceased for good the following summer.

Historic Wagon Road leads to the ruins of the Empire Camp and Empire Mine.

Strikingly beautiful Spring Lake can be accessed from either the Black Rock Pass or Sawtooth Pass Trails. The easiest route leaves the Black Rock Trail near 10,000 feet and contours 0.9 mile to the lake. A more difficult route leaves the unmaintained stretch of the Sawtooth Pass Trail near 11,200 feet and traverses easily to Glacier Pass (approximately 11,800 feet). The crux of the route descends a short but steep cliff (Class 3) to easier slopes below leading to the north shore. Snow on the north side of the pass may require the use of an ice axe.

Two difficult routes exit Big Five Lakes basin. The first climbs over Cyclamen Pass (approximately 11,145 feet) on the Great Western Divide and continues on to Cyclamen and Columbine Lakes. The second ascends to Bilko Pass (approximately 11,480 feet) and around the east side of the divide to Columbine Lake.

Mountaineers have a variety of options as well. Mt. Eisen is Class 1–2 from the Black Rock Pass Trail. A Class 3 route up a couloir on the north side of Needham Mountain leads to easier climbing along the east ridge. Sawtooth Peak is Class 2 from the pass. The southeast ridge of Empire Peak is Class 2 via Glacier Pass. Mineral Peak is Class 2 from Monarch Lakes.

R Wilderness permits are required for overnight stays. Campfires are prohibited above 10,400 feet.

MINERAL KING TRAILHEAD

TRIP 17

Great Western Divide Loop

Ⓜ 𝒫 BP

DISTANCE: 37.7 miles, semiloop

ELEVATION: 7,820'/9,511'/5,560'/10,700'/
9,520'/11,670'/7,124'/
9,511'/7,820',
+13,175'/-13,175'/±26,350'

SEASON: Mid-July to mid-October

USE: Moderate

MAPS: USGS's *Mineral King, Triple
Divide Peak,* and *Lodgepole*
or Tom Harrison Maps'
Mineral King

TRAIL LOG

2.25 Timber Gap
5.0   Black Rock Pass Trail junction
8.3   Redwood Meadow and Atwell-
      Redwood Trail junction
8.5   Bearpaw Trail junction
10.6 Middle Fork Kaweah River
11.6 Little Bearpaw Meadow
12.7 Bearpaw Meadow Campground
12.9 High Sierra Trail junction
14.6 Elizabeth Pass Trail junction
16.4 Upper Hamilton Lake
19.5 Kaweah Gap
22.3 Little Five Lakes Trail junction
22.5 Big Arroyo Trail junction
25.2 Big Five Lakes Trail junction
27.0 Black Rock Pass
30.2 Pinto Lake
32.7 Timber Gap Trail junction

INTRODUCTION: This trip samples all the main features for which the High Sierra is known—giant sequoia groves, flower-filled meadows, rushing creeks, and granite summits. Toss in the usually sunny Sierra weather and you have the complete package.

Solitude should be a nearly constant companion on the initial stretch of a mostly forested route over Timber Gap to Redwood and Little Bearpaw Meadows. Once you reach Bearpaw Meadow and the popular High Sierra Trail (HST), you'll have to deal with a definite increase in foot traffic. However, the scenic rewards of Hamilton Creek canyon, Nine Lakes Basin, and Big Arroyo will more than compensate for any lack of solitude. Farther on, the beautiful Little Five Lakes area is far enough off-the-beaten path to avoid any potential overcrowding, which should be the case for upper Cliff Creek canyon as well.

Although the Timber Gap Trail is one of the easier routes out of Mineral King, a stiff 1,700 feet of elevation gain in 2.25 miles is required to reach the gentler terrain beyond, where picturesque meadows, churning streams, and giant sequoias offer points of interest. Beyond Redwood Meadow is the low point of the journey at a ford of Middle Fork Kaweah River, which may present difficulties early in the season. Stiff climbing leads from there to the Bearpaw Meadow area, which has a developed backpackers' camp, ranger station, and the High Sierra Camp, where guests with reservations can sleep in tent cabins and eat hearty meals. A rolling traverse through River Valley is followed by a stiff ascent to Kaweah Gap and the entry to stunning Nine Lakes Basin just beyond. The HST section continues down the upper part of sweeping Big Arroyo, before you leave the famous trail on a climb to peaceful Little Five Lakes and then continue the ascent to a stunning vista from Black Rock Pass. Descending upper Cliff Creek canyon leads past diminutive Pinto Lake before a reunion with the Timber Gap Trail closes the loop.

DIRECTIONS TO TRAILHEAD: From the east end of Three Rivers, leave Highway 198 and turn onto Mineral King Road. Follow the road past Atwell Mill Campground, Silver City, Cold Springs Campground, and Mineral King Ranger Station (which issues wilderness permits and has food storage areas) to the Sawtooth-Monarch Trailhead parking area, 0.8 mile from the ranger station and 23 miles from Highway 198.

DESCRIPTION: Climb steeply away from the Sawtooth-Monarch Trailhead up a hillside carpeted with sagebrush, manzanita, chinquapin, and gooseberry to a junction with the Timber Gap Trail at 0.6 mile. Turn left at the junction and climb less severely across open slopes, and then follow switchbacks through a copse of red firs providing pockets of welcome shade. Near 9,200 feet, leave the trees and make a long ascending traverse toward Timber Gap. Before reentering red fir forest just below the gap, take in one last view toward Mineral King. Reach the forested saddle of Timber Gap at 2.25 miles from the trailhead.

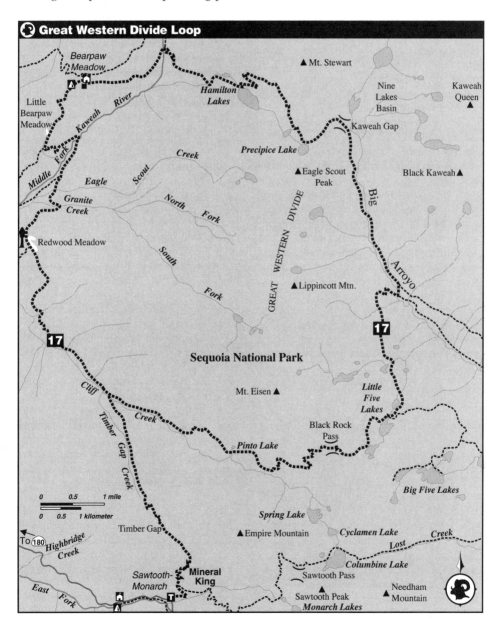

Great Western Divide Loop

Bearpaw Meadow

Little Bearpaw Meadow

Kaweah River

Middle Fork

Hamilton Lakes

▲ Mt. Stewart

Nine Lakes Basin

Kaweah Queen ▲

Kaweah Gap

Scout Creek

Precipice Lake

Eagle

▲Eagle Scout Peak

Black Kaweah▲

Granite Creek

North Fork

Big Arroyo

Redwood Meadow

South Fork

GREAT WESTERN DIVIDE

▲Lippincott Mtn.

17

17

Sequoia National Park

Cliff Creek

Timber Gap Creek

Mt. Eisen ▲

Little Five Lakes

Black Rock Pass

Pinto Lake

Big Five Lakes

0   0.5   1 mile

0   0.5   1 kilometer

Spring Lake

Cyclamen Lake

Lost Creek

Timber Gap

To (180) Highbridge Creek

▲Empire Mountain

Columbine Lake

Sawtooth-Monarch

Mineral King

Sawtooth Pass

Needham Mountain ▲

East Fork

Sawtooth Peak

Monarch Lakes

A forested, switchbacking descent leads away from the gap to a crossing of Timber Gap Creek, where a long swath of flower-bedecked meadow along the banks supplants a mixed forest. Continue down the verdant canyon, quickly crossing back over the main branch and then a number of lushly lined, spring-fed tributaries. Eventually the trail departs the Timber Gap Creek drainage and makes a short climb over the northeast lip of the canyon, before following a switchbacking descent toward Cliff Creek below. At 5 miles, you boulder hop Cliff Creek and come to red fir–shaded campsites (which have a bear box) near a signed junction with the Black Rock Pass Trail.

From the junction, continue ahead down the canyon of Cliff Creek on a moderate descent through a dense forest of pines, firs, cedars, and oaks. The trail initially hugs the east bank of the creek, but after crossing a mud-lined side stream, it favors the forested slope away from the creek. Make a brief return to Cliff Creek at the next crossing of a side stream, but soon veer away again on a mildly descending stretch of trail. Soon, a more moderate descent resumes and leads to the low point of the journey at the crossing of another small tributary.

Climb steeply away from the crossing until a gently ascending traverse wraps around a forested hillside. Sugar and Jeffrey pines join the mixed forest and, where the trail bends into a side canyon, you begin to see the first giant sequoias of the Redwood Meadow Grove.

Suddenly leave the forest and the Big Trees behind, as the trail exits the side canyon and reaches a rocky promontory dotted with manzanita and oaks. Here an impressive view of Moro Rock, Alta Peak, and Tharps Rock unfolds above the canyon of Middle Fork Kaweah River. Beyond this viewpoint, the trail descends moderately through a light mixed forest, with an understory of manzanita and mountain misery. Soon, you find yourself back in thick forest sprinkled with more giant sequoias.

Reach Redwood Meadow, 8.3 miles from the trailhead, and a signed junction with the Atwell-Redwood Trail.

REDWOOD MEADOW

A large log cabin occasionally houses seasonal rangers, who spend part of their summers amid the serenity of Redwood Meadow. Numerous scratch marks on the exterior walls testify to the resident black bear population. Nearby a tack shed, hitching post, and corral contribute to the pastoral ambiance. The namesake meadow is a thin strip of verdant vegetation surrounded by a thick forest of mixed conifers and giant sequoias.

A short stroll through the tree-rimmed meadow leads to some primitive campsites, where a water faucet provides drinking water during the summer. Aside from this faucet, water is hard to come by at Redwood Meadow, especially late in the season. An outhouse is a stone's throw away. Just beyond the campsites, the trail crosses a low wood bridge over a boggy drainage and then comes to a junction of the Bearpaw Trail on the right and a connector to the Middle Fork Trail on the left, 8.5 miles from the trailhead.

Veer right and follow the Bearpaw Trail on a climb through a mixed forest to the crest of a low ridge. Beyond the ridge, traverse a lightly forested hillside of black oaks, incense cedars, red firs, and patches of manzanita with periodic views of Moro Rock, Alta Peak, and some interesting granite domes. A mile from the ranger station, reach the rock chasm of turbulent Granite Creek and an easily negotiated crossing via a stout, wood-plank-and-rail bridge.

Beyond Granite Creek, follow an easy traverse around the nose of an oak-shaded ridge to the crossing of cascading Eagle Scout Creek (possibly a difficult ford early in the season). Pass a small campsite above the far bank and contour over to a junction of the Middle Fork Trail.

Turn right and follow gently graded trail a half mile to the broad ford of Middle

Fork Kaweah River, 10.6 miles from the trailhead. Be sure to check with the Park Service on the condition of this ford before embarking on your trip; it is potentially dangerous when the river is high and swift. The far bank has pleasant campsites shaded by alders and sugar pines.

The Bearpaw Trail turns west beyond the river crossing and makes a stiff, winding climb up the dry, south-facing wall of the canyon through black oaks, red firs, and incense cedars. Near the top of the climb, reach a junction with a lateral to the Middle Fork Trail.

Turn right (north) at the junction, and climb more gently to Little Bearpaw Meadow, 11.6 miles from the trailhead. Skirt the fern-covered meadow and pass secluded campsites next to a gently flowing tributary.

Beyond the serene glade, the trail attacks the slope on a moderate to moderately steep climb through cedars and firs. The mile-long ascent leads to the shady backpackers' campground near Bearpaw Meadow, with numbered sites, bear boxes, pit toilets, and water faucets. Picnic tables and fire pits seem to be the only things missing from the typical auto-accessible campground.

From a signed junction at the edge of the campground, take the right-hand branch leading through the campground 0.2 mile east to the A-framed ranger station and Bearpaw Meadow High Sierra Camp, picturesquely set near the lip of Middle Fork Canyon. Unlike the claustrophobic backpackers' campground, the open setting of Bearpaw Camp offers excellent views of the glacier-scoured surroundings above the canyon, including such features as Eagle Scout Peak and Mt. Stewart on the Great Western Divide, the granite cleft of Hamilton Canyon, and Black Kaweah above Kaweah Gap. Similar to the popular High Sierra Camps of Yosemite, guests with reservations for the camp sleep in tent cabins and enjoy hot meals for breakfast and dinner. Community restrooms have flush toilets and hot showers. For more information, or to make a reservation, consult the website at **www.visitsequoia.com/bearpaw.aspx**.

From the ranger station, follow a descending traverse across the precipitous north wall of River Valley with excellent views across the canyon. At the bottom of Middle Fork canyon, a concrete culvert spans the rowdy river. A short climb away from the river leads to a small bench and a junction with the Elizabeth Pass Trail, 12.2 miles from the trailhead. Decent campsites can be found in the vicinity of the junction.

Away from the junction, a stiff, switchbacking climb ensues through sagebrush, manzanita, and scattered black oaks, which eventually leads around a corner and into Hamilton Creek canyon. The view-packed scenery in this granite sanctuary is absolutely stunning, with the towering face of Angel Wings crowning the north wall, a rival to the better known climbing walls of Yosemite. The white domes of Hamilton Towers tops the ridge on the opposite side of the canyon. Soon, you ford tumbling Hamilton Creek and climb over shards of rock above Lower Hamilton Lake to the outlet of the upper lake, 14 miles from the trailhead.

The northwest shore of Upper Hamilton Lake has excellent campsites, but the basin is a very popular overnight destination, so *don't expect solitude.* The Park Service has instituted a two-night camping limit and

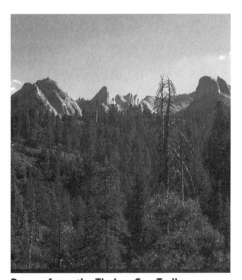

Domes from the Timber Gap Trail

banned campfires in an attempt to minimize the effects of overuse. The scenery is magnificent, and anglers will enjoy the challenge of attempting to land the resident rainbow, brook, and golden trout. Glacier-polished slabs around the shoreline create fine spots for swimmers and sunbathers.

Now you face the 2,500-foot climb to Kaweah Gap. The trail itself is something of an engineering marvel, blasted right out of the rock in many places. From the outlet of Upper Hamilton Lake, zigzag up the north wall of the enormous cirque and then veer south past a tarn on the way up to Precipice Lake, 2.6 miles from Upper Hamilton Lake. The frigid lake reposes at the base of the impressive north face of Eagle Scout Peak. A final 0.75-mile climb past a smattering of miniature tarns leads to Kaweah Gap (approximately 10,700 feet), 17.25 miles from the trailhead. A spectacular view unfolds from Kaweah Gap of the Kaweah Peaks, Nine Lakes Basin, and the canyon of Big Arroyo.

To visit Nine Lakes Basin, drop from Kaweah Gap on a few switchbacks. Leave the HST and head north cross-country to the first lake (approximately 10,455 feet). Off-trail travel north to the upper two lakes is straightforward. To reach the set of lakes to the east you have to cross more difficult terrain that requires more advanced routefinding skills. Whichever lake you decide to visit, the U-shaped basin at the convergence of the Great Western Divide and Kaweah Peaks Ridge, culminating at Triple Divide Peak, presents unparalleled alpine scenery worthy of an extended layover.

From Kaweah Gap, the HST makes a continuous and steady descent to the west of the nascent creek draining Big Arroyo. Just shy of 2 miles from the gap, the trail crosses the creek, and the descent continues through pockets of meadow and granite, crossing numerous side streams along the way. The open terrain permits fine views of Big Arroyo and the multihued Kaweah Peaks to the north. Near a tributary stream draining an unnamed tarn, the trail skirts some campsites and then reaches a junction between the Big Arroyo Trail and the Black

Rock Pass Trail to Little Five Lakes, 3 miles from Kaweah Gap.

Turn right (south) and follow the trail past the Big Arroyo patrol cabin directly east of a meadow along Big Arroyo Creek. Proceed shortly to a junction, where the Big Arroyo Trail heads southeast and your trail to Little Five Lakes veers northwest. Near the junction are some campsites (which have a bear box).

Beyond a ford of Big Arroyo Creek, the trail attacks the wall of the canyon on a 3-mile, moderate to moderately steep, switchbacking climb through light forest cover, which allows fine views of sweeping Big Arroyo. Near the top of the climb, you cross a minor ridge and make a short drop to the crossing of a tributary stream draining Little Five Lakes. One look at the topo map indicates the area was poorly named, as there are many more than five lakes clustered in the two basins sharing the same name. A faint use trail heads upstream to the first set of lakes occupying a cirque beneath Mt. Eisen along the Great Western Divide.

A gentler ascent continues generally south to the second group of lakes, where the main trail bends southwest to pass around the south shore of the lower lake. A short, mild climb leads to a four-way junction near a crossing of the next lake's outlet near the east shore. There are campsites with a bear box along a path to the backcountry patrol cabin.

From the junction, follow the northwest shore of Lake 10476 to a set of rocky switchbacks to an ascending traverse toward the northwest shore of the highest lake, where view-packed campsites will lure overnighters. Anglers can ply the waters of all the Little Five Lakes for brook trout.

As you leave the Little Five Lakes area behind, the trail climbs stiffly toward Black Rock Pass at a notch in the Great Western Divide. Views along the way are quite stunning, but the climax is reached at the pass after a set of final switchbacks. The vista from Black Rock Pass takes in the rugged Kaweahs to the northeast, including Mt. Kaweah, Second Kaweah, Red Kaweah, and Black Kaweah. Peaks seen along the

Sierra Crest include Mt. Whitney above Red Spur and Mt. Langley 5 miles to the south. Ahead is the beautiful open basin of upper Cliff Creek.

A series of rocky switchbacks lead down from the pass across open terrain with stunning scenery from Cyclamen and Spring Lakes occupying a cirque below the Great Western Divide. Farther down-slope, a fine display of wildflowers and a variety of shrubs signal your arrival to more hospitable terrain. Continue past a series of meadows to a use trail on the left leading to campsites (which have a bear box). In the opposite direction lies diminutive Pinto Lake, hidden in a thick pocket of willows. The tiny lake is not much to look at in comparison to the much more dramatic scenery around Cyclamen and Spring Lakes, but the shallow waters offer pleasant swimming.

Continuing down the canyon, you cross a tributary and then zigzag down the slope to eventually come alongside the main stem of Cliff Creek. Head downstream to a large boulder field, where the creek adopts a subterranean course temporarily. Farther down, enter a forest of scattered firs and cross several lush rivulets on the way to a junction with the Timber Gap Trail at the close of the loop section. Campsites nearby offer one last opportunity to sleep under the stars before retracing your steps 5 miles to the trailhead.

O A journey to strikingly beautiful Spring Lake is fairly straightforward from the 10,000-foot level of the Black Rock Pass Trail. From there, contour 0.9 mile across open terrain to the lake.

Mountaineers can accept a challenge to climb Mt. Eisen on a Class 1–2 route from Black Rock Pass.

R A wilderness permit is required for overnight stays. Camping is limited to designated sites at Bearpaw Meadow Campground. Hamilton Lakes has a two-night limit. Campfires are prohibited at Timber Gap, in Bearpaw Meadow, in the Hamilton Lakes and Nine Lakes Basins, and above 10,000 feet in Big Arroyo.

Introduction to the Foothills

Most of the Sierra backcountry is inaccessible during the winter, at least to those who don't wish to don cross-country skis or snowshoes. Fortunately, Sequoia has a low-elevation area with a handful of all-year trails. Hikers in the foothills may enjoy their pursuit no matter what the season. However, summer temperatures on these trails are generally unbearably hot (90°–100°F), and most recreationists seem to spend more time in the water than on the trail. While fall and winter provide wonderful times to enjoy the foothills, spring is perhaps the best season, when winter rains have turned the grassy hillsides a verdant green, wildflowers add a complementary splash of brilliant color, and the trees and shrubs of the oak woodland have sprouted new growth.

Native Americans were the first to enjoy the mostly pleasant climate of the foothills, establishing villages near streams and rivers (evidenced by pictographs and bedrock mortars in a variety of locations). Game was plentiful, as were seeds, nuts, and berries. Today, much of the limited tourist traffic in the foothills is tied to sites highlighting the presence of Native Americans in the park.

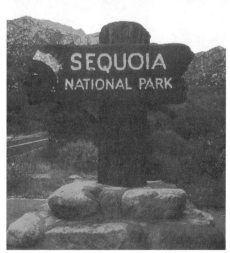

Historic entrance sign

Generally, vegetation in the foothills zone is outside the conifer belt, composed mainly of grasslands, chaparral, and oak woodland. Those unfamiliar with this landscape may consider the area rather scrubby, but more perceptive eyes will see a diverse flora, particularly in riparian areas. While the region's characteristic granite appears sporadically, most of the rock in this zone is metamorphic, lending a decidedly different appearance than that usually associated with the Sierra Nevada. Much of the foothills terrain is not only brush-filled but also steep and virtually inaccessible without the aid of a trail. While lines of motorists scurry through the foothills on their way to the more famous features above, hikers who stop and take the time to will see much more than brushy, dry, rocky, and inhospitable terrain. The foothills region of Sequoia is filled with dramatic rivers, tumbling streams, splendid vistas, and exquisite terrain.

Campgrounds

Campground	Fee	Elevation	Season	Restrooms	Water	Bear Boxes	Phone
Potwisha (3.8 miles from Ash Mountain Entrance)	$18	2,100 feet	All year	Flush	Yes	Yes	Yes
Buckeye Flat	$18	2,800 feet	Late spring to early September	Flush	Yes	Yes	Yes*

*At Hospital Rock

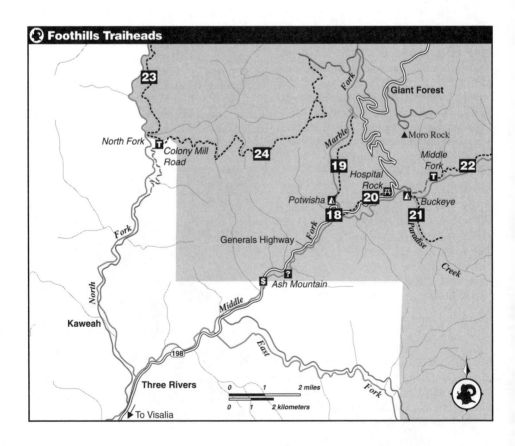

Visitors planning on swimming or wading in the rivers and streams should exercise caution in spring and early summer because conditions can be quite dangerous at times. The low elevations may present additional concerns, including rattlesnakes, ticks, and poison oak.

ACCESS: Year-round access to the foothills is via State Highway 198, which becomes the Generals Highway inside the park.

AMENITIES: The resort-driven community of Three Rivers offers the basic necessities for motor-bound tourists visiting the national parks and Lake Kaweah (managed by US Corps of Army Engineers). Amenities include motels, cafes, restaurants, general stores, a drug store, gas stations, and auto repair shops. Visalia, a larger town 20 miles west, has a correspondingly larger array of services.

RANGER STATION: The Ash Mountain Visitor Center, 0.7 mile east of the entrance station, is Sequoia's year-round headquarters. The visitor center offers a variety of books, maps, and gifts. Visitors can get wilderness permits during normal business hours.

GOOD TO KNOW BEFORE YOU GO: Although the Ash Mountain Entrance is open all year, the Generals Highway between Hospital Rock and the Giant Forest may require chains during winter driving conditions. In addition, the Generals Highway between Sequoia and Kings Canyon is subject to periodic closures during winter storms.

POTWISHA TRAILHEAD

TRIP 18

Potwisha Pictographs Loop

E ◯ DH

DISTANCE: 0.5 mile, loop

ELEVATION: 2,095'/2,070'/2,160', +205'/-205'/±410'

SEASON: All year

USE: Light

MAP: *Giant Forest*

INTRODUCTION: An easy half-mile jaunt suitable for all ages, the Potwisha loop is not much of a hike by most standards. However, an extensive display of bedrock mortars, in which the native Monache ground nuts and seeds, plus a set of pictographs add an interesting historical glimpse into the lifestyles of those who first inhabited this scenic area. During the hot part of the year, sandy beaches and rock slabs along the river provide sunbathers and swimmers with a picturesque setting. A suspension bridge over Middle Fork Kaweah River will be of special interest and a fine vantage from which to watch the river gliding over slabs, tumbling into cataracts, and swirling through delightful pools. Although the trail is easy enough for small children, exercise caution at all times because the river can be treacherous during spring and early summer.

MONACHE ARTISTS

The Monache used bedrock mortars to grind acorns from the native oaks into meal, a staple of their diet. Since only women were involved in this task, anthropologists suggest females drew the nearby pictographs, the meanings of which remain a mystery.

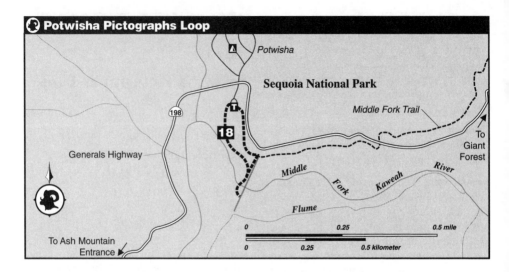

Potwisha Pictographs Loop

Potwisha

Sequoia National Park

Middle Fork Trail

To Giant Forest

Generals Highway

Middle

Fork

Kaweah

River

Flume

To Ash Mountain Entrance

0   0.25   0.5 mile

0   0.25   0.5 kilometer

DIRECTIONS TO TRAILHEAD: Follow the Generals Highway from the Ash Mountain Entrance 3.8 miles to the Potwisha Campground entrance. Turn right onto the road opposite the campground and proceed to the right-hand (west) side of the gravel parking area.

DESCRIPTION: Find the unmarked path and head down toward the river, soon encountering a series of granite slabs, site of numerous bedrock mortars. An overhanging rock to the south has several pictographs on its underside.

Proceed around granite boulders above the river to a wood suspension bridge. On the far side, a series of slabs provide a fine vantage from which to watch the Middle Fork flow through the canyon. The path soon dead-ends above the bridge near an old flume.

Cross back over the bridge and veer to the right on a path headed toward a large-diameter steel pipe. A faint path follows the pipe on a short, steep climb to a junction with the Middle Fork Trail. Turn left at the junction and follow the trail high above the river through oak woodland back to the parking area.

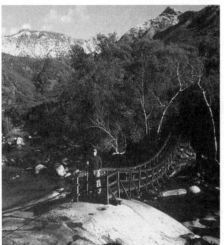

Suspension bridge over Middle Fork Kaweah River

TRIP 19

Marble Falls

Ⓜ ↗ DH

DISTANCE: 6.6 miles, out-and-back

ELEVATION: 2,160'/3,760', +1,750'/-295'/±4,090'

SEASON: All year (best from March to May)

USE: Light

MAP: *Giant Forest*

INTRODUCTION: The Marble Falls Trail offers a year-round opportunity to enjoy the foothills and is particularly fine in spring when the Marble Fork Kaweah River courses and cascades through aptly named Deep Canyon, and swelling meltwater drops through a series of dramatic waterfalls surrounded by glistening marble slabs and boulders. Slopes covered with verdant grasses and an assortment of colorful wildflowers add touches of beauty in the spring as well. Hiking in the foothills poses some concerns uncommon in the high country—rattlesnakes, ticks, and poison oak.

DIRECTIONS TO TRAILHEAD: Follow the Generals Highway 3.8 miles from the Ash Mountain Entrance to the Potwisha Campground entrance. Turn left into the campground and follow the loop road to a dirt access road at the northwest end near site #14. Follow the short access road to the parking area.

DESCRIPTION: Walk up the access road to a wood plank bridge spanning a concrete-lined flume, and continue up a dirt road paralleling the flume to a stream-flow gauge and a fenced control gate. The signed trail begins opposite the gate, 0.2 mile from the parking area.

Leaving the road behind, head uphill on single-track trail via switchbacks through typical foothills woodland accented by seasonal wildflowers. Pay close attention to the vegetation because poison oak is prevalent along the lower part of the trail. Leave the trees behind above the switchbacks, as you proceed across chaparral-covered slopes high above the Marble Fork, climbing around the folds and creases on the east side of Deep Canyon. Views of the turbulent river across the low-growing chaparral are periodically interrupted by forays into small wooded nooks at the crossings of numerous side streams along the way. The Marble Fork provides dramatic scenery in the spring, when the swollen stream cascades down rock steps and swirls through churning pools, producing a raucous thunder that reverberates up the steep walls of the canyon. After crossing a stream that drains the southwest slope of Switchback Peak, the trail heads through woodland back into the main canyon and ascends the hillside to meet the riverbank. The trail suddenly ends amid a jumble of boulders and slabs.

Although the name "Marble Falls" specifically applies to the uppermost falls in Deep Canyon, a series of picturesque falls below extend from the end of the trail

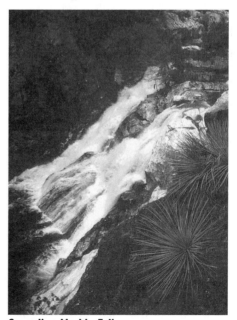

Cascading Marble Falls

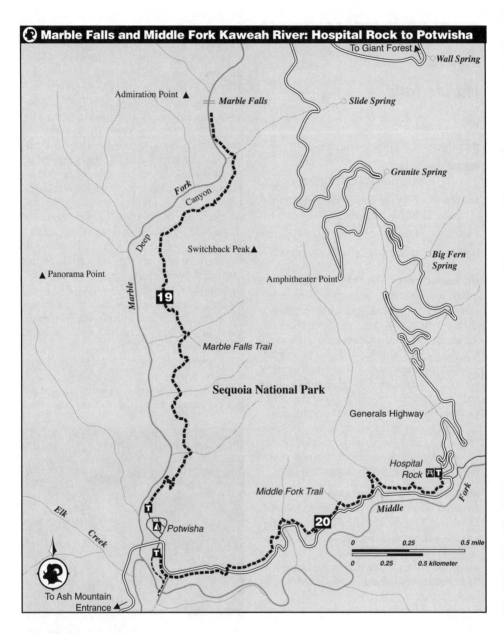

Marble Falls and Middle Fork Kaweah River: Hospital Rock to Potwisha

over a narrow, quarter-mile section of the canyon. Across the cleft, Admiration Point stands guard over the thunderous clamor the river makes as it spills over glistening marble precipices into wildly churning pools. The most convenient vantage point from which to view the lower falls is just below the trail, accessible via short paths leading to a grassy bench. By scrambling over boulders, slabs, and sections of the steep canyon wall, you can make limited progress upstream to additional views, but the terrain can be quite treacherous—*only attempt it if you are skilled in such travel.* The terrain becomes even more difficult farther up the canyon.

HOSPITAL ROCK TRAILHEAD

TRIP 20

Middle Fork Kaweah River: Hospital Rock to Potwisha

Ⓜ / DH

DISTANCE: 2.4 miles, point-to-point

ELEVATION: 2,695'/2,100', +345'/-935'/±2,560'

SEASON: All year (best from September to June)

USE: Light

MAP: *Giant Forest*

see map on p.108

INTRODUCTION: Although unbearably hot in the summer, the Middle Fork Trail offers pleasant hiking the rest of the year. This short section of trail offers fine views of the Middle Fork Kaweah River canyon, as well as periodic glimpses of Moro Rock and Castle Rocks. A fine cross section of foothills vegetation rewards hikers as they pass through zones of oak woodland, chaparral, and grasses. Late winter and early spring bring splashes of color from a pleasant array of wildflowers.

DIRECTIONS TO TRAILHEAD:

START: Follow the Generals Highway to the Hospital Rock parking area, 6.1 miles from the Ash Mountain Entrance.

END: Follow the Generals Highway to the Potwisha Campground entrance, 3.8 miles from the Ash Mountain Entrance.

Turn opposite the campground entrance and proceed to the left-hand (east) side of the gravel parking area, near the Potwisha Campground dump station.

DESCRIPTION: The signed trail begins on the far, uphill side of the Hospital Rock picnic area, near a small concrete and wood structure. Proceed through shady oak woodland away from the picnic area, soon breaking out onto open slopes, where a nearly continuous view down the Middle Fork canyon begins. Follow the undulating trail across the north side of the canyon through mostly open terrain, interrupted occasionally by brief dips into narrow side canyons. Continuing down the canyon, don't forget to turn around every now and then to take in views of Moro Rock and Castle Rocks. Eventually, switchbacks lead down the slope to a crossing of the Generals Highway, 1.75 miles from Hospital Rock.

The trail resumes on the far side of the highway and enters oak woodland. Gently graded tread eventually leads to the end of the trail near the Potwisha Campground's dump station.

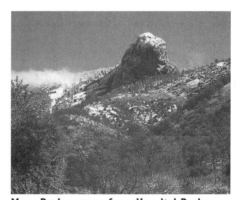

Moro Rock as seen from Hospital Rock

HOSPITAL ROCK TRAILHEAD

TRIP 21

Paradise Creek Trail

Ⓜ ╱ **DH**

DISTANCE: 4.6 miles, out-and-back

ELEVATION: 2,685'/3,385',
+975'/-280'/±2,510'

SEASON: All year

USE: Light

MAP: *Giant Forest*

INTRODUCTION: The Paradise Creek Trail is a little-known gem, providing a relatively temperate hike in the summer and a low-elevation alternative to the snowbound high country during the rest of the year. Dense forest cover with a lush understory

prevents hikers from suffering the intense summer heat common to other foothills trails. Late winter and early spring provides the added bonus of green grass and colorful wildflowers.

After the bridged crossing of Middle Fork Kaweah River, the trail ascends the narrow canyon of Paradise Creek on a mild to moderate 1.5-mile climb to a 15-foot waterfall. Built in the 1920s, the trail originally went all the way to Mineral King. However, after the Mineral King Road was completed, the trail suffered from a lack of use and the upper portion was abandoned in the 1960s.

DIRECTIONS TO TRAILHEAD: Follow the Generals Highway to the Hospital Rock parking lot, 6.1 miles from the Ash Mountain Entrance.

DESCRIPTION: Campers at Buckeye Flat Campground have the luxury of being able

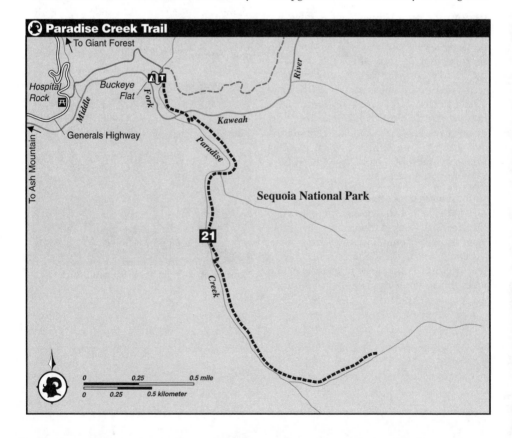

to stroll over to the start of the trail. Everyone else will have to park at Hospital Rock and walk an additional 0.6 mile east on the campground road since day-use parking is prohibited.

From Hospital Rock, cross the Generals Highway and follow the campground access road a half mile to a Y-junction. Veer right, remaining on paved road, and head downhill another 0.1 mile to the entrance to Buckeye Flat Campground. Follow the road ahead to the east side of the campground and the start of the Paradise Creek Trail opposite Campsite #28.

Follow single-track trail through dense oak woodland on gently ascending read, until a short descent leads to a bridge across Middle Fork Kaweah River, 0.9 mile from Hospital Rock. Just past the bridge is an informal junction with paths leading both upstream and downstream along the river. If you have a few extra minutes, detour onto the upstream trail and walk a short distance to a picturesque waterfall emptying into a huge pool surrounded by colorful rock formations. The downstream path leads to a smaller waterfall and a fine swimming hole on Paradise Creek.

From the informal junction, follow the middle trail, which climbs gently via a pair of switchbacks through oak woodland with lush ground cover. High above the river, you have good views of the cataracts and cascades of the Middle Fork below. Soon the trail reaches another informal junction, where the main trail veers left.

Follow the left-hand trail to a crossing of Paradise Creek, 1.9 miles from Hospital Rock, which may be a wet ford early in the season. After 0.1 mile, the trail crosses back over the creek and continues upstream. As the trail gets steeper, the tread becomes fainter, and brush crowds the path. With a little extra effort, determined hikers can proceed to a scenic, 15-foot waterfall on the east tributary of Paradise Creek. The vegetation parts momentarily on the way to the fall, allowing fine views of Paradise Creek canyon and Paradise Ridge.

HOSPITAL ROCK TRAILHEAD

TRIP 22

Middle Fork Kaweah River: Hospital Rock to Panther Creek

Ⓜ ↗ **DH** or **BP**

DISTANCE: 5.5 miles, out-and-back (plus 3.6 miles when road is closed)

ELEVATION: 3,220'/3,875', +1,325'/-935'/±4,520'

SEASON: All year (best from September to June)

USE: Light

MAP: *Giant Forest*

INTRODUCTION: Spring may be the best time to take the trail up Middle Fork Kaweah River. The trail is likely to be free of snow, and mild temperatures, colorful wildflowers, and a swollen river will combine for a fine vernal journey. No matter what the season, stunning views of Moro Rock, Castle Rocks, and the Great Western Divide provide excellent scenery. Good campsites near Panther Creek offer an opportunity for an off-season backpacking trip as well, with the possibility of extending the trip farther up the Middle Fork.

The route of the trail along the south-facing wall of the canyon is exposed to the sun most of the way, which makes for a potentially hot trip—get an early start when fair skies are forecasted. Traveling in the foothills also includes such potential hazards as rattlesnakes, ticks, and poison oak.

When the Buckeye Flat Campground is open, you can drive 1.8 miles on the access road to the official trailhead. However, if the gate is closed at the junction with the Generals Highway, you'll have to park at Hospital Rock and walk an extra 1.8 miles on the road to reach the trailhead.

DIRECTIONS TO TRAILHEAD: Follow the Generals Highway to Hospital Rock, 6.1

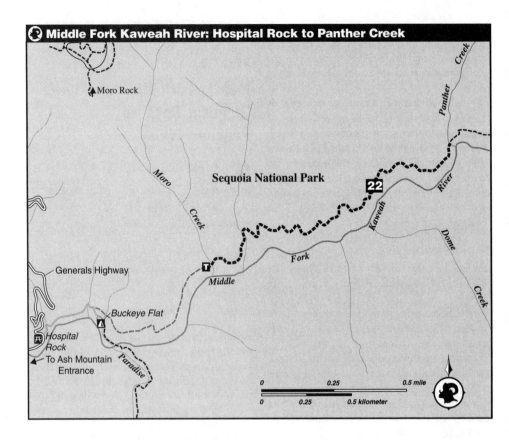

Middle Fork Kaweah River: Hospital Rock to Panther Creek

Moro Rock

Sequoia National Park

22

Moro Creek

Panther Creek

Kaweah River

Dome Creek

Generals Highway

Middle Fork

Buckeye Flat

Hospital Rock

To Ash Mountain Entrance

Paradise

0   0.25   0.5 mile

0   0.25   0.5 kilometer

miles from the Ash Mountain Entrance. If the road is open, turn right (east) and continue another half mile to a Y-junction with the paved Buckeye Flat Campground road. Continue ahead from the junction onto a dirt road and proceed another 0.8 mile to the trailhead.

DESCRIPTION:

FROM HOSPITAL ROCK: Cross the Generals Highway and walk the paved access road for a half mile to a Y-junction with the road to Buckeye Flat Campground. Continue ahead on the left-hand dirt road on a steady climb across a grassy hillside dotted with oaks and lined with wildflowers. Along the way are good views of the cascading and careening Middle Fork Kaweah River below and the Great Western Divide to the east. Eventually you reach the official trailhead, 1.8 miles from the Generals Highway.

FROM THE MIDDLE FORK TRAILHEAD: From the trailhead, descend single-track trail a short distance to a boulder hop of Moro Creek, which may necessitate a ford early in the season. The crossing is an attractive scene, as the alder- and laurel-lined creek dances over a series of slanted rock slabs, backdropped picturesquely by the narrow, V-shaped canyon framing the granodiorite dome of Moro Rock, 3,500 feet above.

From Moro Creek, climb moderately on sandy tread heading up the canyon across open, chaparral-covered slopes. Soon, the trail wraps around into the drainage of an unnamed tributary to an easy crossing of the lively but diminutive stream. Beyond the stream, follow the serpentine course of the Middle Fork on a steady climb, weaving around the folds and creases of the canyon. Keep a lookout for patches of poison oak lining the trail. For the most part, the mighty river is distant enough from the trail to remain hidden by the intervening terrain, but the raucous torrent is close enough to be within earshot constantly. Across the canyon, the spires and pinnacles of Castle Rocks lend a craggy feel to the otherwise shrubby surroundings. Before Panther Creek, three switchbacks lead to a vantage point with an expansive vista including the Great Western Divide, Moro Rock, Castle Rocks, and the turbulent Middle Fork below. Continue to climb moderately until a short, moderately steep descent brings you to Panther Creek.

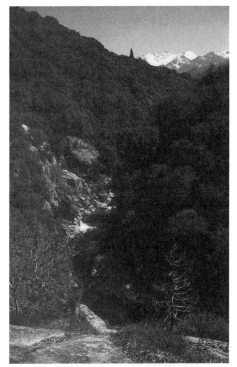

Great Western Divide from the trail

Conveniently placed rocks provide a straightforward boulder hop across the usually shallow but rapidly moving creek, although the crossing may feel a bit intimidating just above the precipitous fall immediately downstream, where the creek hurtles through a narrow chute of rock to plummet 100 feet straight down toward the river. Be extra cautious while crossing and especially if you decide to swim in the inviting pools above the fall. Good campsites can be found on a bench above the far side of the creek, near some slabs near the lip of the canyon. The bench also provides excellent views of the river and the Great Western Divide.

O The Middle Fork Trail continues up the canyon to junctions with trails leading to Little Bearpaw and Redwood Meadows, offering a rare opportunity for an extended, off-season backpack. Beyond Panther Creek, the trail passes through a transition forest of oaks and cedars for 2.5 miles to a junction with the unmaintained Castle Creek Trail. Campsites may be available a short distance down the old trail near Mehrten Creek, or 0.4 mile farther along the Middle Fork. Continuing east, the Middle Fork Trail accesses more campsites near Mehrten Creek and near the bridge across Buck Creek, 2.5 miles from the Castle Creek Trail junction. From there, a 1.8-mile climb leads to a junction with a lateral to Little Bearpaw Meadow. Another mile-long climb is followed by a sustained descent to a crossing of the Middle Fork Kaweah River and a junction with a trail to Redwood Meadow (see Trip 17, page 98).

R A wilderness permit is required for overnight stays.

NORTH FORK TRAILHEAD

TRIP 23

North Fork Trail

Ⓜ ↗ **DH**

DISTANCE: 8.4 miles, out-and-back

ELEVATION: 1,800'/2,355',
+1,415'/-555'/±3,940'

SEASON: All year (best from September to June)

USE: Light

MAP: *Shadequarter Mountain*

INTRODUCTION: Following the route of an old fire road built by the CCC (Civilian Conservation Corps) in the 1930s, this seldom-used trail offers plenty of solitude and splendid views of its namesake canyon. The road once extended nearly 14 miles to Hidden Springs, but today only the first 6 miles are in good enough condition for problem-free hiking. While a scorcher in the summer, this trip offers a splendid off-season hiking opportunity.

DIRECTIONS TO TRAILHEAD: Follow Highway 198 to Three Rivers and head north on North Fork Drive, immediately crossing a bridge over Middle Fork Kaweah River. Continue through the community of Kaweah, where the road narrows and starts a winding climb up the canyon. At 6 miles from the highway, you enter the BLM's North Fork Recreation Area and proceed another 1.5 miles to the end of the pavement and onto dirt road. At a Y-junction with the Colony Mill Road, 10 miles from the highway, veer left and head downhill for 0.7 mile to the Sequoia National Park boundary. Park your vehicle on a broad flat at the end of the road.

DESCRIPTION: From the parking area, cross a wood-beam bridge over Yucca Creek and continue up an old roadbed above the north bank of the creek, crossing a grassy slope dotted with oaks. At 0.3 mile, reach an unmarked junction with a short trail on the right leading to Yucca Flat. The flat has seen several occupants over the years, including Native Americans, Kaweah colonists, and ranchers before eventual purchase by the Park Service.

Steeper climbing leads away from Yucca Creek and up a series of hillsides. In the midst of the climb, a short use trail leads to a pair of concrete bunkers, which the CCC used to store explosives. Continuing to ascend, pass through an old steel gate and head up grassy slopes carpeted with wildflowers in season. Where the grade eases, pass through another gate and then come above the main canyon of North Fork Kaweah River. Now roughly paralleling the river, the trail traverses the folds and creases on the east side of the canyon, periodically veering into small, forested side canyons along the way. The open topography allows for good views of the canyon and Burnt 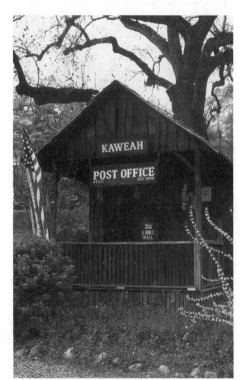 Point to the west.

Historic Kaweah Post Office

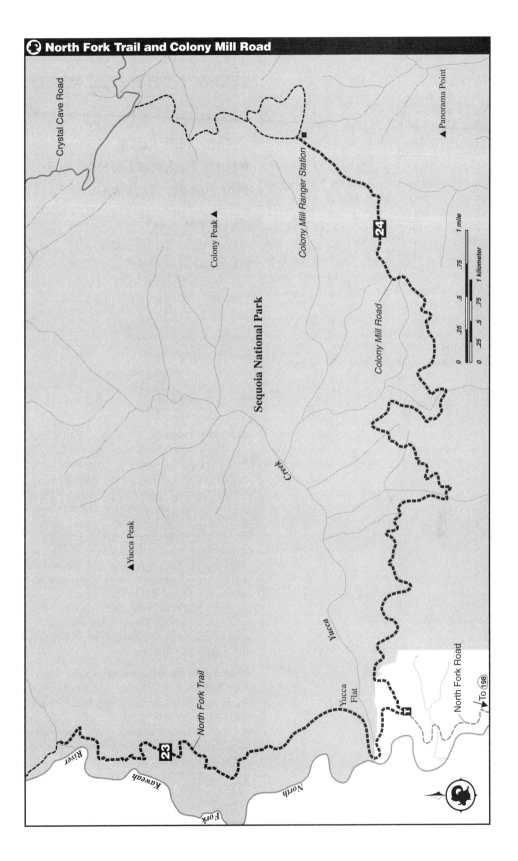

Crystal Cave Road

Panorama Point ▲

Colony Peak ▲

Colony Mill Ranger Station

Sequoia National Park

24

Colony Mill Road

Creek

0   .25   .5   .75   1 mile
0   .25   .5   .75   1 kilometer

▲ Yucca Peak

Yucca

Yucca
Flat

North

North Fork Trail

23

Kaweah

River

Fork

North Fork Road

To 198

1

Reach an unnamed creek, 3.8 miles from the trailhead, where sloping granite slabs offer a convenient place for a rest stop. Continue another half mile on gently graded tread to a crossing of Burnt Creek in a shady nook, where the creek flows through a culvert beneath the old roadbed. The pleasant grade continues for another couple of miles, with fine views of the canyon along the way. Eventually, brush crowds the trail and the tread becomes less distinct as it climbs steeply away from the river and up Pine Ridge and then down to Hidden Spring.

TRIP 24

Colony Mill Road: North Fork to Colony Mill Ranger Station

Ⓜ ✗ **DH** or **BP**

DISTANCE: 16 miles, out-and-back

ELEVATION: 2,360'/5,445', +5,170'/-1,085'/±12,510'

SEASON: March to November

USE: Light

MAPS: *Shadequarter Mountain* and *Giant Forest*

see map on p.115

INTRODUCTION: Modern-day hikers can enjoy a dose of history along the Colony Mill Road, while experiencing fine views and the diverse foliage of the foothills zone. Chaparral, woodland, and riparian flora provide plenty of vegetative diversity over the first 6.5 miles of trail before entering the starkly contrasting mixed coniferous forest belt below the ranger station. The low elevation provides fine early and late season hiking; scorching daytime temperatures are common during the summer. Spring is possibly the best time for a visit, when colorful wildflowers are in bloom. Plan for a short stop at the historic Kaweah Post Office on the way to the trailhead.

DIRECTIONS TO TRAILHEAD: Follow Highway 198 to Three Rivers and head north on North Fork Drive, immediately crossing a bridge over Middle Fork Kaweah River. Continue through the community of Kaweah, where the road narrows and starts a winding climb up the canyon. At 6 miles from the highway, you enter the BLM's North Fork Recreation Area and proceed another 1.5 miles to the end of the pavement and onto dirt road. At a Y-junction 10 miles from the highway, veer right and head uphill on the narrow Colony Mill Road for 0.4 mile to a closed gate at the park boundary. If space is available, park your vehicle near the gate. Otherwise, you'll have to park near the Y-junction and walk the additional 0.4 mile to the gate.

DESCRIPTION: Pass through the pedestrian bypass at the locked gate and follow the old roadbed of the Colony Mill Road on a steady climb through typical foothills vegetation. Except for a narrow footpath, the roadbed is now covered with grasses, small plants, and seasonal wildflowers. The well-graded road follows the folds and creases of Yucca Creek canyon, well above the level of the creek. Periodic gaps in the deciduous forest lining the road allow for views down to Yucca Flat and up toward forested Colony Peak.

At 0.6 mile, reach the first of many tributary streams and seasonal rivulets that feed Yucca Creek. Due to the excellent construction of the Colony Mill Road, all the streams pass below the surface of the road through culverts. Another 0.6 mile leads to

COLONY MILL ROAD

Perhaps no other route through Sequoia National Park is more replete with history than the Colony Mill Road. In 1885, a group of San Francisco–based radicals formed the Kaweah Colony in an attempt to create a utopian society based on socialist principles. They established a group of community land claims in the giant sequoia groves and constructed a wagon road from the area above Three Rivers to the Giant Forest plateau. They planned to transport timber from the groves to a mill and then ship the lumber to market for sale. The projected profits from the lumber would then finance their utopian dream.

From a base near the present community of Kaweah, the colonists began work on their road, using hand tools. Despite the lack of modern machinery, they performed an admirable job of construction, evidenced by the road's excellent grade and fine quality of workmanship in the many hand-stacked retaining walls. After four years, the colonists completed the road through chaparral and foothills woodland to just inside the mixed coniferous forest zone. On a small flat at 5,400 feet, they erected a steam-powered, portable sawmill, which operated for a relatively brief period, milling a rather modest quantity of lumber.

A number of factors combined to dash the dream of the Kaweah Colony, including a growing concern among ranchers and preservationists over destruction of the forest, government-disputed land claims, and internal squabbles. Legal battles made the mill a short-lived proposition, which was abandoned by the colonists, who then quickly attempted to regroup by leasing Atwell's mill near Mineral King. Additional disputes with the government over the new mill eventually deflated the last of the colonists' resolve, and by 1892 the Kaweah Colony was formally dissolved.

Although the Kaweah Colony had a short run, their road lived on for many years. Upon creation of the park, the US Cavalry extended the road from the mill site into the Giant Forest in 1903. For the next 23 years, the Colony Mill Road served as the only access for visitors to the giant sequoia groves. The narrow road allowed only one-way traffic, with vehicles traveling by convoy from the Kaweah Post Office, past the entrance station at Colony Mill, and then into the Giant Forest. With completion of the Generals Highway in 1926, use of the old road started to diminish. Since 1969, only the section between the Giant Forest and Crystal Cave has been open to vehicular traffic, with the remaining 10 miles restricted to foot traffic.

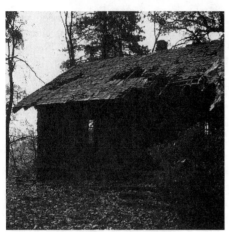

The old Colony Mill Ranger Station

the densely forested side canyon of a spring-fed stream, where a small concrete room with a metal door is built into the hillside on the uphill side of the road. A larger rock structure nearby, missing its roof, was used to store explosives during construction.

Away from the stream, the vegetation diminishes considerably, allowing more good views of the canyon until the trail reenters dense foliage on a winding, easterly course. Near the 2-mile mark, the road swings south and enters the canyon of Maple Creek, where a dense tangle of maples and alders produces plenty of shade on the way to the crossing of the creek at 2.5 miles. Follow the road out of the canyon and around the nose of the north ridge of point 4234. Well below the crest of Ash Peaks Ridge, the road curves around to cross a tributary of Cedar Creek, 4.7 miles from the trailhead.

Still heading roughly east, the road makes an ascending traverse across the northwest face of Ash Peaks Ridge above the canyon of Cedar Creek. Eventually, the road draws near to Cedar Creek, where a few of the namesake conifers make an appearance, the first evergreens seen along

the trail so far. Wrap around a hill and soon pass over a branch of the creek, where another small concrete room is built into the hillside. Beyond the creek, the road climbs steadily toward a saddle on the crest of Ash Peaks Ridge, from where you have an excellent view down the canyon of Elk Creek.

After an easy stroll along the ridgecrest, the road starts climbing again across a moderately forested hillside of ponderosa pines and incense cedars—a stark contrast to the foothills woodland seen previously. Stride easily across the crest of Ash Peaks Ridge once again, this time while admiring views down the precipitous canyon of Marble Fork Kaweah River. More climbing leads to a junction, where a seldom-used road veers left (north) and ascends the west side of point 5878.

Bear right from the junction and continue up the Colony Mill Road past overturned outhouses to the dilapidated Colony Mill Ranger Station, near the old mill site. Few visitors reach the old ranger station anymore, which has been left to crumble and decay in relative obscurity. The view from the old porch down Marble Fork to Potwisha Campground and the Middle Fork Kaweah River is still impressive, although probably not as grand as in the old days when the surrounding vegetation was less mature. Although it was a lonesome outpost, rangers who served here had excellent accommodations, including indoor plumbing with hot running water, to go along with the fine views. Nowadays, the few backpackers who stay here overnight will find a fire pit and perhaps a stack of wood but no water nearby.

O With shuttle arrangements, hikers can continue along the Colony Mill Road for another 2 miles and reach the Crystal Cave Road (see Trip 25, page 121).

R A wilderness permit is required for overnight stays.

Introduction to the Giant Forest

Upon seeing the splendor of a plateau covered with an abundance of giant sequoias, famed naturalist John Muir dubbed this area the "Giant Forest." His appellation certainly rings true; four of the five largest sequoias in the world reside here (the General Sherman, Washington, President, and Lincoln Trees), along with hundreds of other deserving specimens. Muir's adulation wasn't for the Big Trees alone; he also declared Crescent Meadow to be "the gem of the Sierra." Nowhere else in the range are so many verdant, flower-filled meadows found within a single sequoia grove. A greater sight than the full profile of a towering sequoia from across a beautiful meadow is hard to imagine, and the Giant Forest offers many such scenes.

Another feature of the Giant Forest plateau is the gentle terrain, which is unlike most of the rest of the parks' topography. An extensive network of trails conveniently covers the plateau, offering hikers a plethora of opportunities for exploration of the area. Aside from the popular General Sherman, Congress, and Crescent Meadow Trails, it's possible to enjoy the Big Trees and picturesque meadows in relative solitude. On many of the area's trails, hikers may humbly stand beneath the towering monarchs amid serene surroundings. Along with the meadows and sequoias, the Giant Forest offers far-reaching vistas and plenty of wildlife.

The trees and meadows of the Giant Forest fascinated white men from the moment they first saw them, which led to both good and bad consequences. Ultimately, the Big Trees received only a portion of the protection they deserved, but not before

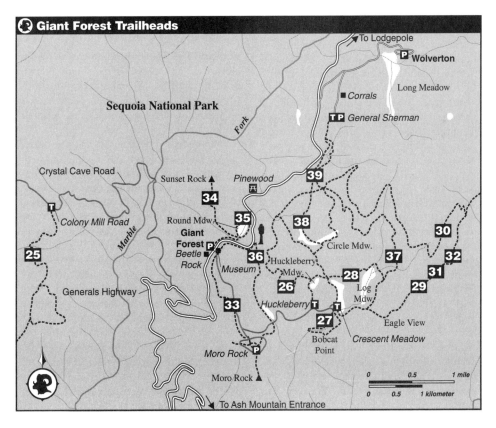

Giant Forest Trailheads

To Lodgepole

Wolverton

Sequoia National Park

Long Meadow

Corrals

General Sherman

Crystal Cave Road

Sunset Rock

Pinewood

34

39

Colony Mill Road

Round Mdw.

35

38

30

Giant Forest

Circle Mdw.

25

Beetle Rock

36

37

32

Museum

Huckleberry Mdw.

28

31

26

Log Mdw.

29

Generals Highway

33

Huckleberry

27

Eagle View

Bobcat Point

Crescent Meadow

Moro Rock

Moro Rock

0   0.5   1 mile

0   0.5   1 kilometer

To Ash Mountain Entrance

overcoming serious threats from both logging and grazing. Once the lumbermen, sheepherders, and cattlemen were driven from the newly created park, a subtler foe emerged—development. To accommodate the increasing interest of visitors in the Big Trees, campgrounds, lodges, and commercial enterprises sprung up in the Giant Forest; a number of administrative buildings were also erected. As the focal point of Sequoia National Park, visitors poured into the area in increasing numbers, and their presence had a negative impact on the environmental health of the Giant Forest. The proliferation of artificial structures testified to the area's increasing peril.

Although many were quick to recognize the destructive influence of excessive tourism on the Giant Forest, what to do about their concern was another matter entirely. As early as 1929, Park Superintendent John White considered ridding the Giant Forest of all artificial improvements to restore the area's health, but such visionaries represented a small minority at that time. Concessionaires obviously opposed such a radical idea, and the public saw these facilities as an enhancement to their experience. By the 1950s, commercial structures in the Giant Forest numbered more than 400; the Park Service had a dozen buildings, plus campgrounds, a picnic area, and numerous support facilities, including sewage plants, water cisterns, and an amphitheater. Traffic jams were nearly constant in summer. The battle over reigning in development in the Giant Forest would rage on for a good part of the 20th century.

Beginning in 1962, the Park Service took steps to minimize their own influence on the Giant Forest by closing the Firewood Campground. The visitor center was replaced by the current facility at Lodgepole in 1966. The gas station and post office were relocated four years later. The remaining three campgrounds, Paradise, Sunset Rock, and Sugar Pine, were dismantled in 1971, along with Hazelwood Picnic Area. Maintenance facilities were eventually relocated to Red Fir. The Park Service had reduced their presence in the

Giant Forest to restrooms, an information station, and one cabin. However, commercial presence was as strong as ever, with no end in sight.

Prompted by research on the detrimental effects of development on giant sequoia groves, a growing environmental awareness of the general public, and economics, the Park Service set in motion a plan to restore health to the Giant Forest. Over the course of several decades, all viable commercial facilities were eventually relocated to Lodgepole and Wuksachi, and the remaining dilapidated structures and needless asphalt were removed. In summer 2002, the doors of the newly redesigned Giant Forest Museum and Beetle Rock Environmental Education Center opened to the public. Improved parking facilities and rehabilitated trails also opened. Less obvious improvements of the Giant Forest restoration included soil restoration, regrading, revegetation, and fire management. Thanks to these measures, generations of future admirers will be able to enjoy a revitalized Giant Forest.

ACCESS: The Generals Highway provides motor vehicle access to the Giant Forest. The museum is 17 miles from the Ash Mountain Entrance, much of which travels up a winding and steep climb from Hospital Rock (vehicles longer than 22 feet are *not* recommended). From the north, the museum is 29 miles from the Y-junction with the Kings Canyon Highway. The road from Ash Mountain Entrance to the Giant Forest is open all year, but motorists must carry chains during the winter. The section of the Generals Highway from the Kings Canyon Highway junction is subject to periodic closures during winter storms.

The Moro Rock-Crescent Meadow Road leaves the Generals Highway near the museum and heads southeast to a variety of trailheads. Congestion on this road and elsewhere in the Giant Forest during the summer has led to the implementation of a free shuttle bus system, with three separate routes providing access to Crescent Meadow, Moro Rock, the Giant Forest Museum, the General Sherman Tree, Lodgepole,

Wuksachi, and Dorst Campground. Consult the park's website for more information.

The 6.7-mile Crystal Cave Road departs the Generals Highway 2 miles south of the museum, providing access to Crystal Cave (which offers tours) and the upper Colony Mill Road Trailhead.

AMENITIES: The Giant Forest Museum has exhibits and a bookstore. The Beetle Rock Environmental Education Center, operated by the Sequoia Natural History Association, is located down a short access road opposite the museum. Lodgepole and Wuksachi, 4.5 and 6 miles north respectively, offer visitor services.

CAMPGROUNDS: The nearest campground is at Lodgepole.

RANGER STATION: The nearest ranger station is at Lodgepole.

GOOD TO KNOW BEFORE YOU GO: The extensive network of trails crisscrossing the Giant Forest plateau is exclusively for dayhiking. The only backpacking route follows the High Sierra Trail eastbound from Crescent Meadow, with the first legal camping at Panther Creek, 2.5 miles from the trailhead.

CRYSTAL CAVE ROAD TRAILHEAD

TRIP 25

Colony Mill Road: Crystal Cave Road to Colony Mill Ranger Station

Ⓜ ↗ DH

DISTANCE: 4 miles, out-and-back (9 miles if Crystal Cave Road is closed)

ELEVATION: 5,300'/5,610', +865'/-245'/±2,220'

SEASON: May to November

USE: Light

MAP: *Giant Forest*

INTRODUCTION: History buffs and solitude seekers will reap big rewards on this short hike to the Colony Mill Ranger Station. From 1886 to 1890, as part of their dream of a utopian society, the Kaweah colonists hand built the Colony Mill Road through the rugged western hills of Sequoia. Modern-day hikers can walk a portion of the old road, still in remarkably good condition, from Crystal Cave Road to the ranger station near the site of an old mill.

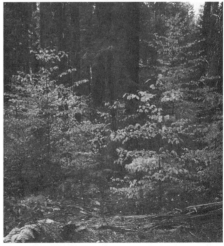

Dogwoods in autumn

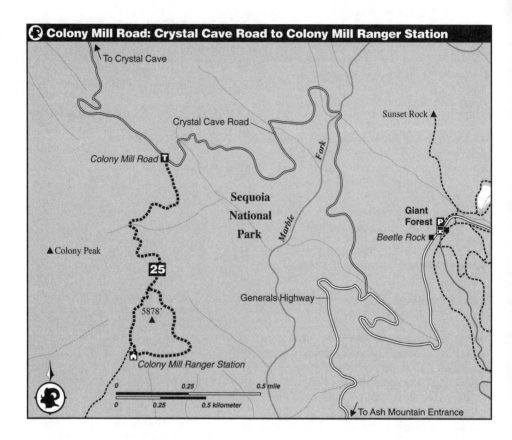

Colony Mill Road: Crystal Cave Road to Colony Mill Ranger Station

To Crystal Cave

Crystal Cave Road

Sunset Rock ▲

Colony Mill Road 🚹

Fork

Sequoia
National
Park

Marble

Giant
Forest 🅿
Beetle Rock ▲

▲ Colony Peak

25

Generals Highway

5878'
▲

Colony Mill Ranger Station

0   0.25   0.5 mile
0   0.25   0.5 kilometer

To Ash Mountain Entrance

DIRECTIONS TO TRAILHEAD: The Crystal Cave Road, 2 miles south of the Giant Forest Museum, is subject to daily and seasonal closures. From mid-May to late October, a gate immediately past the Marble Fork Bridge opens in the morning and then closes in the late afternoon, allowing motorists with reservations for cave tours to pass. Hikers must plan their trip to either correspond to the hours the road is open, or park at the bridge and walk an extra 2.5 miles to the trailhead.

DESCRIPTION:

FROM MARBLE FORK BRIDGE: Follow the easy grade of the paved road under the shade of mixed forest, weaving around hillsides and dipping into small side canyons, where lushly lined streams trickle down the slope. Reach Colony Mill Road on the left, 2.5 miles from the bridge.

COLONY MILL

The Kaweah Colonists' goal was to construct a road from Three Rivers to a mill near marketable timber. They erected a steam-driven mill named Ajax, which ultimately produced very little lumber. In 1913, well after the colonists' dream was dashed, the US Cavalry extended the road from the defunct mill to the Giant Forest. The road served as the main access to the Giant Forest until the Generals Highway was completed in 1926. The Park Service built a ranger station near the old mill site to take advantage of the far-ranging view but, like the mill, the structure was eventually abandoned.

FROM CRYSTAL CAVE ROAD TRAILHEAD: Follow the old road through dense foliage of thimbleberry and maple beneath a mixed forest that includes dogwood. Climb mildly to moderately on the well-graded old roadbed. Reach a fork, 1.5 miles from the Crystal Cave Road, with a brush-filled roadbed heading uphill to the right.

Remaining on the Colony Mill Road, veer left and continue climbing to a saddle, then follow a gently descending traverse across a hillside. Along this traverse, the trees part just enough to allow fine views down the steep canyon of Marble Fork Kaweah River. Continue as the road bends west and soon arrives at a small flat and the abandoned Colony Mill Ranger Station, 2 miles from the Crystal Cave Road.

Few visitors reach the old ranger station anymore, which has been left to crumble and decay in relative obscurity. The view from the old porch down Marble Fork to Potwisha Campground and the Middle Fork Kaweah River is still impressive, although probably not as grand as in the old days when the surrounding vegetation was less mature. Although it was a lonesome outpost, rangers who served here had excellent accommodations, including indoor plumbing with hot running water, to go along with the fine views.

CRESCENT MEADOW TRAILHEAD

TRIP 26

Huckleberry Meadow Loop

E ♫ **DH**

DISTANCE: 3.75 miles, loop

ELEVATION: 6,700'/6,970'/6,700', +840'/-840'/±1,680'

SEASON: June to November

USE: Moderate

MAPS: USGS's *Giant Forest* and *Lodgepole* or SNHA's *Giant Forest*

INTRODUCTION: This pleasant loop sees little traffic, sandwiched between two of the Giant Forest's more popular trails, Crescent Meadow Trail on the south and Congress Trail to the north. The route samples three delightful meadows, Huckleberry, Circle, and Crescent, and several of the most prominent giant sequoias, including the Washington Tree, the world's second largest. A log cabin built in the 1880s and bedrock mortars at the site of a Native American village provide some historical interest. Options abound for extending the trip beyond the 3.75 miles described below.

DIRECTIONS TO TRAILHEAD: Take the free shuttle bus via Route 2 to Crescent Meadow. From there, walk 0.3 mile back down the road to the trailhead. Rather than return to the trailhead, you could follow the trail on the west side of Crescent Meadow to the shuttle bus stop at the Crescent Meadow parking area.

Private vehicles should take the narrow Crescent Meadow Road from the Generals Highway near the museum and proceed 1.2 miles to the Moro Rock junction. Continue 1 mile to the small parking area for the Huckleberry Trail, 0.3 mile before Crescent Meadow.

DESCRIPTION: Through a mixed forest of giant sequoias, white firs, sugar pines, and

Huckleberry Meadow Loop

To Lodgepole ►

Washington Tree

Round Meadow

Generals Highway

Alta Trail

Circle Meadow

P

Museum

Giant Forest

To Ash Mountain

Sequoia National Park

Squatters Cabin

Huckleberry Meadow

Huckleberry Trail

Crescent Meadow

Crescent Meadow Road

26

Crescent Meadow

P T

Huckleberry Meadow T P

0   0.25   0.5 mile

0   0.25   0.5 kilometer

---

dogwoods, follow the Huckleberry Trail on a mild climb to the Dead Giant, one of the few examples of a sequoia succumbing to a forest fire. The thick bark of giant sequoias usually provides adequate protection from all but the most intense fires. A short distance beyond, pass diminutive Huckleberry Meadow, carpeted with verdant grasses and decorated by splashes of color from assorted wildflowers. Reach Squatters Cabin at the far edge of the meadow, shaded by towering trees. Reach a junction just beyond the cabin, 0.3 mile from the trailhead.

Bear left at the junction and make a winding ascent to the crest of a low ridge, where Jeffrey pines and manzanita thrive in the drier conditions. Descend moderately from the ridge, returning to the damper surroundings of a mixed forest with a ground cover of azaleas, wildflowers, and ferns.

Meet the Alta Trail at a well-signed junction, 1.25 miles from the trailhead.

Turn right (north) and follow the Alta Trail on a mild, half-mile climb past an abandoned 0.3-mile spur to the Rimrock Trail on the left. A short distance farther, a sign points the way to some bedrock mortars, where Native Americans once ground

SQUATTERS CABIN

Squatters Cabin is a one-room log structure with a split-shake roof containing a rock fireplace and a single window. An unidentified man intent on filing a claim on the adjoining land built the cabin in the 1880s, but was forced to leave when he realized that Hale Tharp already owned the property.

acorns and seeds. Nearby, the trail crosses Little Deer Creek, a reliable source of water until late summer, and proceeds to another junction, 2 miles from the trailhead.

Leaving the Alta Trail and following signed directions for the Washington Tree, gently ascend an azalea-lined trail to recross Little Deer Creek, bordered by a narrow swath of lush foliage. Beyond the creek, you may notice a profusion of young sequoias, beneficiaries of a prescribed burn in the late 1970s. Nearby, a signed, short lateral leads to the base of the Washington Tree, with a volume of 47,850 cubic feet, second in size only to General Sherman. In 2002 Washington measured 255 feet tall with a circumference of 101 feet.

Return to the main trail and follow a moderate ascent over a low rise, followed by a short drop to a junction near the edge of Circle Meadow, 2.5 miles from the trailhead. Before continuing on the right-hand trail, take the short side trip on the left-hand trail to Bears Bathtub.

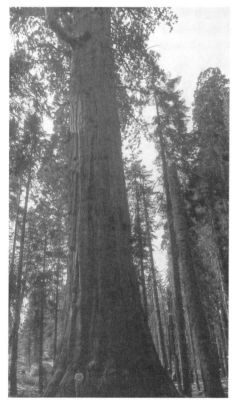

The Washington Tree

BEARS BATHTUB

Bears Bathtub consists of two sequoias that have grown together. Winter snows and rain fill a fire-scarred hollow inside the trees with dank water. An implausible legend tells the tale of an old-timer who witnessed a bear wallowing in the water.

Head southeast along the fringe of Circle Meadow, and then make a short climb to the crest of a hill and the next junction, a quarter mile from the previous one. Continue southeast on a 0.3-mile descent to the north tip of Crescent Meadow and a junction with the Crescent Meadow Loop at 3.1 miles. (Shuttle bus riders should head south from here around the west side of the meadow to the Crescent Meadow parking lot).

Turn right (west) and follow a nearly level course, eventually passing around the north edge of Huckleberry Meadow on the way to the first junction near Squatters Cabin. From there, turn left and retrace your steps 0.3 mile to the trailhead.

CRESCENT MEADOW TRAILHEAD

TRIP 27

Bobcat Point Loop

E ↻ **DH**

DISTANCE: 1.25 miles, loop

ELEVATION: 6,720'/6,530'/6,720',
+255'/-255'/±510'

SEASON: May to November

USE: Light

MAPS: USGS's *Lodgepole* and *Giant Forest* or SNHA's *Giant Forest*

INTRODUCTION: Crescent Meadow is a busy hub of activity on a typical summer day, with a bevy of tourists picnicking, sightseeing, or strolling along the nearby paths. Despite the minimal distance, this trip, combining the Bobcat Point and Sugar Pine Trails, leads away from the crowds. You won't see flower-filled meadows or towering sequoias on this loop, but you will have incredible views of Middle Fork Kaweah River canyon, Moro Rock, and Castle Rocks from the viewpoints of Kaweah Vista and Bobcat Point. For those interested in Native American life, the trail passes a couple of locations where women

once ground acorns and seeds in bedrock mortars. A visit to the top of Moro Rock is a straightforward extension of this trip.

DIRECTIONS TO TRAILHEAD: Take the free shuttle bus via Route 2 to Crescent Meadow. Visitors driving private vehicles should take the narrow Crescent Meadow Road from the Generals Highway near the museum and proceed 1.2 miles to the Moro Rock junction. Continue 1.3 miles to the end of the road at the Crescent Meadow parking area.

DESCRIPTION: Start your adventure on the High Sierra Trail (HST), which begins near the restroom at the east end of the Crescent Meadow parking lot. Cross a pair of short wood bridges over Crescent Creek, and soon reach a junction with the Crescent Meadow Trail on the left. Remain on the HST for approximately 25 yards to a second junction.

Turn right (south) on the fork signed for Bobcat Point, and climb a lightly forested hillside. Then follow the trail as it bends west, drops into a saddle, and then climbs along a ridge high above the Middle Fork Kaweah River. Emerging from the forest at the rock outcrop of Kaweah Vista, a splendid view unfolds of the 3,000-foot deep canyon below and the Great Western Divide to the east. A short distance farther, the trail

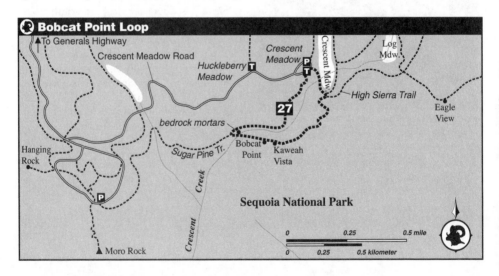

Bobcat Point Loop

▲ To Generals Highway
Crescent Meadow Road
Huckleberry Meadow
Crescent Meadow **P**
Log Mdw.
High Sierra Trail
Eagle View
bedrock mortars
27
Sugar Pine Tr.
Bobcat Point
Kaweah Vista
Hanging Rock
P
Crescent Creek
Sequoia National Park
▲ Moro Rock

0   0.25   0.5 mile
0   0.25   0.5 kilometer

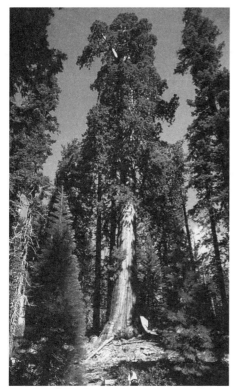

A majestic giant sequoia

leads to Bobcat Point, 0.6 mile from the trailhead. Directly southwest, a mere 0.75 mile away, stands the impressive granite dome of Moro Rock. Across the yawning chasm of the Middle Fork, the crags and spires of Castle Rocks are quite impressive as well.

Turning away from Bobcat Point, head back into the trees and cross Crescent Creek, which flows picturesquely over a broad, sloping slab of granite. Nearby are several bedrock mortars worth inspecting. Shortly beyond the creek is a junction of the Sugar Pine Trail, which offers an easy 0.9-mile traverse to the base of Moro Rock, from where a quarter-mile climb up rock stairs leads to a superb view.

To return to Crescent Meadow, bear right at the junction and make a steady climb through light forest, soon encountering a short spur to the bedrock mortars. From there, a gentle ascent leads through mixed forest, including a number of stately sugar pines, to the end of the loop at Crescent Meadow Road, near the west end of the parking area.

SUGAR PINES

Although the Giant Forest was named for the largest living tree on the planet, the giant sequoia, the area is also home to the largest species of pine as well. The huge cones on the forest floor, some as long as 20 inches, signify the presence of the stately sugar pine. Reaching heights of more than 200 feet, the sugar pine grows in the montane zone, and some individuals live as long as 600 years.

TRIP 28

Crescent and Log Meadows Loop

Ⓔ ◯ **DH**

DISTANCE: 2.2 miles, loop

ELEVATION: 6,720'/6,900'/6,720', +435'/-435'/±870'

SEASON: June to November

USE: Heavy

MAPS: USGS's *Lodgepole* and *Giant Forest* or SNHA's *Giant Forest*

INTRODUCTION: Although the Crescent Meadow Trail is one of the busiest paths in the Giant Forest, two flower-filled meadows and numerous notable giant sequoias make this loop worth the crowds. Early to midsummer is the best season to view the verdant sedges and grasses of the meadows, highlighted by a colorful palette of wildflowers. However, the majesty of the sequoias is always in season. Add in a visit to Tharps Log—the oldest structure in the park—and you have the quintessential Giant Forest experience.

DIRECTIONS TO TRAILHEAD: Take the free shuttle bus via Route 2 to Crescent Meadow. Visitors driving private vehicles should take the narrow Crescent Meadow Road from the Generals Highway near the museum and proceed 1.2 miles to the Moro Rock junction. Continue 1.3 miles to the end of the road at the Crescent Meadow parking area.

DESCRIPTION: Start your adventure on the High Sierra Trail (HST), which begins near the restroom at the east end of the Crescent Meadow parking lot. Cross a pair of short wood bridges over Crescent Creek, and soon reach a junction with the Crescent Meadow Trail on the left. Remain on the HST for approximately 25 yards to a second junction, the right-hand fork signed for Bobcat Point. Beyond the second junction, the tread turns to dirt and makes a gentle ascent across the north side of a low hill. Pass a few scattered sequoias on the way to a junction near the Burial Tree in a forested saddle, a half mile from the trailhead.

Turn left (northwest) from the junction and soon drop to a junction with the Log Meadow Loop Trail near the southeast edge of Log Meadow. Head north from the junction, strolling along the east edge of the meadow, a grass- and flower-filled glade ringed by giant sequoias and other conifers. Proceed on gently graded tread lined with

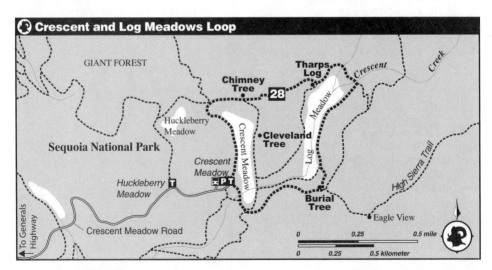

Crescent and Log Meadows Loop

GIANT FOREST

Tharps Log

Chimney Tree

28

Huckleberry Meadow

Cleveland Tree

Sequoia National Park

Crescent Meadow

Crescent Meadow

Log Meadow

Huckleberry Meadow

Burial Tree

Crescent Meadow Road

Eagle View

High Sierra Trail

Crescent Creek

To Generals Highway

0   0.25   0.5 mile

0   0.25   0.5 kilometer

ferns and azaleas to the north end of this lovely dell and a T-junction with the Trail of the Sequoias, 1 mile from the trailhead.

Continue straight ahead from the junction, step over a sliver of a stream to a forested flat, and then soon come to a second stream crossing on a wood-plank bridge, where a number of stately sequoias line the drainage. Heading southwest around the north fringe of Log Meadow, you soon encounter Tharps Log, reposing in a small clearing. Nearby is a junction with the Tharps Log Trail, 1.3 miles from the trailhead.

At the junction near Tharps Log, turn right (northwest) toward the Chimney Tree. Climbing away from Log Meadow, you ascend some stairs hewn out of a fallen sequoia and continue climbing to the top of a low ridge separating Log and Crescent Meadows. From the ridge, a gentle descent leads to a pair of trail junctions. At the first fork, a short lateral heads over to the base of the Chimney Tree, allowing visitors to stand inside the fire-hollowed snag of a dead sequoia. This giant apparently met its doom at the hands of a careless camper in 1919. About 25 feet beyond the lateral, reach the second junction with the east portion of the Crescent Meadow Loop Trail.

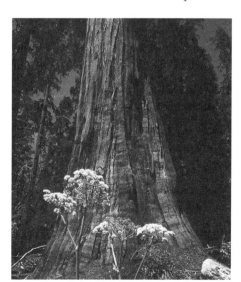

Giant sequoias and wildflowers

HALE D. THARP AND THARPS LOG

Gaining a perspective of the true size of a giant sequoia is quite difficult while the tree is standing. When one of the giants topples from old age and spans across the forest floor, visitors can gain a better feel for the immensity of the Big Trees. Tharps Log is just such a tree, large enough for the hollowed out interior to have been used as a summer cabin in the late 1880s. Modern-day visitors may view the restored cabin, complete with a rock fireplace, bed, plank table, and rough-hewn benches and chairs. Interpretive signs provide some bits of history, along with a warning to respect the historical nature of the structure. Benches positioned around the clearing provide places to linger.

Tharps Log recalls a simpler time. Michigan native Hale D. Tharp originally settled near Three Rivers in 1856, where he quickly befriended the native Yokuts, who told their new friend tales of giant trees. Two years later, Tharp was guided by way of the Middle Fork and Moro Rock to Log Meadow, credited as the first white man to see the Giant Forest. A rancher and cattleman, Tharp eventually homesteaded Log Meadow, driving his cattle into the mountains each summer to graze upon the lush meadows. He used the namesake log as a cabin from 1861 to 1890. The restored Tharps Log remains the oldest artificial edifice in the park.

Bear right at the junction and skirt the north side of Crescent Meadow (a short detour on the left-hand trail leads to the Cleveland Tree). Continue westbound to a Y-junction, 1.75 miles from the trailhead.

Turn left (south) and proceed along the west edge of picturesque Crescent Meadow for a half mile to return to the Crescent Meadow parking lot.

TRIP 29

High Sierra Trail: Crescent Meadow to Panther Creek

E ⟋ **DH**

DISTANCE: 5.4 miles, out-and-back

ELEVATION: 6,720'/7,045'/6,650', +850'/-800'/±1,650'

SEASON: Late April to November

USE: Moderate

MAPS: USGS's *Lodgepole* and *Giant Forest* or SNHA's *Giant Forest*

INTRODUCTION: The High Sierra Trail (HST) is one of the better known trails in the park, taking backpackers from the Big Trees (giant sequoias) to the big mountain (Mt. Whitney). Dayhikers can enjoy the initial segment of the HST from Crescent Meadow to Panther Creek, with grand views of the Great Western Divide, Middle Fork Kaweah River, and surrounding landmarks along the way. Built by the NPS between 1927 and 1932, the HST has a quite pleasant grade, and this section's southern exposure makes it an excellent spring or fall trip. Summer hikers will want to get an early start to beat the heat.

DIRECTIONS TO TRAILHEAD: Take the free shuttle bus via Route 2 to Crescent Meadow. Visitors driving private vehicles should take the narrow Crescent Meadow Road from the Generals Highway near the museum and proceed 1.2 miles to the Moro Rock junction. Continue 1.3 miles to the end of the road at the Crescent Meadow parking area.

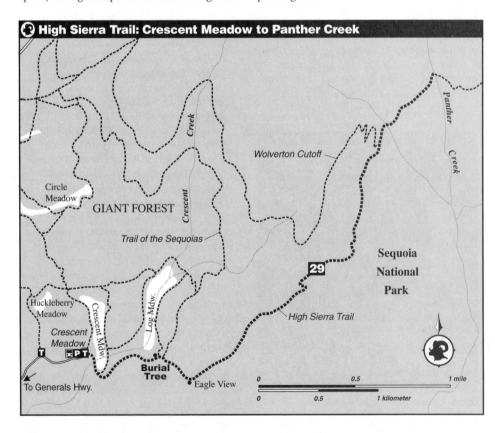

High Sierra Trail: Crescent Meadow to Panther Creek

DESCRIPTION: To start your adventure on the High Sierra Trail, begin near the restroom at the east end of the Crescent Meadow parking lot. Cross a pair of short wood bridges over Crescent Creek and soon reach a junction with the Crescent Meadow Trail on the left. Remain on the HST for approximately 25 yards to a second junction, the right-hand fork signed for Bobcat Point. Beyond the second junction, the tread turns to dirt and makes a gentle ascent across the north side of a low hill. Pass a few scattered sequoias on the way to a junction near the Burial Tree in a forested saddle, a half mile from the trailhead.

Continue eastbound from the junction, as the trail swings across an open hillside high above the Middle Fork Kaweah River. Nearly level hiking leads to aptly named

> **BUCKEYE FIRE**
>
> In October 1988, a chaparral-covered slope near the Leaning Tree was the site of the Buckeye Fire, ignited by a discarded cigarette at the bottom of the canyon. At a cost of $2.5 million and with the efforts of 1,200 firefighters, the weeklong blaze was extinguished, but not before consuming more than 3,000 acres. A policy of controlled burning was credited with slowing the advance of the fire into the Giant Forest.

Eagle View at 0.75 mile. From this aerie 3,500 feet above the river, you have a grand view of the canyon, Moro Rock, Castle Rocks, and the glacier-sculpted peaks of the Great Western Divide.

Traverse the south-facing hillside, where open areas with grand views alternate with pockets of light, mixed forest, including black oaks, white firs, Jeffrey pines, and incense cedars. A series of four switchbacks interrupts the otherwise gently graded trail on the way to the high point of the journey near the 2-mile mark. From there, a general descent leads through light forest and past a short rock wall to a junction with the Wolverton Cutoff Trail, 2.5 miles from the trailhead.

From the junction, you can hear Panther Creek roaring. An easy 0.2-mile stroll leads to the banks of this refreshing stream, where a ribbon of water spills over moss-covered rocks and down a steep chasm tangled with logs and lush vegetation. Backpackers with extra vigor can continue farther up the HST, past the multiple branches of Panther Creek to the first legal campsites near Mehrten Creek, 3.5 miles from the trailhead (see Trip 31, page 134).

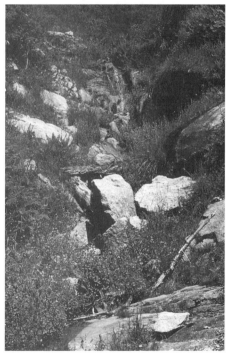

Panther Creek

TRIP 30

Giant Forest East Loop

Ⓜ 🔍 **DH**

DISTANCE: 8.5 miles, loop

ELEVATION: 6,720'/7,600'/6,720', +2,370'/-2,370'/±4,740'

SEASON: May to November

USE: Light to moderate

MAPS: USGS's *Lodgepole* and *Giant Forest* or SNHA's *Giant Forest*

INTRODUCTION: This trip uses the extensive network of trails crisscrossing the Giant Forest plateau to create a loop showcasing the best the area has to offer. Along the way,

you'll see plenty of the iconic giant sequoias, a pair of picturesque meadows, and grand views of Moro Rock, Castle Rocks, the Great Western Divide, and Middle Fork Kaweah River from Eagle View. A portion of the loop leads travelers on a serene journey through a seldom-seen section of the Giant Forest, passing numerous magnificent examples of the Big Trees.

While most of the loop follows gently graded trail, a 1-mile climb up the little-used Wolverton Cutoff Trail is steep and can be scorching during hot afternoons. Water is scarce along this route, especially late in the season; stash an extra bottle or two in your pack.

DIRECTIONS TO TRAILHEAD: Take the free shuttle bus via Route 2 to Crescent Meadow. Visitors driving private vehicles should take the narrow Crescent Meadow Road from the Generals Highway near the

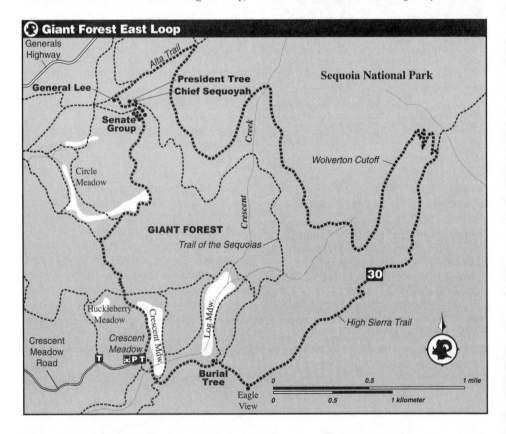

Giant Forest East Loop

museum and proceed 1.2 miles to the Moro Rock junction. Continue 1.3 miles to the end of the road at the Crescent Meadow parking area.

DESCRIPTION: Start your adventure on the High Sierra Trail (HST), which begins near the restroom at the east end of the Crescent Meadow parking lot. Cross a pair of short wood bridges over Crescent Creek, and soon reach a junction with the Crescent Meadow Trail on the left. Remain on the HST for approximately 25 yards to a second junction; the right-hand fork is signed for Bobcat Point. Continuing ahead beyond the second junction, the tread turns to dirt and makes a gentle ascent across the north side of a low hill. Pass a few scattered sequoias on the way to a junction near the Burial Tree in a forested saddle, a half mile from the trailhead.

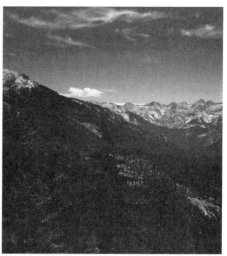

Alta Peak and the Great Western Divide

Continue eastbound from the junction, as the trail swings across an open hillside high above the Middle Fork Kaweah River. Nearly level hiking leads to aptly named Eagle View at 0.75 mile. From this aerie 3,500 feet above the river, you have a grand view of the canyon, Moro Rock, Castle Rocks, and the glacier-sculpted peaks of the Great Western Divide.

Traverse the south-facing hillside, where open areas with grand views alternate with pockets of light, mixed forest, including black oaks, white firs, Jeffrey pines, and incense cedars. A series of four switchbacks interrupts the otherwise gently graded trail on the way to the high point of the journey near the 2-mile mark. From there, a general descent leads through light forest and past a short rock wall to a junction with the Wolverton Cutoff Trail, 2.5 miles from the trailhead.

Leaving the HST behind, start a 1.25-mile, 800-foot, switchbacking climb to the top of a ridge through a forest of red and white firs. Nearing the crest, the trees part enough to allow views of Alta Peak, the Great Western Divide, and Castle Rocks. Just past some granite humps on the crest, the trail descends across the edge of the Giant Forest into the presence of the noble

monarchs. Gently descending tread passes many fine examples of the Big Trees, as well as a pair of tiny seasonal rivulets. Near the 5-mile mark, the trail curves around a meadow and crosses Crescent Creek on a log footbridge.

For the next mile, the trail arcs around peak 7758, passes more interesting sequoias, and crosses some diminutive brooks. A short descent leads to a junction with the Alta Trail near a pocket meadow carpeted with ferns and lupines, 6.2 miles from the trailhead.

Turn left (southwest) onto the Alta Trail and follow a moderate, 0.4-mile descent past more splendid sequoias to a junction of the highly popular Congress Trail. Although it adds an extra 0.4 mile to the trip, a jaunt around the southern end of the Congress Trail loop leads to a handful of notable sequoia landmarks, including the Senate and House Groups and the President Tree, the world's fourth largest giant sequoia. However you choose to continue, the Alta and Congress Trails reconverge 0.2 mile west at a five-way junction near the McKinley Tree.

From the five-way junction, turn left (south) and soon reach a series of astonishing Giant Forest features. The first is the Room Tree, a very large sequoia with a small opening leading into a roomy, fire-hollowed base. Just beyond is the Founders Group, an attractive collection of a dozen impressive sequoias named to honor those who were instrumental in the establishment of Sequoia National Park. Next, you step over a rivulet coursing through a narrow swath of Circle Meadow, which is more representative of a horseshoe than a true circle. On the far side of the meadow is Cattle Cabin, originally used by stockmen who grazed their cattle in the meadows. The trail arcs around the east fringe of Circle Meadow, passing an unsigned lateral heading northwest. Just beyond are the Pillars of Hercules, where the trail passes right between a pair of massive sequoias. Shortly beyond is the Black Arch, a huge, fire-scorched sequoia. A short descent leads to another thin ribbon of Circle Meadow and a junction on the far side with the Trail of the Sequoias on the left, 7.6 miles from the trailhead.

Continue straight ahead (south and then west) from the junction for 0.1 mile to another junction. From there, head southeast for another 0.4 mile to a junction with the Crescent Meadow Trail. Follow the Crescent Meadow Trail for a half mile along the west edge of the meadow to the trailhead.

⬚ Strong hikers can opt for a more strenuous 14-mile loop, continuing on the HST past the Wolverton Cutoff to the Sevenmile Hill Trail, 0.4 mile past Mehrten Creek. From there, a potentially blistering 2-mile, 1,400-foot climb leads to a connection with the Alta Trail, west of Mehrten Meadow. From there, head west past Panther Gap and Red Fir Meadow to join the route described above at the junction with the Wolverton Cutoff Trail.

Hikers can follow the Congress Trail to General Sherman and use the shuttle bus system to return to Crescent Meadow.

CRESCENT MEADOW TRAILHEAD

TRIP 31

Bearpaw Meadow, Hamilton Lakes, and Nine Lakes Basin

Ⓜ ⟋ BP

DISTANCE: 42 miles, out-and-back

ELEVATION: 6,720'/10,600, +7270'/-3390'/±21,320'

SEASON: July to November

USE: Moderate

MAPS: *Lodgepole* and *Triple Divide Peak*

TRAIL LOG

5.5	Mehrten Creek
9.5	Buck Creek
10.5	Bearpaw Meadow Camp
12.2	Elizabeth Pass Trail Junction
14.0	Upper Hamilton Lake
17.3	Kaweah Gap

INTRODUCTION: A weekend trip to Bearpaw Meadow provides plenty of enjoyable scenery. Layover days with a base camp at the campground allow stunningly scenic excursions to impressive mountain landscapes, including Hamilton Lakes basin, which offers stunning views of Angels Wings, Sequoia's biggest rock wall, on the way.

DIRECTIONS TO TRAILHEAD: Take the free shuttle bus via Route 2 to Crescent Meadow. Visitors driving private vehicles should take the narrow Crescent Meadow Road from the Generals Highway near the museum and proceed 1.2 miles to the Moro Rock junction. Continue 1.3 miles to the end of the road at the Crescent Meadow parking area.

DESCRIPTION: Start your adventure on the High Sierra Trail (HST), which begins near the restroom at the east end of the Crescent Meadow parking lot. Cross a pair of short wood bridges over Crescent Creek, and

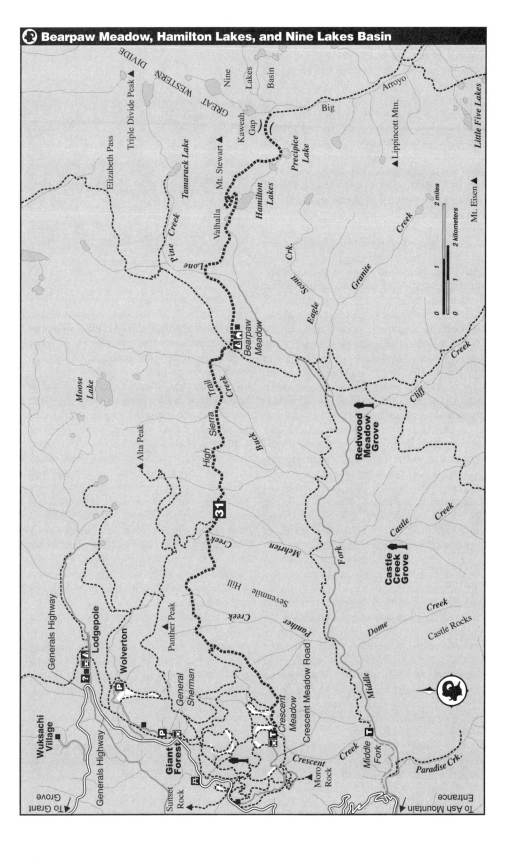

soon reach a junction with the Crescent Meadow Trail on the left. Remain on the HST for approximately 25 yards to a second junction; the right-hand fork is signed for Bobcat Point. Continuing ahead beyond the second junction, the tread turns to dirt and makes a gentle ascent across the north side of a low hill. Pass a few scattered sequoias on the way to a junction near the Burial Tree in a forested saddle, a half mile from the trailhead.

Continue eastbound from the junction, as the trail swings across an open hillside high above the Middle Fork Kaweah River. Nearly level hiking leads to aptly named Eagle View at 0.75 mile. From this aerie 3,500 feet above the river, you have a grand view of the canyon, Moro Rock, Castle Rocks, and the glacier-sculpted peaks of the Great Western Divide.

Traverse the south-facing hillside, where open areas with grand views alternate with pockets of light, mixed forest, including black oaks, white firs, Jeffrey pines, and incense cedars. A series of four switchbacks interrupts the otherwise gently graded trail on the way to the high point of the journey near the 2-mile mark. From there, a general descent leads through light forest and past a short rock wall to a junction with the Wolverton Cutoff Trail, 2.5 miles from the trailhead. From the junction, a short stroll leads to refreshing Panther Creek.

For the next couple miles beyond Panther Creek, the trail undulates in and out of the seams of the creek's tributaries. Beyond the final branch, climb over Sevenmile Hill and continue the ascent for 0.75-mile to Mehrten Creek, 5.5 miles from the trailhead. On the west bank, a use trail climbs steeply up the hillside to the first legal campsites (which have a bear box) on the HST. A third of a mile from Mehrten Creek is a junction with the Sevenmile Trail, which connects to the Alta Trail in another a steep 2.2 miles.

From the junction, a short traverse through light forest leads to the crossing of a tiny branch of Mehrten Creek, followed by a pronounced descent to a crossing of a twin-channeled tributary of Rock Creek.

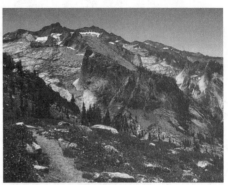

Eagle Scout Peak and vicinity

Occasional breaks in the forest allow fine views of Castle Rocks, Middle Fork canyon, Sugarbowl Dome, and Little Blue Dome, as you continue up the trail, hopping across more refreshing brooks along the way. The next developed campsite (with a bear box) is near the first branch of a twin-channel tributary of Buck Creek, 8.25 miles from the trailhead. Beyond here, the trail bends around the mostly open slope of Buck Canyon and then descends to a bridge over Buck Creek, 9.5 miles from the trailhead.

A switchbacking climb up the east wall of Buck Canyon leads through dense sugar pine and fir forest to the top of a minor ridge and the signed junction of the 200-yard lateral to Bearpaw Meadow Campground. The popular campground has numbered sites under the plentiful shade of dense forest and is equipped with bear boxes, pit toilets, and a faucet with treated water (fires are prohibited).

Approximately 0.2 mile east of the camp and the HST junction is the A-framed ranger station. Nearby Bearpaw Meadow High Sierra Camp is set picturesquely near the lip of Middle Fork Canyon. Unlike the claustrophobic backpackers' campground, the open setting of Bearpaw Camp offers excellent views of the glacier-scoured surroundings above the canyon, including such features as Eagle Scout Peak and Mt. Stewart on the Great Western Divide, the granite cleft of Hamilton Canyon, and Black Kaweah above Kaweah Gap. Similar to the popular High Sierra Camps of Yosemite, guests with reservations sleep in tent cabins and enjoy hot meals for breakfast and dinner. Community restrooms have flush toilets and hot showers. For more information or to make a reservation, consult the website at www.visitsequoia.com/bearpaw.aspx.

[O] A base camp at Bearpaw Meadow allows hikers to make short forays to Hamilton Lakes and Tamarack Lake sans backpacks. A scenic 4.4-mile loop combines the HST with a portion of the Elizabeth Pass Trail and the Over the Hill Trail.

Backpackers in search of more solitude than what's likely available at Hamilton Lakes, can detour 2.2 miles to Tamarack Lake, where lonely campsites nestle beneath a grove of lodgepole pines and Lion Rock and Mt. Steward offer pleasant alpine scenery. A steep 2-mile, off-trail ascent from Tamarack Lake leads to austere Lion Lake, where a pair of Class 2 passes offer passage north to Cloud Canyon over Lion Lake Pass (approximately 11,600 feet), or south to Nine Lakes Basin via Lion Rock Pass (approximately 11,760 feet)

From Nine Lakes Basin, a difficult, Class 2 cross-country route travels over Pants Pass (approximately 12,000 feet) on the way to the Kern-Kaweah River country.

Mountaineers have plenty of options for intermediate and advanced climbs once they are within striking distance of the Great Western Divide and Kaweah Peaks Ridge. From Tamarack Lake, Lion Rock is Class 2–3 from the bowl on the southwest side of the peak. The southwest face of Triple Divide Peak is Class 2–3 from Lion Lake. Nine Lakes Basin is a fine base camp for Class 2 routes up the southwest slope of Lawson Peak or the east side of Mt. Stewart. The Kaweah Peaks offer more technical routes.

[R] A wilderness permit is required for overnight stays. Camping is limited to designated sites at Bearpaw Meadow Campground. Camping is limited to two nights at Hamilton Lakes. Campfires are prohibited at Bearpaw Meadow and Hamilton Lakes and in Nine Lakes Basin.

CRESCENT MEADOW TRAILHEAD

TRIP 32

High Sierra Trail: Crescent Meadow to Whitney Portal

(MS) / BP

DISTANCE: 62 miles, point-to-point

ELEVATION: 6,720'/10,700'/6,720'/ 13,580'/8,360', +18,475'/–16,835'/±35,310'

SEASON: Mid-July to early October

USE: Light (heavy near Crescent Meadow and Mt. Whitney)

MAPS: USGS's *Lodgepole, Triple Divide Peak, Mt. Kaweah, Chagoopa Falls, Mt. Whitney,* and *Mt. Langley* or Tom Harrison Maps' *Mt. Whitney High Country Trail Map*

TRAIL LOG

5.6	Mehrten Creek
10.6	Bearpaw Meadow Camp
17.5	Kaweah Gap
20.0	Little Five Lakes junction
27.25	Moraine Lake
32.25	Kern River Trail junction
34.0	Kern Hot Springs
41.25	Junction Meadow and Colby Pass Trail
45.5	John Muir Trail junction
49.0	John Muir and PCT junction
51.25	Trail Crest
55.25	Trail Camp
62.0	Whitney Portal Trailhead

INTRODUCTION: Although less celebrated than the John Muir Trail (JMT), the High Sierra Trail (HST) is another significant jewel in the long-distance backpacker's crown. Built by the Civilian Conservation Corps in the early 1930s, the trail was the grand scheme of Park Superintendent Colonel John White, who fancied a trail link between Sequoia's two most enchanting

Continued on p. 139

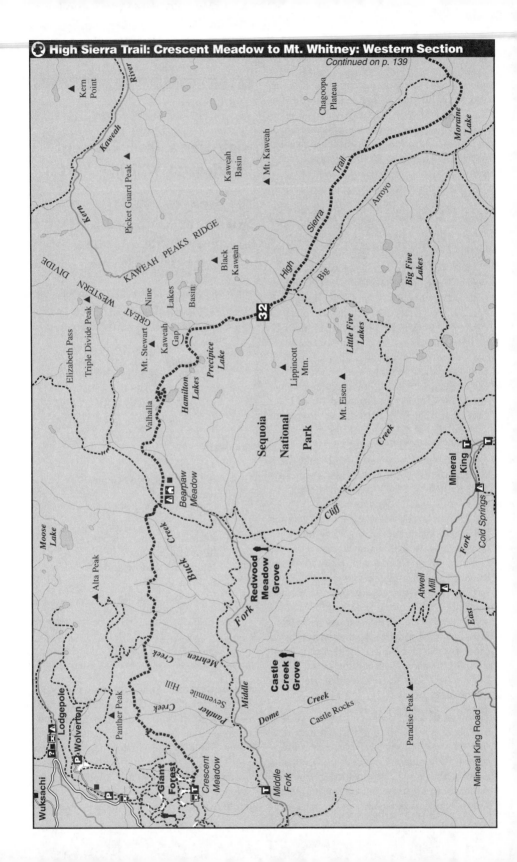

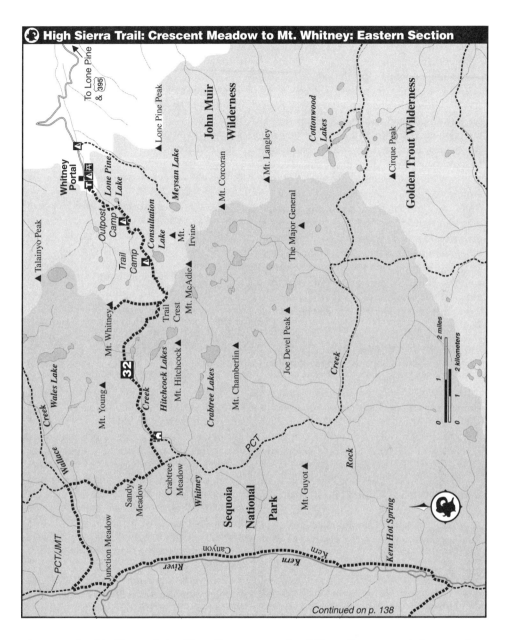

High Sierra Trail: Crescent Meadow to Mt. Whitney: Eastern Section

Continued on p. 138

features, the Big Trees of the Giant Forest and the big mountain, Mt. Whitney. Grand in scope, the trail passes through some of the park's most majestic scenery—the Giant Forest, the alpine beauty of Hamilton Lakes, an expansive vista from Kaweah Gap, the canyon splendor of Big Arroyo, the remote Chagoopa Plateau, the U-shaped trench of Kern Canyon, and the towering heights of Mt. Whitney.

Beginning and ending on some of the region's most heavily traveled trails, the middle portion of the HST is relatively remote, offering solitude-seeking backpackers a high rate of return. The beginning and ending sections at Crescent Meadow and Whitney Portal are a different matter entirely, as hordes of tourists crowd the trails into the Big Trees, and a vast number of summit hopefuls clog the route to Mt. Whitney. Between these two epicenters of activity, peace and quiet usually reign in the heart of Sequoia's backcountry, with the possible exception of Kern Hot Springs, where long-distance hikers often congregate to soak their sore and tired muscles.

As with every long trail, logistics are important. The greatest obstacle to overcome on the HST is the tremendously long shuttle between the two trailheads—a driver willing to drop you off and pick you up at the other end is truly a friend worth keeping. Although most backpackers could complete the 62-mile journey in a week, more time allows hikers to savor all the trail has to offer, including Nine Lakes Basin and Wallace Lake.

DIRECTIONS TO TRAILHEAD:

START: Take the free shuttle bus via Route 2 to Crescent Meadow. Visitors driving private vehicles should take the narrow Crescent Meadow Road from the Generals Highway near the museum and proceed 1.2 miles to the Moro Rock junction. Continue 1.3 miles to the end of the road at the Crescent Meadow parking area.

END: In the heart of Lone Pine, turn west from US 395 onto Whitney Portal Road and drive 13 miles to the overnight parking lot at Whitney Portal. The trailhead area has campgrounds, a picnic area, restrooms, and a small store and cafe.

DESCRIPTION: Start your adventure on the High Sierra Trail (HST), which begins near the restroom at the east end of the Crescent Meadow parking lot. Cross a pair of short wood bridges over Crescent Creek, and soon reach a junction with the Crescent Meadow Trail on the left. Remain on the HST for approximately 25 yards to a second junction; the right-hand fork is signed for Bobcat Point. Continuing ahead beyond the second junction, the tread turns to dirt and makes a gentle ascent across the north side of a low hill. Pass a few scattered

sequoias on the way to a junction near the Burial Tree in a forested saddle, a half mile from the trailhead.

Continue eastbound from the junction, as the trail swings across an open hillside high above the Middle Fork Kaweah River. Nearly level hiking leads to aptly named Eagle View at 0.75 mile. From this aerie 3,500 feet above the river, you have a grand view of the canyon, Moro Rock, Castle Rocks, and the glacier-sculpted peaks of the Great Western Divide.

Traverse the south-facing hillside, where open areas with grand views alternate with pockets of light, mixed forest, including black oaks, white firs, Jeffrey pines, and incense cedars. A series of four switchbacks interrupts the otherwise gently graded trail on the way to the high point of the journey near the 2-mile mark. From there, a general descent leads through light forest and past a short rock wall to a junction with the Wolverton Cutoff Trail, 2.5 miles from trailhead. From the junction, a short stroll leads to refreshing Panther Creek.

For the next couple of miles beyond Panther Creek, the trail undulates in and out of the seams of the creek's tributaries. Beyond the final branch, climb over Sevenmile Hill and continue the ascent for 0.75 mile to Mehrten Creek, 5.5 miles from the trailhead. On the west bank, a use trail climbs steeply up the hillside to the first legal campsites (which have a bear box) on the HST. A third of a mile from Mehrten Creek is a junction with the Sevenmile Trail, which connects to the Alta Trail in another steep 2.2 miles.

From the junction, a short traverse through light forest leads to a crossing of a tiny branch of Mehrten Creek, followed by a pronounced descent to a crossing of a twin-channeled tributary of Rock Creek. Occasional breaks in the forest allow fine views of Castle Rocks, Middle Fork canyon, Sugarbowl Dome, and Little Blue Dome as you continue up the trail, hopping across more refreshing brooks along the way. The next developed campsite (with a bear box) is near the first branch of a twin-channel tributary of Buck Creek, 8.25 miles from the trailhead. Beyond here, the trail bends around the mostly open slope of Buck Canyon and then descends to a bridge over Buck Creek, 9.5 miles from the trailhead.

A switchbacking climb up the east wall of Buck Canyon leads through dense sugar pine and fir forest to the top of a minor ridge and the signed junction of the 200-yard lateral to Bearpaw Meadow Campground. The popular campground has numbered sites under the plentiful shade of dense forest, and is equipped with bear boxes, pit toilets, and a faucet with treated water (fires are prohibited).

Approximately 0.2 mile east of the camp and the HST junction is the A-framed ranger station. Nearby Bearpaw Meadow High Sierra Camp is set picturesquely near the lip of Middle Fork Canyon. Unlike the claustrophobic backpackers' campground, the open setting of Bearpaw Camp offers excellent views of the glacier-scoured surroundings above the canyon, including such features as Eagle Scout Peak and Mt. Stewart on the Great Western Divide, the granite cleft of Hamilton Canyon, and Black Kaweah above Kaweah Gap. Similar to the popular High Sierra Camps of Yosemite, guests with reservations sleep in tent cabins and enjoy hot meals for breakfast and dinner. Community restrooms have flush toilets and hot showers. For more information or to make a reservation, consult the website at **www.visitsequoia.com/bearpaw.aspx**.

From the ranger station, follow a descending traverse across the precipitous north wall of River Valley with excellent views across the canyon. At the bottom of Middle Fork canyon, a concrete culvert spans the rowdy river. A short climb away from the river leads to a small bench and a junction with the Elizabeth Pass Trail, 12.2 miles from the trailhead. Decent campsites can be found in the vicinity of the junction.

Away from the junction, a stiff, switchbacking climb through sagebrush, manzanita, and scattered black oaks ensues and eventually leads around a corner and into Hamilton Creek canyon. The view-packed scenery in this granite sanctuary is absolutely stunning, with the towering face of Angel Wings crowning the north wall, a rival to the better known climbing walls of Yosemite. The white domes of Hamilton Towers tops the ridge on the opposite side of the canyon. Soon, you ford tumbling Hamilton Creek and climb over shards of rock above Lower Hamilton Lake to the outlet of the upper lake, 14 miles from the trailhead.

Excellent campsites can be found above the northwest shore of Upper Hamilton Lake, but the basin is a very popular overnight destination, so *don't expect solitude*. The Park Service has instituted a two-night camping limit and banned campfires to minimize the effects of overuse. The scenery is magnificent and anglers will enjoy the challenge of attempting to land the resident rainbow, brook, and golden trout. Glacier-polished slabs around the shoreline create fine spots for swimmers and sunbathers.

Now you face the 2,500-foot climb to Kaweah Gap. The trail itself is something of an engineering marvel, blasted right out of the rock in many places. From the outlet of Upper Hamilton Lake, zigzag up the north wall of the enormous cirque and then veer south past a tarn on the way up to Precipice Lake, 2.6 miles from Upper Hamilton Lake. The frigid lake reposes at the base of the impressive north face of Eagle Scout Peak. A final 0.75-mile climb past a smattering of miniature tarns leads to Kaweah Gap (approximately 10,700 feet), 17.25 miles from the trailhead. A spectacular view unfolds from Kaweah Gap, with the Kaweah Peaks, Nine Lakes Basin, and the canyon of Big Arroyo providing fine scenery.

SIDE TRIP TO NINE LAKES BASIN: To visit Nine Lakes Basin, drop from Kaweah Gap on a few switchbacks. Leave the HST and head north cross-country to the first lake (approximately 10,455 feet). Off-trail travel north to the upper two lakes is straightforward. The set of lakes to the east is over more difficult terrain requiring more advanced route-finding skills. Whichever lake you decide to visit, the U-shaped basin at the convergence of the Great Western Divide and Kaweah Peaks Ridge, culminating at Triple Divide Peak, presents unparalleled alpine scenery worthy of an extended layover. **END OF SIDE TRIP**

From Kaweah Gap, the HST makes a continuous and steady descent west of the nascent creek draining Big Arroyo. Just shy of 2 miles from the gap, the trail crosses the creek and the continues to descend through pockets of meadow and granite, crossing numerous side streams along the way. The open terrain permits fine views of Big Arroyo and the multihued Kaweah Peaks to the north. Near a tributary stream draining an unnamed tarn, the trail skirts some campsites and then reaches a junction with the Big Arroyo Trail and the Black Rock Pass Trail to Little Five Lakes, 3 miles from Kaweah Gap. The Big Arroyo patrol cabin is just a short way down the trail.

Remaining on the HST, you start a long, sustained climb on a traverse across the northeast wall of the canyon, soon hopping over a healthy stream. The timber in this section of Big Arroyo is sparse, with much of the hillside covered with sagebrush, manzanita, and chinquapin, splashed with color from a bevy of wildflowers, including paintbrush, lupine, and columbine. After crossing several tributaries, pass a small tarn about 6 miles from Kaweah Gap, and begin a gentle descent leading away from the lip of the canyon. Through alternating sections of meadow and lodgepole and foxtail pine forest, you reach a junction in a large meadow with a trail to Moraine Lake, 7.5 miles from Kaweah Gap.

Although the designated route of the HST continues across Chagoopa Plateau, a more scenic route follows the trail to Moraine Lake. Veer right at the junction, leave the meadow behind, and drop through dense stands of foxtail and lodgepole pines. Returning to the edge of Big Arroyo canyon, excellent views of the Great Western Divide will impress even the most jaded hiker. The descent intensifies, eventually reaching the wooded shore of Moraine Lake, 10 miles from Kaweah Gap. Excellent campsites scattered around the south shoreline offer fine views of the Kaweah Peaks.

From Moraine Lake, hop across the outlet, traverse the moraine at the east end of the lake, and then descend to lovely, flower-filled and grass-covered Sky Parlor Meadow. Across the meadow are more fine views of the Kaweah Peaks and the Great Western Divide. Just beyond the ford of Funston Creek, near the east end of the meadow, rejoin the HST at a junction, 28.5 miles from the trailhead.

A moderate, then steep descent leads toward the deep U-shaped Kern Trench below. On the way, white firs and Jeffrey pines replace the lodgepole pines and, farther down, an occasional western juniper or black oak extends above shrub-covered slopes of manzanita and snowbush. Tight, rocky switchbacks follow the tumbling course of Funston Creek, which the trail crosses and then recrosses on the way to the bottom of Kern Trench and a junction of the Kern River Trail, 15 miles and 4,000 vertical feet from Kaweah Gap.

Turn left (north) and follow the Kern River upstream. Drop into a marshy area, make an imperceptible climb across a pair of meadows, and then proceed through Jeffrey pines and incense cedars. After 0.75 mile, you cross Chagoopa Creek and catch glimpses through the trees of Chagoopa Falls, high on the west wall of the canyon.

Gently graded tread leads upstream to a stout bridge spanning Kern River. Continue up the east side of the canyon a short way to a ford of Rock Creek. Shortly beyond the ford and around a point is Kern Hot Spring, 1.75 miles from the junction. Situated near the edge of the rushing river, a crude cement bathtub downstream from the spring is filled with hot water, providing a warm oasis in which to soothe aching and tired muscles. Despite the seemingly remote location, Kern Hot Spring is a magnet for backpackers. The designated backpacker campground (with a bear box) just northeast of the spring feels cramped and overused, offering little in the way of a wilderness experience—those seeking solitude should plan on camping elsewhere.

Away from the spring, the HST leads to a ford of the upper branch of Rock Creek and then proceeds on a gravelly path past some campsites. For the next 7 miles, the trail follows the river up the U-shaped gorge of Kern River beneath the towering rock walls of Kern Trench. Glacial action has left numerous hanging valleys on both sides, where scenic cascades and waterfalls spill down the canyon walls on the way to the river. The trail crosses numerous creeks and rivulets on the northbound route, some of which may be difficult in early season, particularly the ford of the unnamed creek draining Guyot Flat, Whitney Creek, and Wallace Creek. The upstream ascent is gentle for the most part, making for straightforward travel through generally open terrain. Near the ford of Wallace Creek, the trail enters moderate forest cover of mainly Jeffrey pines, with a smattering of lodgepole and western white pines. Continue through the forest to shady campsites (with bear boxes) near Junction Meadow, where you intersect the Colby Pass Trail, 9 miles from the Kern River Trail junction.

From the junction, climb moderately through groves of mixed forest alternating with manzanita- and currant-covered clearings that provide good views of the Kern-Kaweah canyon and Kern River Trench. After 1.2 miles from Junction Meadow, the HST leaves the Kern River Trail and follows an ascending traverse toward Wallace Creek. A mile farther, the trail veers northeast and follows Wallace Creek toward a junction with the Pacific Crest Trail (PCT) and JMT. A moderate, mile-long ascent leads to a ford of Wright Creek, followed by a 1.1-mile climb to the junction, 4.2 miles from Junction Meadow.

Follow the JMT south 3.4 miles to a junction, where the PCT continues south and the JMT heads east. With the west face of Mt. Whitney in constant view, leave the PCT and make a gentle ascent to the north bank of Whitney Creek and a junction with a lateral to Crabtree Ranger Station, which fords the creek and heads to campsites (which have a bear box).

Following the JMT, ascend along the north bank of Whitney Creek through a smattering of lodgepole and foxtail pines.

About a half mile from the junction, pass some campsites on the way to picturesque Timberline Lake. Although closed to camping, the lake is worthy of an extended visit, especially a vantage point on the south shore, where the bulk of Mt. Whitney is reflected in its placid surface.

Beyond Timberline Lake, the steady ascent continues through an open basin laden with granite slabs and benches. You climb over a flat-topped ridge to Guitar Lake (approximately 11,460 feet), 3.5 miles from the PCT junction, where camping is still allowed in sandy pockets away from the meadow grass. Away from the lake, a pair of tarns offers additional campsites and the last reliable water source before the stiff climb to Trail Crest.

As the grade increases, the Hitchcock Lakes appear to the south, luring knapsackers to a remote location beneath the precipitous north face of Mt. Hitchcock. A series of long-legged switchbacks leads up the steep west face of the Sierra Crest on a steady, 1,500-foot climb to a junction with the Mt. Whitney Trail, 5.5 miles from the PCT junction. A typical summer day will see a plethora of packs reposing against a steep wall of rock nearby, as backpackers jettison them for the final 2-mile climb to Whitney's summit.

SIDE TRIP TO MOUNT WHITNEY: Unless the weather is threatening, to come all this way and not detour the additional 2 miles to the summit would be a lapse in judgment (unless there's say a lightning storm). Climb steadily along the west side of the crest, where the trail periodically enters airy notches that provide acrophobic vistas straight down the east face. Proceed along rocky tread to the final slope below the summit, where the grade increases and several paths angle toward the top. Cairns may aid you but the route is obvious—head for the highest point! The top of the peak is a broad, sloping plateau of jumbled slabs and large boulders, with an indescribable view. **END OF SIDE TRIP**

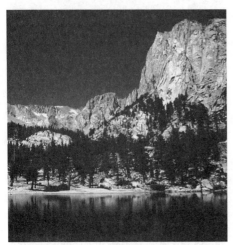

Lone Pine Lake on the Mt. Whitney Trail

From the Mt. Whitney junction, a short climb leads to Trail Crest (approximately 13,650 feet), 8.2 miles from Whitney Portal. Now you must descend the 100 switchbacks to Trail Camp. Zigzag down the rocky slope, which may have snow patches through midseason. A seep about halfway down, oftentimes in the shade, may produce icy conditions as well. Unless you are longing for human contact, you'll most likely want to breeze past Trail Camp; this last legal camping area below Mt. Whitney is usually a hubbub of frenetic activity. If you must camp for the night, sites near Consultation Lake may be slightly less crowded.

Continue your descent through a sea of rock to lovely Trailside Meadow, a verdant strip of meadowlands contrasting starkly with the otherwise rocky terrain. Beyond the meadow, the trail crosses Lone Pine Creek and proceeds downstream. Switchbacks lead down to Mirror Lake (where camping is prohibited) and onward to a crossing of Mirror Creek just prior to reaching Outpost Camp (which has several campsites).

With 4.6 miles to go, cross Lone Pine Creek and stroll through the willow-lined meadows of Bighorn Park. From there, switchbacks descend a rocky slope and a rock-filled wash to a junction with the lateral to Lone Pine Lake. A short way beyond the junction the trail fords Lone Pine Creek and begins a steady, mostly shadeless descent with occasional switchbacks that leads out of the wilderness, across North Fork Lone Pine Creek, and back into forest on the way to the Whitney Portal Trailhead.

O Options for further wanderings from the HST are too numerous to adequately list. Consult Trip 32 (page 137) for options in the Kaweah Gap area and Trip 96 (page 332) for options around Mt. Whitney.

R A wilderness permit is required for overnight stays. Camping is limited to designated sites at Bearpaw Meadow Campground. Camping is limited to two nights at Hamilton Lakes. Campfires are prohibited in Bearpaw Meadow, at Hamilton Lakes, in Nine Lakes Basin, above 10,000 feet in Big Arroyo, and above 10,400 feet in Sequoia.

MT. WHITNEY ZONE: Bear canisters are required, and campfires are prohibited. Camping is prohibited at Mirror Lake or Trailside Meadow. Stock is prohibited. Within the Whitney Zone the Forest Service has instituted mandatory use of WAG (waste alleviation and gelling) bags for disposal of all human waste. Hikers should pick up bags near the Crabtree junction and dispose of them at Whitney Portal Trailhead.

GIANT FOREST TRAILHEADS

TRIP 33

Moro Rock: Soldiers Trail and Moro Rock Loop

Ⓜ 🔎 DH

DISTANCE: 4.4 miles, loop

ELEVATION: 6,395'/6,725'/6,395', +1,475'/-1,475'/±2,950'

SEASON: Late May to November

USE: Moderate (high at Moro Rock)

MAPS: USGS's *Giant Forest* or SNHA's *Giant Forest*

INTRODUCTION: This 4-plus-mile loop across the Giant Forest plateau is definitely the long way to the extraordinary view from the top of the exfoliated granite dome of Moro Rock, but hikers should enjoy a modicum of serenity before reaching the tourist mecca at the midpoint. Every summer day, hundreds of tourists trek via shuttle bus or private automobile along the narrow Crescent Meadow Road to the parking lot, and then huff and puff their way up the quarter-mile stairway climb to the top of Moro Rock. Restrooms, interpretive displays, and steel railings lend a decidedly civilized feel to Moro Rock, counter to what you should find on the rest of this trip. To avoid the biggest crowds, visit in spring or fall.

DIRECTIONS TO TRAILHEAD: Follow the Generals Highway to the large parking area near the Giant Forest Museum.

DESCRIPTION: From the museum, follow the crosswalk over Crescent Meadow Road to the well-signed trailhead, and then gently ascend a hillside through mixed forest along the west edge of the Giant Forest plateau, passing a sprinkling of giant sequoias along the way. At 1.2 miles from the trailhead, as you approach the Moro Rock Road, reach a junction with the Bear Hill Trail. Another 0.2 mile farther, as the trail once again nears

the road, you reach a signed junction with a lateral to Hanging Rock.

🔲 **SIDE TRIP TO HANGING ROCK:** Turn left (southwest) at the junction and make a short climb to the exposed granite slab of Hanging Rock, from where you have fine views of Middle Fork Kaweah River and west to Ash Peaks Ridge. A short scramble up a nearby rock knob provides the added bonus of a close-up of Moro Rock backdropped nicely by the crags of Castle Rocks. **END OF SIDE TRIP**

From the Hanging Rock junction, follow the trail across the Moro Rock Road, and continue another 0.2 mile to a junction with the Soldiers Trail. A short descent leads away from the serenity of the forest to the usual hustle and bustle found at the Moro Rock parking lot. Across the pavement, the highly popular Moro Rock Trail climbs to the top of the granite dome.

As billed, the view from the top of Moro Rock, which juts out into the air above the Middle Fork canyon, is breathtaking. The Giant Forest plateau spreads out in the northern foreground, the characteristic

---

MORO ROCK

In 1861, Hale Tharp and his stepson were the first settlers to climb Moro Rock. A century and a half later, hundreds of sightseers attempt the journey every summer day, ascending 300 vertical feet in a quarter mile on nearly 350 steps. Interpretive displays give tourists opportunities to try and catch their breath, and railings attempt to keep them safely corralled. The steps were constructed in 1931 and subsequently placed in the National Register of Historic Places. The rock was named for a Spanish word for the color of a blue roan mustang belonging to a neighbor of Tharp. Legend claims the horse could often be seen roaming the slopes beneath the granite dome.

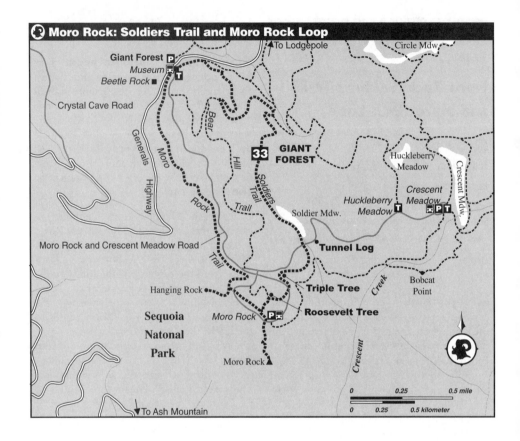

Moro Rock: Soldiers Trail and Moro Rock Loop

crowns of the Big Trees rising above the lesser conifers. The sculpted summits of the Great Western Divide scrape the sky to the east. The deep cleft of Middle Fork Kaweah River 4,000 feet below is also impressive, with the multispired Castle Crags dominating the far wall. Miniature-looking cars can be seen snaking down the Generals Highway, with the Three Rivers community visible farther down the canyon. On clear days, views extend across San Joaquin Valley to the Coast Range; unfortunately, clear days are the rare exception, and smoggy days the rule. In fact, air pollution from the valleys of western California pose one of the biggest threats to the health of the parks. Commonsense dictates that hikes should avoid Moro Rock during thunderstorms and wet or icy periods when the glacier-polished rock is slick.

To resume the loop, retrace your steps to the Soldiers Trail junction above the parking lot. A short, moderate climb up the Soldiers Trail leads to a junction with the Bear Hill Trail, near the symmetrical Roosevelt Tree. Bear right, remaining on the Soldiers Trail, and curve around for 0.2 mile to a diagonal crossing of the Moro Rock Road. Pass the Triple Tree, an unusual sight where three sequoias have grown together. A half mile of gently graded tread leads to a crossing of the Crescent Meadow Road near the Tunnel Log, a massive, unnamed sequoia that fell across the road on December 4, 1937. The next summer, a Civilian Conservation Corps crew cut a hole 17 feet wide by 8 feet deep so that motorists could drive through the downed tree.

Beyond the road, stroll along the edge of picturesque Soldier Meadow, a lush swath

SOLDIER MEADOW

US Cavalry soldiers camped on the knoll above Soldiers Meadow between 1891 and 1913, while charged with protecting the sequoias from loggers and the wildlife from poachers. In addition to these duties, they extended Colony Mill Road from the mill site to the Giant Forest, completing the project in 1903.

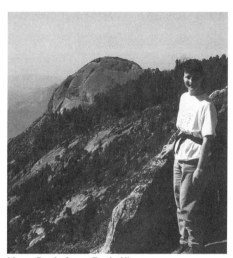

Moro Rock from Eagle View

of vegetation, well watered by a tributary of Crescent Creek.

Leaving Soldier Meadow, climb toward the crest of a low ridge, passing Broken Arrow, a burned, topless sequoia, on the way. A serpentine descent off the ridge leads to a junction with the Alta Trail, shortly followed by a junction with the Hazelwood Nature Trail. Veer right and proceed on the west side of the loop to the paved path paralleling the Generals Highway to the museum.

GIANT FOREST TRAILHEADS

TRIP 34

Sunset Rock

E ✒ **DH**

DISTANCE: 1.6 miles, out-and-back

ELEVATION: 6,370'/6,472', +215'/-115'/±660'

SEASON: May to November

USE: Moderate

MAPS: USGS's *Giant Forest* or SNHA's *Giant Forest*

INTRODUCTION: An easy hike with negligible elevation gain leads hikers to a vista point atop the summit of one of Sequoia's numerous granite domes. Despite the short distance, the trail offers relative peace and quiet, along with good views from the top.

DIRECTIONS TO TRAILHEAD: Follow the Generals Highway to the large parking area near the Giant Forest Museum.

DESCRIPTION: The well-signed Sunset Rock Trail begins across the Generals Highway

from the north end of the museum. Follow paved trail on a short descent through a dense forest of white firs and sugar pines to a wood bridge over Little Deer Creek. Immediately past the bridge, veer left at a junction with a trail bound for Round Meadow, and proceed above the creek before a mild ascent leads away from the stream and past the tiny meadow of Eli's Paradise. Incense cedars, ponderosa pines, and black oaks join the mixed forest on a climb up paved trail to a saddle. From this saddle, an abandoned section of the Sunset Rock Trail descends toward an old trailhead near the Marble Fork Bridge on Crystal Cave Road. However, the short route to the top of the rock proceeds ahead across the broad, exposed granite dome.

While not as dramatic as the one from Moro Rock, the view from Sunset Rock is fine nonetheless. The vista includes the canyon of Marble Fork Kaweah River, Ash Peaks Ridge, Colony Mill, and the companion dome of Little Baldy to the north. When the dome first received its name, the sunsets were undoubtedly quite eye-catching. Nowadays, the mature vegetation and the ubiquitous valley smog have diminished them considerably.

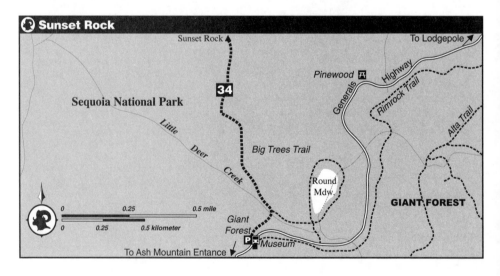

TRIP 35

Big Trees Trail

E **DH**

DISTANCE: 1 mile, loop

ELEVATION: Negligible

SEASON: May to November

USE: Heavy

MAPS: USGS's *Giant Forest* or
SNHA's *Giant Forest*

INTRODUCTION: This paved, wheelchair-accessible nature trail around Round Mead-ow provides visitors a taste of the Giant Forest experience while they learn about the ecology of the area.

DIRECTIONS TO TRAILHEAD: Follow the Generals Highway to the large parking area near the Giant Forest Museum.

DESCRIPTION: The Big Trees Trail circles Round Meadow, providing a fine opportunity to see several giant sequoias across a flower-filled meadow. From the museum, follow signed directions on a paved trail alongside the Generals Highway for a quarter mile to a crossing of the highway. The loop begins on the far side just beyond a crossing of Little Deer Creek. Proceed clockwise around the meadow back to the junction and then retrace your steps to the museum.

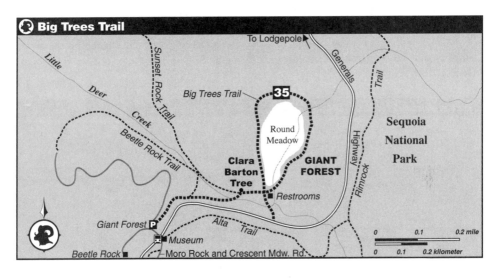

TRIP 36

Hazelwood Nature Trail

E 🔍 **DH**

DISTANCE: 0.5 mile, loop

ELEVATION: Negligible

SEASON: May to November

USE: Heavy

MAPS: USGS's *Giant Forest* or SNHA's *Giant Forest*

INTRODUCTION: An easy loop, the Hazelwood Nature Trail provides a fine introduction to the sequoias of the Giant Forest, with interpretive displays offering information on the human history and ecology of the area.

DIRECTIONS TO TRAILHEAD: Follow the Generals Highway to a small parking area

0.4 mile north of the Giant Forest Museum. If the lot is full, park in the large lot near the museum and follow the paved path signed for the Big Trees Trail for 0.4 mile to the start of the trail.

DESCRIPTION: Heading away from the highway on paved trail, reach a large fallen sequoia and pass through a notch in the tree to reach the loop junction. Follow the right-hand fork, proceeding counterclockwise through mixed forest, where the mighty sequoias dwarf the other conifers. A sprinkling of dogwoods offer creamy white blossoms in early summer and blazing orange leaves in autumn. The trail is lined with azalea, thimbleberry, ferns, wildflowers, and other small plants. At a signed junction with the Alta Trail, bend left, cross a tiny rivulet, and continue the loop through the lovely forested dell. Eventually, the trail veers west to cross a wood bridge over a tributary of Little Deer Creek before reaching the close of the loop. From there, retrace your steps to the trailhead.

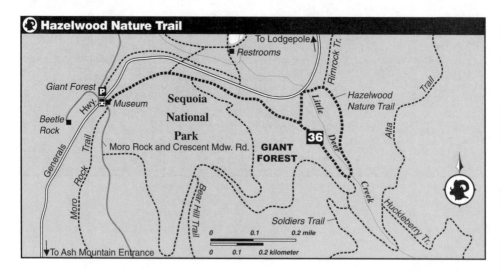

GIANT FOREST TRAILHEADS

TRIP 37

Trail of the Sequoias

M 🔍 **DH**

DISTANCE: 6.1 miles, loop

ELEVATION: 7,050'/6,760'/7,050',
+1,325'/-1,325' ±2,650'

SEASON: May to November

USE: Moderate (heavy on
Congress Trail)

MAPS: USGS's *Giant Forest*
and *Lodgepole* or SNHA's
Giant Forest

INTRODUCTION: This trip offers the opportunity to explore the heart of the Giant Forest in silence and serenity, away from the crowds customary on the more popular Congress and Crescent Meadow Trails. You will see plenty of notable sequoia landmarks on this loop, along with many unnamed giant sequoias and three picturesque meadows.

DIRECTIONS TO TRAILHEAD: Take the free shuttle bus via Route 1 to the General Sherman bus stop. By using the bus, hikers can shave off nearly a mile of hiking to and from the General Sherman parking lot.

Visitors driving private vehicles can follow the Generals Highway to the Wolverton Road, 2.8 miles north of the museum, and then follow the road 0.5 mile to a three-way stop. Turn right and follow a spur road another 0.5 mile to the General Sherman parking lot at the end of the road.

DESCRIPTION: From the General Sherman parking lot, pass through an elaborate wood archway lined with informational placards and descend along a well-graded, paved path with periodic steps toward the General Sherman Tree. Several conveniently placed park benches offer rest stops for tourists unaccustomed to the altitude. Where the path makes a sharp bend, a set

of stairs marks a junction with a seldom-used connector to Lodgepole. Farther on, a wide spot in the trail is stamped with a cross section of the Sherman Tree's base, a graphic representation of this truly massive tree. This spot also offers an unobstructed view of the world's largest tree's profile, distant enough for most cameras to capture the entire tree in one shot. A brief walk leads to a junction with a short trail on the right to General Sherman and the signed Congress Trail on the left, 0.4 mile from the trailhead.

GENERAL SHERMAN TREE

At 275 feet high, 103 feet around at its base, and a volume of 52,508 cubic feet, General Sherman is not only the world's largest tree but also the largest living organism on the planet. At a diameter of seven feet, the largest branch is bigger than the trunks of many conifers. James Wolverton, a pioneer cattleman, who served under the general in the Civil War, named the tree.

Whether arriving by shuttle bus or by walking the trail from the parking lot, find the start of the marked Congress Trail and head downhill to the Learning Tree. Continue across a pair of bridges over tributaries of Sherman Creek. Past the second bridge, reach a lateral on the right, which provides a possible shortcut back to the trailhead. From there, a winding, quarter-mile ascent leads to a four-way junction of the Alta Trail.

Nearing the south end of the loop, the trail passes many notable sequoias, including Chief Sequoyah (29th largest), the Senate and House Groups, and the General Lee and McKinley Trees. Amid the Senate Group, the Trail of the Sequoias branches south.

Following the Trail of the Sequoias, head through the Senate Group and then follow a general descent past a couple of

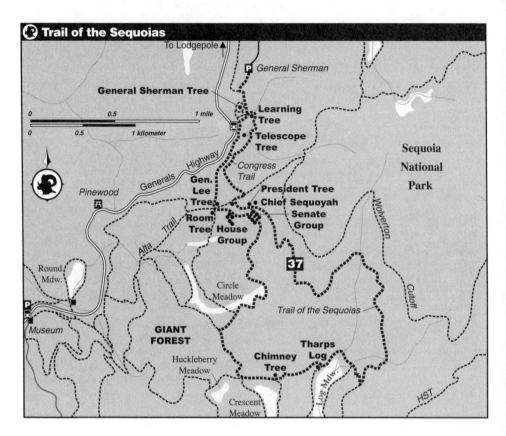

Trail of the Sequoias

scorched giants that at first glance appear to have died but, upon further inspection, are amazingly still alive. Cross a tiny rivulet trickling into the southeast fringe of Circle Meadow, and then follow the trail across the slope above this verdant clearing. Pass an unsigned fork, where a use trail wanders out into the meadow, and reach a signed junction a short way farther with the Circle Meadow Trail, 2.5 miles from the trailhead.

Continue on the Trail of the Sequoias for 0.1 mile to a junction, and veer toward Crescent Meadow. Head south-southeast and descend through moderate forest cover to a pair of Y-junctions, approximately 25 yards apart. Continue southeast at both junctions, following signs for Crescent Meadow and then Tharps Log. Skirt the north edge of verdant Crescent Meadow for 0.2 mile to another pair of junctions

about 10 yards apart. The Chimney Tree, a fire-hollowed giant sequoia, is just up the hill past the second junction. After pondering the effects of fire on the Big Trees, turn right from the second junction and proceed toward Tharps Log. A short, winding climb leads to the crest of a low ridge, and then you descend briefly to Tharps Log at the north end of Log Meadow, 4.5 miles from the trailhead. (For more information about Tharps Log, see Trip 28, page 128).

From a signed junction near Tharps Log, head east around the tip of Log Meadow, cross Crescent Creek on a wood-plank bridge, and then shortly step over a smaller tributary to arrive at a junction with the eastern part of the Log Meadow Loop.

From the junction, climb up a fern-covered hillside to a junction with a seldom-used connector trail, 0.2 mile from the previous junction.

Remain on the Trail of the Sequoias and make a lengthy traverse across a hillside, stepping over a couple of small rivulets along the way and encountering several notable sequoias, including passing through a break in the trunk of a fallen giant. Arc across the drainage of Crescent Creek, and then climb to the top of a ridge, from where you have limited views of the surrounding woodland. Gazing across the mixed coniferous forest, you can see the characteristic sequoia crowns overshadowing other conifers. A half-mile descent leads past more sequoias on the way to a junction with the Congress Trail near the President Tree.

Turn left from the junction, and soon reach the five-way junction with the Alta and Circle Meadow Trails. From the five-way junction, the Congress Trail turns north on a mild descent and weaves through the forest back to the lateral. From there, continue to the vicinity of General Sherman, and either head over to the shuttle bus stop or retrace your steps on the 0.4-mile climb back to the parking area.

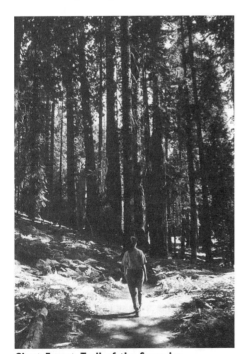

Giant Forest, Trail of the Sequoias

TRIP 38

Circle Meadow Loop

E ☸ **DH**

DISTANCE: 3.8 miles, loop

ELEVATION: 7,050'/6,835'/7,050', +675'/-675' ±1,350'

SEASON: May to November

USE: Moderate (heavy on Congress Trail)

MAPS: USGS's *Giant Forest* and *Lodgepole* or SNHA's *Giant Forest*

INTRODUCTION: A journey of contrasts, the Circle Meadow Loop begins and ends on the heavily used, paved Congress Trail, passing a number of notable sequoias on the way. The middle part of the trip is on infrequently used sections of the Trail of the Sequoias and Circle Meadow Trail.

DIRECTIONS TO TRAILHEAD: Take the free shuttle bus via Route 1 to the General Sherman bus stop. By using the bus, hikers can shave off nearly a mile of hiking to and from the General Sherman parking lot.

Private vehicles can follow the Generals Highway to the Wolverton Road, 2.8 miles north of the museum, and then follow the road 0.5 mile to a three-way stop. Turn right and follow a spur road another 0.5 mile to the General Sherman parking lot at the end of the road.

DESCRIPTION: From the parking lot, pass through an elaborate wood archway lined with informational placards and descend along a well-graded, paved path with periodic steps toward the General Sherman Tree. Several conveniently placed park benches offer rest stops for tourists unaccustomed to the altitude. Where the path makes a sharp bend, a set of stairs marks a junction with a seldom-used connector to Lodgepole.

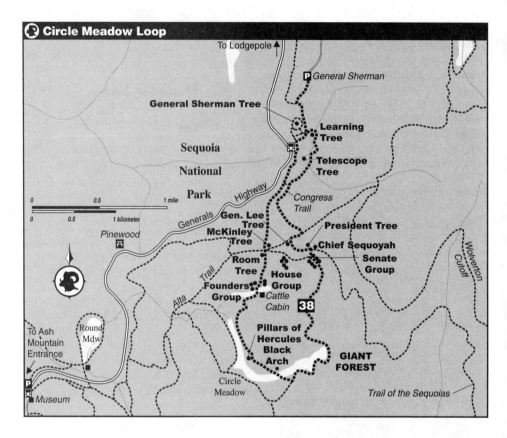

Circle Meadow Loop

To Lodgepole

General Sherman

General Sherman Tree

Learning Tree

Sequoia

National

Park

Telescope Tree

Congress Trail

Highway

Generals

Gen. Lee Tree

McKinley Tree

President Tree

Chief Sequoyah

Room Tree

Senate Group

Trail

House Group

Founders Group

Cattle Cabin

38

Alta

Pinewood

Pillars of Hercules

Black Arch

GIANT FOREST

Round Mdw

To Ash Mountain Entrance

Circle Meadow

Trail of the Sequoias

Museum

Wolverton Cutoff

0   0.5   1 mile

0   0.5   1 kilometer

Farther on, a wide spot in the trail is stamped with a cross section of the Sherman Tree's base, a graphic representation of this truly massive tree. This spot also offers an unobstructed view of the world's largest tree's profile, distant enough for most cameras to capture the entire tree in one shot. A brief walk leads to a junction with a short trail on the right to General Sherman and the signed Congress Trail on the left, 0.4 mile from the trailhead.

Whether you arrive by shuttle bus or by walking the trail from the parking lot, find the start of the marked Congress Trail and head downhill to the Learning Tree. Continue across a pair of bridges over tributaries of Sherman Creek. Past the second bridge, reach a lateral on the right, which provides a shortcut back to the trailhead. From there, a winding, quarter-mile ascent leads to a four-way junction of the Alta Trail.

Nearing the south end of the loop, the trail passes many notable sequoias, including Chief Sequoyah (29th largest), the Senate and House Groups, and the General Lee and McKinley Trees. Amid the Senate Group, the Trail of the Sequoias branches south.

Following the Trail of the Sequoias, head through the Senate Group and then follow a general descent past a couple of scorched giants that at first glance appear to have died but, upon further inspection, are amazingly still alive. Cross a tiny rivulet trickling into the southeast fringe of Circle Meadow and then follow the trail across the slope above this verdant clearing. Pass an unsigned fork, where a use trail wanders out into the meadow, and reach a signed junction a short way farther with the Circle Meadow Trail, 2.5 miles from the trailhead.

Turn right (northwest) onto the Circle Meadow Trail, immediately crossing the

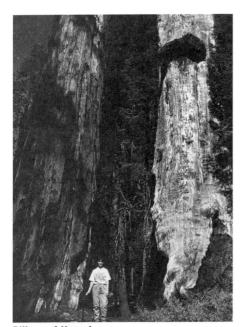

Pillars of Hercules

where the trail passes right between two massive sequoias.

Proceed along the west fringe of Circle Meadow, passing a junction with a little-used trail heading northwest to Cattle Cabin. This structure was built by cattlemen who pastured their stock in the meadows nearby. Just beyond the cabin, step across another tiny rivulet coursing through the northern swath of meadow and then continue through the Founders Group, a stand of a dozen stately sequoias named in honor of citizens who helped establish the park. Not far from the Founders Group is the Room Tree, a giant sequoia with a small entrance in the trunk that leads into a large, hollowed-out section at its base. A short distance farther, you reach a junction of the Circle Meadow, Alta, and Congress Trails.

From the five-way junction, the Congress Trail turns north on a mild descent and weaves through the forest back to the lateral. From there, continue to the vicinity of the General Sherman Tree, and either head over to the shuttle bus stop or retrace your steps on the 0.4-mile climb back to the parking area.

thin ribbon of Circle Meadow. Beyond the meadow, you climb a low hill and reach Black Arch, another interesting scorched giant, and then the Pillars of Hercules,

GIANT FOREST TRAILHEADS

TRIP 39

Congress Trail

E ↻ **DH**

DISTANCE: 3.1 miles, semiloop

ELEVATION: 7,050'/6,830'/7,050', +550'/-550'/±1,100'

SEASON: May to November

USE: Heavy

MAPS: USGS's *Giant Forest* and *Lodgepole* or SNHA's *Giant Forest*

INTRODUCTION: Predictably, the most popular trail in the Giant Forest takes visitors to the biggest giant sequoia in the world,

the General Sherman Tree, as well as many of the other most notable Big Trees in the grove, including the fourth, fifth, and twenty-ninth largest. On this loop you will also see two of the most notable stands of sequoias, the Senate and House Groups. Connecting trails offer the possibility of numerous side trips to even more prominent Big Trees. *Don't expect to experience these monarchs in reverent solitude;* the trail's popularity will dictate otherwise, although the number of tourists drops dramatically the farther hikers travel from the parking area.

DIRECTIONS TO TRAILHEAD: Take the free shuttle bus via Route 1 to the General Sherman bus stop. By using the bus, hikers can shave off nearly a mile of hiking to and from the General Sherman parking lot.

Visitors driving private vehicles can follow the Generals Highway to the Wolverton

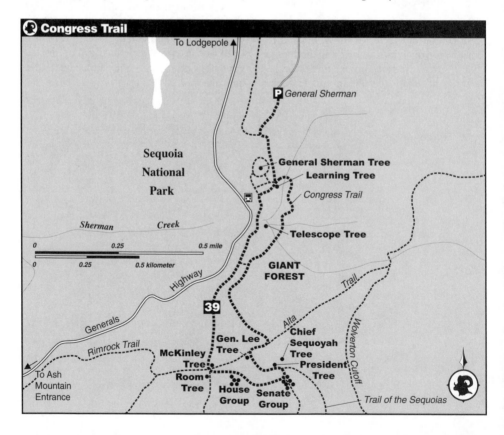

Congress Trail

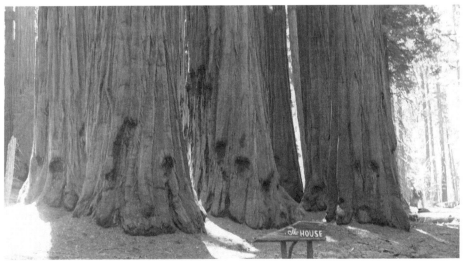

House Group on the Congress Trail

Road, 2.8 miles north of the museum, and then follow the road 0.5 mile to a three-way stop. Turn right and follow a spur road another 0.5 mile to the General Sherman parking lot at the end of the road.

DESCRIPTION: From the parking lot, pass through an elaborate wood archway lined with informational placards and descend along a well-graded, paved path with periodic steps toward the General Sherman Tree. Several conveniently placed park benches offer rest stops for tourists unaccustomed to the altitude. Where the path makes a sharp bend, a set of stairs marks a junction with a seldom-used connector to Lodgepole.

Farther on, a wide spot in the trail is stamped with a cross section of the Sherman Tree's base, a graphic representation of this truly massive tree. This spot also offers an unobstructed view of the world's largest tree's profile, distant enough for most cameras to capture the entire tree in one shot. A brief walk leads to a junction with a short trail on the right to General Sherman and the signed Congress Trail on the left, 0.4 mile from the trailhead.

Whether you arrive by shuttle bus or by walking the trail from the parking lot, find the start of the marked Congress Trail and head downhill to the Learning Tree.

Continue across a pair of bridges over tributaries of Sherman Creek. Past the second bridge, reach a lateral on the right, which provides a possible shortcut back to the trailhead. From there, a winding, quarter-mile ascent leads to a four-way junction of the Alta Trail.

Nearing the south end of the loop, the trail passes many notable sequoias, including Chief Sequoyah (29th largest), the Senate and House Groups, and the General Lee and McKinley Trees. Amid the Senate Group, the Trail of the Sequoias branches south. After another 0.3 mile, reach a five-way junction with the Alta and Circle Meadow Trails near the McKinley Tree. With extra time, these trails access additional sequoia landmarks—the Lincoln and the Cloister Trees are just a short jaunt southwest on the Alta Trail, and the Room Tree, Founders Group, and Cattle Cabin are just south down the Circle Meadow Trail.

From the five-way junction, the Congress Trail turns north on a mild descent and weaves through the forest back to the lateral. From there, continue to the vicinity of the General Sherman Tree, and either head over to the shuttle bus stop or retrace your steps on the 0.4-mile climb back to the parking area.

Introduction to Wolverton, Lodgepole, and Wuksachi

The areas that would one day become Wolverton, Lodgepole, and Wuksachi were of little interest to Native Americans, who preferred more temperate locations nearby, such as the Giant Forest. Nowadays, since the Park Service relocated infrastructure away from the Giant Forest, these areas are bustling centers of activity for many park visitors. Lodgepole serves as the center for information, commercial activity, and camping, while Wuksachi Village is the focal point for lodging, and Wolverton is the principal backcountry gateway.

Lodgepole is located in the picturesque, glacier-scoured Tokopah Valley, near the banks of the Middle Fork Kaweah River,

where steep cliffs rise out of the valley up to granite ridges and peaks. Wuksachi Village is tucked quietly away from the Generals Highway in serene forest along Clover Creek.

Wolverton is the main trailhead for hikers, backpackers, and equestrians entering the backcountry of Sequoia from the western side. The large Wolverton Trailhead parking lot is near flower-bedecked, forest-rimmed Long Meadow, the starting point for trails heading into the mid-elevation forests common to the western Sierra. Several of the park's more popular trails begin from Wolverton and Lodgepole, as do less used routes into more remote areas of the backcountry. Many trails climb into high elevations, which may leave backpackers unaccustomed to such heights short of breath. Offering quiet forest strolls, grand views, wildflower-covered meadows, and alpine lakes cradled in rugged cirques, trails

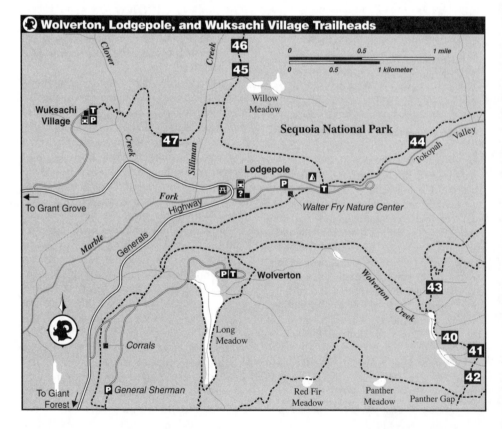

from Wolverton and Lodgepole offer a bounty of options, from short dayhikes to extended backpacks.

ACCESS: All trailheads in this area are easily accessed from the Generals Highway, which is open all year from the Ash Mountain Entrance. Access from the north on the Generals Highway is subject to closure during winter storms.

AMENITIES: Facilities at Lodgepole include a visitor center, market, gift shop, snack bar and deli, laundry, public showers (which are closed in winter), post office, campground, picnic areas, and the Walter Fry Nature Center (also closed in winter).

Wuksachi Village offers all-year, upscale lodging. The village has a main lodge, which houses guest registration, a gift shop, restaurant, lounge, and conference facilities. Three detached buildings have 102 guest rooms. Consult the website at **www.visitsequoia.com** for more information or reservations.

Aside from being primarily a backcountry trailhead, Wolverton offers horseback riding and pack trips during the summer. In winter, Wolverton becomes a snow-play center with two sledding hills. Visitors may rent cross-country skis and snowshoes at Wuksachi Village.

RANGER STATION: Hikers can get wilderness permits and backcountry information from the wilderness permit office next to the visitor center at Lodgepole. A parking permit is required to park overnight at Lodgepole. General information is available at the visitor center.

GOOD TO KNOW BEFORE YOU GO: Groups planning to stay at the Lodgepole Campground the night before starting a backpack trip should be forewarned of the campground's popularity. Reservations are recommended. A parking permit is required to park overnight at Lodgepole and is available from the wilderness permit office next to the visitor center.

Bear boxes are provided at all trailheads, but they are often full during the busiest parts of the summer. Minimize the amount of extra food and scented items you bring on your trip.

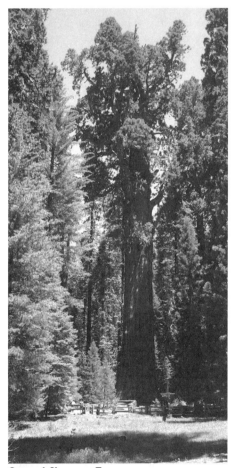

General Sherman Tree

Campground							
Campground	Fee	Elevation	Season	Restrooms	Water	Bear Boxes	Phone
Lodgepole (25.4 miles from Ash Mountain Entrance)	$20	6,700 feet	All year	Flush	Yes	Yes	Yes

TRIP 40

Mehrten and Alta Meadows

Ⓜ ⟋ DH or BP

DISTANCE: 11.8 miles, out-and-back

ELEVATION: 7,270'/9,300',
+2,600'/-570' ±6,340'

SEASON: July to mid-October

USE: Moderate

MAPS: USGS's *Lodgepole* or
SNHA's Lodgepole

TRAIL LOG

1.75 Lakes Trail and Panther Gap
      Trail junction
2.7   Panther Gap
3.9   Mehrten Creek
4.7   Alta Peak Trail junction

INTRODUCTION: Journey through the serenity of a red fir forest to the magnificence of flower-filled meadows and wonderful views of impressive peaks. The 12-mile round-trip is within the range of hikers in good condition, while excellent campsites will lure backpackers who want extra time to fully enjoy the beautiful surroundings. The first cluster of campsites near Mehrten Meadow reposes in the cool shade of forest, a mere 4 miles from the trailhead. The second set along the fringe of Alta Meadow sits beneath the ramparts of Tharps Rock and Alta Peak. Beyond Alta Meadow, a cross-country route to the alpine realm of Moose Lake and The Tableland will tantalize off-trail buffs.

Although the Alta Trail officially begins near the Giant Forest Museum, most trail users will want to access the trail from Wolverton, which saves considerable mileage and elevation gain.

DIRECTIONS TO TRAILHEAD: From the Generals Highway, 1.75 miles south of Lodgepole, turn east at the signed Wolverton junction and follow paved road 1.5 miles to the large parking area (which has restrooms, running water, and bear boxes).

DESCRIPTION: Near a plethora of signs, stairs lead away from the parking area to a wide, single-track trail up a hillside to the crest of a low ridge and a junction with a connector from Lodgepole. Turn right and follow the Lakes Trail, soon passing a junction on the right with a trail around Long Meadow. After the initial ascent, the grade eases to a mild to moderate climb through sparse red fir forest. The ascent continues along Wolverton Creek, which trickles through a strip of verdant, wildflower-filled meadow. Eventually, the trail crosses a spring-fed tributary lined with flowers, including columbine, monkeyflower, leopard lily, aster, and cow parsnip. Reach a junction between the Lakes Trail and Panther Gap Trail at 1.75 miles.

Turn south and follow the Panther Gap Trail through moderate forest cover, roughly paralleling Wolverton Creek and crossing numerous lushly lined tributaries along the way. Eventually, you leave behind the delightful streams and lush foliage, as the trail climbs out of the drainage to a T-junction with the Alta Trail at Panther Gap, 2.7 miles from the trailhead. A short stroll toward the lip of the canyon reveals a commanding view of the canyon of the Middle Fork Kaweah River, Castle Peaks, and summits on the Great Western Divide.

Head east on the Alta Trail, initially following the crest, through distinctly drier slopes of manzanita and ceanothus dotted with Jeffrey and sugar pines. Soon the path veers onto an open, south-facing hillside, with more far-ranging views. After stepping across a spring-fed rivulet, the route follows a series of short switchbacks up to a junction with the Sevenmile Trail, 3.7 miles from the trailhead, which connects to the High Sierra Trail.

From the junction, head into forest cover and drop down to a ford of Mehrten Creek at 3.9 miles. Nearby is Mehrten Meadow Camp, where a few campsites (which have a bear box) are sheltered by red

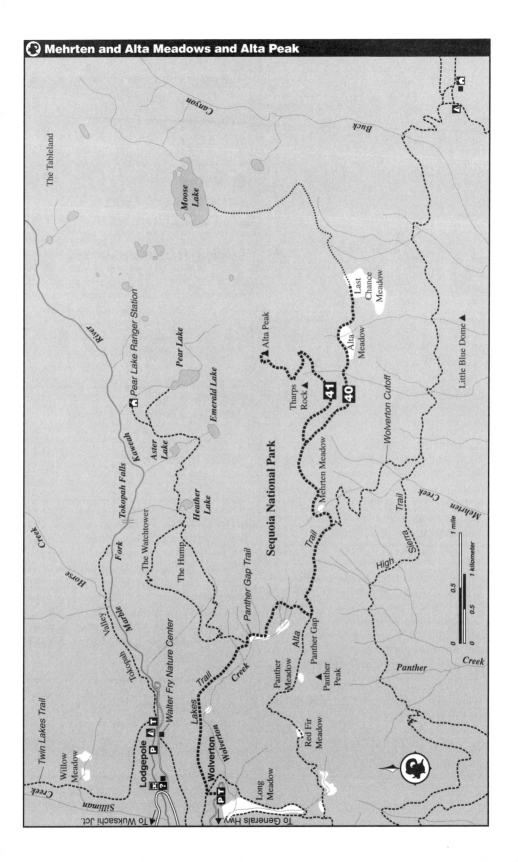

firs. Mehrten Meadow is a narrow, sloping, flower-packed glade well below the trail.

Leave Mehrten Meadow behind and follow a gently ascending traverse across a hillside through patchy fir cover, as Tharps Rock appears through breaks in the forest. Reach a junction with the Alta Peak Trail, 4.7 miles from the trailhead. Backpackers with a base camp at Mehrten or Alta Meadows should consider a climb of Alta Peak (see Trip 41).

From the junction, follow a gentle climb around the forested base of Tharps Rock until you break out of the trees to a wide-ranging view. Beyond a stream crossing, you reach the verdant and extensive clearing of flower-carpeted Alta Meadow. The exquisite beauty of the meadow is complemented by fine views of Tharps Rock, Alta Peak, and the Great Western Divide. Excellent campsites nestle beneath red firs on a low ridge south of the trail. An unmaintained trail continues a short distance through vales and over rivulets to Last Chance Meadow and more remote campsites.

From the vicinity of Last Chance Meadow, a fairly well-known cross-country route connects to Moose Lake and The Tableland beyond. Hikers can follow a faint use trail most of the way to the lake, which heads northeast to an open ridge above Buck Canyon. Follow the ridge northwest to the last of the stunted pines, and then descend boulder-filled slopes north toward the lake. Continue north over rocky terrain to a grassy swale leading to a series of ramps. Climb up the ramp system to a saddle overlooking the south shore, and drop down to the lake. Campsites are spread around the shoreline. Brook trout will entice anglers.

A wilderness permit is required for overnight stays. Campfires are prohibited above 10,400 feet.

WOLVERTON TRAILHEAD

TRIP 41

Alta Peak

S ⚐ DH or BP

DISTANCE: 13.4 miles, out-and-back

ELEVATION: 7,270'/11,204', +4,265'/-330'/±9,190'

SEASON: Mid-July to mid-October

USE: Moderate

MAPS: USGS's *Lodgepole* or SNHA's *Lodgepole*

see map on p.161

TRAIL LOG

1.75 Lakes Trail and Panther Gap Trail junction
2.7 Panther Gap
3.9 Mehrten Creek
4.7 Alta Peak Trail junction
6.7 Alta Peak

INTRODUCTION: The airy summit of Alta Peak is blessed with one of the best views possible from by maintained trail from the west side of Sequoia. A one-day ascent is viable for strong, acclimatized hikers, but lesser mortals can make a two-day summit bid from campsites at Alta or Mehrten Meadows (see Trip 40, page 160). However many days you spend, the supreme summit vista is a worthy reward.

DIRECTIONS TO TRAILHEAD: From the Generals Highway, 1.75 miles south of Lodgepole, turn east at the signed Wolverton junction, and follow paved road 1.5 miles to the large parking area (which has restrooms, running water, and bear boxes).

DESCRIPTION: Near a plethora of signs, stairs lead away from the parking area to a wide, single-track trail up a hillside to the crest of a low ridge and a junction with a connector from Lodgepole. Turn right and follow the Lakes Trail, soon passing a junction on the right with a trail around Long Meadow. After the initial ascent, the grade eases to a mild to moderate climb through sparse red fir forest. The ascent continues along Wolverton Creek, which trickles through a strip of verdant, wildflower-filled meadow. Eventually, the trail crosses a spring-fed tributary lined with flowers, including columbine, monkey-flower, leopard lily, aster, and cow parsnip. Reach a junction between the Lakes Trail and Panther Gap Trail at 1.75 miles.

Turn south and follow the Panther Gap Trail through moderate forest cover, roughly paralleling Wolverton Creek and crossing numerous lushly lined tributaries along the way. Eventually, you leave behind the delightful streams and lush foliage, as the trail climbs out of the drainage to a T-junction with the Alta Trail at Panther Gap, 2.7 miles from the trailhead. A short stroll toward the lip of the canyon reveals a commanding view of the canyon of the Middle Fork Kaweah River, Castle Peaks, and summits on the Great Western Divide.

Head east on the Alta Trail, initially following the crest, through distinctly drier slopes of manzanita and ceanothus dotted with Jeffrey and sugar pines. Soon the path veers onto an open, south-facing hillside, with more far-ranging views. After stepping across a spring-fed rivulet, the route follows a series of short switchbacks up to a junction with the Sevenmile Trail, 3.7 miles from the trailhead, which connects to the High Sierra Trail.

From the junction, head into forest cover and drop down to a ford of Mehrten Creek at 3.9 miles. Nearby is Mehrten Meadow Camp, where a few campsites (which have a bear box) are sheltered by red firs. Mehrten Meadow is a narrow, sloping, flower-packed glade well below the trail.

Leave Mehrten Meadow behind and follow a gently ascending traverse across a hillside through patchy fir cover, as Tharps Rock appears through breaks in the forest.

Reach a junction with the Alta Peak Trail, 4.7 miles from the trailhead.

From the junction, zigzag up a hillside through the intermittent shade from a grove of scattered red firs. Soon you leave the trees on the way to a refreshing, spring-fed, willow- and wildflower-lined stream, where a small campsite nestles above the far bank. Beyond the stream, a long ascending traverse heads across the face of Tharps Rock, passing through more scattered firs and patches of chinquapin. Excellent views abound across the Middle Fork Kaweah River canyon to the terrain of southwest Sequoia, as well as the verdant swath of Alta Meadows directly below and Tharps Rock and Alta Peak above. Near the end of the traverse, you reach the last reliable water source at a pretty little arroyo, filled with heather and wildflowers.

Beyond a switchback, the trail makes a swift climb, zigzagging up the rocky slope above Tharps Rock. A few stunted foxtail pines herald your arrival into the alpine zone, where tufts of ground-hugging vegetation cling to the nearly barren slopes. Over decomposed granite and around boulders, the ascent continues just below the peak's southwest ridge to reach the crest of the summit ridge. A short climb leads to the summit block and a final scramble to the top.

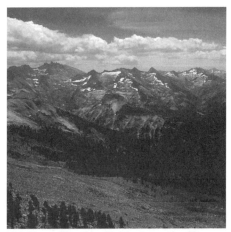

The Great Western Divide from the Alta Peak Trail

To say that the view from Alta Peak is incredible would be an understatement. The lake directly north is Pear Lake, back-dropped by an immense sea of granite rising toward The Tableland. Numerous park landmarks, including the Sierra Crest stretching across the eastern horizon, are visible. Bring a map large enough to help identify the plethora of geographical features. If the normal western haze is absent, consider yourself truly blessed; few have the opportunity to gaze across the farmland of the San Joaquin Valley to the Coast Range through clear skies.

TRIP 42

Panther Gap Loop

M **ℚ** **DH**

DISTANCE: 7 miles, loop

ELEVATION: 7,270'/8,645', +1,720'/-1,720'/±3,440'

SEASON: Early July to mid-October

USE: Light to moderate

MAPS: USGS's *Lodgepole* or SNHA's *Lodgepole*

TRAIL LOG

1.75 Lakes Trail and Panther Gap Trail junction
2.7   Panther Gap
5.1   Long Meadow junction

INTRODUCTION: Grand views, flower-filled meadows, and quiet forests greet you on this loop. The route begins on the popular Lakes Trail and the almost as popular lateral to the Alta Trail, but it veers away from the crowds beyond Panther Gap. Strolling past serene Panther and Red Fir Meadows, you should have the area to yourself. The last leg of the loop passes around pictur-esque Log Meadow, where you will likely see few people, except for some horseback riders from Wolverton Corral.

DIRECTIONS TO TRAILHEAD: From the Gen-erals Highway, 1.75 miles south of Lodge-pole, turn east at the signed Wolverton junction and follow paved road 1.5 miles to the large parking area (which has rest-rooms, running water, and bear boxes).

DESCRIPTION: Near a plethora of signs, stairs lead away from the parking area to a wide, single-track trail up a hillside to the crest of a low ridge and a junction with a connector from Lodgepole. Turn right and follow the Lakes Trail, soon passing a junction on the right with a trail around

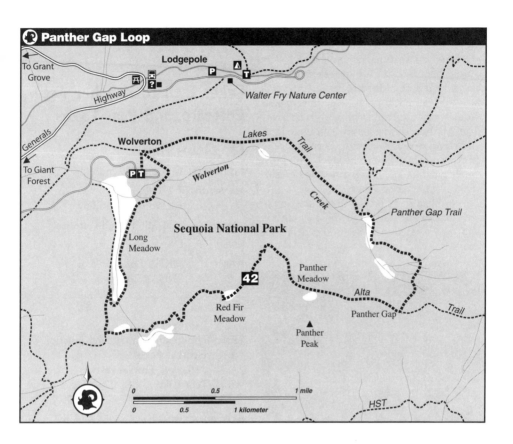

Panther Gap Loop

To Grant Grove

Lodgepole

Highway

Walter Fry Nature Center

Generals

To Giant Forest

Wolverton

Lakes Trail

Wolverton

Creek

Panther Gap Trail

Long Meadow

Sequoia National Park

42

Panther Meadow

Alta

Red Fir Meadow

Panther Gap

Trail

Panther Peak

0   0.5   1 mile

0   0.5   1 kilometer

HST

Long Meadow. After the initial ascent, the grade eases to a mild to moderate climb through sparse red fir forest. The ascent continues along Wolverton Creek, which trickles through a strip of verdant, wildflower-filled meadow. Eventually, the trail crosses a spring-fed tributary lined with flowers, including columbine, monkey-flower, leopard lily, aster, and cow parsnip. Reach a junction between the Lakes Trail and Panther Gap Trail at 1.75 miles.

Turn south and follow the Panther Gap Trail through moderate forest cover, roughly paralleling Wolverton Creek and crossing numerous lushly lined tributaries along the way. Eventually, you leave behind the delightful streams and lush foliage, as the trail climbs out of the drainage to a T-junction with the Alta Trail at Panther Gap, 2.7 miles from the trailhead. A short stroll toward the lip of the canyon reveals a com-

manding view of the Middle Fork Kaweah River canyon, Castle Peaks, and summits on the Great Western Divide.

From Panther Gap, turn west and follow the Alta Trail around the north side of Panther Peak on slightly rising tread through pine forest to diminutive Panther Meadow. From there, an upward traverse leads to the trip's high point, followed by a steep, 0.4-mile descent to Red Fir Meadow at 4.1 miles. Bordered by willows and edged by forest, the serene meadow is a fine spot for viewing wildlife. Continue the descent beyond the meadow to a junction in a saddle, 5.1 miles from the trailhead.

At the junction, leave the Alta Trail and turn north toward Long Meadow. A steep, switchbacking, 0.3-mile descent leads to another junction, where a paucity of signs provides little helpful information about what's ahead since the only direction is for the Alta Trail behind you.

Turn right at the junction and follow a usually dusty path around the south and east sides of Long Meadow, passing through lush foliage and hopping over tiny rivulets on the way. The trail eventually veers away from the meadow, crosses a grassy slope, and then crosses Wolverton Creek twice in pockets of firs. Beyond the creek, you cross an old road and climb up a forested hillside to meet the Lakes Trail at 6.75 miles.

Turn left, walk briefly to the junction of the single-track trail from the parking lot, and then retrace your steps shortly to the trailhead.

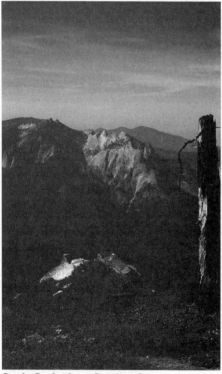

Castle Rocks from Panther Gap

WOLVERTON TRAILHEAD

TRIP 43

Lakes Trail to Heather, Aster, Emerald, and Pear Lakes

Ⓜ ♀ **DH** or **BP**

DISTANCE: 11.5 miles, semiloop

ELEVATION: 7,270'/9,350', +2,795'/-535'/±6,660'

SEASON: Mid-July to mid-October

USE: Heavy

MAPS: USGS's *Lodgepole* or SNHA's *Lodgepole*

TRAIL LOG

1.75 Panther Gap
2.1   Hump and Watchtower junction
3.75 Heather Lake
4.7   Aster and Emerald Lakes
5.75 Pear Lake

INTRODUCTION: Easy access and spectacular scenery combine on one of Sequoia's most popular hiking and backpacking trips. All four lakes are quite picturesque, and hikers will enjoy plenty of outstanding views along the way, including the spectacular vista from the Watchtower, a narrow ledge dynamited out of a sheer cliff forming the canyon wall above Tokopah Valley, 2,000 feet below.

To mitigate the trail's popularity and resulting human impact, the Park Service has implemented camping bans and limits and installed backcountry toilets. Overnight visitors face fierce competition for wilderness permits, especially on weekends. An early start will allow hikers in good condition to complete the nearly 12-mile semiloop in one day, thus avoiding the competition for wilderness permits.

DIRECTIONS TO TRAILHEAD: From the Generals Highway, 1.75 miles south of Lodgepole, turn east at the signed Wolverton

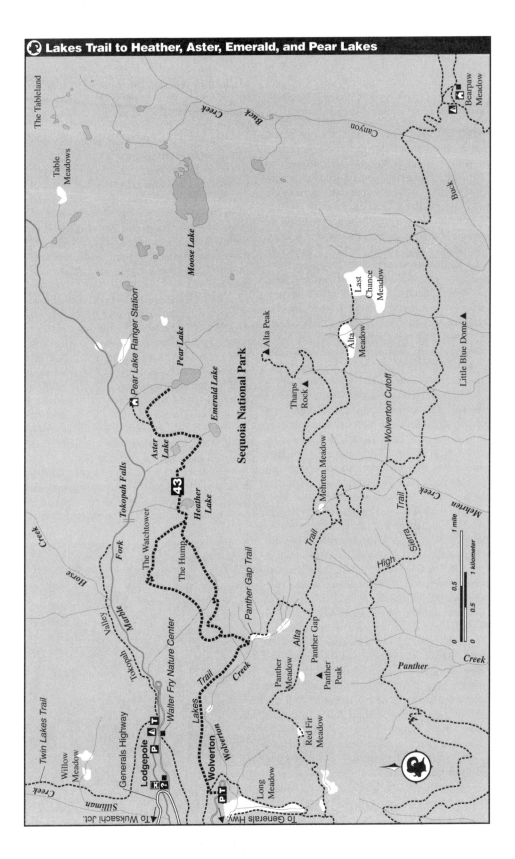

junction, and follow paved road 1.5 miles to the large parking area (which has restrooms, running water, and bear boxes).

DESCRIPTION: Near a plethora of signs, stairs lead away from the parking area to a wide, single-track trail up a hillside to the crest of a low ridge and a junction with a connector from Lodgepole. Turn right and follow the Lakes Trail, soon passing a junction on the right with a trail around Long Meadow. After the initial ascent, the grade eases to a mild to moderate climb through sparse red fir forest. The ascent continues along Wolverton Creek, which trickles through a strip of verdant, wildflower-filled meadow. Eventually, the trail crosses a spring-fed tributary lined with flowers, including columbine, monkeyflower, leopard lily, aster, and cow parsnip. Reach a junction between the Lakes Trail and Panther Gap Trail at 1.75 miles.

Remaining on the Lakes Trail, weave up the hillside and then drop down briefly to a crossing of a flower- and fern-lined tributary of Wolverton Creek. From there, a moderate climb leads to a junction at 2.1 miles, where you have two options for continuing to Heather Lake. The Watchtower Route is by far the more scenic alternative, but acrophobes may feel safer on the Hump Route, which is a quarter mile shorter but gains an additional 200 feet. The Hump Route is not completely devoid of good scenery; its high point offers fine views of Silliman Crest and The Tablelands. The following description follows the Hump Route on the way out and returns via the Watchtower Route, to keep from missing out on any fine scenery.

Veer right at the junction and follow moderate to moderately steep switchbacks through red fir forest. In the midst of the ascent, step across a tiny stream lined by strips of flower-dotted meadow. From the stream, a 0.75-mile climb leads to a fine view from a saddle known as The Hump, 3.4 miles from the trailhead. The vista is easily improved by strolling onto an open hill just past a stand of scattered trees.

A steep descent leads from the saddle down to a small flat, carpeted with pockets of heather and dotted with a smattering of lodgepole pines, where the Hump and Watchtower routes rejoin, 3.6 miles from the trailhead.

Along a brief, gentle descent, you catch a glimpse of Heather Lake below and pass a lateral to an open-air, three-sided, screened pit toilet with a fine view. A short distance beyond the lateral, reach the heather-laced shore of aptly named Heather Lake, 3.75 miles from the trailhead. A few pines once sheltered campsites around the cliff-rimmed shore, but the Park Service closed the area to camping many years ago because of overuse.

From Heather Lake, rocky trail climbs through scattered pines and around boulders out of the basin. Farther on, cross an open granite slope on a gentle grade, with fine views of Alta Peak and across Marble Fork Kaweah River canyon. Wrap around a hillside and drop into the basin holding Emerald and Aster Lakes to a crossing of the meadow-lined stream connecting the two lakes, 4.7 miles from the trailhead. Aster Lake is 0.2 mile northwest and Emerald Lake 0.1 mile southeast.

Between the lakes, an enclosed, three-hole solar toilet provides a more sophisticated convenience than the primitive one near Heather Lake, albeit without the view.

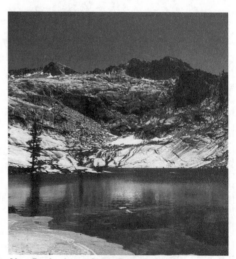

Alta Peak rises above Pear Lake.

Although camping has been banned around Aster Lake, granite slabs around the mostly open shoreline afford fine spots for sunbathing and swimming. Anglers can test their skills on rainbow trout, although fishing pressure at these popular lakes will undoubtedly be high.

Between the trail and Emerald Lake, ten designated campsites (with bear boxes) sheltered by scattered pines offer backpackers the first legal opportunity to camp between here and the trailhead.

Past the campsites, Emerald Lake sits picturesquely below Alta Peak, with steep cliffs bordering the lake on three sides. The inlet cascades dramatically down cliffs above the far shore before gracefully pouring across granite slabs into the lake. Resident brook trout will tempt the angler.

A gently ascending traverse leads from the Aster and Emerald Lakes basin around a spur ridge and into the Pear Lake basin, and small pockets of wildflowers soften the otherwise rocky surroundings. Fine views across the cleft of Marble Fork canyon and Tokopah Valley will capture your attention on the journey around the ridge. Pass the junction with the trail to the ranger station at 5.2 miles, and continue the curving ascent another half mile to the lake.

Rockbound Pear Lake is rimmed by craggy ridges and towered over by the lofty summit of Alta Peak. Widely scattered pines and small tufts of grasses find tenuous footholds in the scarce soil of this stony basin. Similar to Emerald, Pear Lake has a solar toilet and 12 designated campsites near the outlet. Anglers can fish for brook trout.

Once you are ready to leave, retrace your steps back to the junction between the Watchtower and Hump routes. From the junction, bear right and follow the trail on a gentle descent. Soon the trail starts clinging to the side of a nearly vertical cliff, with staggering views straight down to the Marble Fork, churning and careening through Tokopah Valley, the thunderous sound of the river reverberating 2,000 feet up the canyon walls. With all the drama below, don't forget to turn around to catch the view of Silliman Crest and the Kings-Kaweah Divide.

A more moderate descent ensues, eventually leading along a wedge of rock protruding into the canyon (shown as point 8973 on the *Lodgepole* USGS quadrangle). An unofficial scramble route leads bold adventurers from the trail to an extraordinary view from the top of the rock. Away from the wedge of rock, a few switchbacks lead across less precipitous slopes and into light forest. At 1.4 miles from the Watchtower and Hump routes junction, step over a vigorous creek lined with lush foliage and proceed on a moderate, 0.4-mile descent to the west junction of the two routes. From there, retrace your steps back to the trailhead.

While maintained trail ends at Pear Lake, experienced cross-country enthusiasts may continue to Moose Lake and The Tableland.

A wilderness permit is required for overnight stays. Camping is restricted to designated sites near Emerald and Pear Lakes (camping is banned at Heather and Aster Lakes). Campfires are prohibited.

TRIP 44

Tokopah Falls

E / DH

DISTANCE: 3.8 miles out-and-back

ELEVATION: 6,735'/7,335',
+700'/-40'/±1,480'

SEASON: April to late October

USE: Heavy

MAPS: USGS's *Lodgepole* or
SNHA's *Lodgepole*

INTRODUCTION: The Tokopah Falls Trail provides an easy 2-mile hike to a viewpoint of the namesake falls, where a stunning waterfall on the Marble Fork Kaweah River plunges down a steep rock wall at the head of Tokopah Valley. *Tokopah* is a Yokut word meaning "high mountain valley," quite appropriate for this dramatically picturesque vale. Early in the season, when snowmelt swells the river to peak flows, is the best time to view the falls. However, the straightforward hike is quite pleasant in summer and fall as well.

DIRECTIONS TO TRAILHEAD: From the Generals Highway, turn east at the Lodgepole junction, and drive through the campground entrance station to the hiker parking area. Walk along the campground access road to a fork past the Walter Fry Nature Center and restrooms. Veer left at the fork, cross a log bridge over Marble Fork, and find the trailhead on the right just past the bridge.

DESCRIPTION: Head away from the road on gently graded tread through mixed forest of red and white firs, incense cedars, ponderosa pines, and Jeffrey pines. The riverbanks are lined with willows, aspens, and chokecherries. Continue heading upstream along the north bank, sometimes right alongside the churning river and sometimes a fair distance away. The forest is occasionally interrupted by low granite outcrops and small grassy meadows filled with a showy display of wildflowers early in the season. Along the way up the canyon, bridges offer easy crossings of several tributary streams.

Depending on the season, you may hear Tokopah Falls well before you see the mighty cascade. Early in the season, the roar of the snowmelt-filled torrent pouring over the brink of the canyon headwall can be deafening. Eventually, the coniferous forest gives way to elderberry, oak, and manzanita growing amid piles of boulders and large

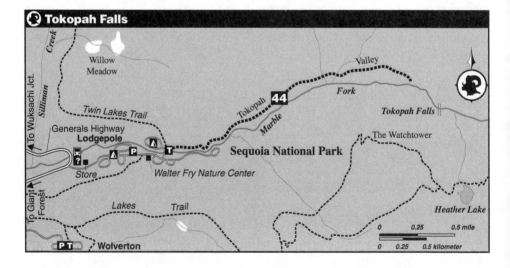

granite blocks. The open terrain allows fine views of the falls ahead and high canyon walls bordering Tokopah Valley. Across the canyon looms the mighty wall of rock known as The Watchtower, which soars 2,000 feet above the valley floor.

The trail climbs a bit more steeply through boulders and piles of granite blocks before terminating near the base of steep cliffs. A sign advises against hiking any farther up the canyon, where slippery and unstable slopes have contributed to a number of fatalities. Ahead, Tokopah Falls creates a majestic display, when a steady stream of water plummets down the steep wall at the head of the canyon.

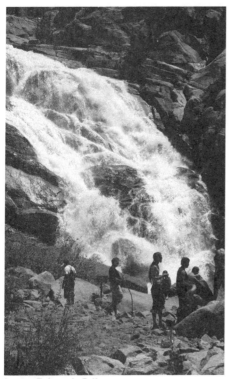

Lower Tokopah Falls

TRIP 45

Twin Lakes

Ⓜ **/** **DH** or **BP**

DISTANCE: 13.5 miles, out-and-back

ELEVATION: 6,735'/9,420',
+3,030'/-285'/±6,630'

SEASON: Late June to mid-October

USE: Moderate

MAPS: USGS's *Lodgepole* and *Mt. Silliman* or SNHA's *Lodgepole*

TRAIL LOG

1.5	Wuksachi Trail junction
2.6	Cahoon Meadow
4.0	Cahoon Gap
4.9	J O Pass junction

INTRODUCTION: The Twin Lakes Trail climbs through mixed forest, past flower-laden meadows, and over gurgling streams to a pair of popular lakes. Despite the name, these two lakes have little in common, aside from their proximity to one another, but they do provide pleasant and picturesque destinations for an overnight backpacking trip. Permits are often at a premium on weekends, and the first mile or so is a scorcher in full sun. It's best to visit the wilderness office and start up the trail as early as you can. Dayhikers who do not feel up to the task of traveling all the way to the lakes and back will find the 2.6-mile journey to Cahoon Meadow a worthy alternative.

DIRECTIONS TO TRAILHEAD: From the Generals Highway, turn east at the Lodgepole junction, and drive through the campground entrance station to the hiker parking area. Walk along the campground access road to a fork past the Walter Fry Nature Center and restrooms. Veer left at the fork, cross a log bridge over Marble Fork, and pass the Tokopah Falls Trailhead to the Twin Lakes Trailhead on the right.

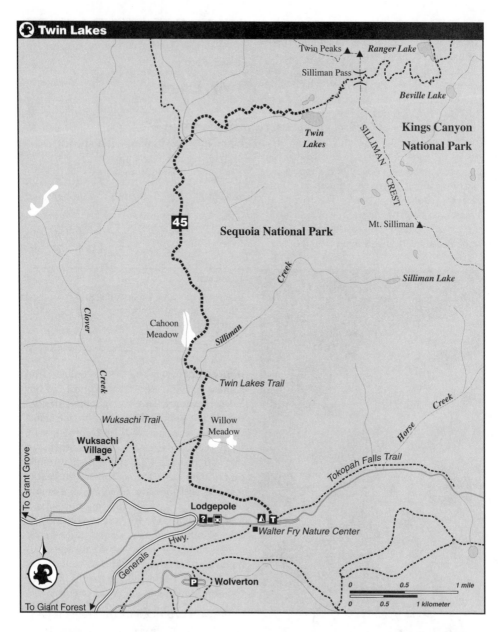

Twin Lakes

Twin Peaks ▲   *Ranger Lake*

Silliman Pass

Beville Lake

Twin Lakes

Kings Canyon National Park

SILLIMAN CREST

45

Sequoia National Park

Creek

Mt. Silliman ▲

Silliman Lake

Clover

Cahoon Meadow

Silliman

Twin Lakes Trail

Creek

Horse   *Creek*

Wuksachi Trail

Willow Meadow

Wuksachi Village

Tokopah Falls Trail

To Grant Grove

Lodgepole

■ *Walter Fry Nature Center*

Generals Hwy.

Wolverton

To Giant Forest ▶

0   0.5   1 mile

0   0.5   1 kilometer

DESCRIPTION: From the trailhead, pass through Lodgepole Campground on a nearly level, rock-lined trail amid mixed forest. Soon, the grade increases as the trail attacks the hillside above the campground. Enter thick red fir and lodgepole pine forest about a mile from the trailhead, where the trail bends north into the Silliman Creek drainage. Cross a tiny, spring-fed brook to a T-junction with the Wuksachi Trail, 1.5 miles from the trailhead.

Beyond the junction, cross a rock-filled wash, the former bed of Silliman Creek, which now flows just over a low ridge to the left. A moderate climb, incorporating rocky switchbacks, leads to the crossing of the main branch of Silliman Creek at 2.25 miles (which may be a difficult ford early in the season). Because the creek is the domestic water supply for Lodgepole, camping, swimming, fishing, and picnicking are prohibited in its vicinity.

Away from Silliman Creek, continue climbing around the nose of a south-facing spur and then head northeast to Cahoon Meadow, 2.6 miles from the trailhead. The pleasant clearing, carpeted with tall grasses and wildflowers, is a favorite haunt of the local deer herd. A few campsites sit beneath tall firs along the fringe of the meadow.

More stiff climbing leads to a lushly lined, spring-fed stream, where lupine, tiger lily, monkeyflower, and aster lend a splash of color to the greenery. From the stream, ascend to a clearing, with fine views across Cahoon Meadow, and continue up-slope, hopping across numerous rivulets lined with brilliantly colored swaths of wildflowers. The uppermost brook drains a fair-size, sloping meadow you pass on the way to Cahoon Gap, 4 miles from the trailhead.

A mild to moderate, 0.6-mile descent from the gap leads alongside East Fork Clover Creek to an easy boulder hop of a tributary and campsites (with a bear box) on the far side. Continue upstream beneath the cover of fir forest another 0.3 mile to a junction with a trail to J O Pass, 4.9 miles from the trailhead, with a few fir-sheltered campsites nearby.

Bear right (northeast) at the junction and continue a mild to moderate ascent along East Fork Clover Creek to a ford, where shooting star, leopard lily, and aster liven the banks. Away from the creek, the grade increases up a hillside, through stands of forest alternating with small clearings. Wildflowers, including leopard lily, shooting star, aster, lupine, corn lily, larkspur, cinquefoil, wallflower, golden senecio, and Mariposa lily, blanket an expansive slope. The grade eventually eases beyond a series of switchbacks. You pass an information sign and catch a glimpse of the larger Twin Lake through the trees, from where an easy stroll leads to the shoreline.

The southern lake is obviously larger, bearing very little resemblance to its smaller neighbor. The smaller lake is completely ringed by thick lodgepole pine and red fir forest. While the larger lake is similarly lined by trees on its north side, the opposite shore is made up of talus slopes and cliffs rising 600 feet above its surface. The rugged towers of Twin Peaks can be seen from spots along the shore of the larger lake. Backpackers will find overused campsites (with bear boxes) on the strip of forested land between the lakes, but less used sites can be found around both shorelines. A pit toilet is located west of the smaller lake. Fishing is fair for brook trout, and swimming in the shallow lakes can be quite pleasant during the usually hot afternoons.

Extended backpacks could be easily arranged by using the trail system in Jennie Lakes Wilderness and the southeastern corner of Kings Canyon National Park.

From Silliman Pass northeast of Twin Lakes, rock climbers can tackle short routes on Twin Peaks. Mountaineers can follow a Class 2 route on Mt. Silliman by traversing from the pass to the east ridge and following it to the summit.

A wilderness permit is required for overnight stays. Campfires are prohibited at Twin Lakes.

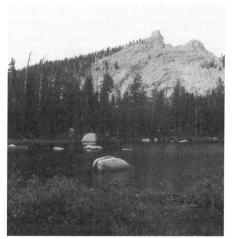

The larger Twin Lake

TRIP 46

Kings-Kaweah Divide Loop

M ↻ **BPx**

DISTANCE: 52 miles, loop

ELEVATION: 6,735'/10,185'/7,095'/
11,370'/6,735',
+14,100'/-14,100' ±28,200'

SEASON: Mid-July to October

USE: Light

MAPS: *Lodgepole, Mt. Silliman,
Sphinx Lakes,* and *Triple
Divide Peak*

TRAIL LOG

6.75	Twin Lakes
11.3	Lost Lake junction
14.9	Comanche Meadow
16.5	Sugarloaf Meadow Camp
21.0	Roaring River
28.0	Upper Ranger Meadow
31.5	Elizabeth Pass
34.1	Tamarack Lake junction
36.25	Bearpaw Meadow
43.0	Alta Trail junction

INTRODUCTION: This moderate 50-mile-plus loop allows backpackers to sample a cross section of the characteristic southern Sierra grandeur of the western side of Sequoia and Kings Canyon National Parks. The trip crosses a wide range of elevations and environments, including mid-elevation forest and subalpine and alpine zones.

The topography is equally diverse with a bounty of beautiful lakes, flower-laden meadows, glaciated canyons, and high alpine basins. Views of soaring peaks, precipitous canyon walls, and airy spires augment the incredible scenery. The potential for solitude is an added bonus; you will likely see few other backpackers between Twin Lakes and Bearpaw Meadow.

Since the loop crosses the Kings-Kaweah Divide at two high passes, Silliman and

Elizabeth, it requires a hearty effort. If you have extra days, you can easily plan forays to other locales.

DIRECTIONS TO TRAILHEAD: From the Generals Highway, turn east at the Lodgepole junction, and drive through the campground entrance station to the hiker parking area. Walk along the campground access road to a fork past the Walter Fry Nature Center and restrooms. Veer left at the fork, cross a log bridge over Marble Fork, and pass the Tokopah Falls Trailhead to the Twin Lakes Trailhead on the right.

DESCRIPTION: From the trailhead, pass through Lodgepole Campground on a nearly level, rock-lined trail amid mixed forest. Soon, the grade increases as the trail attacks the hillside above the campground. Enter thick red fir and lodgepole pine forest about a mile from the trailhead, where the trail bends north into the Silliman Creek drainage. Cross a tiny, spring-fed brook to a T-junction with the Wuksachi Trail, 1.5 miles from the trailhead.

Beyond the junction, cross a rock-filled wash, the former bed of Silliman Creek, which now flows over a low ridge to the left. A moderate climb, incorporating rocky switchbacks, leads to the crossing of the main branch of Silliman Creek at 2.25 miles (which may be a difficult ford early in the season). Because the creek is the domestic water supply for Lodgepole, camping, swimming, fishing, and picnicking are prohibited in its vicinity.

Away from Silliman Creek, continue climbing around the nose of a south-facing spur and then head northeast to Cahoon Meadow, 2.6 miles from the trailhead. The pleasant clearing, carpeted with tall grasses and wildflowers, is a favorite haunt of the local deer herd. A few campsites sit beneath tall firs along the fringe of the meadow.

More stiff climbing leads to a lushly lined, spring-fed stream, where lupine, tiger lily, monkeyflower, and aster lend a splash of color to the greenery. From the stream, ascend to a clearing, with fine views across Cahoon Meadow, and continue up-slope, hopping across numerous rivulets lined with brilliantly colored swaths of wildflowers. The uppermost brook drains a fair-size, sloping meadow you pass on the way to Cahoon Gap, 4 miles from the trailhead.

A mild to moderate, 0.6-mile descent from the gap leads alongside East Fork Clover Creek to an easy boulder hop of a tributary and campsites (with a bear box) on the far side. Continue upstream beneath the cover of fir forest another 0.3 mile to a junction with a trail to J O Pass, 4.9 miles from the trailhead, with a few fir-sheltered campsites nearby.

Bear right (northeast) at the junction and continue a mild to moderate ascent along East Fork Clover Creek to a ford, where shooting star, leopard lily, and aster liven the banks. Away from the creek, the grade increases up a hillside, through stands of forest alternating with small clearings. Wildflowers, including leopard lily, shooting star, aster, lupine, corn lily, larkspur, cinquefoil, wallflower, golden senecio, and Mariposa lily, blanket an expansive slope. The grade eventually eases beyond a series of switchbacks. You pass an information sign and catch a glimpse of the larger Twin Lake through the trees, from where an easy stroll leads to the shoreline.

The southern lake is obviously larger, bearing very little resemblance to its smaller neighbor. The smaller lake is completely ringed by thick lodgepole pine and red fir forest and, while the larger lake is similarly lined by trees on its north side, the opposite shore is made up of talus slopes and cliffs rising 600 feet above its surface. The rugged towers of Twin Peaks can be seen from spots along the shore of the larger lake. Backpackers will find overused campsites (with bear boxes) on the strip of forested land between the lakes, but less used sites can be found around both shorelines. A pit toilet is located west of the smaller lake. Fishing is fair for brook trout, and swimming in the shallow lakes can be quite pleasant during the usually hot afternoons.

From Twin Lakes, a series of switchbacks lead up a steep hillside on a winding, 700-foot climb. The trail crosses back and forth over the diminutive inlet of Twin Lakes, providing welcome opportunities to slake your thirst during the stiff ascent. Between sporadic stands of lodgepole pines views of the lakes below and Twin Peaks above improve. The grade eases on the approach to the crest and Silliman Pass, which marks the boundary between Sequoia and Kings Canyon National Parks at 7.8 miles. Widely scattered trees allow fine views of Mt. Silliman, the Great Western Divide, The Tableland, and Sugarloaf Creek below. If not for the ever present smog in San Joaquin Valley, the westward view would be equally impressive.

Steep switchbacks lead down the far side of the pass, with good views of the Kings River country, including Tehipite Dome and the Monarch Divide, along the way. Farther on, the blue surfaces of Beville and Ranger Lakes spring into view. The serpentine descent eventually eases on the floor of the lakes' basin, as you reach a junction in a stand of lodgepoles, 9.5 miles from the trailhead, where a faint path on the right branches toward Beville Lake. The grass-rimmed lake offers fine views of Mt. Silliman, but campsites are marginal.

Continue ahead from the junction for a short distance to another junction, this one with a very short lateral heading north over a low rise to Ranger Lake. Just before the lake, a posted map alerts backpackers to the location of five designated campsites (with bear boxes). A cabin nearby provides quarters for a seasonal ranger. Anglers can

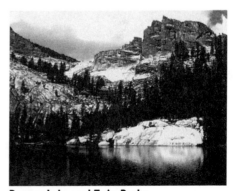

Ranger Lake and Twin Peaks

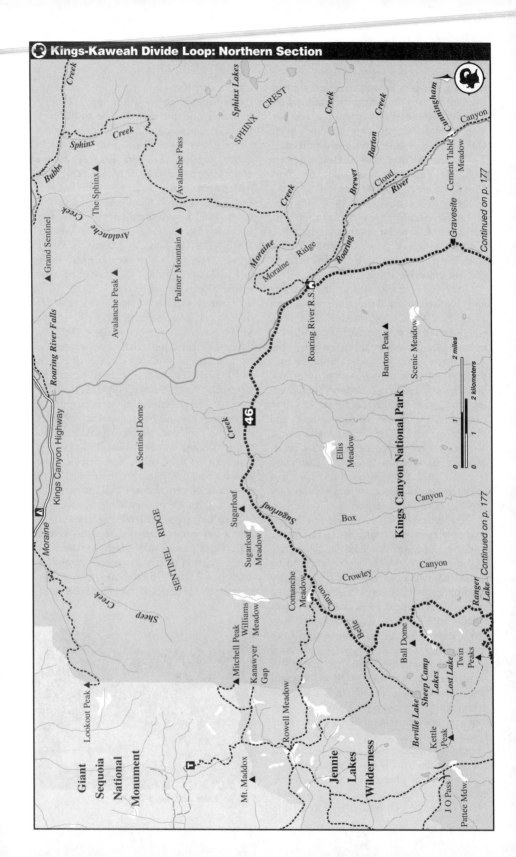

Continued on p. 177

Continued on p. 177

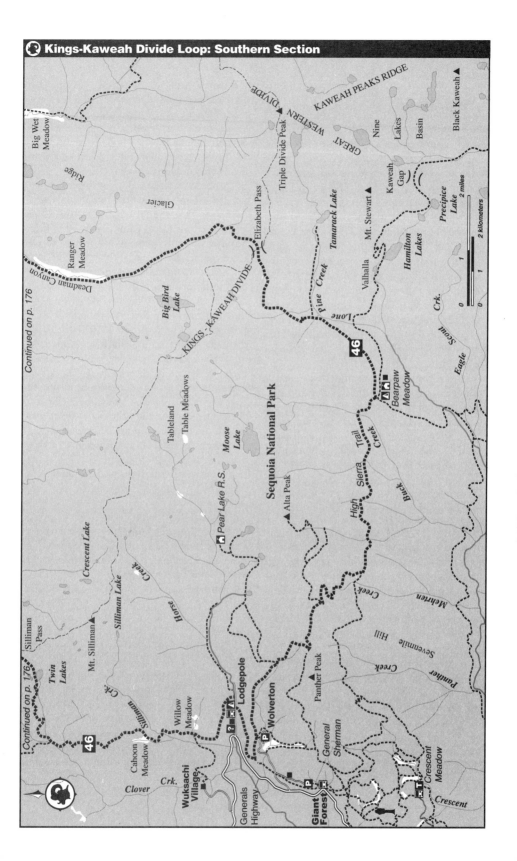

Kings-Kaweah Divide Loop: Southern Section

Continued on p. 176

Continued on p. 176

KAWEAH PEAKS RIDGE

Black Kaweah ▲

Big Wet Meadow

Nine Lakes Basin

Ridge

GREAT WESTERN DIVIDE

Glacier

Triple Divide Peak ▲

Kaweah Gap

Precipice Lake

Ranger Meadow

Elizabeth Pass

Tamarack Lake

Mt. Stewart ▲

Valhalla

Hamilton Lakes

2 miles

Deadman Canyon

Big Bird Lake

Pine Creek

2 kilometers

KINGS - KAWEAH DIVIDE

Lone

Eagle

Scout Crk.

46

Tableland

Table Meadows

Sequoia National Park

Bearpaw Meadow

Moose Lake

Pear Lake R.S.

▲ Alta Peak

Sierra Trail

High Creek

Buck

46

Crescent Lake

Silliman Lake

Creek

Horse

Creek

Mehrten

Creek

Silliman Pass

Twin Lakes

Mt. Silliman ▲

Sevenmile Hill

Panther Peak ▲

Panther Creek

46

Cahoon Meadow

Willow Meadow

Lodgepole

Wolverton

General Sherman

Crescent Meadow

Clover Crk.

Wuksachi Village

Generals Highway

Giant Forest

Crescent

ply the waters for rainbow trout around the lodgepole-encircled lake.

From the Ranger Lake junction, proceed over slabs, around boulders, and beneath widely scattered pines on a general descent, interrupted briefly by a short climb to the crest of a low ridge. Drop off the ridge, continue past a verdant pocket meadow, cross a flower-lined stream, and reach a junction with a trail to Lost Lake, 11.3 miles from the trailhead. The half-mile trail to the lake follows the fringe of a meadow before climbing a forested slope to the north shore. Picturesque Lost Lake is backdropped by the rugged cliffs of Twin Peaks and the Silliman Crest. Camping is limited to three designated campsites on the north side, since the rest of the shore has been closed for restoration. Anglers can fish for brook trout.

From the Lost Lake junction, cross a bridge over the lushly lined outlet and proceed through fir forest around the southeast flank of Ball Dome to the top of a ridge. Descend from the ridge, initially down a meadow vale, to the floor of Belle Canyon and a broad ford of Sugarloaf Creek. On the far bank is a junction with a trail to Seville Lake and Rowell Meadow, 13.1 miles from the trailhead.

○ **SIDE TRIP TO SEVILLE LAKE:** Turn east at the junction, step across a tributary of Sugarloaf Creek, and follow a gently graded path upstream through forested Belle Canyon. Eventually, the cliffs of the Kings-Kaweah Divide forming the lake's cirque appear above the treetops. Reach the north shore of lovely Seville Lake, 1.25 miles from the junction.

Granite cliffs rise above the south shore, culminating at the summit of 10,041-foot Kettle Peak. Lodgepole pines and red firs rim the marshy shoreline, shading a number of pleasant campsites. A bevy of rainbow and brook trout is sure to tempt anglers. **END OF SIDE TRIP**

Turn right (northeast) from the Seville Lake junction to follow a gently graded descent across a tributary and head down the north bank of Sugarloaf Creek. Step across a pleasant side stream, about a mile from the junction, which offers a refreshing locale for a rest stop. Continue the easy descent for another 0.4 mile to a junction, 14.6 miles from the trailhead, where a trail heads west toward Rowell Meadow.

Proceed another 0.3 mile from the junction to aspen- and willow-lined Comanche Meadow. Near the far edge of the meadow, a short path leads to campsites (with a bear box). Use trails provide access to water from the nearby creek.

From Comanche Meadow, continue downhill through lush foliage to cross a stream draining Williams Meadow. Pass into the markedly drier surroundings of a Jeffrey pine forest, site of a 1974 fire. Pass through a gate in a drift fence and drop into broad Sugarloaf Valley, with fine views through scattered trees and over clumps of manzanita of the prominent granite hump for which the valley is named. Gently graded trail across the valley floor leads to a junction of a side trail at 16.5 miles. Down this short path is a pine-shaded camping area (with a bear box and hitching post) just south of wildflower-laden Sugarloaf Meadow. A small stream nearby provides water.

Beyond the camp lateral, cross a side stream and proceed on gently graded, dusty tread through Sugarloaf Valley along the base of Sugarloaf to a ford of Sugarloaf Creek, the lowest point of the loop. Plan on getting at least your feet wet here, even during low water periods in late summer. The far bank has a couple of primitive campsites.

From the ford of Sugarloaf Creek, gently graded tread heads through denser forest and across minor rivulets to tumbling Ferguson Creek. A steep, half-mile climb from there leads to the top of a manzanita-covered and pine-dotted moraine that forms the lip of Roaring River canyon. The view from includes Palmer Mountain, the Sphinx Crest, and summits along the north end of the Great Western Divide. Living up to its name, the tumultuous river below is clearly audible.

From the moraine, a 0.75-mile descent brings you to the floor of the canyon. Pass through a gate in a drift fence and begin a steady climb up the drainage, sometimes right alongside frothy Roaring River tumbling down the canyon. Just past another fence, cross a side stream and reach the grassy clearing of fenced Scaffold Meadow, followed by a T-junction near the solar-powered Roaring River Ranger Station, 22 miles from the trailhead. Numerous campsites (with bear boxes) line the riverbanks.

From the ranger cabin, head up the canyon a short distance to a fork in the trail. The more distinct path on the left leads to additional campsites for both backpackers and equestrians; the fainter right-hand path is the Elizabeth Pass Trail.

Remaining on the west side of the river, follow the Elizabeth Pass Trail on a short, steep climb, followed by a more gently graded ascent through a light forest of red firs, Jeffrey pines, and incense cedars. Pass through a three-pole gate, and continue upstream to campsites near the ford of Deadman Canyon Creek, 1.6 miles from the junction.

Beyond the creek, cross a wildflower-covered meadow while enjoying good views of the steep cliffs and granite walls of the canyon. For the next 1.5 miles, the landscape alternates between groves of mixed forest and pockets of clearing, where good views of the glacier-scoured canyon complement colorful wildflowers. Sporadic swaths of young aspens testify to the numerous avalanches that have roared down the canyon walls.

Pass through a long meadow, where the creek glides sinuously through grasses and flowers. A use trail accesses campsites at the near end of the meadow, and a short way beyond is the gravesite for which the canyon received its name.

Ford the creek again, and then continue upstream on a gently graded ascent around boulders and through wildflowers and shrubs to a picturesque scene, where the creek spills down a series of slabs. Past another drift fence, you ascend moderately through more lush foliage to a stand of

DEADMAN CANYON

Before the current designation, the canyon was known as Copper Canyon, for a copper mine near the head. An old sign cryptically inscribed HERE REPOSES ALFRED MONIERE, SHEEPHERDER, MOUNTAIN MAN, 18–1887, marks the grave. Little else is known about the deceased, which has fueled a variety of interesting tales. One version has the Basque shepherd murdered, while another has him taking ill and passing away before his partner could make the two-week round-trip to Fresno and back for a doctor. Whatever the cause of death, a more beautiful final resting place is hard to imagine; the meadow is blessed with a sweeping panorama of the granite cathedral. Aspens and pines dot the meadow, and columbine, delphinium, daisy, Mexican hat, penstemon, pennyroyal, and shooting star are among the numerous flower species gracing the surroundings.

lodgepole pines and firs where the grade eases. Break out of the trees into the extensive grasslands of Ranger Meadow, where the steep canyon walls and peaks at its head combine to create a spectacular view across the flower-bedecked meadow.

Stroll to the far end of the meadow, and begin a moderate ascent through scattered lodgepole pines to cross a lushly lined tributary. Continue the steady climb across rocky slopes dotted with heather to a ford of the vigorous main channel of the creek. A moderate to moderately steep climb leads through a rock garden and through another drift fence to the edge of Upper Ranger Meadow. Just off the trail to the right in a grove of pines are a couple of good campsites, 6.1 miles from the Roaring River junction.

◎ **CROSS-COUNTRY SIDE TRIP TO BIG BIRD LAKE:** From the campsites in Upper Ranger

Meadow, cross the main channel of the creek and climb up a steep hillside, staying well to the left of the deep cleft of the outlet of Big Bird Lake. Sections of a boot-beaten path may be evident, but if they are not, the route is straightforward although quite steep. Work your way up to a bench overlooking the lake and several small ponds to the north, and then drop easily to the lakeshore. Big Bird Lake is long and narrow, cradled in a U-shaped alpine cirque below the crest of the Kings-Kaweah Divide. A few wind-battered lodgepole pines cling tenuously to the sparse soil around the lake, affording little protection from the elements to campsites on sandy flats above the north shore. The view down Deadman Canyon from the lake is quite stunning. **END OF SIDE TRIP**

Follow the gently graded trail in Upper Ranger Meadow through sagebrush, grasses, sedges, and wildflowers to where the grade increases and the trail draws near the creek, which is lined with low-growing willows and clumps of flowers. Approaching the canyon headwall, the trail climbs more steeply and starts switchbacking up a rocky slope. After crossing the creek, the trail veers southwest to ascend a talus- and boulder-filled cirque on an interminable set of switchbacks. Finally, the immediate goal comes into view, as you zigzag up dirt trail to fine views at Elizabeth Pass, 9.4 miles from the Roaring River junction.

Although the 2,100-foot ascent is now behind you, a perhaps more difficult challenge awaits, as you begin a 3,300-foot, knee-wrenching descent to the Tamarack Lake Trail junction. Initially, good views of Moose and Lost Lakes from just below the pass may help to cheer you, as may a profusion of wildflowers on the more hospitable slopes below. Farther down, views of Lion Rock, Mt. Stewart, and Eagle Scout Peak issue a siren call to backpackers and mountaineers with extra time for side trips up the Tamarack Lake and High Sierra Trails. The switchbacks eventually end, and the grade eases on the approach to the Tamarack Lake junction, 2.7 miles from the pass and 12.1 miles from the Roaring River junction.

SIDE TRIP TO TAMARACK LAKE: To visit Tamarack Lake, turn east from the junction, and cross a boulder field to a ford of Lonely Lake's outlet. Just past the ford, a use trail leads shortly to campsites. Soon the grade increases, climbing above a scenic stair-step falls to sloping Lone Pine Meadow, backdropped regally by Lion Rock and Mt. Stewart, as well as a bounty of unnamed rock towers and ramparts on the canyon rim. Continue climbing, initially through a tangle of grasses, ferns, and flowers, followed by the drier vegetation of manzanita and sagebrush. Reach the pleasant surroundings of Tamarack Meadow, stroll through wildflowers to the far end, and cross triple-branched Tamarack Creek. A short climb from there leads to Tamarack Lake, 1.8 miles from the junction. The picturesque lake nestles in an impressive rock amphitheater, capped by Mt. Stewart and Lion Rock. Plenty of campsites are scattered around the lake. Brook trout will tantalize anglers. **END OF SIDE TRIP**

From the Tamarack Lake junction, make a short, gently graded descent to a junction with the Over the Hill Trail (your route)

ELIZABETH PASS

Elizabeth Pass was once known as Turtle Pass, named for a rock about four feet long near its east side, which bears a striking resemblance to the reptile. In 1905, author Stewart Edward White, along with his wife and another man, traveled up Deadman Canyon, crossed the Kings-Kaweah Divide at the pass, and then descended steep cliffs to Lone Pine Meadow. Their adventure was originally chronicled in *Outing* magazine, and later in White's book *The Pass*. The name of the pass was subsequently changed to Elizabeth in honor of White's wife.

and a connecting trail to the High Sierra Trail (HST).

Veer right onto the Over the Hill Trail, and climb stiffly up the northwest wall of Middle Fork Kaweah River canyon. Where the slope is open, fine views abound to the east, initially of the rugged terrain surrounding Lone Pine Creek canyon and farther on, after an intervening stretch of forest, of similarly dramatic terrain up Hamilton Creek drainage. The grade eases on a traverse around the brow of a ridge, passing through lush vegetation and then thickening fir forest. After 2.1 miles, reach a T-junction with the HST. The ranger station and Bearpaw High Sierra Camp are just 200 yards to the left (east), while the lateral to Bearpaw Meadows backpacker camp is about the same distance to the right (west).

The next leg of the journey follows the famed HST. Begin on a switchbacking descent through a forest of sugar pines and firs to a bridge over Buck Creek. From there, ascend the mostly open slopes of Buck Canyon, and then bend around to the crossing of a twin-branched tributary with fine campsites nearby (with a bear box). A long, rolling traverse leads across the north wall of Middle Fork Kaweah River canyon, crossing several refreshing brooks along the way. Excellent views of the canyon and Little Blue Dome, Sugarbowl Dome, and Castle Rocks appear through periodic breaks in the forest. Reach the Sevenmile Hill junction, 4.6 miles from Bearpaw Meadow.

Turn right (northwest) from the junction and follow the Sevenmile Hill Trail on a steep, half-mile climb through thick stands of white fir and incense cedar to a crossing of Mehrten Creek. Continue the unrelenting ascent past the creek, weaving uphill through Jeffrey pines and manzanita to the crossing of two invigorated branches of the creek. The grade eventually eases where the trail bends west and traverses back over the creek and some rills. Beyond the traverse, a series of switchbacks lead up to a junction with the Alta Trail, 2.1 miles from and 1,300 feet above the HST junction. Campsites at Mehrten Meadow are just a short, quarter-mile descent east of the junction.

Turn west onto the Alta Trail at the junction and descend a series of short-legged switchbacks to a spring-fed rivulet. Proceed across a south-facing, open hillside, enjoying views of Middle Fork Kaweah River canyon on the way to a T-junction at Panther Gap, 1 mile from the previous junction.

Leaving the Alta Trail at Panther Gap, head north on a short, moderate descent into the Wolverton Creek drainage. Reaching the valley floor, proceed past meadows, lush foliage, and wildflower-lined tributaries, following the creek downstream. Nearly a mile from Panther Gap, reach a junction with the Lakes Trail.

Turn left (west) and follow the Lakes Trail for 1.6 miles, roughly paralleling Wolverton Creek, first northwest and then west on a mild to moderate descent to a pair of T-junctions. From the first junction, a trail heads southeast to circle around Long Meadow; from the second junction, a trail heads south to the Wolverton trailhead. Continue ahead (west) at both junctions, and follow a half-mile descent toward Wolverton Creek. Just before the creek, turn right onto an old roadbed, and follow the road on a 1.25-mile descent to the parking area at Lodgepole.

This trip offers several options for returning to trailheads other than Lodgepole. You could use the shuttle bus, arrange for someone to pick you up, or travel west on the HST to any of a variety of trailheads in the Giant Forest.

Hikers with more time can extend this trip in numerous ways. Perhaps the most attractive would be visiting Hamilton Lakes or Nine Lakes Basin via the HST.

A wilderness permit is required for overnight stays. Campfires are prohibited at Twin Lakes and Tamarack Lake, in Bearpaw Meadow, and above 10,400 feet. Camping is restricted to designated sites at Ranger Lake and Lost Lake and in Bearpaw Meadow.

WUKSACHI TRAILHEAD

TRIP 47

Wuksachi Trail

Ⓜ ↗ **DH**

DISTANCE: 3 miles, out-and-back

ELEVATION: 7,025'/6,890'/7,230',
+220'/-430'/±1,300'

SEASON: Late June to mid-October

USE: Light

MAPS: USGS's *Lodgepole* or
SNHA's *Lodgepole*

INTRODUCTION: Built primarily for guests staying at Wuksachi Lodge, the Wuksachi Trail is a secluded forest walk that connects the village to the Twin Lakes Trail. Along the way, hikers cross a pair of impressive bridges over Clover and Silliman Creeks. By using the shuttle bus, you can enjoy a 3-mile, one-way hike from Wuksachi to Lodgepole via the Twin Lakes Trail.

DIRECTIONS TO TRAILHEAD: From the Generals Highway, 1.5 miles north of the Lodgepole junction, turn north toward Wuksachi Village. Follow paved road past the village center to the farthest parking lot, and park near the trailhead at the far end.

DESCRIPTION: A small sign marked TWIN LAKES 7.3, LODGEPOLE 3.1 is all that marks the trailhead. Head into moderately thick fir forest, soon following three switchbacks down-slope to a bridge across Clover Creek, which flows through a rocky gorge into a series of delightful pools. Beyond the bridge, another set of switchbacks climbs up the forested slope, followed by an arcing traverse around the nose of a ridge separating the Clover and Silliman Creeks drainages. The traverse passes through drier vegetation of Jeffrey pines and manzanita, where the forest thins enough briefly to allow a view across the Lodgepole area to Wolverton Ridge.

Curve into the Silliman Creek drainage, and drop down to a crossing of the creek on another stout bridge. Since Silliman Creek is the domestic water supply for Lodgepole, swimming, camping, fishing, and picnicking are prohibited. Gently graded trail follows a tributary draining Willow Meadow to a junction of the Twin Lakes Trail.

Rather than backtrack to Wuksachi Village, you could turn right (south) at the junction, follow the Twin Lakes Trail 1.5 miles to Lodgepole, and then catch the Route 3 shuttle bus back to the village.

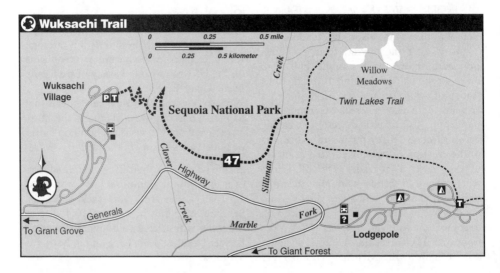

Introduction to Dorst Creek

The main attraction of this heavily wooded area is Dorst Creek Campground, from where a handful of trails lead dayhikers on wooded journeys through some of the quietest sections of Sequoia. Covered primarily with red and white firs, the Dorst Creek area houses some excellent giant sequoia groves as well, including the most easily accessed stand, Lost Grove, 2.5 miles north of Dorst Campground and just off the Generals Highway. In contrast, one of the best collections of the Big Trees in either Sequoia or Kings Canyon is found within Muir Grove, tucked quietly away from the road down a serene 2-mile trail. Trees are not the only feature found around Dorst Creek; a 1.75-mile path to the top of Little Baldy offers a fine vista.

Dorst Creek and Campground were named for Joseph Haddox Dorst (1852–1916), captain of the 4th Calvary, who was the first superintendent of Sequoia National Park.

ACCESS: Dorst Creek has straightforward access from the Generals Highway during

Campground

Campground	Fee	Elevation	Season	Restrooms	Water	Bear Boxes	Phone
Dorst Creek (28.9 miles from Ash Mountain Entrance)	$20	6,800 feet	Late June through Labor Day	Flush	Yes	Yes	Yes

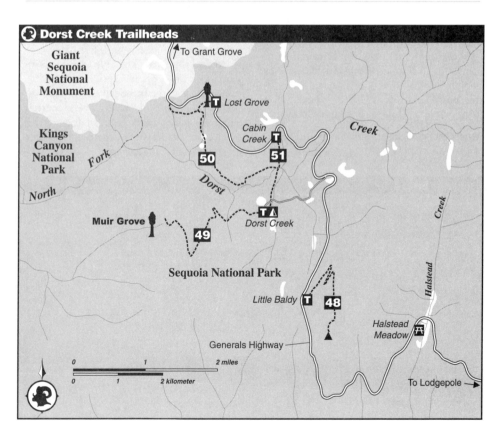

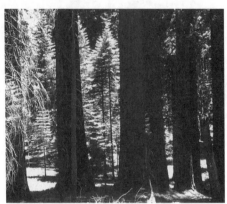

Circle Grove, Muir Grove Trail

TRIP 48

Little Baldy

M / DH

DISTANCE: 3.5 miles, out-and-back

ELEVATION: 7,335'/8,044',
+735'/-85'/±1,640'

SEASON: June to mid-October

USE: Moderate

MAP: *Giant Forest*

spring, summer, and fall. Snow may close this section of the Generals Highway during winter storms, between the Y-intersection with Highway 180 and a gate just north of Wuksachi. Dorst Creek Campground is 28.9 miles from the Ash Mountain Entrance and 17.3 miles from the Y-intersection.

AMENITIES: Lodgepole provides the closest services to Dorst Creek at 8.1 miles. Grant Grove is 17.6 miles northwest. The closest lodging to the south is at Wuksachi and to the north is at Stony Creek Village, Montecitio Sequoia Lodge, or Grant Grove.

RANGER STATION: Lodgepole and Grant Grove are the nearest ranger stations.

INTRODUCTION: An excellent vista requiring less than a 4-mile hike should be enough to lure any self-respecting hiker with two to four hours to spare. The moderate climb to the top of Little Baldy follows a well-graded trail to what is arguably one of western Sequoia's supreme views. So wide ranging is this vista that the Park Service used to maintain a fire lookout on Little Baldy.

Make sure you start your hike with plenty of water because none is available anywhere near the trailhead or on the trail. Despite the lack of water, a few parties spend the night each year on top of this granite dome, drawn by the incomparable sunsets and fine stargazing.

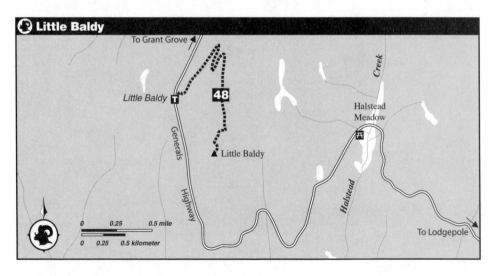

DIRECTIONS TO TRAILHEAD: Follow the Generals Highway to Little Baldy Saddle, 6.6 miles north of Lodgepole and 17 miles south of the Y-intersection with Highway 180. Park your vehicle along the shoulder as space allows.

DESCRIPTION: Begin by walking up a lightly forested hillside composed mainly of red firs with a smattering of Jeffrey pines. After a pair of switchbacks, proceed on a steady, moderate climb, as the trail slices northeast across the steep hillside, roughly paralleling the highway below. Sporadic gaps in the forest allow glimpses of Big Baldy to the northwest and the craggy spires of Chimney Rock directly ahead. Farther up the hillside, three more switchbacks lead to gently graded hiking along the ridgecrest through pockets of forest and manzanita and oak. A short, rocky climb takes you to the top and the extraordinary view.

From the summit, a splendid vista unfolds of the Great Western Divide to the east, plus Castle Rocks and the valley of Mineral King to the southeast. Southwest is a rugged, remote section of Sequoia, where a once-prominent network of trails has now mostly disappeared, succumbing to a lack of maintenance and encroaching brush.

DORST CREEK TRAILHEADS

TRIP 49

Muir Grove

M ↗ **DH**

DISTANCE: 4.2 miles, out-and-back

ELEVATION: 6,715'/6,800', +530'/-515'/±2,090'

SEASON: June through October

USE: Light

MAP: *Muir Grove*

INTRODUCTION: A rare gem, Muir Grove is tucked away from the hordes of tourists who frequent the more popular giant sequoia groves. The 1-mile drive from the Generals Highway through Dorst Campground, combined with the 2-mile hike to the grove seems enough to deter the general public, allowing willing hikers to stand among the Big Trees in relative seclusion. If John Muir himself were still alive to see the natural features bearing his name, he almost certainly would enjoy the peace and quiet of this grove of stately trees.

DIRECTIONS TO TRAILHEAD: Follow the Generals Highway to the entrance to Dorst Campground, 17.3 miles southeast of the Y-intersection with Highway 180 and 8 miles northwest of Lodgepole. Proceed through the campground approximately 0.8 mile, turn onto the road to the group campground, and continue to the trailhead parking area near the northeast end of parking area B.

DESCRIPTION: Walk back down the access road from the parking area to the start of single-track trail near a small metal sign marking the trailhead. Immediately cross a delightful tributary of Dorst Creek on a log bridge, and follow gently descending tread to a signed junction with a connector heading north to Dorst Creek.

Turn sharply left at the junction and traverse around a hillside, staying well

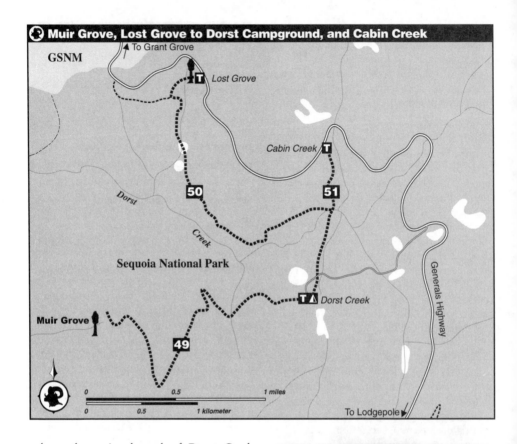

Muir Grove, Lost Grove to Dorst Campground, and Cabin Creek

GSNM

To Grant Grove

T Lost Grove

Cabin Creek T

50

51

Dorst

Creek

Sequoia National Park

Muir Grove

49

T △ Dorst Creek

Generals Highway

0   0.5   1 miles

0   0.5   1 kilometer

To Lodgepole

above the main channel of Dorst Creek to the crossing of another tributary at 0.6 mile from the trailhead. A moderate descent augmented by a pair of switchbacks follows, leading to the crest of a ridge and an exposed granite hump, from where there are fine views of Chimney Rock, Big Baldy, and the densely forested drainages of Stony and Dorst Creeks. The confluence of these two streams, amid rugged and virtually inaccessible terrain, is the birthplace of the North Fork Kaweah River. Careful observation should reveal giant sequoia crowns rising above lesser conifers directly across the canyon.

From the viewpoint, proceed in and out of a mixed forest composed of firs, pines, and cedars on a slightly undulating traverse to the crossing of a flower-lined stream, 1.5 miles from the trailhead. From there, follow gently ascending tread to the top of a ridge,

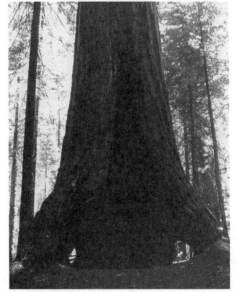

Cave Tree in Muir Grove

passing pockets of azalea and small groves of dogwood along the way.

Shortly after cresting the ridge, you reach the first of the Big Trees, a pair of burned remnants and a massive sequoia standing just off the trail. A short distance farther is perhaps the highlight of Muir Grove, a circle of a dozen or so giant sequoias arranged in a nearly symmetrical pattern. Standing within this ring of Goliaths creates a feeling of reverent awe, aptly fitting for such a grand cathedral. Short, faint paths wander away to other sequoias scattered around the grove, but the old trail that once continued on to Skagway Grove, Hidden Springs, and North Fork Kaweah River is overgrown and very difficult to follow.

DORST CREEK TRAILHEADS

TRIP 50

Lost Grove to Dorst Campground

E / **DH**

DISTANCE: 2.3 miles, point-to-point

ELEVATION: 6,645'/6,245'/6,665', +555'/-545'/±1,000'

SEASON: May to mid-October

USE: Light

MAP: *Muir Grove*

see map on p.186

INTRODUCTION: This pleasant hike begins at Lost Grove, where hundreds of giant sequoias live within a 50-plus-acre sanctuary. Unfortunately, the Lost Grove Trail visits only a fraction of the grove's many sequoias and quickly leaves the stately monarchs behind, visiting refreshing streams, rills, and verdant pocket meadows on the way to Dorst Campground.

Relatively quiet year-round, after Dorst Campground closes for the season after Labor Day, this trip may offer a large dose of solitude, but it requires nearly an extra mile of walking on the campground road to reach a vehicle-accessible end point at the campground entrance on the Generals Highway. For a fine trip extension, an unmarked path just prior to the campground provides a short connection to the Muir Grove Trail (see Trip 49, page 185).

No one seems to remember how Lost Grove became lost in the first place, or how it was found again. Prior to the creation of Kings Canyon National Park in 1940, Lost Grove served as the entrance station to Sequoia.

DIRECTIONS TO TRAILHEAD:

START: Follow the Generals Highway to the Lost Grove parking area, 10.2 miles from Lodgepole and 14.7 miles from the Y-intersection with Highway 180.

END: Follow the Generals Highway to the entrance to Dorst Campground, 17.3 miles southeast of the Y-intersection with Highway 180 and 8 miles northwest of Lodgepole. Proceed through the campground approximately 0.8 mile, turn onto the road to the group campground, and continue to the trailhead parking area near the northeast end of parking area B.

DESCRIPTION: The signed trail begins below the south side of the highway, near a restroom building. First, zigzag steeply down the fern-carpeted hillside through mixed forest containing a nice assemblage of giant sequoias. Soon cross a tiny tributary of Dorst Creek and reach an unsigned junction at 0.3 mile. The seldom-used trail to the right ends after a half mile at the Generals Highway, near the park boundary.

Continue downhill from the junction, passing through more ferns and some azaleas and walking alongside the tributary for a spell, before hopping over a rivulet near a small pocket meadow. Soon cross a pair of tiny brooks near the upper end of a thin band of meadow, and after a short while, leave the lush ground cover behind. An ascending traverse through drier vegetation follows, leading to a junction with the Cabin Creek Trail, 2 miles from the Lost Grove Trailhead.

A short drop from the junction leads to willow-lined Dorst Creek, which has some boulders and logs that hikers can use to cross. Use caution here in early season when the stream is swollen with meltwater. Beyond the creek, climb a short slope and pass above an appealing little tributary that the trail follows to Dorst Campground. A short, moderate climb leads to an unsigned junction with a path on the right, a connector to the Muir Grove Trail a quarter mile below the campground.

From the junction, continue climbing a short distance to the ending trailhead at Dorst Campground.

DORST CREEK TRAILHEADS

TRIP 51

Cabin Creek Trail

 / DH

DISTANCE: 0.8 mile, point-to-point

ELEVATION: 6,710'/6,545'/6,665', +165'/-120'/±285'

SEASON: May to mid-October

USE: Light

MAP: *Muir Grove*

see map on p.186

INTRODUCTION: The short trail down Cabin Creek and on to Dorst Campground won't knock your socks off with stunning views, but for an easy stroll through a serene forest with few people it can't be beat. If you happen to be camping at Dorst Campground, this short trip is a fine diversion.

DIRECTIONS TO TRAILHEAD:

START: Follow the Generals Highway to Cabin Creek, 9.1 miles from Lodgepole and 14.1 miles from the Y-intersection with Highway 180.

END: Follow the Generals Highway to the entrance to Dorst Campground, 17.3 miles southeast of the Y-intersection with Highway 180 and 8 miles northwest of Lodgepole. Proceed through the campground approximately 0.8 mile, turn onto the road to the group campground, and continue to the trailhead parking area near the northeast end of parking area B.

DESCRIPTION: Find the beginning of the unmarked trail just below the turnout on the south shoulder, just west of the bridge. Head downstream through light, mixed forest along the course of Cabin Creek, which puts on a frothy display in early summer. Nearly a half mile from the highway, reach a junction with the Lost Grove Trail on the right, and continue descending briefly to the low point of the journey at willow-lined Dorst Creek. The creek offers good pools for fishing or swimming.

Beyond the creek, climb up a short slope and pass above an appealing little tributary that the trail follows to Dorst Campground. A short, moderate climb leads to an unsigned junction with a path on the right, a connector to the Muir Grove Trail a quarter mile below the campground.

From the junction, continue climbing a short distance to the ending trailhead at Dorst Campground.

Introduction to Giant Sequoia National Monument and Jennie Lakes Wilderness

A relatively small parcel of Sequoia National Forest sits to the northwest of Sequoia National Park, virtually surrounding the thin, westernmost finger of Kings Canyon National Park. A 10,500-acre section of the forest was designated in 1984 as the Jennie Lakes Wilderness. Most of the remaining acreage was declared part of Giant Sequoia National Monument in 2000.

Jennie Lakes Wilderness is a compact slice of land, somewhat forgotten in the shadow of the more famous parks. The

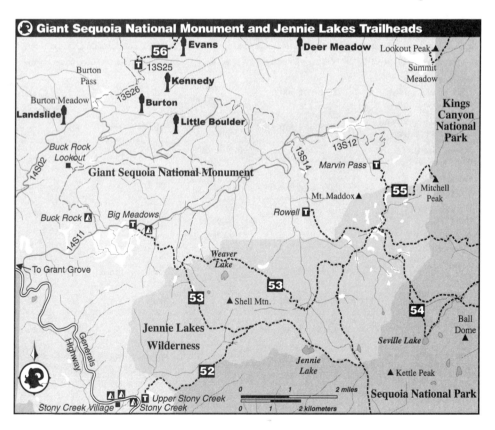

Giant Sequoia National Monument and Jennie Lakes Trailheads

area is lightly used providing dayhikers and backpackers with plenty of opportunities on 26 miles of maintained trail. A fine network of connecting trails provides access into the parks' backcountry. Despite the wilderness's small size, its topography is quite diverse, with a fine mixture of scenic lakes, serene forest, rushing streams, grassy meadows, and craggy peaks. Early season offers the added bonus of an excellent display of wildflowers.

Giant Sequoia National Monument is an eclectic mixture of development and neglected forest. While backcountry excursions are virtually nonexistent, a few little-used hiking trails lead to some interesting features. Hopefully, as time passes, roads will be closed, logging curtailed, and funding increased in order to improve recreational opportunities within the monument.

ACCESS: The most direct entry to these Forest Service lands is via Highway 180

(Kings Canyon Highway), which is open year-round to the Hume junction (10.3 miles north of the Y-intersection with the Generals Highway). From spring through fall, Hume Lake can be accessed from the Generals Highway at Quail Flat via Tenmile Road, or from Kings Canyon Highway at Hume Junction via Hume Road. Secondary roads branching out from both Highway 180 and the Generals Highway provide access to trailheads. The Generals Highway is subject to winter closures during storms from the Y-intersection to a gate north of Wuksachi.

AMENITIES: Grant Grove, with a range of services, is relatively close to most of the trailheads in this section. Facilities open to the public at Hume Lake include a general store with gas pumps, a gift shop, snack bar, and boat rentals. Montecito Sequoia Lodge, off the Generals Highway 8.9 miles south-east of the Y-intersection, offers year-round

Campgrounds

Campground (all are USFS)	Fee	Elevation	Season	Restrooms	Water	Bear Boxes	Phone
Stony Creek (28.9 miles from Ash Mountain Entrance)	$20	6,800 feet	Mid-May to late September	Flush	Yes	Yes	Yes
Upper Stony Creek (Generals Highway)	$16	6,450 feet	Mid-May to late September	Vault	Yes	Yes	Yes
Horse Camp (Big Meadows Road)	Free	7,600 feet	May to early October	Vault	No	Yes	No
Buck Rock (FS 13S04)	Free	7,600 feet	May to early September	Vault	No	Yes	No
Big Meadows (Big Meadows Road)	Free	7,600 feet	May to early October	Vault	No	Yes	No
Tenmile (Tenmile Road)	$16	5,800 feet	Late May to late September	Vault	No	Yes	No
Landslide (Tenmile Road)	$16	5,800 feet	Late May to late September	Vault	No	Yes	No
Logger Flat (Tenmile Road)	$123	5,300 feet	Mid-May to mid-September	Vault	Yes	Yes	No
Aspen Hollow Group (Tenmile Road)	$225	5,300 feet	Mid-May to mid-September	Vault	Yes	Yes	No
Hume Lake (Hume Road)	$20	5,200 feet	Mid-May to late September	Flush	Yes	Yes	Yes
Princess (Hwy. 180)	$18	5,900 feet	Mid-May to early September	Vault	Yes	Yes	No

lodging (800-227-9900, **www.montecitose-quoia.com**). Stony Creek Village, 12.5 miles southeast of the Y-intersection, has motel-style accommodations and a general store, open between mid-May and mid-October (866-522-6966, **www.sequoia-kingscanyon.com**).

RANGER STATION: The nearest Sequoia National Forest ranger station is the Hume Lake Ranger District, located in Dunlap off Highway 180. Wilderness permits are not required for overnight stays, unless you plan to enter the parks. Forest Service personnel can issue a wilderness permit for groups originating in the national forest and subsequently entering the parks. You must have a valid campfire permit if you plan to have a campfire within Sequoia National Forest; stop in at any USFS ranger station to get one.

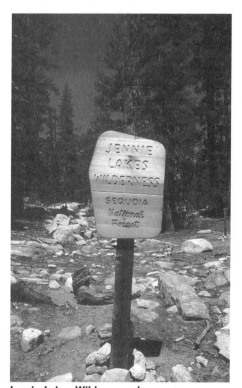

Jennie Lakes Wilderness sign

TRIP 52

Stony Creek Trail to Jennie Lake

S ↗ **DH or BP**

DISTANCE: 11.5 miles, out-and-back

ELEVATION: 6,575'/9,185'/9,015', +2,875'/-405'/±6,560'

SEASON: Mid-June to early October

USE: Light

MAPS: USGS's *Muir Grove* or USFS's *A Guide to the Monarch Wilderness & Jennie Lakes Wilderness*

INTRODUCTION: Jennie Lakes Wilderness is a nearly forgotten parcel of the western Sierra tucked between two popular national parks. The Generals Highway provides straightforward access to this gem via the Upper Stony Creek Trailhead. However, once the trail begins, the easy part ends at the start of a stiff, 4.25-mile climb to appropriately named Poop Out Pass. The upper part of the steep ascent offers fine views of the surrounding terrain, which may make the pain and suffering a bit more bearable. An early start is highly recommended to avoid the midday heat during the climb. Beyond the pass, the final 1.5-mile forested journey to Jennie Lake is much more pleasant and the lake is a fine reward for the labor involved in getting there.

DIRECTIONS TO TRAILHEAD: Follow the Generals Highway to the turnoff for Upper Stony Creek Campground, 11.3 miles southeast of the Y-intersection with Highway 180 and 12.2 miles northwest of Lodgepole. Proceed to the upper end of the campground and the small parking area near the Stony Creek Trailhead. A walk-in section of the campground provides a first-night option for backpackers who want to get an early start the next morning.

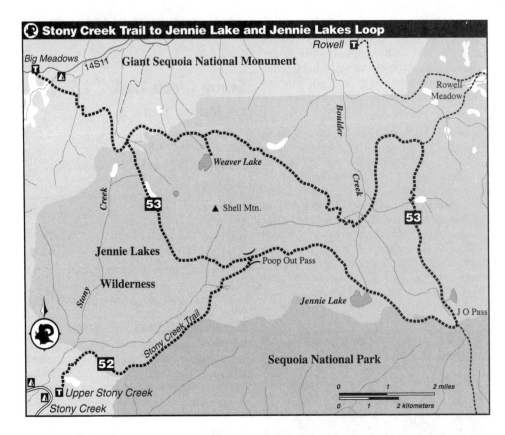

Stony Creek Trail to Jennie Lake and Jennie Lakes Loop

DESCRIPTION: From the get-go, the Stony Creek Trail attacks the slopes above with a vengeance on a continuous, moderate to moderately steep climb through a scattered to light forest of red firs, with a smattering of western white and Jeffrey pines. Although the trail bears the name Stony Creek, it spends very little time near the stream and instead climbs high above the floor of the canyon. A half mile from the campground, you cross into the signed Jennie Lakes Wilderness.

The long, steady ascent continues, as the trail weaves along the boundary between Sierra National Forest and Kings Canyon National Park. The roar of a nearby waterfall, where Stony Creek spills precipitously over a slab of granite, becomes more pronounced with the gain in elevation. Unfortunately, the forest cover never allows a good view of this picturesque cascade,

forcing would-be admirers to forsake the trail and head across a steep hillside to gain a better vantage. Farther up the trail, the Kings-Kaweah Divide springs into view from an exposed, rocky ridge.

Discernible tread disappears for a short stretch, but by simply following the rocky ridgecrest you can regain the trail higher up the slope. Returning to forest cover, the grade finally eases where the trail bends away from the crest and heads over to a crossing of twin-channeled Stony Creek, 3.25 miles from the trailhead. Away from the creek, you soon leave behind the pleasantly graded stretch of trail, and the stiff ascent resumes through mixed forest. Reach a T-junction, 0.6 mile from the creek, with the Jennie Lake Trail from Big Meadow.

Veer right at the junction, and make an easier climb to the forested saddle of Poop Out Pass (9,140 feet), aptly named in light of the previously steep climb. The pass offers no view, but a 0.8-mile, 450-foot, straightforward ascent of nearby Shell Mountain to the northwest offers rewarding vistas from the 9,594-foot summit.

Gratefully leaving the climbing behind, drop moderately from the pass to a switch-back and then follow a mostly gentle, mile-long descending traverse across exfoliated granodiorite slopes, with occasional views of rugged peaks. A final, gently rising ascent through the trees leads to a junction at 5.7 miles from the trailhead.

Turn right (south) and follow a short spur to the north shore of lovely Jennie Lake. Jennie, named in 1897 by S. L. N. Ellis of the Sierra Forest Preserve for his wife, is a kidney-shaped lake cradled in a basin at the talus-covered foot of an exfoliated granite peak with a pyramid-shaped summit. A light forest of lodgepole pines and red firs shelters campsites along the lake's outlet. Swimmers can take a refreshing dip, and anglers can test their skills on the resident rainbow trout.

Jennie Lakes Wilderness has a fine network of trails offering a variety of possibilities for extending a trip. A straightforward extension follows the description in Trip 53. Other trails offer connections leading into the adjoining parks.

Wilderness permits are not required and campfires are legal.

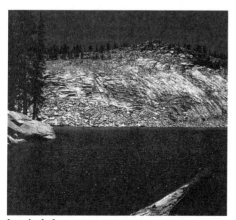

Jennie Lake

BIG MEADOWS ROAD TRAILHEADS

TRIP 53

Jennie Lakes Loop

M **↺** **BP**

DISTANCE: 17.8 miles, loop

ELEVATION: 7,615'/9,645', +4,135'/-4,135'/±8,270'

SEASON: Mid-June to early October

USE: Light

MAPS: USGS's *Muir Grove* and *Mt. Silliman* or USFS's *A Guide to the Monarch Wilderness & Jennie Lakes Wilderness*

see map on p.192

TRAIL LOG

2.0	Loop junction
3.1	Weaver Lake junction
7.5	Rowell Meadow Trail junction
10.1	J O Pass
11.5	Jennie Lake junction
13.4	Poop Out Pass and Stony Creek Trail junction
15.8	Loop junction

INTRODUCTION: Pleasant lakes with craggy backdrops, rushing streams, grassy meadows, and shady forests lure backpackers away from the more glamorous national parks and into lightly used Jennie Lakes Wilderness. The 13-mile Jennie Lakes Loop is perhaps the ultimate way to experience the 10,500-acre wilderness, well suited for a weekend journey, although extra days could easily be spent languishing along the shores of either Jennie or Weaver Lakes. Throw in some good views from various points along the loop and you have the makings for a wonderful backpacking adventure.

DIRECTIONS TO TRAILHEAD: Leave the Generals Highway, 6.4 miles southeast of the Y-intersection with Highway 180, and follow Big Meadows Road northeast 3.5 miles to the Big Meadows Trailhead. Park your vehicle in the trailhead parking lot (which has vault toilets and a phone).

DESCRIPTION: Near the restroom, a sign points the way up a wooded hillside and across the paved access road to the top of a low rise. Drop down the far side to a plank bridge spanning sluggish Big Meadows Creek and then follow the sandy, gently graded tread of the Jennie Lake Trail on a traverse around a granite hump. Come alongside a delightful, spring-fed tributary, and proceed through a mixed forest of red firs, lodgepole pines, and Jeffrey pines to a crossing of the tributary via some large boulders. From there, a moderate climb leads around an exposed ridge with a good view of the Monarch Divide and Shell Mountain. Continue arcing around the ridge to verdant Fox Meadow, and then climb to a junction near a stream, 2 miles from the trailhead, where the loop portion of the journey begins.

Head straight across the stream into Jennie Lake Wilderness, and follow the trail through scattered to light forest alternating with shrub-covered clearings to a junction with the short lateral to Weaver Lake, 3.1 miles from the trailhead.

Turn right at the junction and wind uphill through mixed forest and boulders for 0.2 mile to Weaver Lake. The shoreline, shaded by lodgepole pines and firs, harbor a boulder-studded forest floor carpeted with patches of azalea, red heather, and Labrador tea. The white granite of Shell Mountain creates a splendid backdrop, mirrored in the lake's placid surface. An array of campsites pepper the shoreline of this easily reached lake; the ones in small groves of trees on the south side are usually the least crowded. Anglers can fish for brook trout, but the lake obviously receives a lot of pressure. When your visit is complete, return to the junction with the Jennie Lake Trail.

From the junction, veer right (northeast) and follow less-used tread on a moderate climb toward Rowell Meadow. Reach a pair

of forested saddles and head down from the second one, gently at first and then more abruptly, to the head of Boulder Creek canyon and multiple crossings of its tributaries. Away from the last tributary, a moderate climb angles up the west-facing wall of the canyon. Shade from a scattered to light forest greets you, where the trail bends east over the crest of a ridge and then drops to a Y-junction with the Rowell Meadow Trail, 7.5 miles from the trailhead.

You angle sharply right at the junction and head south on a gentle climb to the crest of a rise. Descend gently and then moderately from the rise, enjoying occasional glimpses of Shell Mountain through the trees. Cross a lushly lined tributary of Boulder Creek, and begin a lengthy climb past slabs and boulders and over a small rivulet draining a hidden pond 0.1 mile off the trail. Eventually, the ascent leads to forested J O Pass and a junction, 10.1 miles from the trailhead.

J O PASS

As the tale goes, S. L. N. Ellis (who also named Jennie Lake for his wife) of the Sierra Forest Reserve named the pass for John Wesley Warren, who reportedly started to carve his name on a nearby tree but only completed the first two letters.

From the pass, bend right (west) to follow the crest of an undulating ridge for a while, before switchbacks lead down a forested hillside, with filtered views of Jennie Lake below. Reach the very short lateral to the lake after 1.4 miles from the pass.

Larger than Weaver Lake, Jennie Lake is also backdropped by impressive granite cliffs and rimmed by a light red fir and lodgepole pine forest. Campsites can be found on either side of the driftwood-choked outlet. Anglers may have better luck here than at Weaver, since Jennie Lake is twice as far from a trailhead.

From the Jennie Lake junction, a gentle descent is followed by an ascending traverse around exfoliated granodiorite slopes through a scattered forest, with good views of the Monarch Divide. A steep, winding climb leads up to Poop Out Pass, followed by a short descent to a Y-junction with the Stony Creek Trail, 13.4 miles from the trailhead.

Veer right at the junction, and continue to descend moderately across the south side of Shell Mountain to a crossing of a nascent, twin-channeled tributary of Stony Creek. Beyond the stream, a mild descent around the nose of a ridge leads to a traverse across the west side of Shell Mountain through mostly open terrain, allowing excellent views of Big Baldy, Chimney Rock, and the San Joaquin Valley. Head back into the trees, cross a lushly lined, spring-fed brook, and embark on a more moderate descent, which leads past a second rivulet on the way to verdant Poison Meadow. Beyond the meadow, cross another brook and the wilderness boundary, and reach the close of the loop at the junction, 15.8 miles from the trailhead.

From the junction, retrace your steps 2 miles to the Big Meadows Trailhead.

With an extensive network of connecting trails, extending trips into the adjoining national parks is straightforward.

Wilderness permits are not required. Campfires are permitted within Jennie Lakes Wilderness.

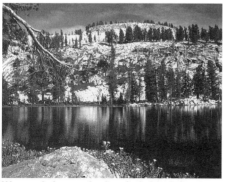

Weaver Lake on the Jennie Lakes Loop

BIG MEADOWS ROAD TRAILHEADS

TRIP 54

Seville Lake

M / **DH** or **BP**

DISTANCE: 13.2 miles, out-and-back

ELEVATION: 7,925'/9,145'/8,410', +1,455'/-955'/±4820'

SEASON: July to mid-October

USE: Light

MAPS: USGS's *Muir Grove* and *Mt. Silliman* or USFS's *A Guide to the Monarch Wilderness & Jennie Lakes Wilderness*

INTRODUCTION: A little-used trail through Jennie Lakes Wilderness leads to a secluded lake just inside the west boundary of Kings Canyon National Park. The trail passes verdant meadows and flower-lined streams on the way to cirque-bound Seville Lake, nestled beneath the rugged cliffs of the Kings-Kaweah Divide. Pleasant campsites and good fishing offer fine rewards for the labor.

DIRECTIONS TO TRAILHEAD: Leave the Generals Highway, 6.4 miles southeast of the Y-intersection with Highway 180, and follow Big Meadows Road northeast 8.5 miles to the signed turnoff for the Rowell Meadow Trailhead. Drive south 2 miles to the campground loop and park your vehicle as space allows. The free walk-in campground has fire pits and a vault toilet but not picnic tables.

DESCRIPTION: Find the start of the trail opposite the trailhead signboard at the lower end of the campground loop road and begin climbing up a heavily vegetated slope of grasses, wildflowers, and shrubs, including Labrador tea, currant, manzanita, and chinquapin. The foliage lessens a bit near some switchbacks, and then the trail enters a mixed forest of red firs, lodgepole pines, and Jeffrey pines. Cross the Jennie

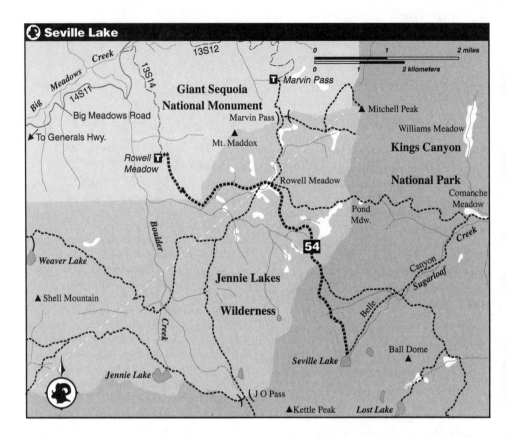

Lakes Wilderness boundary, climb around the nose of a ridge, and come alongside a tributary of Rowell Creek. Eventually, the trail crosses the stream and proceeds on gently graded tread to a three-way junction, 2 miles from the trailhead.

Continue straight ahead from the junction, passing flower-bedecked Rowell Meadow on the right. A faint path branches to a snow-survey cabin just before a crossing of Rowell Creek on a wood plank bridge. Immediately beyond the creek are some campsites. Reach another junction at the far edge of the meadow, 0.3 mile from the previous one.

Bear right (southeast) at the junction, and follow a gentle climb through lodgepole pine forest to a crossing of flower-lined Gammon Creek. Away from the creek, a more moderate ascent leads to the crest of a forested ridge and the boundary of Kings Canyon National Park at 4 miles.

Descend moderately steeply from the ridge on dusty tread through the trees to a tiny brook and a meadowland filled with wildflowers, including lupine, blue lips, and columbine. Raised sections of trail span a particularly marshy section of this lovely dell. Beyond, the descent resumes and leads to a junction, 6.4 miles from the trailhead.

Turn right (east) at the junction and cross a tributary of Sugarloaf Creek. Gently graded tread leads through mixed forest, following the course of the creek upstream through Belle Canyon. Farther on, the cliffs of the Kings-Kaweah Divide appear over the treetops, signaling the approach to Seville Lake's cirque. Soon you reach the north shore of the lovely lake, one of the group of lakes known as Sheep Camp Lakes.

Granite cliffs rise above the far shore of the lake, culminating at 10,041-foot Kettle Peak, on the crest of the Kings-Kaweah Divide. The marshy shoreline is rimmed with lodgepole pines and red firs, which shade a number of pleasant campsites. Plenty of rainbow and brook trout should tempt anglers.

O A base camp at Seville Lake offers off-trail enthusiasts the chance to explore the other Sheep Camp Lakes. Kettle Peak is a straightforward scramble.

Rather than simply returning the way you came, you could follow a semiloop back through Comanche Meadow.

R A wilderness permit is required for overnight stays in Kings Canyon. Campfires are permitted.

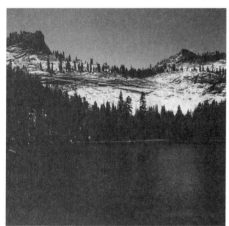

Seville Lake

BIG MEADOWS ROAD TRAILHEADS

TRIP 55

Mitchell Peak

M ↗ **BP**

DISTANCE: 6.5 miles, out-and-back

ELEVATION: 8,330'/10,365', +2,090'/-365,'/±4,910'

SEASON: July to mid-October

USE: Light

MAPS: USGS's *Mt. Silliman* or USFS's *A Guide to the Monarch Wilderness & Jennie Lakes Wilderness*

INTRODUCTION: Mitchell Peak, straddling the border between Jennie Lakes Wilderness and Kings Canyon National Park, provides one of the finest viewpoints accessible to hikers on the west side of the area. Seemingly, such a grand vista would attract hordes of devotees, but the summit sees few visitors.

DIRECTIONS TO TRAILHEAD: Leave the Generals Highway, 6.4 miles southeast of the Y-intersection with Highway 180, and follow Big Meadows Road northeast 9.7 miles to the signed turnoff for the Marvin Pass Trailhead. Turn onto single-lane, dirt road and travel 2.5 miles to the signed trailhead, remaining on the main road at all intersections.

DESCRIPTION: Head past a trailhead register and proceed uphill on single-track tread through a mixed forest of white firs, lodgepole pines, and western white pines, along with an assortment of shrubs, including chinquapin, manzanita, and currant. A moderately steep climb leads to the top of a ridge, where the ascent eases and then proceeds to a junction with a lateral to Sequoia High Sierra Camp, a hike-in resort 0.3 mile to the east.

Proceed ahead from the junction, immediately crossing a small fern- and flower-lined rivulet. Pass above a pocket of lush

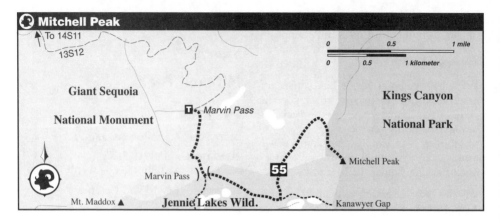

foliage dotted with an array of wildflowers, including shooting star, corn lily, buttercup, and monkeyflower. Away from the lush surroundings, the steady ascent continues via switchbacks to the signed wilderness boundary and a junction at Marvin Pass, 1 mile from the trailhead.

From the pass, head southeast on the Kanawyer Gap Trail across the south side of a ridge through scattered to light forest and shrubs and boulders. Lupine and paintbrush add splashes of color in early season. A gentle traverse leads to a junction in a swath of chinquapin, 0.7 mile from Marvin Pass.

Turn left (north) and ascend a mostly open slope back to and across the ridgecrest. Veer northeast on an ascending traverse across the northwest side of Mitchell Peak through a light forest of red firs, western white pines, and Jeffrey pines. Eventually, the grade increases on a winding climb toward the blocky summit. Leaving the last of the trees behind, weave southeast among boulders to a commanding view from the top of Mitchell Peak.

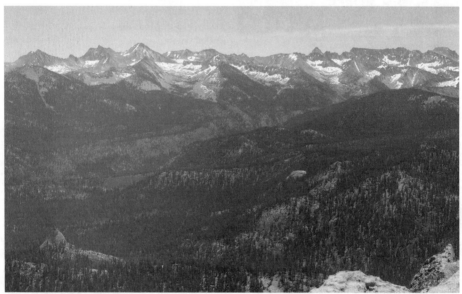

View from Mitchell Peak

Perhaps the most impressive sight from the summit is the foreground terrain plummeting steeply northeast into the vast chasm of Kings Canyon, backdropped majestically by the rising profile of the Monarch Divide. Enjoy the vast array of visible Sierra summits, including the Palisades and Mt. Goddard along the northeast horizon, a multiplicity of peaks along the Great Western Divide, and the multihued Kaweah Peaks to the southeast. Remnants of the old fire lookout are scattered about, a silent reminder that rangers once had the privilege of this view on a daily basis.

KENNEDY MEADOW TRAILHEAD

TRIP 56

Evans Grove

M ♀ **DH**

DISTANCE: 4 miles, semiloop

ELEVATION: 7,430'/6,750', +595'/-920'/±3,030'

SEASON: Early June to mid-October

USE: Light

MAP: *Wren Peak*

INTRODUCTION: A virtually forgotten trail in a remote section of Giant Sequoia National Monument allows hikers to stand among the monarchs of the forest in serenity and solitude, providing a much less crowded alternative to the more popular groves within the national parks. Although

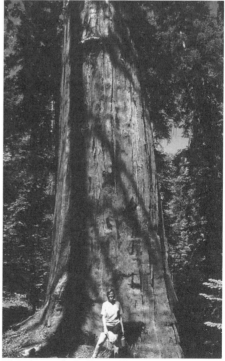

Giant sequoia in Evans Grove

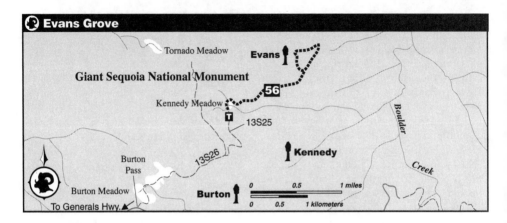

heavily logged in the early 20th century, the Evans Grove still contains more than 500 specimens and is one of the larger sequoia groves.

DIRECTIONS TO TRAILHEAD: Follow the Generals Highway to Quail Flat, 3.4 miles southeast of the Y-intersection with Highway 180, and head northeast on paved, single-lane FS Road 14S02, which is one of four roads branching away from the flat. Continue for 5.1 miles to a junction, and turn left onto FS Road 13S26, heeding signed directions for the Kennedy Meadow Trailhead. Reach a junction after 1.4 miles, and turn right onto FS Road 13S25. Continue another 0.5 mile to the parking area in a wide clearing.

DESCRIPTION: Follow an old dirt road through scattered firs to a culvert draining a spring-fed tributary of Boulder Creek, climb away from the stream on single-track trail through an old gate, and then ascend to the crest of a manzanita-covered ridge. The ridge offers fine views to the east of Shell Mountain and the surrounding terrain. Continue along the ridgecrest until a pronounced descent leads back into forest cover. Soon, giant sequoias start to appear as the trail winds down to a junction, just over a mile from the trailhead.

Veer left at the junction and follow a downhill grade through the Big Trees. After the short, steep descent, the trail intersects an old road. Turn right and follow the road, lined with thimbleberry, lupine, and paintbrush, for 0.3 mile to the next junction, where you leave the road and climb up single-track trail past more sequoias. A 0.3-mile climb closes the loop section. From there, retrace your steps back to the trailhead.

Introduction to Redwood Mountain

When General Grant and Sequoia were established as national parks in 1890, the Redwood Mountain Grove was not included. Ninety years passed before federal protection was extended to include this land in Kings Canyon National Park. Nowadays, the grove is a vital national treasure—the largest intact grove of giant sequoias in the world. In spite of such stature, the grove receives far fewer visitors than expected, probably because of access via an inauspicious, unsigned dirt road leading to the trailhead. Hikers and backpackers will find numerous magnificent monarchs in a secluded setting within Redwood Mountain Grove. A pair of vista points, Big Baldy and Buena Vista Peak, in this section are accessed by two relatively short trails leading to excellent westward views.

ACCESS: The Generals Highway provides access to Redwood Mountain and the surrounding area during spring, summer, and fall. Snow may temporarily close the highway during winter between the Y-intersection with Highway 180 and a gate north of Wuksachi. The road to Redwood Saddle leaves the Generals Highway at Quail Flat, 4.7 miles from the Y-intersection and 41.3 miles from the Ash Mountain Entrance.

AMENITIES: Grant Grove offers the nearest park services. Lodging is also available at Montecito Sequoia Lodge and Stony Creek Village on the Generals Highway. Hume Lake, with a general store, gas pumps, a snack bar, picnic area, and campground is north of Quail Flat via Tenmile Road.

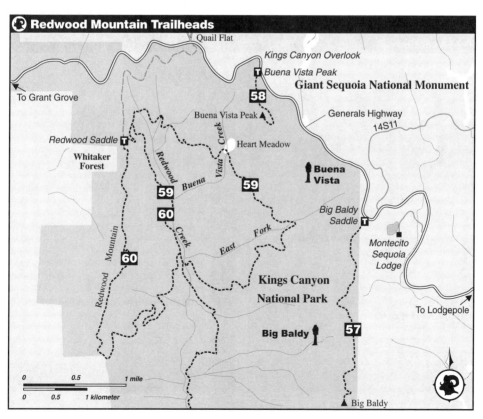

CAMPGROUNDS: The nearest Park Service campgrounds are near Grant Grove and at Dorst Creek. Forest Service campgrounds are located at Stony Creek on the Generals Highway and along the Big Meadows and Tenmile Roads. (See the Giant Sequoia National Monument and Grant Grove introductions, pp. 189 and 210, for campgrounds near Redwood Mountain.)

RANGER STATIONS: Grant Grove and Lodgepole are the nearest ranger stations.

TRIP 57

Big Baldy

M ↗ **DH**

DISTANCE: 4.4 miles, out-and-back

ELEVATION: 7,630'/8,209', +975'/-445'/±2,840'

SEASON: June to mid-October

USE: Light

MAP: *General Grant Grove*

INTRODUCTION: A number of granite domes rise from the western mountains providing inspirational views of the Sierra Nevada and San Joaquin Valley. The 8,909-foot-high dome of Big Baldy is no exception, offering

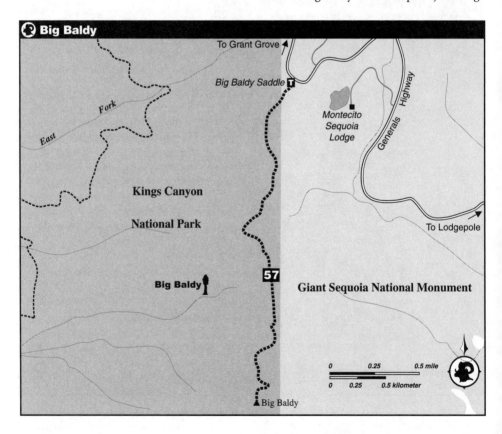

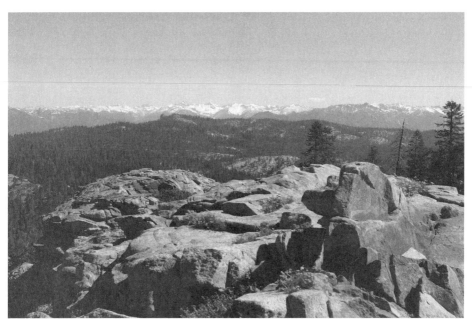

View from Big Baldy

a 360-degree view, a fine reward for the 2.2-mile hike. Remember to pack plenty of water because there is none near the trailhead or along the route.

DIRECTIONS TO TRAILHEAD: Follow the Generals Highway to the trailhead, 6.3 miles east of the Y-intersection of Highway 180 and 16.9 miles northwest of Lodgepole. Park your vehicle along the shoulder of the highway as space allows.

DESCRIPTION: Find the start of the trail near a wood trailhead sign on the west side of the highway and walk away from the road through sparse fir forest, soon crossing the Kings Canyon National Park boundary. The trail generally follows near the crest of a ridge that bends south on a gently undulating route. Near the half-mile mark, atop a granite outcrop, a break in the trees offers

a fine spot for a view down into Redwood Canyon.

For the next 1.5 miles, continue along the ridge, passing in and out of light, mixed forest. Breaks in the trees offer tantalizing glimpses of the surrounding terrain—fine precursors to the unobstructed view awaiting you at the top. Approaching the summit, pass above a TV tower and a concrete-block building to the final, winding climb up over rocks to the crest of the exposed dome.

As billed, the view from Big Baldy is grand. To the east, beyond Little Baldy, are the serrated summits of peaks along the Kings-Kaweah and Great Western Divides. Westward, the view across Redwood Canyon and Mountain to the foothills and San Joaquin Valley will depend on the haziness of the sky. Rare, clear days offer a view all the way to the coastal hills.

GENERALS HIGHWAY TRAILHEADS

TRIP 58

Buena Vista Peak

Ⓔ ⁄ DH

DISTANCE: 2 miles, out-and-back

ELEVATION: 7,230'/7,605',
+975'/-445'/±2,840'

SEASON: May to November

USE: Moderate to heavy

MAP: *General Grant Grove*

INTRODUCTION: A short hike leads to the top of Buena Vista Peak and a fine view of the western part of Kings Canyon National Park. The relatively easy 1-mile trail, combined with easy access from the Generals Highway, makes this a very popular hike with tourists. Even the ubiquitous, overweight, artery-blocked, video-carrying sightseer seems readily willing to accept the challenge of ascending the trail to the summit. However, don't allow the potential for crowds to deter you; the short climb is an enjoyable way to spend an hour or two, and the view will be quite rewarding, particularly just after the atmosphere has been cleansed by a recent rain shower.

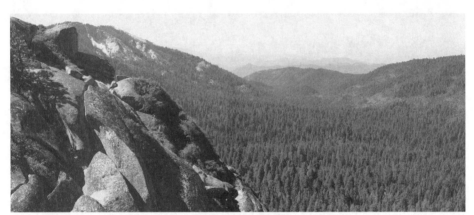

View of Redwood Mountain Grove from top of Buena Vista Peak

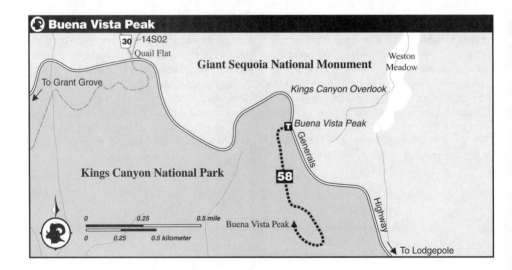

DIRECTIONS TO TRAILHEAD: Follow the Generals Highway to the trailhead, 5.8 miles east of the Y-intersection of Highway 180, directly across from the Kings Canyon Overlook.

DESCRIPTION: Follow a dirt path on a moderate climb through mostly open terrain dotted with large boulders, clumps of manzanita, and an occasional incense cedar or fir. Drawing nearer to the domelike summit, scamper over granite slabs and follow an ascending traverse around the east side of a ridge through light fir forest, where a series of switchbacks up the southeast ridge leads to the top of Buena Vista Peak.

On a rare smogless day, the view west can be quite splendid, extending all the way across San Joaquin Valley to the coastal hills. During periods of less idyllic atmospheric conditions, summiteers can still enjoy the view of nearby landmarks, including Redwood Mountain, Mt. Baldy, Buck Rock, and the deep cleft of Kings Canyon to the northeast.

REDWOOD MOUNTAIN TRAILHEAD

TRIP 59

Redwood Mountain Grove: Hart Trail Loop

M **Q** **DH** or **BP**

DISTANCE: 7.25 miles, loop

ELEVATION: 6,250'/6,445'/5,485'/6,250', +2,065'/-2,065'/±4,130'

SEASON: Late April to November

USE: Light

MAP: *General Grant Grove*

TRAIL LOG

1.9	Hart Meadow
2.4	Fallen Tunnel Tree
3.0	East Fork Redwood Creek and Hart Tree
4.75	Fallen Goliath
5.25	Redwood Creek Trail junction

INTRODUCTION: The Redwood Mountain Grove represents the largest intact grove of giant sequoias in the world. Such a distinction would seemingly make this area a tourist magnet, yet the trails are lightly used. Without a paved road to the trailhead, a plethora of signs pointing the way, or a motorized tram similar to Yosemite's conveyance through Mariposa Grove, this grove of magnificent trees can be experienced sans crowds. Walking among the towering monarchs in relative tranquility and basking in the presence of the world's largest living trees without hordes of tourists can be a transcendent experience on this 7-plus-mile-loop through the grove's eastern side. For those looking for even more time with the Big Trees, a nearly 9-mile loop is possible (see options below).

The giant sequoias are usually more than enough reward, but the Hart Trail Loop offers much more. Along the way, you encounter lush riparian habitats, where wildflowers and ferns line the banks of

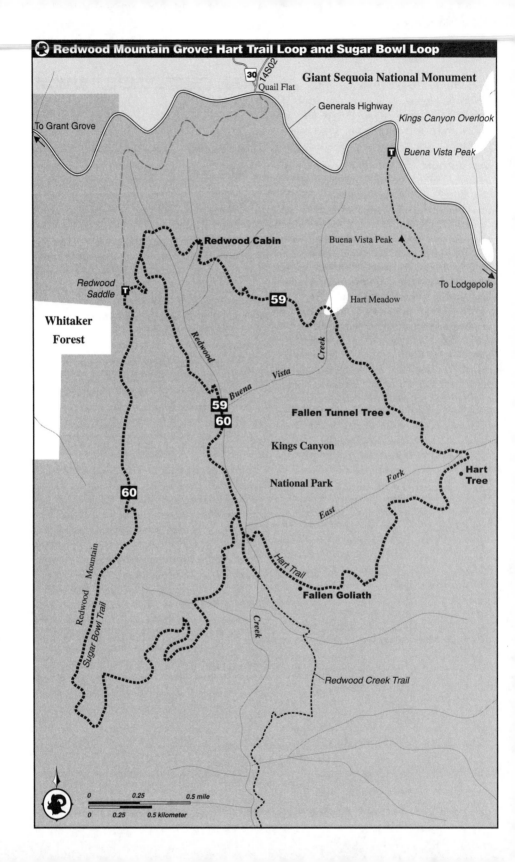

a number of enchanting tributaries of Redwood Creek. Although the majority of the trip is spent in the cool shade of the forest, on occasion the trees part enough to reveal pleasant views of the surrounding terrain. Hart Meadow is a fine example, where the stunning west face of Buena Vista Peak offers an excellent backdrop to the verdant meadow. Backpackers may enjoy a good selection of campsites farther down Redwood Creek.

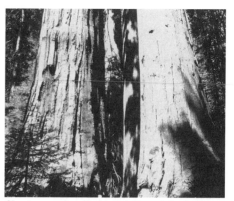

Giant sequoias, Redwood Mountain Grove

DIRECTIONS TO TRAILHEAD: Follow the Generals Highway to Quail Flat, 3.4 miles from the Y-intersection with Highway 180. From Quail Flat, directly opposite Tenmile Road, turn south and follow a single-lane dirt road with turnouts for 1.7 miles to a Y-junction. Bear left at the junction and immediately enter the large parking area at Redwood Saddle.

DESCRIPTION: From near the trailhead signboard, follow the left-hand trail north on a winding descent along the course of an old roadbed into a mixed forest of giant sequoias and firs. Reach a small ravine and a junction, 0.3 mile from the trailhead, where you bear left, proceeding under the cool shade of forest on soft, dirt tread through lush ground cover. Wind down to an easy boulder hop of a wildflower- and fern-lined tributary of Redwood Creek, followed by a gentle, 0.3-mile climb to the next wildflower-lined rivulet. Just on the other side of this delightful stream sits Redwood Cabin.

Beyond Redwood Cabin, the gentle climb continues for 0.2 mile to the next

stream crossing, beyond which the grade increases and you leave most of the redwoods behind. Gaps in the forest offer occasional glimpses of Redwood Mountain to the west. Hop across a tiny seasonal stream and climb up to a granite outcrop, from where there are unobstructed views of Redwood Mountain across the canyon and the bare rock summit of Big Baldy to the southeast. Gentle climbing away from the outcrop leads to the fringe of Hart Meadow, 1.9 miles from the trailhead, the sloping glade picturesquely backdropped by the west face of Buena Vista Peak. On the way around the meadow, step across the twin channels of Buena Vista Creek before bidding adieu to this pastoral scene.

Away from the meadow, follow a general descent back into forest cover, where giant sequoias return. After a half mile, reach the Fallen Tunnel Tree, so named because the trail heads straight through the hollowed core of a sequoia. The mostly gentle decline continues, eventually leading alongside a trickling seasonal stream and then proceeds to East Fork Redwood Creek, 3 miles from the trailhead. The lushly lined creek spills over moss-covered rocks into delightful pools, creating a lovely forest scene. A brief climb from the creek brings you to a junction with a short, steep spur to the Hart Tree, one of the 20 largest sequoias. Black scars 30 to 40 feet up the trunk testify to the tree's ability to have survived numerous fires in the past.

> ### REDWOOD CABIN
>
> The "cabin" is in actuality a fallen giant sequoia, naturally hollowed out (in part by fire) and fashioned into a cabin by some enterprising human in the late 1930s. Rock fireplaces used to occupy both ends. Nowadays, the remains of Redwood Cabin provide an interesting curiosity for both young and old.

A gentle stroll from the Hart Tree spur leads to a tiny seasonal stream, where a thin ribbon of water cascades down a rocky cleft into an appealing pool surrounded by lush plants and wildflowers. Continue on a gentle descent through mixed forest before entering a clearing filled with drier vegetation. Back in the trees, the mild descent eventually becomes moderate on the way to a signed junction with a side trail that wanders around the Fallen Goliath, an immense, downed sequoia. Another half mile leads down to the crossing of Redwood Creek. The crossing may prove difficult early in the season. Just across the creek is a junction with the Redwood Creek Trail, 5.25 miles from the trailhead. Backpackers in need of overnight accommodations should turn left (south) at the junction and head downstream along Redwood Creek to campsites farther down the canyon.

From the junction, turn right (north) and follow the lushly lined Redwood Creek Trail upstream on a mild climb beneath towering sequoias. Soon reach a signed junction with the Sugar Bowl Trail on the left (see Trip 60). The beautifully scenic hike continues upstream past more magnificent sequoias for another 0.75 mile until the trail forsakes the creek in favor of an ascent across the hillside above. Reach the close of the loop at a junction between the Redwood Creek and Hart Tree Trails at 6.9 miles. From there, retrace your steps 0.3 mile to the trailhead at Redwood Saddle.

By combining the Hart Tree and Sugar Bowl Trails, you can create a slightly longer loop, totaling 8.9 miles. At the junction of the Redwood Creek and Sugar Bowl Trails, 5.3 miles from the trailhead, turn left (south) and follow the Sugar Bowl Trail as described in Trip 60 back to Redwood Saddle.

A wilderness permit is required for overnight stays. Campfires are prohibited in Redwood Canyon. Camping is limited to two nights and prohibited within 1.5 miles of the trailhead. Group size is limited to 10.

REDWOOD MOUNTAIN TRAILHEAD

TRIP 60

Redwood Mountain Grove: Sugar Bowl Loop

M ↻ **DH** or **BP**

DISTANCE: 6.6 miles, loop

ELEVATION: 6,250'/5,520'/6,995'/6,250', +2,130'/-2,130'/±4,260'

SEASON: Late April to November

USE: Light

MAP: *General Grant Grove*

see map on p.206

TRAIL LOG

2.0   Sugar Bowl Trail junction
4.75 Redwood Mountain high point

INTRODUCTION: Even though Redwood Mountain holds the largest intact grove of giant sequoias, tourist traffic is fairly light, enabling hikers to enjoy the Big Trees without much company. This trip, which follows the west loop through the grove, lacks the number of noteworthy individual trees of the east loop described in Trip 59 (page 205). However, it has plenty of stately trees along with an interesting work in progress—a hillside covered with Christmas tree–size young sequoias on the site of an old burn. Biologists have learned a great deal about the relationship between sequoias and fire through experimental burns performed in research areas within the Redwood Mountain Grove.

Other features on this trip include delightful Redwood Creek, where the pleasant stream tumbles down a canyon carpeted with lush foliage and towering sequoias. Backpackers can wander farther downstream to fine streamside campsites. Away from the creek, the route climbs to the crest of Redwood Mountain, with excellent vistas of nearby landmarks, including Buena Vista Peak and Big Baldy.

DIRECTIONS TO TRAILHEAD: Follow the Generals Highway to Quail Flat, 3.4 miles from the Y-intersection with Highway 180. From Quail Flat, directly opposite Tenmile Road, turn south and follow a single-lane dirt road with turnouts for 1.7 miles to a Y-junction. Bear left at the junction and immediately enter the large parking area at Redwood Saddle.

DESCRIPTION: From near the trailhead signboard, follow the left-hand trail north on a winding descent along the course of an old roadbed into a mixed forest of giant sequoias and firs. Reach a small ravine and a junction, 0.3 mile from the trailhead, where you bear right and follow the gently graded Redwood Creek Trail briefly before a more moderate descent leads down into the canyon. Wind down to meet the enchanting creek at 1.25 miles and proceed downstream through lush vegetation and below a number of stately sequoias. The trail stays close to the creek for a while, veers away briefly, and then returns to the stream bank before reaching a junction with the Sugar Bowl Trail, 2 miles from

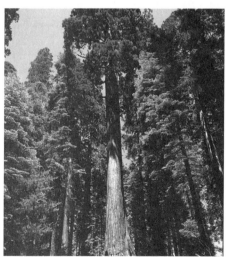
Redwood Mountain Grove, largest intact grove of stately giant sequoias

the trailhead. Backpackers should continue ahead on the Redwood Creek Trail to access campsites farther down the canyon.

Turn right at the junction and climb moderately up the hillside. After a pair of short-legged switchbacks, ascend a hillside covered with myriad young sequoias amid a few widely spaced old giants. A fine view of Big Baldy across the canyon appears over the tops of the short trees. Reach the crossing of a seasonal stream at 2.5 miles, where thick forest cover provides some welcome shade. Beyond the stream, head back out into the open and continue climbing, following a series of switchbacks up a hillside carpeted with drier vegetation of manzanita, oaks, and ponderosa pines. This section of trail offers improving views of Big Baldy, Buena Vista Peak, and the surrounding terrain. Reach the crest of Redwood Mountain near the 4-mile mark, where the grade eases.

The trail turns north and follows the ridge into the cover of mixed forest, where giant sequoias once again tower over the lesser conifers. Traveling among the monarchs on soft tread, you may notice the disappearance of the Big Trees near the east end of the ridge, a reminder that sequoias require specialized conditions to grow and survive. Most likely, the soil doesn't receive, or at least husband, a suitable amount of moisture. Climb mildly for 0.75 mile to the high point of the loop, weaving in and out of forest cover along the way. Intermittent clearings allow splendid views across Redwood Creek canyon of Big Baldy and Buena Vista Peak. Beyond the high point, a gentle, 1.75-mile descent through mixed forest leads back to the close of the loop at Redwood Saddle.

By combining the Sugar Bowl and Hart Trails, you could create a slightly longer loop of 8.9 miles (see Trip 54, page 195).

A wilderness permit is required for overnight stays. Campfires are prohibited in Redwood Canyon. Camping is limited to two nights and is prohibited within 1.5 miles of the trailhead. Group size is limited to 10.

Introduction to Grant Grove

Grant Grove's giant sequoias were some of the first to be seen by early Californians. The grove was also one of the first to receive limited federal protection, when in 1890 four sections of land were set aside as General Grant National Park in the same bill establishing Yosemite and Sequoia National Parks. The expanse of parkland seen today did not come into being until 1940, during the creation of Kings Canyon National Park. The private inholding of Wilsonia near Grant Grove is the lone piece of property the government failed to acquire from old land claims filed in the late 1800s, despite a reasonable purchase offer of $19 per acre in 1913.

The focal point of Grant Grove has always been the General Grant Tree, the third largest sequoia at 46,608 cubic feet, with a height of more than 268 feet and the largest base diameter, 40.3 feet, of any sequoia. Named by Lucretia Baker in 1867 for Ulysses S. Grant, commanding general of the Union Army during the Civil War and subsequently the 18th president, the tree was "discovered" by Joseph Hardin Thomas in 1862 (undoubtedly, the tree had been seen before by members of the local Monache tribe). In the 1920s, President Calvin Coolidge declared the tree to be "The Nation's Christmas Tree," and in the 1950s, President Dwight D. Eisenhower proclaimed it a "living national shrine," in memory of Americans who had perished during wars. Today, hundreds of visitors pay tribute to the grand giant every day from spring through fall.

While there are virtually no backpacking opportunities around Grant Grove, the excellent network of trails crisscrossing the

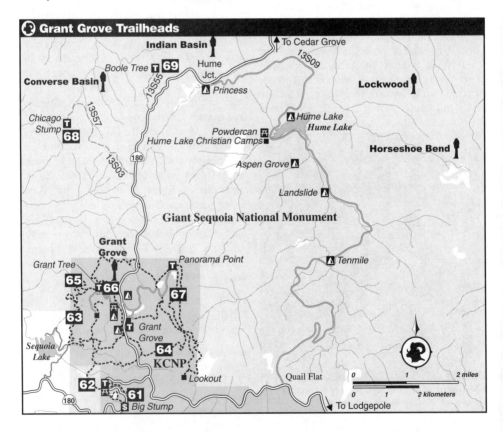

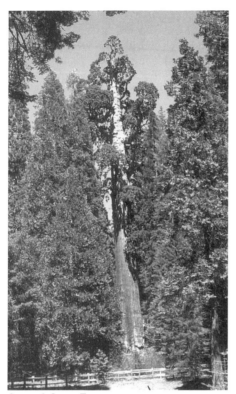

General Grant Tree

grove affords plenty of dayhiking opportunities. Aside from the obvious attraction of the Big Trees, hikers can enjoy quiet forest strolls accented by lovely meadows, wide-ranging viewpoints, dramatic waterfalls, and dancing streams. The Big Stump Trail

provides a bit of history as well. Although the General Grant Tree Trail is often packed with tourists, many of the other trails within the grove are lightly used, inviting hikers to experience the majesty of the Big Trees in relative seclusion.

ACCESS: The General Grant area has straightforward access year-round from Highway 180 (Kings Canyon Highway). From the Y-intersection with the Generals Highway, Grant Grove Village is a mere 0.9 mile north.

AMENITIES: Grant Grove Village offers a wide range of services, including a visitor center, restaurant, general store and gift shop, post office, and public showers. Lodging runs the gamut from the rustic cabins of Grant Grove to lodge rooms and suites at John Muir Lodge (866-522-6966, **www. sequoia-kingscanyon.com**).

RANGER STATION: Wilderness permits and backcountry information are available at the Grant Grove Visitor Center.

GOOD TO KNOW BEFORE YOU GO: Water is scarce on many of the trails within Grant Grove, particularly as the summer progresses. Make sure you are carrying plenty of water when setting out on the trail. With elevations ranging from 5,400 to 7,600 feet, Grant Grove typically sheds its winter snow well before the adjacent backcountry, which provides hiking opportunities early in the season.

Campgrounds							
Campground	Fee	Elevation	Season	Restrooms	Water	Bear Boxes	Phone
Azalea	$18	6,500 feet	All year	Flush	Yes	Yes	Yes
Crystal Springs	$18	6,500 feet	Late May to mid-September	Flush	Yes	Yes	Yes
Sunset	$18	6,500 feet	Late May to mid-September	Flush	Yes	Yes	Yes

TRIP 61

Big Stump Grove

E ◯ **DH**

DISTANCE: 2 miles, loop

ELEVATION: 6,355'/6,155'/6,405',
+325'/-325'/±650'

SEASON: Late May to November

USE: Moderate to heavy

MAPS: USGS's *General Grant Grove*
or SNHA's *Grant Grove*

INTRODUCTION: Experience a slice of history on this loop, which exposes visitors to the ethic of a bygone era of the late 1800s, when resources in the western US seemed inexhaustible. Loggers were drawn to the sequoia groves with the lure of jobs and big-time profits. Although the lumber from sequoias eventually proved to be too brittle for commercial applications, just about every Big Tree in this grove was sacrificed. Modern-day visitors will bear witness to the results: Countless giant stumps are a vivid reminder of shortsightedness. What could have been one of the most impressive groves

of sequoias is instead a graveyard of fallen monarchs.

Although the Big Stump Trail is quite popular with tourists, few go beyond the loop around Big Stump Meadow, leaving the greater part of the trail to the willing souls who don't mind a 2-mile walk.

DIRECTIONS TO TRAILHEAD: Follow Highway 180 (Kings Canyon Highway) to the Big Stump Picnic Area parking lot near the relocated entrance station.

DESCRIPTION: The trail begins near a restroom building on the south side of the parking area. From there, head downhill on a wide, well-graded path through pockets of manzanita and a mixed forest of incense cedars, Jeffrey pines, sugar pines, and firs. Soon, encounter the first notable sequoia, the Resurrection Tree, a topless sequoia still thriving despite having been struck by lightning. The winding descent leads down to the west junction with the loop around Big Stump Meadow, 0.3 mile from the parking area.

Veer left at the junction and circle the meadow, site of the abandoned Smith Comstock Mill, which occupied the clearing in the late 1800s. A number of large sequoia stumps and piles of redwood sawdust litter the otherwise pristine clearing. Partway around the meadow, come to the Burnt

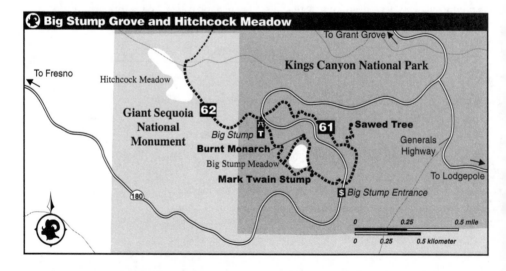

Monarch, a huge sequoia that succumbed to fire but remains erect. Just beyond are two young sequoias, planted in 1888 by Jesse Pattee, a lumberjack who lived in a nearby cabin. A cursory glance at this pair of sequoias reveals their limited stature in comparison to the massive stumps nearby. Just past a short lateral to the Feather Bed (see sidebar) is the east junction.

> **FEATHER BEDS**
>
> Since the brittle sequoias tend to burst into pieces when felled, loggers would dig a trench and line it with boughs to cushion the blow and keep the Big Tree intact. The feather beds of Big Stump Meadow are overgrown with a tangle of willows and shrubs, a jumble that belies its former purpose.

Before continuing on the main trail, turn right (west) and walk around the south side of Big Stump Meadow to a small brook and the Shattered Giant. Rather than using the standard logging practice of the day, loggers dropped this particular tree down-slope and watched the sequoia fragment into hundreds of useless pieces, which still lie in waste in the streambed. After marveling at the results of this mishap, retrace your steps back to the east junction.

From the east junction of the loop around Big Stump Meadow, head across a bridge and soon reach the Mark Twain Stump.

Away from the Mark Twain Stump, the trail leads through a narrow swath of meadow to Highway 180, 1 mile from the trailhead. Follow an angling crosswalk over the highway and to the resumption of trail on the far side. A moderate climb proceeds through mixed forest that roughly parallels the highway. After a bridge across a tiny brook, reach a junction with a short but steep lateral to the Sawed Tree. Loggers attempted to cut down this massive sequoia but eventually gave up, perhaps because they tired of the prolonged labor. Since the

> **MARK TWAIN STUMP**
>
> Instead of being chopped down for lumber in 1891, this tree was meticulously disassembled and transported for exhibition at the American Museum of Natural History and the British Museum in London. Thirteen days of chopping, sawing, and wedging were necessary to drop the tree. Nowadays, a stairway takes visitors to the top of the stump, where they gain a better appreciation for the immensity of this giant sequoia.

bark wasn't completely severed, life-giving nutrients continued to travel up the tree.

Back on the main trail, continue the ascent, passing more sequoia stumps along the way. Soon, the grade eases and the trail veers southwest toward the highway, where a tunnel takes hikers safely to the other side and a junction with the Hitchcock Meadow Trail. Turn left here and climb up a hill to close the loop at the Big Stump parking lot.

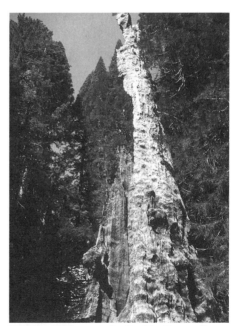

The Burnt Monarch in the Big Stump Grove

GRANT GROVE TRAILHEADS

TRIP 62

Hitchcock Meadow

E ↗ **DH**

DISTANCE: 1.2 miles, out-and-back

ELEVATION: 6,360'/6,090', +20'/-290'/±620'

SEASON: Late May to November

USE: Light

MAPS: USGS's *General Grant Grove* or SNHA's *Grant Grove*

see map on p.212

INTRODUCTION: A very short hike to a picturesque meadow on an infrequently used trail will tempt visitors away from the more popular nearby Big Stump Grove (see Trip 61, page 212). The trail passes several sequoia stumps, victims of excessive logging in the late 1800s. With shuttle arrangements, hikers can continue north from Hitchcock Meadow and then follow connectors to Grant Grove.

DIRECTIONS TO TRAILHEAD: Follow Highway 180 (Kings Canyon Highway) to the Big Stump Picnic Area parking lot.

DESCRIPTION: The trail begins at the northeast end of the parking area, immediately descending to a junction with the Big Stump Loop. Veer left at the junction, and descend moderately through light mixed forest, passing a number of giant sequoia stumps along the way. The nearly continuous descent leads shortly to Hitchcock Meadow, a thin ribbon of luxurious grasses, sedges, plants, and wildflowers along a small stream flowing northwest into nearby Sequoia Lake. More sequoia stumps can be seen scattered around the fringe of the meadow.

By continuing northbound for 0.75 mile from Hitchcock Meadow, you intersect the South Boundary Trail, which could be followed 1.2 miles to a union with the Azalea Trail and then onward to Grant Grove. Perhaps a more interesting trip extension would be to continue north another 0.7 mile from the South Boundary Trail junction to the Sunset Trail and then on to Grant Grove (see Trip 63, page 215).

GRANT GROVE TRAILHEADS

TRIP 63

Sunset Loop Trail

Ⓜ ↻ DH

DISTANCE: 5.75 miles, loop

ELEVATION: 6,650'/5,440'/6,650,
+1,885'/-1,885'/±3,770'

SEASON: Late May to mid-October

USE: Light

MAPS: USGS's *General Grant Grove*
or SNHA's *Grant Grove*

INTRODUCTION: Waterfalls, vistas, and Big Trees are the chief attractions along this loop through the west fringe of Grant Grove. While busloads of tourists rub elbows with one another on the ever popular General Grant Tree Trail, hikers can revel in the relative quiet and solitude found nearby on the Sunset Trail. Late spring and early summer are the times to see Viola and Ella Falls, when snowmelt has swelled Sequoia Creek.

DIRECTIONS TO TRAILHEAD: Follow Highway 180 (Kings Canyon Highway) to Grant Grove Village, 1.5 miles north of the Y-intersection with the Generals Highway. Park your vehicle in the visitor center parking lot.

DESCRIPTION: Cross to the west side of Highway 180 using the crosswalk directly opposite the visitor center, and follow a very short section of trail downhill to a signed junction. Turn left and follow the trail through light forest as it parallels the highway across the Sunset Campground access road to a T-junction, 0.3 mile from the trailhead. Where the Azalea Trail continues ahead, your route bears right and follows

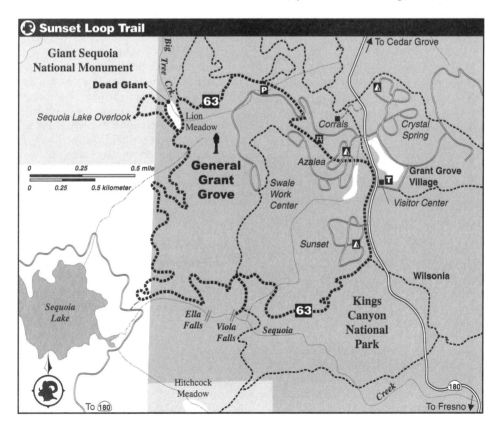

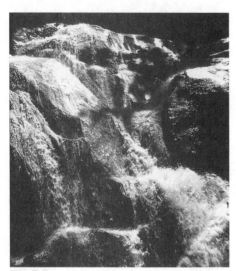

Ella Falls

the Sunset Trail over a low hill, followed by a short, gentle descent on indistinct tread to a swale. A short climb over another low rise leads to a small clearing, where manzanita lines the trail.

Away from the clearing, begin a protracted descent, weaving down a hillside over slabs and around boulders through a light, mixed forest to a bridge over a tributary of Sequoia Creek. Reach a signed four-way junction with a road from the Swale Work Center, 1.5 miles from the trailhead.

◻ **SIDE TRIP TO VIOLA FALLS:** Turn left at the junction, and follow the old road on a mild decline through the trees for 0.2 mile, where the road curves east. Here a small sign marked VIOLA FALLS directs foot traffic straight ahead onto single-track trail that soon comes alongside Sequoia Creek. The narrow path ends at the base of a hill, from where you work your way to an overlook directly above the falls. Don't expect a rival to the famous falls of Yosemite; Viola Falls is a series of short cataracts that pour swiftly down a narrow channel and into swirling pools scoured out of solid rock. Seasonal wildflowers add a touch of color to the stream banks. After admiring the falls, retrace your steps back to the junction. **END OF SIDE TRIP**

From the four-way junction, proceed straight ahead on a steady descent through light to moderate forest cover. A series of switchbacks leads across a seasonal stream, over a seep, and down to Ella Falls, 2 miles from the trailhead. While Viola Falls may have seemed a bit tame, Ella presents the sights and sounds expected of a significant waterfall, especially early in the season when Sequoia Creek plunges raucously down a sheer face and into a whirling pool, before continuing a cacophonous journey toward Sequoia Lake below.

Away from Ella Falls, proceed another quarter mile to a junction near the boundary between the park and the private property of a YMCA camp bordering Sequoia Lake. Historically, the YMCA has granted hikers permission to continue ahead from the junction to an overlook of the lake, provided they stay on the trail and do not enter the camp.

Remaining on the Sunset Trail, follow a faint path angling away to the right signed GRANT TREE. Climb moderately steeply up to an old road, which used to be the entrance road into the park from Sequoia Lake until the Kings Canyon Highway replaced it in 1939. Turn right onto the road, and begin the long climb back to Grant Grove, following broken asphalt on a steady, winding ascent through the partial shade of a mixed forest. Pass a road on the left coming up from Sequoia Lake near the 3-mile mark and an unmarked, single-track trail, also on the left, a quarter mile farther. Continue climbing to the top of a hill to the signed junction with the Dead Giant Loop to Sequoia Overlook, 4 miles from the trailhead.

◻ **SIDE TRIP TO DEAD GIANT AND SEQUOIA LAKE OVERLOOK:** From the junction, take the lower trail across a lightly forested hillside above verdant Lion Meadow. A short distance past the meadow is the Dead Giant, a very large sequoia that met an untimely demise at the hands of axe-wielding loggers. Careful inspection reveals axe marks encircling the trunk, effectively destroying the cambium layer and interrupting the flow of nutrients up the tree. Without life-giving sustenance, the sequoia eventually died, leaving behind a visible memorial to the age-old adage: Nature's greatest enemy is man himself.

Beyond the Dead Giant, climb to the crest of an open ridge, and follow this spine southwest to an unmarked junction. Continue straight ahead for a short distance to where the ridge starts to drop away, arriving at Sequoia Lake Overlook. Although the attractive lake appears natural, Sequoia Lake was created as a millpond in the late 1800s, supplying water for a flume that transported lumber to Sanger in San Joaquin Valley. Today, the lake is home to several summer camps.

After fully enjoying the view, backtrack the short distance to the junction and proceed eastbound on the return leg of the loop, soon arriving back at the old road. **END OF SIDE TRIP**

From the Dead Giant junction, resume the climb along the old roadbed, passing Lion Meadow and reaching the west junction with the North Grove Trail a quarter mile farther (see Trip 65, page 219). Another 0.3-mile climb leads past the east junction and on to the edge of a large parking lot for the popular General Grant Tree complex. Head past the start of the General Grant Tree Trail, and find the single-track tread at the far side of the parking lot. Nearby is a stand of five stately sequoias known as the Happy Family.

Follow alongside a split-rail fence just left of the delightful rivulet of Big Tree Creek, soon cross a plank bridge over this tiny brook, and stroll past the Michigan Tree, a huge, fallen sequoia reposing in broken sections beside the trail. Continues to a crossing of the Grant Tree access road, make a short climb, and then follow a stream through light forest past the Columbine Picnic Area and into Azalea Campground. Pass through the campground, crossing several access roads and a plank bridge over the creek and then climbing a hillside to the junction across from the visitor center. Turn left (uphill), to retrace your steps across the highway and return to the visitor center parking lot.

GRANT GROVE TRAILHEADS

TRIP 64

Azalea and Manzanita Trails Loop

Ⓜ ◯ DH

DISTANCE: 4.6 miles, loop

ELEVATION: 6,650'/7,495'/6,650, +1,200'/-1,200'/±2,400'

SEASON: Mid-June to mid-October

USE: Moderate

MAPS: USGS's *General Grant Grove* or SNHA's *Grant Grove*

INTRODUCTION: A short, pleasant hike on a moderately used trail samples a wide variety of terrain, from azalea- and fern-lined brooks to dry, manzanita-covered hillsides.

DIRECTIONS TO TRAILHEAD: Follow Highway 180 (Kings Canyon Highway) to Grant Grove Village, 1.5 miles north of the Y-intersection with the Generals Highway. Park your vehicle in the visitor center parking lot.

DESCRIPTION: Follow the crosswalk directly opposite the visitor center to the west side of Highway 180 and follow a very short section of trail downhill to a signed junction. Turn left and follow the trail through light forest as it parallels the highway across the Sunset Campground access road to a T-junction, 0.3 mile from the trailhead. Where the Sunset Trail turns right, your route continues ahead and proceeds through scattered to light forest, roughly paralleling the highway. Walk across the highway near the half-mile mark, climb up a low hill, and then descend to a lushly lined seasonal stream.

A gentle descent within earshot of the highway traffic leads to the crossing of another pleasant stream and then across the road into the private area of Wilsonia. Look for the trail a short distance down the road, and then follow single-track trail on a gentle descent to the crossing of

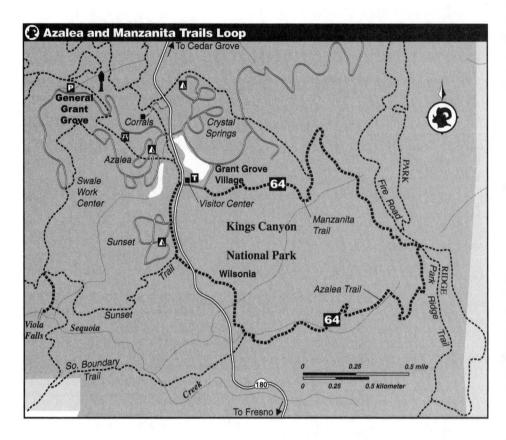

Azalea and Manzanita Trails Loop

another picturesque little stream. A short distance farther, reach a junction with the South Boundary Trail, 0.9 mile from the trailhead.

Bend left and climb moderately through patches of azalea, ignoring the unsightly clutter of cabins and power lines of Wilsonia. Ascend moderately for the next mile, strolling alongside the attractive stream you crossed earlier and eventually leaving the signs of civilization behind. Along the way toward Park Ridge, the trail crosses the creek a couple more times on wood bridges. Eventually, the trail climbs out of the drainage and switchbacks up to the crest of Park Ridge. Reach a signed junction with the Manzanita and Park Ridge Trails and an extremely short lateral to the Park Ridge Fire Road, 2.5 miles from the trailhead (a round-trip to the Park Ridge Lookout will add 2 miles to the total distance).

Bear left (northwest) at the junction and follow the nearly level tread of the Manzanita Trail, paralleling the fire road briefly before bending away on a gentle descent across the west side of Park Ridge. On sandy tread, break out into the open on manzanita-covered slopes dotted with widely scattered conifers. Farther on, the trees almost totally disappear, which allows fine westward views, at least when the valley

DEAD TREES

Cursory observation reveals a number of dead white firs bordering the manzanita-covered slopes. Although fires have affected the Park Ridge area in the past, these trees fell victim to a tussock moth infestation in the mid-1990s.

haze permits. Eventually, you leave the open slopes behind in a stand of dead conifers on the way to a Y-junction, 3.3 miles from the trailhead.

From the junction, angle back downslope to the left, and continue the descent into thickening forest cover. After 0.3 mile, reach a junction with a lateral to Crystal Springs Campground, and continue straight ahead, arcing around a large water tank to an access road. Follow this road downhill toward some cabins used for employee housing to where a single-track trail veers off to the left and passes around the cabins. Soon the trail ends at a service road, which your route follows back to Grant Grove Village and the visitor center parking area.

GRANT GROVE TRAILHEADS

TRIP 65

North Grove Loop

E Q DH

DISTANCE: 1.5 miles, loop

ELEVATION: 6,320'/5,965'/6,320', +355'/-355'/±710'

SEASON: Late May to mid-October

USE: Light

MAPS: USGS's *General Grant Grove* or SNHA's *Grant Grove*

INTRODUCTION: A reasonably short trail leads hikers away from the hubbub surrounding General Grant Tree down into the secluded North Grove of giant sequoias. Initially, the route follows a paved road that once served as the main entrance into the park from Sequoia Lake. Nowadays, the cars are gone and so are the majority of tourists. Those with extra time and energy could easily add the 0.75-mile Dead Giant Loop or the much longer Sunset Loop to this trip.

DIRECTIONS TO TRAILHEAD: Follow Highway 180 (Kings Canyon Highway) to Grant Grove Village, and continue to the left-hand

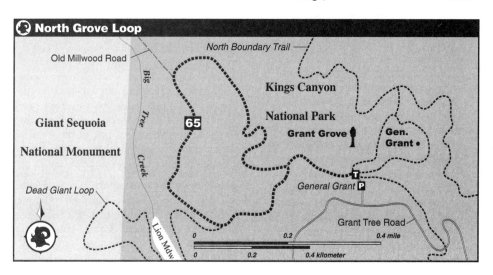

turn onto the General Grant Tree Road. Follow this road 0.7 mile to the large parking area.

DESCRIPTION: Head west from the parking lot, through the RV and bus parking area, and then to the closed road at the far end. Follow this road for 0.1 mile to a signed junction with the North Grove Trail. Leaving the road, turn right (west) and begin a moderate, winding descent through mixed forest. Eventually, the trail draws near a trickling stream on the left, which provides enough moisture to sustain a number of large sequoias, as well as an assortment of shrubs and seasonal wildflowers. Where the descent bottoms out, the trail veers west and merges with an overgrown wagon road.

Your immediate task is to regain all the lost elevation on the way back toward the old entrance road. Eventually, you leave the magnificent sequoias behind for other conifers. Just past the 1-mile mark, the grade eases where the trail intersects the old road. From this junction, the Dead Giant Loop is only a quarter mile to the right (see Trip 63, page 215). To return to the parking lot, turn left and follow the road to the first intersection. From there, retrace your steps to the parking lot.

OLD WAGON ROAD

Lumbermen used to travel this road to Millwood, site of two mills built in 1889 by the Sanger Lumber Company. They also built a 54-mile flume for transporting lumber to the San Joaquin Valley. Just beyond the old road is a rare sight—a mature giant sequoia that succumbed to fire. Most sequoias of this size are able to withstand the ravages of the average forest fire quite well. In fact, their reproductive cycle benefits from such calamities. Heat from the fire opens up the cones, allowing seeds to fall to the ground. To see a sequoia of this size unable to survive a fire is rare.

TRIP 66

General Grant Tree Trail

E ↻ **DH**

DISTANCE: 0.5 mile, loop

ELEVATION: 6,320'/6,415'/6,320', +100'/-100'/±200'

SEASON: Mid-May to mid-October

USE: Heavy

MAPS: USGS's *General Grant Grove* or SNHA's *Grant Grove* or *General Grant Tree Trail*

INTRODUCTION: At a height of 267 feet and a base diameter of more than 40 feet, the General Grant Tree is the third largest sequoia in existence. Additional prestige is attached to the Grant Grove area since it is the oldest section of Kings Canyon National Park, set aside originally in 1890 as General Grant National Park in the same bill that established Yosemite as a national park and greatly enlarged Sequoia. Such notoriety results in Grant Grove being one of the park's most popular tourist attractions. While the General Grant Tree Trail takes visitors to the base of the namesake tree and past an assortment of other giants, the resulting crowds create an atmosphere reminiscent of a theme park.

The best bet for minimizing the effects of the tourist season (Memorial Day weekend to Labor Day) is to pay homage to the Grant Tree early in the morning or late in the afternoon. Crowds aside, the General Grant Tree Trail allows visitors to experience the awe-inspiring majesty of one of the world's largest living creatures in one of the finest groves of giant sequoias on the planet.

DIRECTIONS TO TRAILHEAD: Follow Highway 180 (Kings Canyon Highway) to Grant Grove Village, and continue to the left-hand turn onto the General Grant Tree Road. Follow this road 0.7 mile to the large parking area.

DESCRIPTION: The Park Service requests that visitors proceed on a counterclockwise circuit around the grove, winding up to the centerpiece, the General Grant Tree. Pick up a pamphlet at the trailhead to learn more about all the notable sites you will pass. A short climb from there leads past the Gamlin Cabin, and then a gentle descent leads beside more giant sequoias on the circuit back to the trailhead. Interpretive signs along the way provide interesting tidbits about the Big Trees.

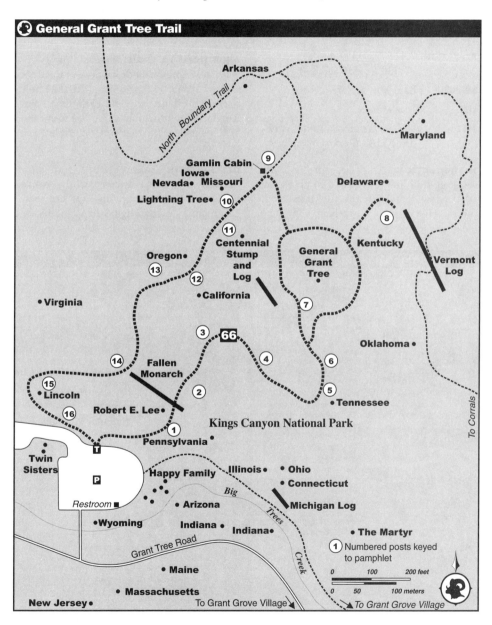

GRANT GROVE TRAILHEADS

TRIP 67

Park Ridge Lookout

E ↻ DH

DISTANCE: 5.6 miles, loop

ELEVATION: 7,415'/7,600'/7,415', +1,430'/-1,430'/±2,860'

SEASON: Late May to late October

USE: Moderate

MAPS: USGS's *General Grant Grove* or SNHA's *Grant Grove*

INTRODUCTION: This pleasant loop uses a hiking trail and a fire road to access one of the few remaining fire lookouts in the Sierra. Hikers are to excellent views, not only at the lookout of the Great Western Divide and San Joaquin Valley (when haze permits), but also near the trailhead at Panorama Point, where visitors can marvel at the extraordinary vista of numerous Sierra summits. Alternating between mixed forest and open clearings, the route is gently graded, following Park Ridge from the trailhead all the way to the lookout.

DIRECTIONS TO TRAILHEAD: Follow Highway 180 (Kings Canyon Highway) to Grant Grove Village, and continue north 0.25 mile to the right-hand turn onto Panorama Point Road. Follow this road 2.3 miles to its end at a parking area (with picnic tables and restrooms).

DESCRIPTION: Follow paved trail bordered by a split-rail fence for 300 yards to Panorama Point, where an excellent view encompasses many High Sierra landmarks,

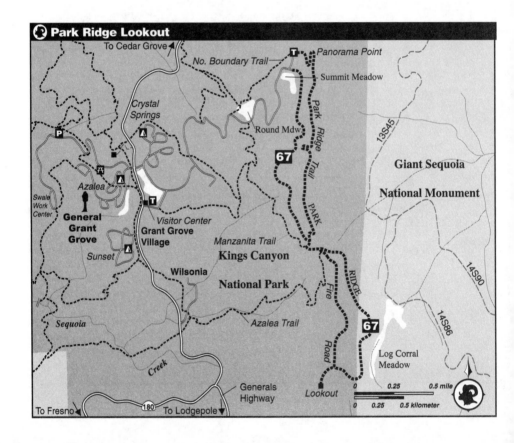

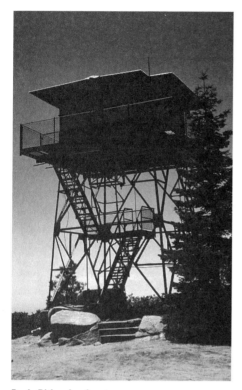

Park Ridge Lookout

including the Monarch Divide, Great Western Divide, and Sierra Crest peaks. A sign identifies many of the more significant features.

Leaving the vast majority of tourists behind, head away from Panorama Point on a winding climb in and out of scattered to light forest with an understory of manzanita and azalea. Scarred trunks on many of the conifers testify to a recent fire. Occasionally, the forest parts enough to allow good views of the Monarch Divide to the northeast, the Great Western Divide to the southeast, and west toward the San Joaquin Valley. A little more than a mile from the trailhead, reach the crest of a knoll, and then descend moderately to a junction with the fire road, 1.6 miles from the trailhead.

Follow the road for about 50 yards to a signed junction, and proceed straight ahead on single-track trail toward the lookout. Follow the undulating trail for another mile to another junction with the fire road, and then follow the road for about 250 yards to Park Ridge Lookout, 2.75 miles from the trailhead. Transformers, power poles, communication towers, weather equipment, and a concrete building litter the edge of Park Ridge. Despite the artificial clutter, the view from the lookout—from the San Joaquin Valley to the Great Western Divide and points in between—is quite rewarding.

After fully enjoying the view from Park Ridge, retrace your steps 250 yards to the junction between the road and single-track trail and then follow the gently graded road through a light, mixed forest, wrapping around the hillside above Log Corral Meadow. At 1.3 miles from the lookout, reach the junction where you first met the fire road. Continue on the road, passing fire-scarred conifers and crossing an open, shrub-covered hillside. A final, half-mile descent leads past a meadow to a closed gate. From the gate, walk a short section of paved road back to the parking lot.

TRIP 68

Chicago Stump

E ⟋ **DH**

DISTANCE: 0.6 mile, out-and-back

ELEVATION: 6,645'/6,610', negligible

SEASON: Late May to November

USE: Light

MAP: *Hume*

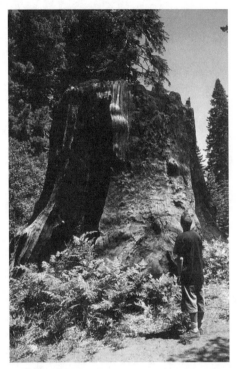

Chicago Stump

INTRODUCTION: A short and easy hike leads to one of the more interesting curiosities in Giant Sequoia National Monument. In 1893, the General Noble Tree, one of the supreme monarchs of Converse Basin, was felled, cut into segments, shipped east, and then reassembled for the Chicago World's Fair. The public met the Noble Tree with widespread skepticism, dubbing it the "California Hoax," and doubting the actual existence of a species as big as the giant sequoia. Along with the rest of the largest sequoias in Converse Basin, the Noble Tree succumbed to loggers, with the stump the only thing left to remind us of its former glory.

DIRECTIONS TO TRAILHEAD: Follow Highway 180 (Kings Canyon Highway) 3 miles north of Grant Grove Village to Cherry Gap, and turn left onto FS Road 13S03. Drive through a gate and past a large wood

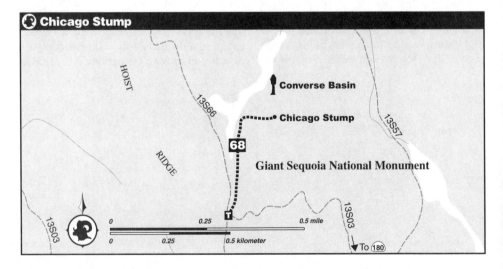

sign recounting the history of Converse Basin, and continue north for 2 miles to the signed trailhead. Park your vehicle on the right-hand side of the road in a small parking area.

DESCRIPTION: Hike down an old roadbed through Jeffrey pines and shrubs to the end of a long, verdant meadow bordered by red firs, azaleas, ferns, and a number of young sequoias. Proceed down the road to a fork, and follow either path to Chicago Stump, where informational signs provide the history of the fallen tree.

NOBLE TREE

This giant sequoia is estimated to be the largest ever felled, requiring 19 men with outstretched arms to encircle its base. Although lumberjacks needed only several days to fell the old monarch, it took the tree 3,200 years to reach such a size. Modern-day hikers will gaze at the stump in awe of the former enormity of the now-truncated tree, secure in the knowledge that future giants are federally protected from meeting a similar fate.

CONVERSE BASIN TRAILHEADS

TRIP 69

Boole Tree

E ○ DH

DISTANCE: 2.25 miles, loop

ELEVATION: 6,265'/6,765', +740'/-740'/±1,480'

SEASON: Late May to November

USE: Light

MAP: *Hume*

INTRODUCTION: Occasionally, size has its advantages; such was the case for the Boole Tree. While hundreds of giant sequoias met the axe in Converse Basin, this lone survivor received a stay of execution because of its immense size. Originally identified as the third largest sequoia in existence, the Boole Tree was spared the fate of its less fortunate neighbors. Although this impressive monarch has the largest base circumference of any sequoia (313 feet), a height of 269 feet and a volume of 47,472 cubic feet ultimately ranked the tree as the eighth largest. Ironically, the tree was named for the mill superintendent of Converse Basin, Frank

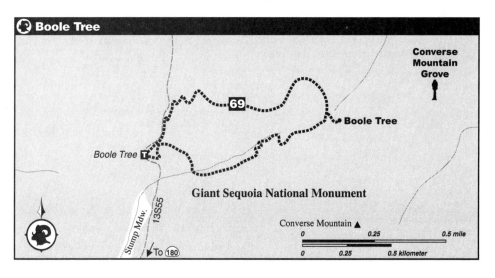

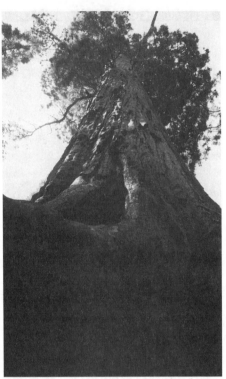

Boole Tree, eighth largest giant sequoia in the world

firs; and incense cedars. Although relatively short, the trail passes through a variety of flora and terrain. In addition, a ridgecrest vantage offers an excellent view of the Kings River area.

DIRECTIONS TO TRAILHEAD: Follow Highway 180 (Kings Canyon Highway) 4.25 miles north of Grant Grove Village to FS Road 13S55. Head north for 0.25 mile to a three-way junction and proceed straight ahead through Stump Meadow to a large trailhead parking area (which has a vault toilet and picnic tables), 2.5 miles from Highway 180.

DESCRIPTION: Pass through a gate in a wood fence, and walk uphill away from the parking area beneath a thick canopy of mixed forest. Climb moderately up wood steps and switchbacks, and then descend briefly to a T-junction, where a very short descent leads to the Boole Tree, 0.9 mile from the parking lot. After admiring this giant of the forest, retrace your steps to the junction.

Boole, who oversaw the demise of the other sequoias in the basin.

Hikers not only have the privilege of seeing such a notable sequoia, but at a little more than 2 miles, this loop offers the opportunity to see seven other conifer species, including lodgepole, western white, Jeffrey, and sugar pines; red and white

Head away from the junction and ascend a hillside to a viewpoint overlooking the deep gorge of the Kings River. Notice the change in the foliage, as the drier vegetation of manzanita, mountain misery, and scattered Jeffrey pines covers the hilltop. Heading west away from the viewpoint, the trail follows a ridge downhill to a series of switchbacks, with more views of the Kings River country along the way. Continue the descent, as the trail swings southwest and leads back to the parking area.

Introduction to Cedar Grove

The South Fork Kings River canyon, one of the deepest gorges in North America, is an undeniably spectacular sight, luring admirers from far and wide. Rivaling Yosemite Valley in many ways, Kings Canyon boasts towering granite walls, monolithic spires, and photogenic meadows. The Whitney Survey published the first written account of the canyon, which described the area as follows:

> The canyon here is very much like the Yosemite. It is a valley from half a mile to a mile wide at the bottom, about eleven miles long and closed at the lower end by a deep and inaccessible ravine like that below the Yosemite, but deeper and more precipitous. It expands above and branches at its head, and is everywhere surrounded and walled in by grand precipices, broken here and there by side canyons, resembling the Yosemite in its main features. The Kings River canyon rivals and even surpasses the Yosemite in altitude of its surrounding cliffs, but it has no features as striking as Half Dome, or Tutucanula (El Capitan), nor has it the stupendous waterfalls which make that valley quite unrivaled in beauty.

While a second place finish to Yosemite in magnificence may be an arguable matter, devotees of Kings Canyon gladly concede the lower ranking in number of tourist visits, especially by the camera-toting, polyester-clad, bus-riding variety.

Not solely a picturesque feature, Kings Canyon is also a gateway to some of the High Sierra's finest backcountry scenery, issuing a siren call to hikers and backpackers from around the world. Myriad trails radiate from Kings Canyon, most all of them requiring stiff climbs of great elevation change in order to reach the high country beyond. The prospect of a major ascent doesn't seem to deter too many recreationists from heading out from Roads End, especially on the Woods Creek and Bubbs Creek Trails, which hikers often combine with a section of the John Muir Trail as part of the popular Rae Lakes Loop. Wilderness permits for these trails are often at a premium, especially on busy summer weekends. Other routes from Kings Canyon are often quiet and lonely, offering true wilderness experiences that are both scenic and serene.

ACCESS: Paved, two-lane Kings Canyon Highway (Highway 180) provides the sole vehicle access to Kings Canyon. Plan on a one-hour drive from the Big Stump Entrance since sections of the road are steep and winding. The highway, open beyond the Hume Junction from late April to mid-November, terminates at appropriately named Roads End. From the Y-intersection with the Generals Highway, the Kings Canyon Highway continues past Grant Grove Village, passes out of Kings Canyon National Park and into Sequoia National Forest, reaching the high point at Cherry Gap at 5.8 miles.

The Hume Junction, 10.3 miles from the Y, provides access to picnic areas and campgrounds around the lake, as well as to Hume Lake Christian Camps (which

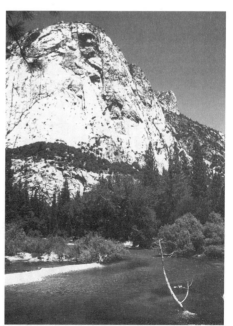

South Fork Kings River backdropped by massive North Dome

has a general store, gift shop, snack bar, gasoline, boat rentals, and lodging). Beyond the Hume Junction, a long, winding descent plummets toward South Fork Kings River, reenters the park, and then follows the river upstream to Cedar Grove and Roads End.

AMENITIES: Park facilities at Cedar Grove include a visitor center, general store and gift shop, snack bar, laundromat, pub-

lic showers, and pack station. Motel-style lodging is available at Cedar Grove Lodge (866-522-6966, **www.sequoia-kingscanyon. com**). Outside the park, 17.5 miles from the Y, rustic Kings Canyon Lodge offers cabin rentals, dining, ice cream, and gasoline (559-335-2405).

RANGER STATION: Wilderness permits, bear canister rentals, backcountry information,

Campgrounds							
Campground	**Fee**	**Elevation**	**Season**	**Restrooms**	**Water**	**Bear Boxes**	**Phone**
Sentinel	$18	4,600 feet	Late April into October	Flush	Yes	Yes	Yes
Sheep Creek	$18	4,600 feet	Mid-May to late September	Vault	Yes	Yes	Yes
Canyon View	$18	4,600 feet	May to October	Flush	Yes	Yes	Yes
Moraine	$18	4,600 feet	May to October	Vault	Yes	Yes	Yes

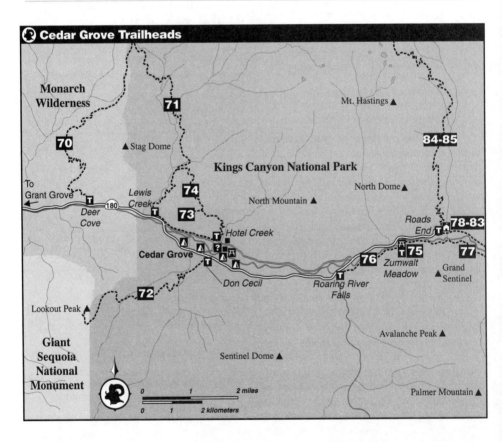

and a small assortment of books and maps are available from seasonal rangers at the permit station near Roads End.

GOOD TO KNOW BEFORE YOU GO: The low elevation combined with the reflectivity of the granite walls of Kings Canyon can turn the typical sunny Sierra afternoon into a hot box during summer. Hikers and backpackers should plan on early starts for climbs out of the canyon, especially on south-facing trails and trails with little to no forest cover.

As in other areas of the parks, do *not* leave food and scented items in vehicles overnight in Kings Canyon. Bears are often active at night. Food lockers are available at trailheads, but reducing such items before you arrive will help to minimize the amount of space you need.

Although hardly considered a bona fide hike, the extremely short stroll to Roaring River Falls should not be missed, especially in early season when the river is swollen with snowmelt.

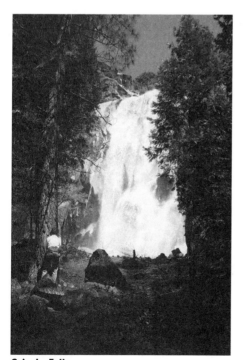

Grizzly Falls

DEER COVE TRAILHEAD

TRIP 70

Deer Cove Trail

Ⓜ ↗ DH

DISTANCE: 6.8 miles, out-and-back

ELEVATION: 4,425'/6,525', +2,720'/-620'/±6,680'

SEASON: May to late November

USE: Light

MAP: *Cedar Grove*

INTRODUCTION: The nearly forgotten Deer Cove Trail within Monarch Wilderness offers hikers an opportunity to escape the crowds in the neighboring park on a relatively short ascent to a vantage point offering pleasant views of Monarch Divide and Kings Canyon. The low elevation and south-facing hillsides combine to make this a good early or late season trip. Summer hikers will have to get a very early start to beat the heat. Although a network of trails penetrates deep into the Monarch Wilderness beyond, they receive very little maintenance and may be difficult to follow.

DIRECTIONS TO TRAILHEAD: Follow Kings Canyon Highway into Kings Canyon. The trailhead is on the north side of the road, about 31.5 miles from the Y-intersection with the Generals Highway and 0.9 mile west of the park boundary.

DESCRIPTION: The trail leaves the highway shoulder and heads uphill through a mixed forest of Jeffrey pines, white firs, and black oaks, with a ground cover principally of manzanita. Soon the trail crosses the wilderness boundary, and the forest becomes scattered on a moderate to moderately steep climb that diagonals up a south-facing hillside to the lip of Deer Cove canyon. A seemingly interminable series of switchbacks leads up the slope well above Deer Cove Creek, before entering thick forest and

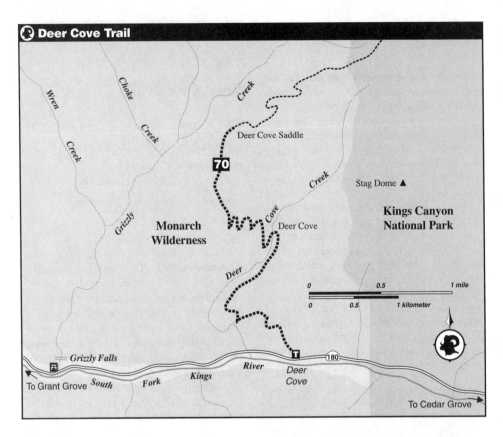

Deer Cove Trail

descending to a crossing of the creek, 1.75 miles from the trailhead.

From the creek, climb out of dense forest and head southwest up a slope. Soon, the trail veers north, then west, following switchbacks up a lightly forested hillside. Alternating views of the Monarch Divide to the north and Kings Canyon to the east appear through gaps in the trees. A long, ascending traverse leads to Deer Cove Saddle and a junction, 3.5 miles from the trailhead.

From the saddle, a short descent leads to a primitive campsite near Grizzly Creek.

TRIP 71

East Kennedy Lake

Ⓢ ↗ BP

DISTANCE: 22 miles, out-and-back

ELEVATION: 4,575'/10,800'/10,160', +7,280'/-1,690'/±17,940'

SEASON: July to mid-October

USE: Light

MAPS: USGS's *Cedar Grove* and *Slide Bluffs* or Tom Harrison Maps' *Kings Canyon High Country Trail Map*

TRAIL LOG

6.2   Frypan Meadow
10.1   Kennedy Pass
11.0   East Kennedy Lake

INTRODUCTION: Any route across the Monarch Divide, which separates the yawning gorges of South Fork and Middle Fork Kings River, is a significant physical challenge because of the tremendous elevation gain. The Lewis Creek Trail is no exception, requiring a stiff, 6,225-foot, 10-mile climb to Kennedy Pass. The south-facing trail starts low, climbs steeply, and is exposed to the sun the majority of the way—even with an early start the ascent can be a grueling scorcher. Despite the conditions, the scenery is superb and usually can be experienced sans crowds; the trail sees far fewer visitors than the Paradise Valley and Bubbs Creek Trails.

East Kennedy Lake is an alpine gem that is sure to please the most critical backcountry aficionado. West Kennedy Lake is easily accessible. Plus a straightforward cross-country route from East Kennedy Lake through the Volcanic Lakes to Granite Pass will tempt off-trail enthusiasts with the possibility of a semiloop trip.

DIRECTIONS TO TRAILHEAD: Follow Kings Canyon Highway into Kings Canyon, and find the Lewis Creek Trailhead on the north shoulder of Kings Canyon Highway, 0.4 mile east of the park boundary and 1.3 miles west of the Cedar Grove turnoff.

DESCRIPTION: Like most trails out of Kings Canyon, the Lewis Creek Trail climbs stiffly away from the canyon floor on a grueling, switchbacking ascent. Through mixed forest, the trail makes a continuous 1.75-mile climb along the east wall of Lewis Creek canyon to a junction with the Hotel Creek Trail.

From the junction, drop into a side canyon, and travel northeast upstream to a crossing. Beyond the stream, a stretch of uneven climbing leads back to the main canyon well above the level of the creek, where patches of canyon live oak offer intermittent shade. Drop down briefly to a crossing of Comb Creek, 3.5 miles from the trailhead, 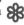 with campsites nearby.

The ascent continues well away from Lewis Creek, as mountain misery, manzanita, and the charred trunks of scattered Jeffrey pines cover the once fire-swept slope. A mile or so of steady climbing from Comb Creek leads back to and across Lewis Creek. Continue the ascent away from the crossing for another 1.5 miles, passing through scattered to light forest and reaching a junction with an infrequently used trail heading south to Wildman Meadow, 6.2 miles from the trailhead.

A short span of gently graded trail leads back to the west branch of the creek and the lush flora of Frypan Meadow, where two campsites (with a bear box) nestle beneath towering white firs. At the far end of the meadow, an overgrown, unmaintained path heads west toward Grizzly Lake.

Away from Frypan Meadow, proceed through dense timber, stepping over multiple braids of Lewis Creek, before switchbacking out of the trees, followed by a long, ascending traverse across the southeast-facing slope of Kennedy Mountain. The mostly open hillside is covered with young aspens, shrubs, and wildflowers, well watered by a number of seeps oozing down the hillside. The combination of verdant foliage and expansive views of the Great Western and

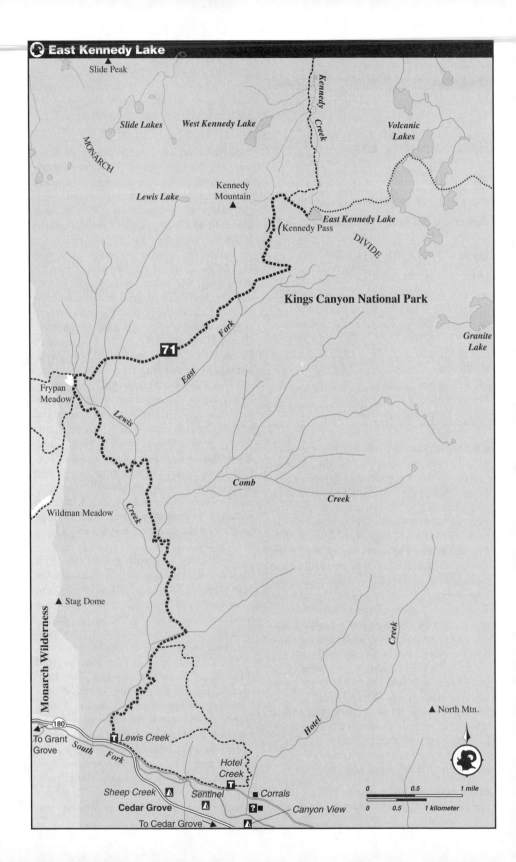

Kings-Kaweah Divides provides exquisite scenery as picturesque as any in the Sierra.

After fighting through the trailside vegetation, cross a willow- and flower-lined tributary of East Fork Lewis Creek, and begin a series of switchbacks toward the pass through scattered lodgepole and whitebark pines. Zigzag up to Kennedy Pass, 10.1 miles from the trailhead, standing between two of the deepest canyons in North America, the Middle Fork and South Fork of the Kings River. The incredible view includes an array of Sierra summits along with the two deep gorges.

From Kennedy Pass, the trail zigzags down sandy slopes amid boulders and rocks to a shallow, steep gully, where the inordinately steep trail is indistinct in parts and rough in others. Descend the gully to more short-legged switchbacks leading downslope to the 10,000-foot level, approximately 0.6 mile from the pass. To reach East Kennedy Lake, leave the trail here and head around the north side of a small tarn northeast of the pass, climb over a rise, and reach the west shore of East Kennedy Lake.

Alpine in nature, East Kennedy Lake, backdropped by a massive cirque wall rising above the surface to the crest of the Monarch Divide, has a foreboding presence. Nearly surrounded by steep cliffs, the shoreline is virtually inaccessible. Exposed, windswept campsites can be found above the west shore in tiny pockets of sand. The view north down Kennedy Canyon to the deep gorge of the Middle Fork is breathtaking.

O The Kennedy Pass Trail continues downstream to a short, off-trail romp up West Fork Kennedy Creek to seldom-visited West

---

ANOTHER ROBERT KENNEDY

The lakes, pass, and canyon were all named for Robert Kennedy—not the former presidential candidate and brother of President John F. Kennedy, but a sheep rancher from Fresno.

Kennedy Lake. Farther down the canyon, the tread deteriorates even more, but some parties still follow the old route over Dead Pine Ridge to Volcanic Lakes. A much more direct cross-country route follows the north side of East Kennedy Lake over rocky terrain to a grassy gully above the east shore and then northeast up the gully to an obvious saddle (approximately 10,900 feet).

From the saddle, descend loose talus to Lake 10199, from where exploration of Volcanic Lakes is straightforward. To reach Granite Pass, from the southern tip of Lake 10199, follow the inlet upstream, cross the stream below the next highest lake (approximately 10,350 feet), and then curve around to the south, passing between Lake 10288 and Lake 10284. Climb a grassy gully on the east side of the basin to the top of a ridge and then head across easy terrain to the Copper Creek Trail near Granite Pass. From there, follow the trail to Roads End (shuttle required to return to Lewis Creek Trailhead).

The ascent of Kennedy Mountain from Kennedy Pass is Class 1–2.

R A wilderness permit is required for overnight stays. Campfires are prohibited above 10,000 feet.

TRIP 72

Don Cecil Trail to Lookout Peak

MS ↗ **DH**

DISTANCE: 10 miles, out-and-back

ELEVATION: 4,665'/8,485,'
+4,000'/-225'/±8,450'

SEASON: June to mid-October

USE: Light

MAPS: USGS's *Cedar Grove* or Tom Harrison Maps' *Kings Canyon High Country Trail Map*

INTRODUCTION: The 5-mile climb up to the top of Lookout Peak affords hikers a bird's-eye view of Kings Canyon and an impressive vista of the peaks and ridges forming the backcountry beyond. A few tourists will hike the first mile up to the cool grotto of Sheep Creek, but most of the remaining 4 miles are lightly used, despite the rewarding vista from the site of a former lookout. The steady, nearly 4,000-foot climb is probably enough of a disincentive to dissuade the average park visitor, but hikers in reasonable condition should be able to complete the ascent in a few hours. Start early so that you will finish climbing before the heat of the day, which can be quite oppressive on the average summer afternoon.

DIRECTIONS TO TRAILHEAD: Follow Kings Canyon Highway into Kings Canyon. The trailhead is on the south side of the road, about 0.15 mile east of the Cedar Grove turnoff.

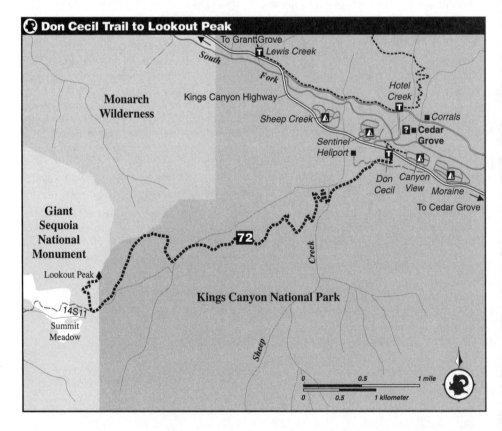

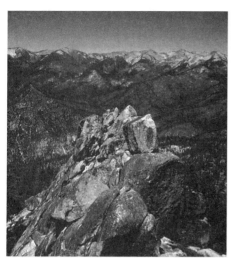

The Monarch Divide from Lookout Peak

DESCRIPTION: The trail begins climbing the south wall of the canyon on a moderately steep grade through a light, mixed forest of black oaks, incense cedars, ponderosa pines, and white firs. Soon the trail bends west to cross an access road for a heliport, resumes its stiff ascent, and then drops to Sheep Creek at 0.9 mile, where the cool and refreshing waters cascade picturesquely down a series of rock slabs. Since Sheep Creek is the domestic water supply for Cedar Grove, do *not* contaminate the water in any way.

Beyond the creek, a series of switchbacks lead through scattered forest, with periodic breaks allowing good views of Kings Canyon below, the Monarch Divide across the canyon, and Sierra summits to the east—precursors to the much more excellent view awaiting at the top of Lookout Peak. The forest thickens a bit on the approach

to the west branch of Sheep Creek, which is lined with a verdant assortment of wild- flowers, ferns, and small plants. After a short stroll alongside the pleasant stream, cross the creek on a flat-topped log.

After following the north bank for a while, the trail veers away from the creek and climbs across the east slope below Lookout Peak through more drought-tolerant vegetation. A protracted ascent leads to a saddle at the boundary between the park and lands of Sequoia National Forest. Beyond the boundary, the condition of the trail deteriorates a bit; a faint path leads up to the crest of the peak's west ridge and then follows the ridge to the summit. In the absence of well-defined tread, cairns may help to guide you, but the general route up the ridge is obvious. The path becomes more distinct again, as the trail dips shortly, winds across a shrub-covered slope, and then zigzags toward the top. Pick your way around large slabs and over boulders to emerge triumphantly on top of Lookout Peak.

The view from the summit is quite dra- matic. Nearly 4,000 feet straight below is South Fork Kings River, tumbling through the rugged and rocky gorge of Kings Canyon. Across the canyon to the north, Monarch Divide cuts a jagged profile across the usually azure Sierra sky. Looking east, the peaks of the High Sierra span the horizon. If you're fortunate enough to be here on a rare, clear day, even the view west across the San Joaquin Valley is impressive.

◙ By traveling west along the course of an old road from the saddle at the park boundary, you can reach Summit Meadow, which harbors a spectacular wildflower display in early summer.

CEDAR GROVE TRAILHEADS

TRIP 73

Cedar Grove Overlook

MS ↗ **DH**

DISTANCE: 4.8 miles, out-and-back

ELEVATION: 4,675'/6,085',
+1,525'/-115'/±3,300'

SEASON: May to November

USE: Light

MAPS: USGS's *Cedar Grove* or
SNHA's *Cedar Grove* or Tom
Harrison Maps' *Kings Canyon
High Country Trail Map*

INTRODUCTION: One of the most scenic chasms in the Sierra, Kings Canyon is also one of the deepest gorges in North America, reaching a depth of 8,000 feet from Spanish Mountain just outside the park boundary. To gain the extraordinary views from the canyon's rim, hikers must surmount the steep walls via one of a handful of correspondingly steep trails. The trail to Cedar Grove Overlook is no exception, gaining more than 1,500 feet in nearly 2.5 miles.

However, the effort is well rewarded with expansive views of Kings Canyon and the Monarch Divide. The ascent can be a scorcher during the typically sunny and hot afternoons—get an early start if possible. Unfortunately, photographers will find the best light in late afternoon, when the sun is well to the west.

DIRECTIONS TO TRAILHEAD: Follow Kings Canyon Highway into Kings Canyon and to the Cedar Grove turnoff, 34 miles from the Y-intersection with the Generals Highway.

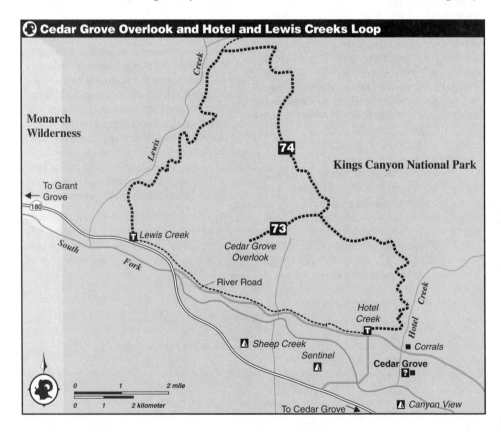
Cedar Grove Overlook and Hotel and Lewis Creeks Loop

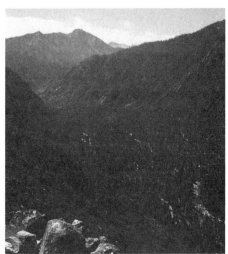

Kings Canyon from Cedar Grove Overlook

Follow signs to the pack station and turn right, 0.5 mile from the highway. Immediately after the turn, locate a small parking area on the left for the Hotel Creek Trailhead.

DESCRIPTION: Climb moderately steeply on the Hotel Creek Trail up a hillside to a junction with a trail from the pack station. Continue climbing through a mixed forest of oaks, pines, and firs, now within earshot of Hotel Creek. Soon reach a spur head-ing shortly down to the creek, and follow the main trail on a series of switchbacks through scattered oaks and pines. After a half mile, the trees are left behind, as the remainder of the stiff climb continues across chaparral-covered slopes. The switchbacks eventually end where the trail turns west and follows gently graded tread away from the creek, a welcome change following the lengthy climb. Beyond a crossing of a seasonal stream, a moderate, half-mile ascent leads to a junction, 1.9 miles from the trailhead.

Turn left (west) at the junction and follow gently descending tread through scattered pines, with views to the north of the Monarch Divide. After a quarter mile, reach a low spot on a ridge, and then start a gently rising climb to Cedar Grove Overlook at a granite knob near the end of the ridge. From the overlook, you can gaze straight down to Cedar Grove, 1,500 feet below. The bird's-eye view of South Fork Kings River is expansive, from the western foothills to beyond the confluence of Bubbs Creek. To the north, the Monarch Divide cuts a dramatic profile across the Sierra sky.

After fully enjoying the awesome view, retrace your steps to the trailhead.

CEDAR GROVE TRAILHEADS

TRIP 74

Hotel and Lewis Creeks Loop

 MS ↻ or / **DH**

DISTANCE: 6.4 miles, out-and-back

5 miles, point-to-point

ELEVATION: 4,675'/6,225'/4,675', +2,100'/-2,100'/±4,200'

4,675'/6,225'/4,560', +1,970'/-2,090/'±4,060'

SEASON: May to November

USE: Light

MAPS: USGS's *Cedar Grove* or SNHA's *Cedar Grove* or Tom Harrison Maps' *Kings Canyon High Country Trail Map*

↑
see
map on
p.236

TRAIL LOG

1.9   Cedar Grove Overlook junction
3.25 Lewis Creek Trail junction
5.0   Lewis Creek Trailhead
6.4   Hotel Creek Trailhead

INTRODUCTION: One of the most scenic chasms in the Sierra, Kings Canyon is also one of the deepest gorges in North America, reaching a depth of 8,000 feet from Spanish Mountain just outside the park boundary. To gain the extraordinary views from the canyon's rim, hikers must surmount the steep walls via one of a handful of correspondingly steep trails. The trail to Cedar Grove Overlook is no exception, gaining more than 1,500 feet in nearly 2.5 miles.

However, the effort is well rewarded with expansive views of Kings Canyon and the Monarch Divide. The ascent can be a scorcher during the typically sunny and hot

afternoons—get an early start if possible. Unfortunately, photographers will find the best light in late afternoon, when the sun is well to the west.

DIRECTIONS TO TRAILHEAD:
START: Follow Kings Canyon Highway into Kings Canyon and to the Cedar Grove turnoff, 34 miles from the Y-intersection with the Generals Highway. Follow signs to the pack station and turn right, 0.5 mile from the highway. Immediately after the turn, locate a small parking area on the left for the Hotel Creek Trailhead.

END: If you are arranging a shuttle, find the Lewis Creek Trailhead on the north shoulder of Kings Canyon Highway, 0.4 mile east of the park boundary and 1.3 miles west of the Cedar Grove turnoff.

DESCRIPTION: Climb moderately steeply on the Hotel Creek Trail up a hillside to a junction with a trail from the pack station. Continue climbing through a mixed forest of oaks, pines, and firs, now within earshot of Hotel Creek. Soon reach a spur heading shortly down to the creek, and follow the main trail on a series of switchbacks through scattered oaks and pines.

After a half mile, the trees are left behind, as the stiff climb continues across chaparral-covered slopes. The switchbacks eventually end where the trail turns west and follows gently graded tread away from the creek, a welcome change following the lengthy climb. Beyond a crossing of a seasonal stream, a moderate, half-mile ascent leads to a junction, 1.9 miles from the trailhead.

⊡ **SIDE TRIP TO CEDAR GROVE OVERLOOK:** Turn left (west) at the junction and follow gently descending tread through scattered pines, with views to the north of the Monarch Divide. After a quarter mile, reach a low spot on a ridge and then start a gently rising climb to Cedar Grove Overlook at a granite knob near the end of the ridge. From the overlook, you gaze straight down to Cedar Grove, 1,500 feet below. The bird's-eye view of South Fork Kings River is expansive, from the western foothills to beyond the confluence of Bubbs Creek. To the north, the Monarch Divide cuts a dramatic profile across the Sierra sky. **END OF SIDE TRIP**

From the overlook junction, make a gentle descent through a forest of scattered Jeffrey pines, where paintbrush and lupine brighten the floor in early season. After crossing a pair of seasonal drainages, follow a moderate climb toward the high point of the trip at the top of a ridge. Along the way, the mostly open terrain affords good views of Monarch Divide. From the ridge, the long descent back to the floor of Kings Canyon begins through light forest, paralleling a tributary of Lewis Creek. Reach a signed junction with the Lewis Creek Trail, 3.25 miles from the trailhead.

Turn left (southwest) passing through Jeffrey pines in various stages of succession following the periodic fires common in this region. High above Lewis Creek, follow numerous switchbacks down the canyon, alternating between brief sections of light shade from a mixed forest and exposed slopes covered with chaparral. Eventually, the lengthy descent ends at the Lewis Creek Trailhead, 5 miles from the Hotel Creek Trailhead.

If you did not make shuttle arrangements, you must hike a little-used trail back to the Hotel Creek Trailhead. Head southeast, paralleling River Road. The 1.4-mile trail undulates needlessly across the hillside above the level road, but provides the most direct return to the trailhead.

ROADS END TRAILHEADS

TRIP 75

Zumwalt Meadow Nature Trail

E ↻ DH

DISTANCE: 1.5 miles, loop

ELEVATION: 5,000'/5,050', +100'/-100'/±200'

SEASON: May to November

USE: Heavy

MAPS: USGS's *The Sphinx* or SNHA's *Cedar Grove* or *Zumwalt Meadow Nature Trail*

INTRODUCTION: The easy 1.5-mile loop around Zumwalt Meadow offers a leisurely way to become acquainted with the ecology

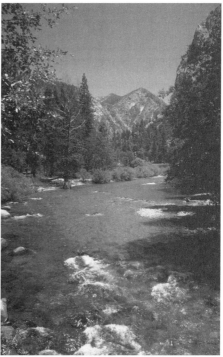

South Fork Kings River from Zumwalt Meadow Bridge

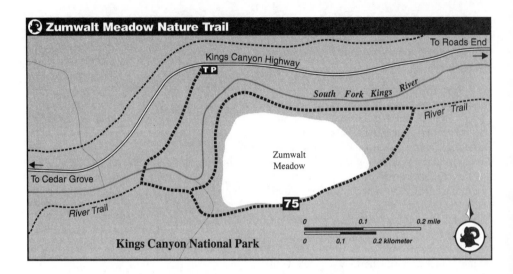

of Kings Canyon. An inexpensive pamphlet, filled with interesting tidbits about the area's natural history and sold at the trailhead, is a fine complement to the circuit around the meadow. The loop offers plenty of fine scenery as well, with fine views of Zumwalt Meadow, South Fork Kings River, and the geologic features of Kings Canyon, including Grand Sentinel and North Dome.

DIRECTIONS TO TRAILHEAD: Follow Kings Canyon Highway into Kings Canyon and to the parking area on the south side of the highway, 4.25 miles past the Cedar Grove turnoff.

DESCRIPTION: Stop first at the trailhead signboard to pick up a pamphlet keyed to the numbered posts along the self-guided trail. From there, follow a wide path to a suspension bridge over South Fork Kings River with a fine view across the water of Zumwalt Meadow and Grand Sentinel. Continue past the bridge a very short distance to a junction with the River Trail, and turn left to head upstream to a junction of the loop around the meadow. Proceed straight ahead, leaving the forest canopy behind and climbing briefly across an exposed section of talus above the meadow, with good views across Zumwalt Meadow of the river and canyon from this slightly higher vantage.

Turn left at the next junction, follow the grassy fringe of the meadow around to the riverbank, and then follow the winding river downstream to close the loop. From there, retrace your steps to the trailhead.

TRIP 76

River Trail

E ⟋ or ⟋ **DH**

DISTANCE: 5 miles, out-and-back

2.5 miles, point-to-point

ELEVATION: 5,040'/4,850'/5,040',
+35'/-225'/±520'

5,040'/4,850', +35'/-225'/±260'

SEASON: May to November

USE: Heavy

MAPS: USGS's *The Sphinx* or SNHA's
Cedar Grove

INTRODUCTION: The River Trail provides hikers an easy opportunity to experience the unique environment along South Fork Kings River. The towering granite walls of Grand Sentinel and North Dome—features that rival the more renowned works of Yosemite—complement the pleasant scenery along the riverbank. With shuttle arrangements, the gently descending trail offers a one-way journey between Roads End and Roaring River Falls. Even without a shuttle, the dis-

tance is short enough to allow most hikers time enough to go out and back.

DIRECTIONS TO TRAILHEAD:

START: Follow Kings Canyon Highway into Kings Canyon and to the day-use parking area at Roads End, 5 miles past the Cedar Grove turnoff.

END: If you are arranging a shuttle, find the Roaring River Falls parking area on the south shoulder of Kings Canyon Highway, 2.8 miles west of the Cedar Grove turnoff.

DESCRIPTION: Find the start of the trail immediately southwest of the day-use parking lot, near a trailhead sign. Follow the path through mixed forest and lush ground cover to a steel-and-wood bridge across South Fork Kings River, from where during the summer hikers will likely see numerous swimmers and anglers in the river or along the banks. On the far side of the bridge is a three-way junction with the Kanawyer Loop Trail on the left and the continuation of the River Trail on the right.

Turn right at the junction, and head downstream toward Zumwalt Meadow, passing a mixture of giant boulders and broken rock deposited at the base of the Grand Sentinel, its vertical walls rising nearly 3,500 feet above. A gentle descent leads through mixed forest along the riverbank to a junction near the grassy clearing

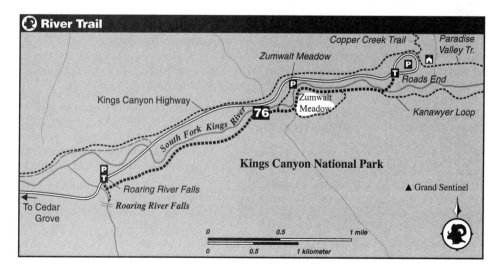

of Zumwalt Meadow, 0.6 mile from Roads End. At this junction, you can follow either branch of the Zumwalt Meadow Nature Trail; the paths will converge again beyond the west edge of the meadow, 0.4 mile downstream.

Near where the paths converge, there is a fine view across the canyon of North Dome, a granite monolith towering 3,600 feet above the floor of Kings Canyon, nearly as high as Yosemite's El Capitan. Soon after the two paths reunite, the Zumwalt Meadow Nature Trail branches north, crosses a bridge over the river, and soon reaches the parking lot.

Remaining on the River Trail, proceed downstream toward Roaring River Falls through mixed forest and past another boulder field. The gently descending trail leads to a junction at 2.4 miles with the extremely short Roaring River Falls Trail on the left. This short side journey is definitely worth the little extra time necessary to reach the viewpoint, especially early in the season when the falls truly lives up to its name. Immediately past the junction, the trail terminates at the parking area along the highway shoulder.

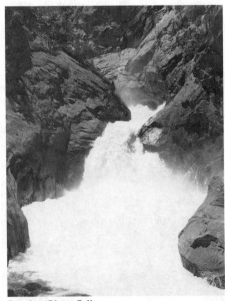

Roaring River Falls

ROADS END TRAILHEADS

TRIP 77

Kanawyer Loop Trail

E ↻ **DH**

DISTANCE: 4.7 miles, loop

ELEVATION: 5,045'/5,175'/5,045', +265'/-265'/±530'

SEASON: May to November

USE: Heavy

MAPS: USGS's *The Sphinx* or SNHA's *Cedar Grove*

INTRODUCTION: Roads End is a very popular trailhead for the army of recreationists bound for the heart of the southern Sierra. Undoubtedly, you will share the first half of this loop with plenty of fellow dayhikers, backpackers, and equestrians headed for popular destinations via the Paradise Valley and Bubbs Creek Trails. On the second half the number of troops should fall off dramatically, raising the opportunity for solitude. The Kanawyer Loop is an easy stroll along the nearly level floor of Kings Canyon, making it a trip for just about anyone. Be prepared for hot summertime temperatures at these elevations, but relief is never too far away with the prospect of a refreshing dip in South Fork Kings River.

DIRECTIONS TO TRAILHEAD: Follow Kings Canyon Highway into Kings Canyon and to the day-use parking area at Roads End, 5 miles past the Cedar Grove turnoff.

DESCRIPTION: The well-signed trail begins at the east edge of the paved turnaround, near the wilderness permit station. Follow wide, sandy, gently ascending tread, roughly paralleling South Fork Kings River, through a mixed forest of incense cedars, ponderosa pines, black oaks, sugar pines, and white firs. Soon cross a wood bridge over Copper Creek, and proceed up the canyon into thinning forest cover, which allows views of the impressive granite walls forming the canyon. Soon enter cool forest on the way to a signed Y-junction with the Paradise Valley Trail, 1.9 miles from the trailhead.

Head right (south) at the junction and immediately cross a bridge over the river, just downstream from the confluence of Bubbs Creek. Past the bridge, reach a junction with the Bubbs Creek Trail.

Turn right (southwest) at the junction, cross Avalanche Creek on a pair of logs, and continue on gently graded tread through dense forest. Pass a small meadow and then draw nearer to the river. Occasionally, the forest parts enough to allow grand views of the canyon walls. A short climb through a boulder field leads to a junction with the River Trail near a bridge across the river. Turn right here, cross the bridge, and then gently ascend through thick forest and lush ground cover back to the parking lot at Roads End.

ROADS END TRAILHEADS

TRIP 78

Sphinx Creek

Ⓜ ↗ **DH** or **BP**

DISTANCE: 12.4 miles, out-and-back

ELEVATION: 5,045'/8,575', +3,745'/-215'/±7,920'

SEASON: Mid-June to November

USE: Moderate

MAPS: USGS's *The Sphinx* or Tom Harrison Maps' *Kearsarge Pass-Rae Lakes Loop Trail Map*

TRAIL LOG

1.9 Paradise Valley Trail junction
2.0 Bubbs Creek and Kanawyer Trails junction
3.5 Sphinx Creek Camp and Sphinx Creek Trail junction

INTRODUCTION: The stiff climb from the floor of Kings Canyon to Sphinx Creek may deter the casual hiker, but the wonderful scenery is exceedingly rewarding for those with enough stamina to survive the

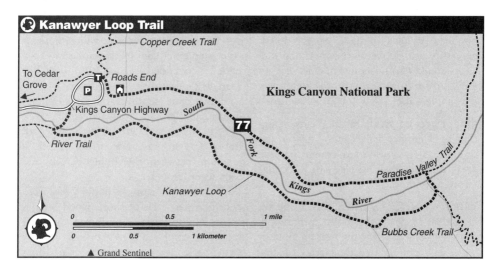

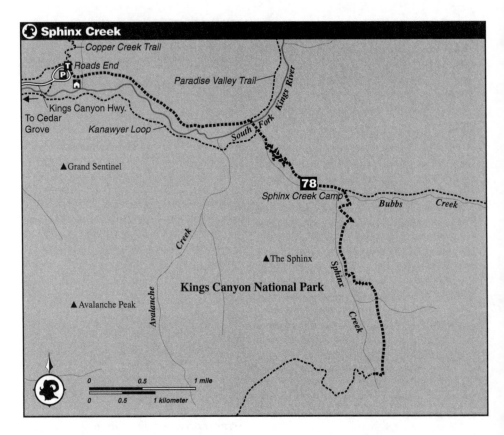

Sphinx Creek

Copper Creek Trail
Roads End
Paradise Valley Trail
Kings River
South Fork
Kings Canyon Hwy.
To Cedar Grove
Kanawyer Loop
▲Grand Sentinel
78
Sphinx Creek Camp
Bubbs Creek
Creek
Sphinx
▲The Sphinx
Kings Canyon National Park
▲ Avalanche Peak
Avalanche
Creek
0   0.5   1 mile
0   0.5   1 kilometer

rugged ascent. Fortunately, most recreationists embarking from Roads End are bound for places other than Sphinx Creek, which makes this trip even more attractive to those looking to escape the customary crowds. Get an early start since this trail's low elevation and the lack of shade on the ascent makes it a real cooker in the afternoon sun. Cross-country enthusiasts will enjoy a 2- to 3-mile, off-trail extension to the highly scenic Sphinx Lakes.

DIRECTIONS TO TRAILHEAD: Follow Kings Canyon Highway into Kings Canyon and to either the day-use or overnight parking areas at Roads End, 5 miles past the Cedar Grove turnoff.

DESCRIPTION: The well-signed trail begins at the east edge of the paved turnaround, near the wilderness permit station. Follow wide, sandy, gently ascending tread, roughly paralleling South Fork Kings River, through a mixed forest of incense cedars, ponderosa pines, black oaks, sugar pines, and white firs. Soon cross a wood bridge over Copper Creek and proceed up the canyon into thinning forest cover, which allows views of the impressive granite walls forming the canyon. Soon enter cool forest on the way to a signed Y-junction with the Paradise Valley Trail, 1.9 miles from the trailhead.

Head right (south) at the junction, and immediately cross a bridge over the river, just downstream from the confluence of Bubbs Creek. Past the bridge, reach a junction between the Bubbs Creek and Kanawyer Loop Trails.

Turn upstream on the Bubbs Creek Trail and follow a series of short, wood bridges across multiple braids of Bubbs Creek. A moderate climb leads to the first of many switchbacks away from the floor of Kings

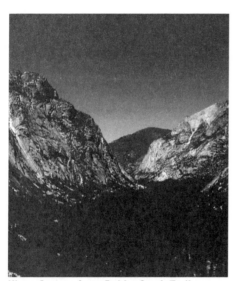

Kings Canyon from Bubbs Creek Trail

Canyon and up the Bubbs Creek drainage. Through gaps in the scrubby forest are excellent views of the canyon, the dramatic rock pinnacle of The Sphinx, and, in early season, a spectacular cascade on Bubbs Creek. Take a break from the switchbacks, where the trail ascends the east side of the canyon, well above the level of the creek. Continuing the moderate climb, pass through an area where conifers cover the slope. At 3.5 miles, reach Sphinx Creek Camp and a junction with the Sphinx Creek Trail. Both sides of Bubbs Creek have excellent campsites (with bear boxes) here, the first legal camping area beyond the trailhead. A pit toilet is above the north bank.

From the junction, cross Bubbs Creek on a log-and-plank bridge to the south bank, and begin a stiff, switchbacking ascent up Sphinx Creek canyon, where widely scattered conifers offer little shade. Higher up the drainage, white firs eventually provide some small respite from the summer sun, but the moderate to moderately steep climb continues unabated. Fine views of the mountainous terrain may temporarily distract you from the grueling ascent.

High above Sphinx Creek, the grade eventually eases near the 5.5-mile mark, where a short drop follows a half mile of mildly ascending tread to a ford of the creek. On the far side, a lush forest floor carpeted with grasses and wildflowers graces the scattered campsites of Upper Sphinx Creek Camp.

An unmaintained path once followed Sphinx Creek up to Sphinx Creek Lakes. A moderately difficult cross-country route still follows traces of the old path up a canyon to a series of lakes. These quite attractive lakes, tucked beneath Sphinx Ridge at about 10,500 feet, offer scenic campsites and good fishing. From the lakes, Class 2 routes lead up to the summits of Mt. Brewer and Cross Mountain.

A wilderness permit is required for overnight stays. Camping is prohibited for the first 3.5 miles between the trailhead and Sphinx Creek Camp. Bear canisters are required. Campfires are prohibited above 10,400 feet.

TRIP 79

Circle of Solitude: Great Western and Kings-Kern Divides Loop

MS ↺ BP

DISTANCE: 68 miles, loop

ELEVATION: 5,045'/10,040'/7,420'/
12,000'/8,080'/13,180'/5,045',
+18,700'/-18,700'/±37,400'

SEASON: Mid-July to early October

USE: Light

MAPS: *The Sphinx, Sphinx Lakes,
Triple Divide Peak,
Mt. Kaweah, Mt. Brewer,
Mt. Williamson,* and
Mt. Clarence King

TRAIL LOG

6.2	Sphinx Creek
8.5	Avalanche Pass
14.2	Roaring River Ranger Station
18.5	Cement Table Meadow
20.5	Upper ford of Roaring River
22.0	Colby Lake
32.1	Junction Meadow and High Sierra Trail junction
40.7	Lake South America junction
48.5	Forester Pass
56.0	Bubbs Creek Trail junction
58.5	Junction Meadow

INTRODUCTION: A treasure trove of scenic wonders awaits backpackers on this extended loop through the heart of Kings Canyon and Sequoia National Parks backcountry. Wildflower-filled meadows, serene forests, scenic alpine lakes, glacier-carved canyons, and dramatic peaks are here in abundance. Beginning near 5,000 feet in Kings Canyon, the circuit eventually crosses three high passes—Avalanche (10,040 feet), Colby (12,000 feet), and Forester (13,160

feet)—before returning to the trailhead. Such a wide range of elevation provides plenty of diversity, from foothills woodland to alpine and just about everything else in between.

Much of the route passes through some of the most scenic and least visited areas of backcountry within the parks. Past the Sphinx Creek junction, foot traffic drops off dramatically until the John Muir and Bubbs Creek Trails. So remote are the Sphinx Creek, Cloud Canyon, Kern-Kaweah, and upper Kern Canyon regions that the route has been dubbed the "Circle of Solitude."

This route's vast elevation changes and the primitive condition of some stretches of trail make it appropriate only for seasoned backpackers who are in good shape. Experienced cross-country enthusiasts may explore the possibility of an off-trail route over Harrison Pass (Class 2) and down East Creek canyon as an alternative to the well-used John Muir Trail (JMT) over Forester Pass. Such a route is more in keeping with the secluded nature of the loop but requires a much higher degree of skill and experience than the straightforward route along the JMT and Bubbs Creek Trail. Both routes are included in this description. You can choose a cornucopia of options for extending your journey.

DIRECTIONS TO TRAILHEAD: Follow Kings Canyon Highway into Kings Canyon and to either of the overnight parking areas at Roads End, 5 miles past the Cedar Grove turnoff.

DESCRIPTION: The well-signed trail begins at the east edge of the paved turnaround, near the wilderness permit station. Follow wide, sandy, gently ascending tread, roughly paralleling South Fork Kings River, through a mixed forest of incense cedars, ponderosa pines, black oaks, sugar pines, and white firs. Soon cross a wood bridge over Copper Creek and proceed up the canyon into thinning forest cover, which allows views of the impressive granite walls forming the canyon. Soon enter cool forest on the way to a signed Y-junction with Paradise Valley Trail, 1.9 miles from the trailhead.

Head right (south) at the junction and immediately cross a bridge over the river, just downstream from the confluence of Bubbs Creek. Past the bridge, reach a junction between the Bubbs Creek and Kanawyer Loop Trails.

Turn up the Bubbs Creek Trail, and follow a series of short, wood bridges across multiple braids of Bubbs Creek. A moderate climb leads to the first of many switchbacks leading away from the floor of Kings Canyon and up the Bubbs Creek drainage. Through gaps in the scrubby forest you will have excellent views of the canyon, the dramatic rock pinnacle of The Sphinx, and, in early season, a spectacular cascade on Bubbs Creek. Take a break from the switchbacks, where the trail ascends the east side of the canyon, well above the level of the creek. Continuing the moderate climb, pass through an area where conifers cover the slope. At 3.5 miles, reach Sphinx Creek Camp and a junction with the Sphinx Creek Trail. Both sides of Bubbs Creek have excellent campsites (with bear boxes), the first legal camping area beyond the trailhead. A pit toilet is above the north bank.

From the junction, cross Bubbs Creek on a log-and-plank bridge to the south bank, and begin a stiff, switchbacking ascent up Sphinx Creek canyon, where widely scattered conifers offer little shade. Higher up the drainage, white firs eventually provide some small respite from the summer sun, but the moderate to moderately steep climb continues unabated. Fine views of the mountainous terrain provide temporary distractions from the grueling ascent. High above Sphinx Creek, the grade eventually eases near the 5.5-mile mark, where a short drop follows a half mile of mildly ascending tread to a ford of the creek. On the far side, a lush forest floor carpeted with grasses and wildflowers graces the scattered campsites of Upper Sphinx Creek Camp.

Leave the verdant creekside refuge of Upper Sphinx Creek Camp and climb over a series of forested ridges with minor stream gullies in between. Western white pines,

red firs, and lodgepole pines shade the trail on an extended moderate climb toward Avalanche Pass. You will have good views of Palmer Mountain through occasional gaps in the forest. Reach Avalanche Pass at 8.6 miles from the trailhead, where foxtail pines obscure any possible views.

Descend from the pass via occasional switchbacks, with views of Glacier Ridge and Silliman Crest across wildflower-covered clearings to a nascent tributary of Moraine Creek. Through scattered lodgepole pines, aspens, and western junipers, head down alongside the cavorting creek amid lush pockets of foliage, where wildflowers include penstemon, gentian, larkspur, paintbrush, pennyroyal, daisy, leopard lily, and Bigelow sneezeweed. Along the way, you hop over numerous tiny rivulets bordered by narrow swaths of similarly verdant flora. Leave the tributary behind, and continue a southbound descent of a forested hillside, interrupted by a pocket meadow, to the V-shaped canyon of Moraine Creek. Veer southwest and proceed down the canyon, passing a solitary campsite near the creek. The trail bends around the nose of the hill and leads to a crossing of vigorous Moraine Creek, 12 miles from the trailhead, aided by a number of downed logs.

Paralleling Moraine Ridge, follow the trail northwest through scattered pines and firs, with evidence of a former fire along the way. Eventually, climb up and over the broad crest of Moraine Ridge, where a fine view of Roaring River and Deadman Canyon unfolds. A steep, zigzagging descent on rocky tread through scrubby manzanita and widely scattered Jeffrey pines leads to a long, descending traverse toward Roaring River.

Approaching the river, pass a corral and some campsites on the way to a three-way junction, 14.3 miles from the trailhead. Your route, the Colby Pass Trail, continues up the east side of the river, while the other path heads over a bridge across the river to the Roaring River Ranger Station, additional campsites, and another three-way junction with trails to Deadman Canyon and Sugarloaf Valley.

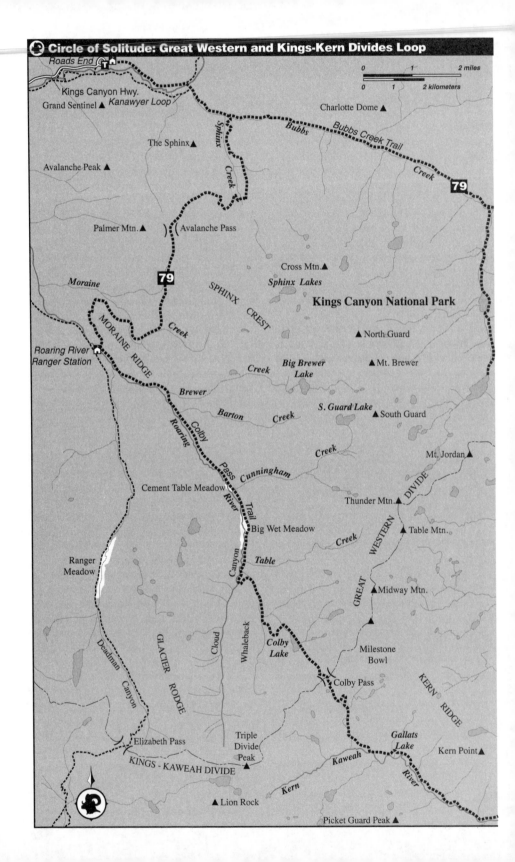

0   1   2 miles

0   1   2 kilometers

Roads End ⛺ T

Kings Canyon Hwy.

Grand Sentinel ▲ *Kanawyer Loop*

Charlotte Dome ▲

The Sphinx ▲

Sphinx

Creek

Bubbs   Bubbs Creek Trail

Avalanche Peak ▲

Creek

79

Palmer Mtn. ▲   ) (Avalanche Pass

Moraine

Cross Mtn. ▲

Sphinx Lakes

Kings Canyon National Park

SPHINX CREST

79

Creek

MORAINE RIDGE

▲ North Guard

Creek

Big Brewer Lake

▲ Mt. Brewer

Roaring River Ranger Station 🏠

Brewer

Barton   *Creek*

S. Guard Lake

▲ South Guard

Mt. Jordan ▲

Roaring

Colby

Creek

Pass

Cunningham

Cement Table Meadow

River

Big Wet Meadow

Table   Creek

Thunder Mtn. ▲

WESTERN

▲ Table Mtn.

DIVIDE

Ranger Meadow

Canyon

Trail

Table

GREAT

▲ Midway Mtn.

▲

Cloud

Whaleback

Colby Lake

Milestone Bowl

Deadman

GLACIER RIDGE

KERN RIDGE

Canyon

Elizabeth Pass

Triple Divide Peak

▲

Colby Pass

Gallats Lake

Kern Point ▲

KINGS - KAWEAH DIVIDE

Kaweah

River

🧭

Kern

▲ Lion Rock

Picket Guard Peak ▲

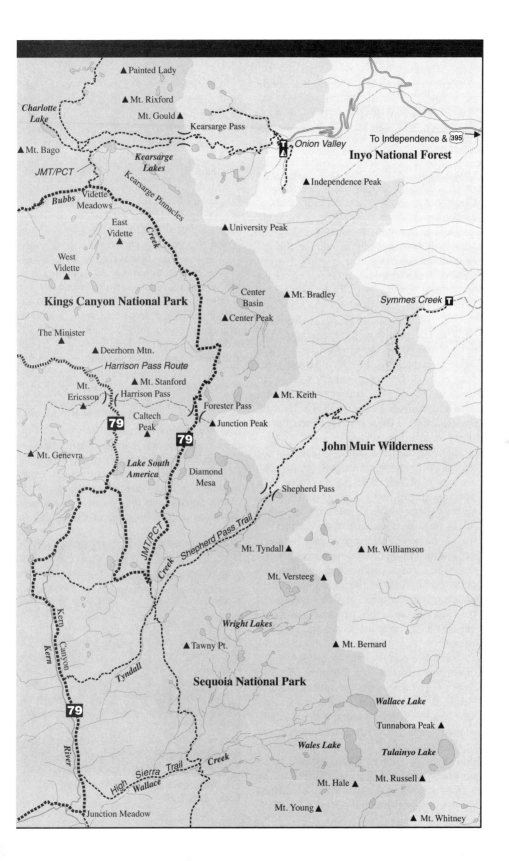

From the junction, follow the gently ascending Colby Pass Trail along the east side of tumbling Roaring River through scattered Jeffrey pines. Soon, a more moderate climb ensues, passing above a patch of meadow, through a gate in a drift fence, and into a light forest of lodgepole pines and red firs. Make a boulder hop over Brewer Creek and then cross the twin channels of Barton Creek a half mile farther. Continuing into Cloud Canyon, forested stands alternate with lush pockets of foliage for the next couple of miles. Climb gently toward Cement Table Meadow, an expansive clearing where the Roaring River becomes a tame, meandering brook weaving sinuously through grasses, sedges, and an array of wildflowers, including lupine, leopard lily, daisy, delphinium, shooting star, buttercup, columbine, paintbrush, and monkeyflower. Just past a three-pole gate, cross broad Cunningham Creek, and reach campsites with a hitching post nearby, 18.6 miles from the trailhead. There are additional campsites farther up the meadow.

Beyond Cement Table Meadow, the trail starts climbing again, passing through a mixture of lodgepole pines, aspens, and lush clearings. As you emerge from an extensive aspen grove, you have an absolutely stunning view of the statuesque formation named Whaleback across the green expanse of Big Wet Meadow. Curve around the south fringe of the meadow beneath pines, mesmerized by the incredible scenery of the upper canyon. Near the far end of the meadow, a couple of campsites nestle beneath lodgepole pines near a seasonal stream.

Ahead, a somewhat confusing stretch of trail leads down to a significant ford of Roaring River, near the confluence of Table Creek. Beyond the ford, climb moderately steeply up a hillside, passing a shady campsite, to where the grade eases and the trail bends back toward the river. Several yards off the trail is Shorty's Cabin, a rustic structure built by Shorty Lovelace (1886–1963), a trapper who established a line of shelters for use during the winter season.

Continuing, step across a wood platform above a spring-fed pool and come to the upper ford of the river, 6.2 miles from the ranger station. Spacious campsites are scattered beneath pines near the ford. One campsite, "Grand Palace Hotel," was named for a sheepherder's carving on a nearby pine, referencing the plush San Francisco hotel. Previously, a trail followed the west side of the river farther up Cloud Canyon, but the path has long been abandoned (see options, page 255).

Leaving the relatively mellow grade of the trail through Cloud Canyon, follow a much steeper ascent that attacks the northern spine of Whaleback. Numerous switchbacks lead across the spine, above a tributary, and up a side canyon. About 0.75 mile from the ford, boulder hop a creek, and head upstream through open, rocky terrain, broken by patches of grasses, wildflowers, heather, willow, and an occasional dwarf lodgepole pine. Continue climbing up the side canyon, crossing back and forth over the creek a few times. Views ahead of the Great Western Divide and behind down Cloud Canyon seemingly improve with each step. Eventually, the trail veers away from the creek to climb directly up the east wall of the canyon, and then follows an ascending traverse to a crossing of Colby Lake's

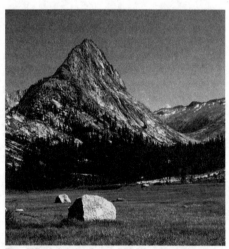

The Whaleback above Big Wet Meadow, Colby Pass Trail

outlet. A short stroll beside the outlet leads to the north shore of the lake, 8.75 miles from the ranger station.

A few campsites at the near end of the lake squeeze onto small pockets of soil between acres of rocky shoreline. If you don't object to sleeping on granite slabs, you'll have a plethora of campsites to choose from. The deep lake is a scenic gem, cradled by a large cirque beneath the craggy crest of the Great Western Divide. Anglers may drool over the sizable brook and rainbow trout gliding through the crystal-clear water.

The trail heads above the east shore of the lake to a willow-lined inlet, where a serious ascent toward Colby Pass begins. Switchbacks lead over rocky slopes to a ravine, which you ascend steeply to a cirque. A final zigzagging climb up a narrow chute culminates at 12,000-foot Colby Pass, 10.3 miles from the ranger station and 24.6 miles from the trailhead. The view from the pass is sublime, especially of the multihued Kaweah Peaks.

From Colby Pass, head down a sandy slope past a rock-rimmed tarn, and descend into a series of bowls, stepping over sprightly rivulets along the way. Excellent views of the Kern-Kaweah watershed and Kaweah Peaks Ridge adorn the descent. Eventually, scattered lodgepole pines start to reappear in the vicinity of a verdant meadow. A steeper descent over sandy soil and rock leads down into Kern-Kaweah River canyon.

The grade mercifully eases along the floor of the canyon, as the trail wanders amid lush ground cover beneath scattered to light timber. However, the mellow nature of the trail is short-lived, as the path begins a steeper decline along the now-tumbling Kern-Kaweah River, which races downstream through a series of cataracts. In due course, the grade eases once again on the approach to expansive Gallats Lake, which in all but early season will resemble more of a wet meadow bisected by a meandering brook than a bona fide lake. A couple of primitive campsites can be found along the fringe of the lake (or meadow), with tiny tributaries nearby.

Leaving the broad clearing of Gallats Lake, the trail resumes a more moderate descent over granite slabs, where the river charmingly cascades through rock clefts and slithers across slabs. Pass across a couple of avalanche swaths in scattered to light forest. The trail is sunk in a deep granite canyon, sandwiched between Kern Point at the end of Kern Ridge to the north and Picket Guard Peak to the south. The river starts to meander again on the aspen-lined approach to small, meadow-rimmed Rockslide Lake. Peaks of the Great Western Divide start to appear above the surrounding hills. Just beyond the lake, a few good campsites along the river nestle beneath lodgepole pines.

More arid vegetation of sagebrush and manzanita lines the trail where the canyon begins to narrow, which forces the trail to make an angling ascent across a hillside and up a series of tight, steep switchbacks out of a hanging valley to a narrow gap known as Kern-Kaweah Pass. Drop from the pass into a narrow ravine, and wind down a rocky trail between tall cliffs to a shrub-covered hillside. Deteriorating tread leads through sagebrush, currant, chinquapin, manzanita, willows, and assorted wildflowers to a set of switchbacks descending toward Junction Meadow. Reaching the floor of Kern River canyon, amble across multiple fords of the river and its tributaries—the main ford can be quite difficult early in the season. Through a thickening forest of pines and cedars, continue across the flat to a junction with the High Sierra Trail (HST), 7.5 miles from Colby Pass. A short distance south on the HST is a camping area (with a bear box) shaded by pines and next to a small stream.

At the junction, turn left (north) and follow the HST on a moderate climb through Jeffrey, ponderosa, and western white pines to a clearing, with excellent views of the Kern-Kaweah cleft and within earshot of the thundering river. More climbing leads up the canyon through a light forest of pines and aspens and eventually to a fine vista of the U-shaped Kern Trench. Reach a junction where the HST turns east, 1.1 miles from Junction Meadow.

Continue ahead up Kern Canyon through more pines, passing a number of good campsites on benches overlooking the river. On a mild to moderate ascent, follow the course of the river past more campsites to a ford of Tyndall Creek, which may be difficult in early season. At 3 miles from Junction Meadow, a small cairn marks a junction with the Tyndall Creek Trail heading northeast.

Continuing up Kern Canyon, pass additional campsites and then climb more steeply above a picturesque waterfall. The grade temporarily eases above the fall but soon intensifies where the trail attempts to match the gradient of the cascading river. In and out of forest cover, proceed upstream to a flower-carpeted glade, where columbine, aster, paintbrush, and groundsel add splashes of color. Step across a tiny stream, and start climbing steeply up a series of switchbacks to a crossing of a significant creek draining several unnamed tarns above (which have campsites). Beyond the creek the ascent resumes, scaling a hillside covered with granite slabs and then climbing over the lip of the upper Kern Plateau. The grade eventually eases on a gentle ascent over slabs and through scattered pines beside the river. Just before a large tarn at the base of some steep cliffs, pass an unmarked route to Milestone Basin (see options, page 255). Campsites on the south shore near the outlet offer good views. East of the tarn, reach a junction with a trail heading east to the JMT, 5.6 miles from Junction Meadow.

On sandy tread, proceed upstream with improving views of upper Kern River basin and the surrounding peaks, passing several picturesque tarns and equally scenic meadows along the way. A more exquisite and remote basin in the Sierra is hard to imagine, as the upper Kern Basin has everything one would want, including seemingly limitless possibilities for off-trail hideaways. Gently ascend slabs of granite through widely scattered whitebark and lodgepole pines and pockets of vegetation. Steeper climbing over rock ribs, outcroppings, and

gullies leads to a signed junction with a lateral to Lake South America, 8.6 miles from Junction Meadow.

Turn north at the junction, and stroll over to the far edge of a small tarn before dropping sharply to the south shore of austere Lake South America. Flanked by an amphitheater of peaks, including Mt. Genevra, Mt. Ericsson, and Caltech Peak, the lonely lake offers incredible alpine scenery. The few campsites scattered around the windswept shore in pockets of soil appear adequate for the small number of backpackers willing to venture this far off the beaten path. Golden trout will test the skill of anglers.

From Lake South America, backpackers have two principal options for returning to Roads End. Experienced cross-country enthusiasts can follow a mostly straightforward route over Harrison Pass but must accept the challenge of a difficult, Class 2 descent down the north side of the pass (see page 254 for a description of that route). Hikers who want to stick to maintained trails should follow the lengthier route of the JMT over Forester Pass to the Bubbs Creek Trail.

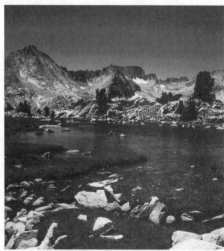

Remote Lake South America near the Kern River headwaters

FORESTER PASS ROUTE: From the junction of the lateral to Lake South America, head southeast up and over a low ridge to a long meadow basin with a pair of tarns at each end. Gently descending tread leads across the lengthy clearing to the far end, where a short, rising climb is followed by a similar descent to a T-junction, 2.25 miles from the previous one.

Turn left (east) at the junction, and descend through the scenic terrain of the upper Tyndall Creek basin rimmed by peaks of the Sierra Crest for about a mile to a junction with the JMT, just beyond a tarn with excellent campsites.

Turn left (north) onto the JMT, and proceed on a mild to moderate climb above timberline through open terrain, which offers excellent views of the upper basin. Pass some lovely tarns and step across trickling streams on the way to the base of the headwall below Forester Pass. As with many High Sierra passes, a viable route over the headwall seems unlikely until the switchbacking ascent begins. The trail is something of an engineering marvel, literally blasted out of the sheer rock face—*sections of the climb will not appeal to acrophobes.* Finally reach a narrow gap in the Kings-Kaweah Divide at Forester Pass at the boundary between Kings Canyon and Sequoia National Parks, 16.5 miles from Junction Meadow. The wide-ranging view from the pass of myriad peaks in almost every direction is quite amazing.

After you have witnessed the precipitous terrain on the south side of Forester Pass, the north side seems a piece of cake, descending smooth, sandy tread on switchbacks to the top of a rock rib above a tarn in the head of the canyon. Proceed to the end of the rib, enjoying excellent views along the way, and then follow an angling descent to a crossing of Bubbs Creek just below the tarn. Continue the winding, rocky descent, fording the creek several more times, as the trail bends west and drops into more hospitable terrain. In a grove of pines, just beyond the fire boundary, pass a couple of poor campsites tiered down the steep slope. More switchbacks lead into a light forest

of scattered lodgepole and whitebark pines, past small pockets of verdant, wildflower-dotted meadows, and through clumps of willow to a ford of Center Basin Creek. Past the ford are better campsites (with a bear box) and a junction with the Center Basin Trail, 4.5 miles from the pass. A side trip to Golden Bear Lake up the Center Basin Trail is a worthy endeavor.

In and out of scattered to light lodgepole pine forest, continue the descent along the course of tumbling Bubbs Creek, sandwiched between the towering pinnacle of East Vidette on the west and the rugged spine of the Kearsarge Pinnacles to the east. Hop across a number of tributaries on the way to Upper Vidette Meadow and a number of overused campsites beneath pines along the creek. Beyond the meadow, pass a lateral to a horse packer's camp, and continue to the popular Vidette Meadows campsites (with bear boxes), which cater to JMT thru-hikers and Rae Lakes Loop backpackers. After a pair of stream crossings, reach a three-way junction with the Bubbs Creek Trail, 7.7 miles from Forester Pass.

Turn away from the JMT, and head west on Bubbs Creek Trail on a short descent to the north edge of expansive Lower Vidette Meadow. Overnighters will find excellent, but heavily used, campsites (with a bear box) nestled beneath lodgepole pines along the meadow's fringe.

Leaving the gently graded trail along the meadow behind, follow a more pronounced descent as the now tumbling creek plunges down the gorge. Momentarily break out into the open, where a large hump of granite provides an excellent vantage from which to survey the surrounding terrain. Head back into forest cover, and continue down the canyon, stepping over a number of lushly lined freshets along the way. The forest breaks enough on occasion to allow views of the dramatic topography above East Creek canyon, including Mt. Brewer, North Guard, and Mt. Farquhar. Farther down Bubbs Creek, picturesque waterfalls and cascades provide additional visual treats. The stiff descent eventually eases near the edge of grassy, fern-filled, wildflower-covered

Junction Meadow. Stroll across the meadow to a signed, three-way junction of the East Creek Trail, 2.3 miles from the JMT junction. Campsites can be found shortly down this trail on either side of a ford of Bubbs Creek, and farther west on the Bubbs Creek Trail past the horse camp.

HARRISON PASS ROUTE: Beyond Lake South America, the cross-country route through the upper Kern River basin is relatively straightforward. Follow the west shore of the lake, and then head directly north on a gentle grade up an open and broad valley. Near the head, a boot-beaten path becomes more evident and then climbs steeply up the headwall to the crest of the Kings-Kern Divide at Harrison Pass (approximately 12,720 feet), which is well east of the actual low point of the saddle. A partially obscured view to the north includes Mt. Goddard and the Palisades. A better vista to the south includes the hulk of Mt. Guyot, Kaweah Peaks Ridge, and Milestone Mountain.

The north side of the pass is the crux of the route. Steep and loose rock make the descent a bit difficult and potentially dangerous. In some years, ice and snow may cover the precipitous slope well into summer, further complicating the descent. Depending on the conditions and your party's experience, a rope and ice axes may be needed. From Harrison Pass, cautiously descend a chute to less difficult terrain below, and then angle toward the uppermost tarn below. Cross the outlet and bend west across the stream between the next two tarns. Climb over a knoll, drop down alongside the outlet of the third tarn, and follow the stream into the trees and then to a meadow. Cross the creek to the north bank, and continue down the canyon, following cairns over a low rise and down to charming campsites at Golden Lake (approximately 10,960 feet). Beyond the lake, the route follows the outlet to traces of an old and dusty trail that eventually switchbacks down a hillside to a junction with an unmaintained section of the East Creek Trail.

Reaching this point and bypassing beautiful Lake Reflection would be a shame, so turn upstream (southwest) and follow a gentle ascent through pockets of willows past a small lake to the north shore of the windswept lake, Scenic campsites are scattered around the far shore. After your visit to Lake Reflection, return to the junction.

From the junction, head north downstream along East Creek canyon through scattered stands of lodgepole and foxtail pines. Just after stepping over a side stream, reach the shore of grass-rimmed East Lake, sandwiched between towering granite peaks. After the rock-filled terrain of the last few miles, the more pastoral surroundings of the lake are a welcome change. Good campsites line the south and north shores and, unlike for many subalpine lakes in the parks, campfires are allowed.

Leaving East Lake, continue downstream on a gentle to moderate descent. Beyond the crossing of a fern-lined tributary, the grade becomes steeper, and the trail switchbacks down the east wall of the canyon through dense pine forest. Follow the course of vigorous East Creek to a ford, 1.4 miles below East Lake, and then continue the descent along the west bank, switchbacking down the canyon through a light forest of red firs, western white pines, lodgepole pines, and aspens. Reaching the floor of Bubbs Creek canyon, pass some secluded campsites, and come to the ford of Bubbs Creek, which could be difficult early in the season. Beyond the ford, stroll through the lush foliage of Junction Meadow to a junction with the Bubbs Creek Trail, 1.9 miles from East Lake.

Whichever route got you to the Bubbs Creek Trail junction, head away from Junction Meadow on a moderate descent alongside turbulent Bubbs Creek, passing through the moderate cover of a white fir forest. After nearly 2 miles of steady descent, the creek mellows and the grade eases through an aspen grove with a floor of ferns on the way to a log crossing over Charlotte Creek. Nearby, a short lateral leads to campsites near Bubbs Creek, where fishing for rainbow, brook, and brown trout is reportedly good.

Gently graded trail continues for a while beyond Charlotte Creek, as you hop across a trio of side streams and stroll through shoulder-high ferns. Then Bubbs Creek resumes its tumultuous course down the gorge. A steady, moderate descent follows the course of the creek for the next several miles. Farther down the canyon, moderate forest gives way to a light covering of trees, composed mainly of Jeffrey pines, with lesser amounts of firs, incense cedars, and black oaks. Reach Sp hinx Creek Camp and a junction of the Sphinx Creek Trail, 8.25 miles from the JMT, which closes the loop. From there, retrace your steps 3.5 miles back to the trailhead at Roads End.

[O] The only limit to trip routes in this area is your own imagination. Where the Colby Pass Trail crosses Roaring River to climb toward the lake, an abandoned trail, once referred to as the Coppermine Trail, continues up Cloud Canyon. Traces of the old trail still exist, but the unmaintained path is now considered a cross-country route. Proceed upstream to the head of the canyon, where you could veer southeast to Glacier Lake or west over Glacier Ridge to Coppermine Pass (11,960 feet, 0.3 mile north of Peak 12345). From the pass, traverse west above the abandoned Oakland Mine to the Elizabeth Pass Trail. From upper Cloud Canyon, Lion Lake Pass (approximately 11,600 feet) provides access to Lion Lake, and Triple Divide Pass (approximately 12,200 feet) and a high

route to the upper Kern-Kaweah country. Both passes are Class 2.

Milestone Basin can be reached via a cross-country route leaving the Colby Pass Trail approximately 1 mile southeast of the pass. From upper Milestone Bowl, a route over Milestone Pass (approximately 12,960 feet, 0.2 mile southeast of Milestone Peak) provides a Class 2 connection through Milestone Basin—via an abandoned trail down Milestone Creek—to the Kern River Trail, about 200 yards south of an unnamed tarn (approximately 10,635 feet), just west of a junction with a connector to the JMT.

The upper Kern Basin offers plenty of interesting nooks for off-trail exploration. Three alternative crossings of the Kern-Kaweah Divide include Lucys Foot Pass (approximately 12,400 feet), Ericson Pass (approximately 12,560 feet), and Millys Foot Pass (approximately 12,240 feet)—all Class 2).

Visitors to upper Cloud Canyon can ascend Triple Divide Peak by a variety of Class 2 and 3 routes. From Milestone Bowl, Milestone Mountain is Class 2 from the south. From Milestone Creek, the east ridge of Midway Mountain is Class 2. Peaks of the Great Western Divide and Kings-Kern Divide offer numerous intermediate climbs.

[R] A wilderness permit is required for overnight stays. Camping is prohibited for the first 3.5 miles between the trailhead and Sphinx Creek Camp. Bear canisters are required. Campfires are prohibited above 10,400 feet.

TRIP 80

East Lake and Lake Reflection

Ⓜ ⟋ **BP**

DISTANCE: 27 miles, out-and-back

ELEVATION: 5,045'/10,300', +5,420'/-410'/±11,660'

SEASON: Mid-July to early October

USE: Light

MAPS: *The Sphinx, Mt. Clarence King,* and *Mt. Brewer*

TRAIL LOG

3.5	Sphinx Creek Camp
6.7	Charlotte Creek
9.6	Junction Meadow
11.6	East Lake
13.5	Lake Reflection

INTRODUCTION: Of the 25 backpackers allowed to leave Roads End each day on the Bubbs Creek Trail, most are bound for the popular Rae Lakes Loop, bypassing the incredible scenery up the nearly forgotten side canyon of East Creek. While most of these loopers usually spend from four to five days completing their circuit, they could easily instead enjoy the serene environs of East Lake, Lake Reflection, and the upper basin beyond. From a stunningly picturesque base camp at Lake Reflection, mountaineers have a bounty of impressive summits to scale. Even anglers will be tempted by rumors of good-size trout. Whatever their motivation, backpackers will be rewarded with incomparable alpine scenery.

DIRECTIONS TO TRAILHEAD: Follow Kings Canyon Highway into Kings Canyon and to either of the overnight parking areas at Roads End, 5 miles past the Cedar Grove turnoff.

DESCRIPTION: The well-signed trail begins at the east edge of the paved turnaround, near the wilderness permit station. Follow wide, sandy, gently ascending tread, roughly paralleling South Fork Kings River, through a mixed forest of incense cedars, ponderosa pines, black oaks, sugar pines, and white firs. Soon cross a wood bridge over Copper Creek and proceed up the canyon into thinning forest cover, which allows views 👁 of the impressive granite walls forming the canyon. Soon enter cool forest on the way to a signed Y-junction with Paradise Valley Trail, 1.9 miles from the trailhead.

Head right (south) at the junction, and immediately cross a bridge over the river, just downstream from the confluence of Bubbs Creek. Past the bridge, reach a junction between the Bubbs Creek and Kanawyer Loop Trails.

Turn up the Bubbs Creek Trail, and follow a series of short, wood bridges across multiple braids of Bubbs Creek. A moderate climb leads to the first of many switchbacks leading away from the floor of Kings Canyon and up the Bubbs Creek drainage. Through gaps in the scrubby forest, you will have excellent views of the canyon, the dramatic rock pinnacle of The Sphinx, and, in early season, a spectacular cascade on Bubbs Creek. Take a break from the switchbacks, where the trail ascends the east side of the canyon, well above the level of the creek. Continuing the moderate climb, pass through an area where conifers cover the slope. At 3.5 miles, reach Sphinx Creek Camp and a junction with the Sphinx Creek Trail. Both sides of Bubbs Creek have excellent campsites (with bear boxes), the first 🄛 legal camping area beyond the trailhead. A pit toilet is above the north bank.

From Sphinx Creek Camp, proceed east on the Bubbs Creek Trail, passing in and out of a mixed forest of black oaks, Jeffrey and ponderosa pines, white firs, and incense cedars, with an understory of ferns and shrubs. Well past a trio of tiny brooks, ford Charlotte Creek and immediately reach a lateral, 6.7 miles from the trailhead, to pleasant, tree-shaded campsites on the 🄛 north bank of Bubbs Creek, where fishing is reportedly fair for brown, brook, and rainbow trout.

Alternating stretches of lush foliage and dry slopes make up the next couple of miles, as the trail makes a steady ascent up the canyon. Mt. Bago looms above the north wall through periodic gaps in the forest. The grade eventually eases, passing campsites, through a gate in a drift fence, and by the horse camp on the way to verdant Junction Meadow, carpeted with grasses, ferns, and wildflowers, and a junction with the East Creek Trail, 9.7 miles from the trailhead. Down the East Creek Trail are several good campsites on either side of Bubbs Creek.

From the junction, turn right (southeast) and proceed through the dense foliage of the meadow to the ford of Bubbs Creek, which may be difficult early in the season. From there, begin a steep climb up East Creek canyon via switchbacks, through a light forest covering of lodgepole and western white pines, red firs, and aspens. Views of the surrounding terrain improve with the gain in elevation. About a half mile from the Bubbs Creek, ford East Creek and continue climbing along the east bank of the vigorous stream. The climb becomes steeper where the trail enters thicker pine forest, switchbacking up the east wall of the canyon, until the grade eases beyond a fern-lined tributary draining an unnamed tarn to the east. A moderate, half-mile ascent leads to a brief, pleasant stroll just prior to the arrival at East Lake, 11.6 miles from Roads End.

Sandwiched between towering granite peaks, grass-rimmed East Lake is a pleasant sight. There are good campsites above the south and north shores, and campfires are permitted at this elevation.

Follow the trail around the east side of East Lake, step across an inlet from a side canyon, and then start climbing through

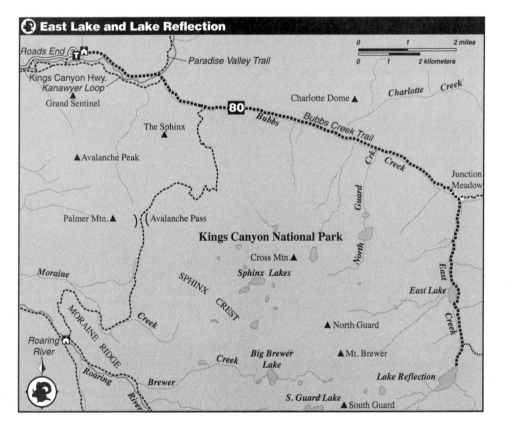

East Lake and Lake Reflection

Roads End
Kings Canyon Hwy.
Kanawyer Loop
Grand Sentinel
The Sphinx
Avalanche Peak
Palmer Mtn.
Avalanche Pass
Moraine
Roaring River
MORAINE RIDGE
Roaring
Brewer
River
SPHINX CREST
Creek
Paradise Valley Trail
Charlotte Dome
Charlotte Creek
Bubbs
Bubbs Creek Trail
Guard Crk.
Creek
Kings Canyon National Park
Cross Mtn.
Sphinx Lakes
Big Brewer Lake
Creek
North Guard
Mt. Brewer
S. Guard Lake
South Guard
Junction Meadow
North Guard
East Creek
East Lake
Lake Reflection
0   1   2 miles
0   1   2 kilometers
80

scattered stands of lodgepole and foxtail pines. Approximately a mile from the lake, near a talus slide, an abandoned trail to Harrison Pass ascends eastward (see options below). After negotiating the talus slide, pass some campsites along the creek, and gently ascend through pockets of meadow and willow. Just past a tarn, come to the shore of windswept Lake Reflection, where campsites are scattered around the south shore. Anglers should delight in fishing for good-size rainbow and golden trout.

[O] Options for further wanderings abound. Unless noted, all of the following passes are rated Class 2.

Two routes connect East Creek to South Guard Lake. The Brewer Pass route follows Ouzel Creek from the East Lake to the pass (approximately 12,640 feet, 0.5 mile south of Mt. Brewer). From there, drop to South Guard Lake. From Lake Reflection, an easy Class 1 route follows an old trail over Longley Pass (approximately 12,400 feet) to the lake.

The Thunder Pass route proceeds from Lake Reflection along the easternmost inlet, past a series of tarns, and up a snowfield (an ice axe may be necessary) to the pass (approximately 12,660 feet, 0.25 mile east of Thunder Mountain). From the pass, descend easier terrain to upper Kern basin.

The Harrison Pass route is a relatively well-known cross-country route from East Lake over Kings-Kern Divide and down to Lake South America (see Trip 79, page 246). Additional routes cross the Kings-Kern Divide at Millys Foot, Lucys Foot, Ericson, and Andys Foot Passes.

The Deerhorn Saddle route leaves the Harrison Pass route to climb over a saddle (approximately 12,560 feet, 0.4 mile southeast of Deerhorn Mountain), providing access to upper Vidette Creek.

A bevy of peaks accessible from East Creek canyon will tantalize mountaineers. There are intermediate routes on North Guard, Mt. Brewer, South Guard, Thunder Mountain, Mt. Jordan, Mt. Genevra, Mt. Ericson, Gregorys Monument, Mt. Stanford, The Minister, and Deerhorn Mountain.

[R] A wilderness permit is required for overnight stays. Camping is prohibited for the first 3.5 miles between the trailhead and Sphinx Creek Camp. Bear canisters are required. Campfires are prohibited above 10,400 feet.

TRIP 81

Charlotte Lake

Ⓜ ↗ BP

DISTANCE: 29 miles, out-and-back

ELEVATION: 5,045'/10,774',
+5,890'/-535'/±12,850'

SEASON: Mid-July to early October

USE: Heavy

MAPS: USGS's *The Sphinx* and
Mt. Clarence King or
Tom Harrison Maps'
*Kearsarge Pass-Rae Lakes
Loop Trail Map*

TRAIL LOG

3.6	Sphinx Creek Camp
6.8	Charlotte Creek
9.7	Junction Meadow
12.1	John Muir Trail junction
13.5	Charlotte Lake Trail junction

INTRODUCTION: Charlotte Lake offers a pleasant atmosphere for overnight stays in the heart of Kings Canyon's backcountry. However, because of the area's popularity, backpackers are limited by park regulations to a two-night stay. The lake is not only a fine destination, but JMT thru-hikers and backpackers doing the Rae Lakes Loop will find the lake a convenient overnight stop. Because of the distance and moderate climb from Roads End, most parties will opt for a first-night's camp somewhere along Bubbs Creek, such as Sphinx Creek Camp, Junction Meadow, or Vidette Meadow. Cross-country enthusiasts with extra time could follow the route of an abandoned trail from Charlotte Lake to isolated Gardiner Basin and then back to the Bubbs Creek Trail via Charlotte Creek (see options, page 261).

DIRECTIONS TO TRAILHEAD: Follow Kings Canyon Highway into Kings Canyon and to either of the overnight parking areas at Roads End, 5 miles past the Cedar Grove turnoff.

DESCRIPTION: The well-signed trail begins at the east edge of the paved turnaround, near the wilderness permit station. Follow wide, sandy, gently ascending tread, roughly paralleling South Fork Kings River, through a mixed forest of incense cedars, ponderosa pines, black oaks, sugar pines, and white firs. Soon cross a wood bridge over Copper Creek and proceed up the canyon into thinning forest cover, which allows views of the impressive granite walls forming the canyon. Soon enter cool forest on the way to a signed Y-junction with Paradise Valley Trail, 1.9 miles from the trailhead.

Head right (south) at the junction, and immediately cross a bridge over the river, just downstream from the confluence of Bubbs Creek. Past the bridge, reach a junction between the Bubbs Creek and Kanawyer Loop Trails.

Turn up the Bubbs Creek Trail, and follow a series of short, wood bridges across multiple braids of Bubbs Creek. A moderate climb leads to the first of many switchbacks leading away from the floor of Kings Canyon and up the Bubbs Creek drainage. Through gaps in the scrubby forest, you will have excellent views of the canyon, the dramatic rock pinnacle of The Sphinx, and, in early season, a spectacular cascade on Bubbs Creek. Take a break from the switchbacks, where the trail ascends the east side of the canyon, well above the level of the creek. Continuing the moderate climb, pass through an area where conifers cover the slope. At 3.5 miles, reach Sphinx Creek Camp and a junction with the Sphinx Creek Trail. Both sides of Bubbs Creek have excellent campsites (with bear boxes), the first legal camping area beyond the trailhead. A pit toilet is above the north bank.

From Sphinx Creek Camp, proceed east on the Bubbs Creek Trail, passing in and out of a mixed forest of black oaks, Jeffrey and ponderosa pines, white firs, and incense cedars, with an understory of ferns and shrubs. Well past a trio of tiny brooks, ford Charlotte Creek and immediately reach

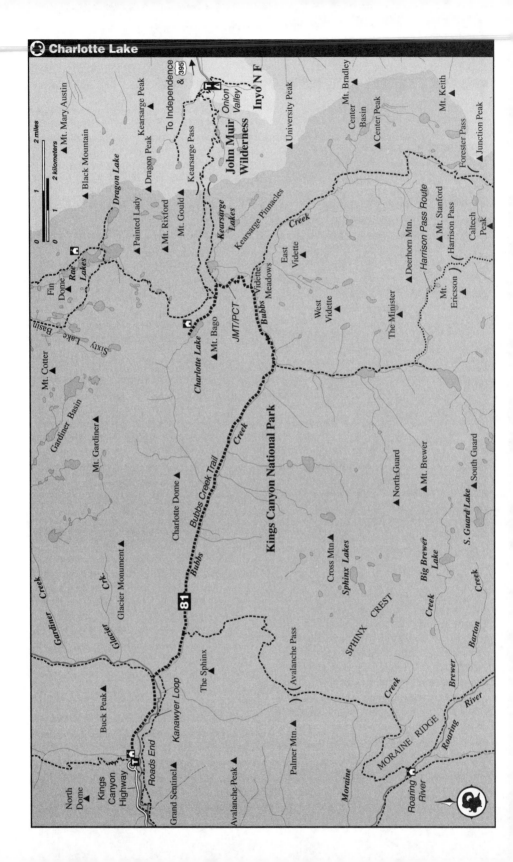

a lateral, 6.7 miles from the trailhead, to pleasant, tree-shaded campsites on the north bank of Bubbs Creek, where fishing is reportedly fair for brown, brook, and rainbow trout.

Alternating stretches of lush foliage and dry slopes make up the next couple of miles, as the trail makes a steady ascent up the canyon. Mt. Bago looms above the north wall through periodic gaps in the forest. The grade eventually eases, passing campsites, through a gate in a drift fence, and by the horse camp on the way to verdant Junction Meadow, carpeted with grasses, ferns, and wildflowers, and a junction with the East Creek Trail, 9.7 miles from the trailhead. There are several good campsites on either side of Bubbs Creek down the East Creek Trail.

From the junction, a short section of gentle tread leads east upstream through Bubbs Creek canyon. Steeper switchbacks follow, passing through alternate sections of forest and open terrain. Along the way, a picturesque stretch of Bubbs Creek, cascading over sloping slabs in dramatic fashion, provides an excellent rest spot. Farther on, openings in the forest grant fine views of the canyon walls and the towering peaks above. The grade eventually eases alongside the verdant expanse of Lower Vidette Meadow.

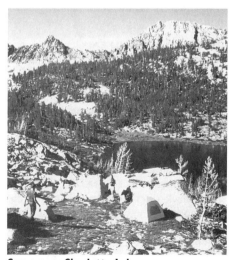

Camp near Charlotte Lake

Pastoral campsites near the meadow's fringe will tempt backpackers. Just beyond the meadow, in a stand of conifers, reach a signed three-way junction with the JMT, 12.1 miles from Roads End.

Turn left (north) onto the JMT, and make a moderate, switchbacking climb up the north wall of Bubbs Creek canyon, with good views of the dramatic Kearsarge Pinnacles to the east. Equally impressive is the vista behind of the Videttes and Deerhorn Mountain. After a pair of crossings over Bullfrog Lake's outlet, come to a three-way junction with the Bullfrog Lake Trail on the right. (Bullfrog Lake is one of the most picturesque lakes in the area and well worth the time to visit, but camping has been banned there for decades because of overuse.)

From the junction, a series of short-legged switchbacks lead up a lightly forested rise to a broad, sandy flat and a signed, four-way junction, 1.5 miles from the Bubbs Creek junction, with the Kearsarge Pass Trail heading northeast and the Charlotte Lake Trail heading west. (This junction is not correctly shown on the USGS map.)

Leaving the JMT, turn left onto the Charlotte Lake Trail, and wind downhill through light pine forest for 0.8 mile to the northeast shore of Charlotte Lake. Plenty of pine-shaded campsites are spread around the northeast shore, with a small ranger cabin and outhouse near the midpoint and a bear box farther northwest. There are a few less used and more open campsites on the south and southwest sides of the lake. The serene lake is cradled in a deep bowl between forested hills, with brilliant sunsets often displayed through the V-shaped notch of the outlet. Fishing for rainbow and brook trout is fair.

An abandoned trail (shown on the USGS map) leaves Charlotte Lake, heads northwest along the outlet, climbs west above the creek, and then veers away northwest toward Gardiner Pass (approximately 11,200 feet). The route then descends the steep north side of the pass and drops into a side canyon of Gardiner Creek. From a

9,534-foot lake, ascend a rise, drop steeply to the main branch of Gardiner Creek, and then turn east upstream. After about 0.75 mile, the route climbs south and then traverses east before ascending southeast into Gardiner Basin.

Two exits can be used to return to Roads End. The first leaves the upper basin, climbs to Sixty Lake Col, drops into Sixty Lakes Basin, and merges with a use trail providing straightforward access to the JMT near the highest Rae Lake. The second possible exit retraces the route down Gardiner Creek and over Gardiner Pass to Charlotte Creek. Easy travel downstream along Charlotte Creek leads to the Bubbs Creek Trail.

R A wilderness permit is required for overnight stays. Camping is prohibited for the first 3.5 miles between the trailhead and Sphinx Creek Camp. Bear canisters are required. Campfires are prohibited above 10,000 feet.

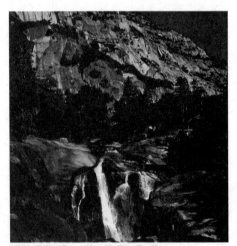

Mist Falls, Paradise Valley Trail

ROADS END TRAILHEADS

TRIP 82

Mist Falls

M ✔ **DH**

DISTANCE: 7.8 miles, out-and-back

ELEVATION: 5,045'/5,810', +765'/negligible/+1,530'

SEASON: May to late October

USE: Heavy

MAPS: USGS's *The Sphinx* or Tom Harrison Maps' *Kearsarge Pass-Rae Lakes Loop Trail Map*

INTRODUCTION: Anyone who visits Kings Canyon should make the nearly 4-mile trek to Mist Falls, especially early in the season when the falls are at full force. The first half of the journey is on relatively flat trail, and the second half climbs at a reasonable grade, allowing both experienced hikers and tourists in reasonable shape the opportunity to see the majestic falls and feel the driving spray near the base. *The trail is popular, not only with dayhikers, but also with backpackers bound on the ever popular Rae Lakes Loop; don't expect a high degree of solitude.*

DIRECTIONS TO TRAILHEAD: Follow Kings Canyon Highway into Kings Canyon and to the overnight parking areas at Roads End, 5 miles past the Cedar Grove turnoff.

DESCRIPTION: The well-signed trail begins at the east edge of the paved turnaround, near the wilderness permit station. Follow wide, sandy, gently ascending tread, roughly paralleling South Fork Kings River, through a mixed forest of incense cedars, ponderosa pines, black oaks, sugar pines, and white firs. Soon cross a wood bridge over Copper Creek, and proceed up the canyon into thinning forest cover, which allows views of the impressive granite walls forming the canyon. Soon enter cool forest on the way

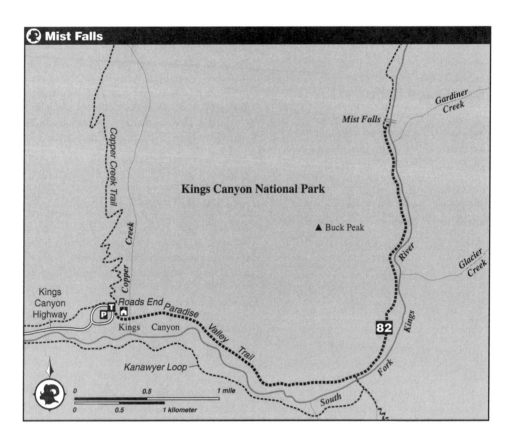

Mist Falls

Gardiner Creek

Mist Falls

Kings Canyon National Park

▲ Buck Peak

Copper Creek Trail

River

Glacier Creek

Copper Creek

Kings Canyon Highway

Roads End

P T A

Paradise

Kings   Canyon

Valley   Trail

82

Kings

Fork

Kanawyer Loop

South

0   0.5   1 mile

0   0.5   1 kilometer

to a signed Y-junction with Bubbs Creek Trail, 1.9 miles from the trailhead.

Veer left at the junction, and ascend through a mixed forest of alders, black oaks, canyon live oaks, incense cedars, white firs, and ponderosa pines. Sunny slopes are covered with manzanita and mountain mahogany, while ferns and thimbleberries thrive in the damper, shady soils. Follow the course of South Fork Kings River past delightful pools and tumbling cascades, while arcing around the base of Buck Peak, which, along with The Sphinx and Avalanche Peak on the opposite side of the canyon, plays hide-and-seek through gaps in the forest cover. Ascending rock slabs and steps, continue up the narrow chasm with periodic views of the dramatic canyon topography. After a

long, forested stretch, you begin to hear the thunderous roar emanating from Mist Falls. Soon, you reach a use trail branching to the right, which leads toward the river and a scramble over large boulders to a view of the falls near their base.

Aptly named Mist Falls tumbles over a precipitous cliff and smashes into the boulders and rocks at its base. A spray of mist catapults down the canyon, coating everything in its path. Even later in summer, when days are characteristically hot, the area around the falls is cool and moist. As with most Sierra waterfalls, Mist Falls is best appreciated in early summer, when the river is swollen with snowmelt and the falls are pouring hard and fast. By mid- to late summer, the falls become fairly tame.

ROADS END TRAILHEADS

TRIP 83

Rae Lakes Loop

Ⓜ Ⓠ BP

DISTANCE: 39 miles, loop

ELEVATION: 5,045'/11,960'/5,045', +7,500'/-7,500'/+15,000'

SEASON: Mid-July to mid-October

USE: Heavy

MAPS: USGS's *The Sphinx* and *Mt. Clarence King* or Tom Harrison Maps' *Kearsarge Pass-Rae Lakes Loop Trail Map*

TRAIL LOG

5.8	Lower Paradise Valley
7.3	Middle Paradise Valley
8.4	Upper Paradise Valley
12.0	Castle Domes Meadow
13.5	Woods Creek crossing and John Muir Trail junction
17.3	Baxter Pass Trail junction and Dollar Lake
20.3	Sixty Lakes Basin junction
24.3	Charlotte Lake and Kearsarge Pass junction
26.8	Bubbs Creek Trail junction and Lower Vidette Meadow
35.3	Sphinx Creek Camp

INTRODUCTION: Many consider the Rae Lakes Loop the quintessential High Sierra trek. Certainly the route is among the most popular. Thousands of backpackers flock to the area every summer, routinely filling the daily quota for wilderness permits. The Rae Lakes area is blessed with subalpine scenery as fine as any in the Sierra, with crystalline lakes reflecting an array of glacier-sculpted domes and jagged peaks. Jaunts into the mountain splendor of the neighboring Sixty Lakes Basin offer more chances for discovering serenity away from the main trail.

Such popularity has resulted in certain consequences affecting anyone traveling to the Rae Lakes. Long ago, black bears in this area figured out ways to acquire hanging food, and now all backpackers must use canisters. A two-night camping limit applies to all lakes in the Rae Lakes vicinity, including Arrowhead, Dollar, and Charlotte.

DIRECTIONS TO TRAILHEAD: Follow Kings Canyon Highway into Kings Canyon and to the overnight parking areas at Roads End, 5 miles past the Cedar Grove turnoff.

DESCRIPTION: The well-signed trail begins at the east edge of the paved turnaround, near the wilderness permit station. Follow wide, sandy, gently ascending tread, roughly paralleling South Fork Kings River, through a mixed forest of incense cedars, ponderosa pines, black oaks, sugar pines, and white firs. Soon cross a wood bridge over Copper Creek, and proceed up the canyon into thinning forest cover, which allows views 👁 of the impressive granite walls forming the canyon. Soon enter cool forest on the way to a signed Y-junction with the Bubbs Creek Trail, 1.9 miles from the trailhead.

Veer left at the junction, and ascend through a mixed forest of alders, black oaks, canyon live oaks, incense cedars, white firs, and ponderosa pines. Sunny slopes are covered with manzanita and mountain mahogany, while ferns and thimbleberries thrive in the damper, shady soils. Follow the course of South Fork Kings River past delightful pools and tumbling cascades, while arcing around the base of Buck Peak, which, along with The Sphinx and Avalanche Peak on the opposite side of the canyon, plays hide-and-seek through gaps in the forest cover. Ascending rock slabs and steps, continue up the narrow chasm with periodic views of the dramatic canyon topography. After a long, forested stretch, you begin to hear the thunderous roar emanating from Mist Falls. Soon, you reach a use trail branching to the right, which leads toward the river and a scramble over large boulders to a view of the falls near their base.

Aptly named Mist Falls tumbles over a precipitous cliff and smashes into the boulders and rocks at its base. A spray of mist catapults down the canyon, coating everything in its path. Even later in summer, when days are characteristically hot, the area around the falls is cool and moist. As with most Sierra waterfalls, Mist Falls is best appreciated in early summer, when the river is swollen with snowmelt and the falls are pouring hard and fast. By mid- to late summer, the falls become fairly tame.

From Mist Falls, continue upstream on a moderate climb following the course of the river up the canyon. One section of the river is quite picturesque, where the water dances over granite slabs before tumbling into a sculpted pool. Follow the well-used trail past large boulders and up rock-stepped switchbacks, with occasional views of the canyon and the towering peaks above. Just before the lip of Paradise Valley, the grade eases on the way into a mixed forest of red firs, lodgepole and Jeffrey pines, stands of aspen, and an occasional western juniper. A tangle of driftwood chokes the slow-moving river, heralding your arrival at the lower end of the valley. A short distance ahead, is Lower Paradise Valley Camp, 5.8 miles from Roads End. The camp has designated sites, a pit toilet, and bear boxes.

Continue through Paradise Valley on a gentle stroll alongside the river through a mixed forest to Middle Paradise Valley Camp, 7.25 miles from the trailhead, where more designated campsites (with bear boxes) provide overnight possibilities.

Proceed upstream on gently graded trail through stands of conifers alternating with clearings with grand views of the steep-walled South Fork Canyon. After a while, a more moderate ascent ensues, followed by a stretch of nearly level tread across a flower-filled meadow. At 8.4 miles, reach the final camping area in the valley at Upper Paradise Valley Camp, with more designated campsites and bear boxes.

Immediately beyond the camp, a system of logs allows for a straightforward crossing to the east bank of South Fork Kings River, just upstream from the confluence of Woods Creek. This crossing may be difficult early in the season. The first half mile beyond the crossing is a gentle climb away from Woods Creek, but then the trail draws nearer to the creek and begins a moderate climb up the steep-walled valley for the next couple of miles. Along the way, periodic avalanches have swept the slope, allowing good views of the granite canyon walls and domes above. After the crossings of two side streams, emerge into Castle Domes Meadow, where campsites (with a bear box) can be found near the east edge, 12 miles from the trailhead.

Beyond the meadow, gently ascending tread heads east toward a junction with the JMT through forest made up mostly of lodgepole pines. Reach the well-signed JMT junction, 13.5 miles from the trailhead. Just up a hillside, about 150 yards to the north, is an open air pit toilet.

Turn right (south) at the junction, and soon arrive at roaring Woods Creek. Fortunately, a suspension bridge, built in 1988, provides a welcome alternative to an otherwise difficult ford. Bridges built across the creek in the past were subject to periodic washouts. Cross the lively bridge, one person at a time, and reach the overused campsites above the south bank (with bear boxes). Although the area has numerous fire rings, finding enough wood for a fire will be an increasing challenge as the season progresses at this extremely popular overnight destination.

Away from the Woods Creek crossing, curve around the north end of King Spur, and begin a moderate climb up the lightly forested canyon of South Fork Woods Creek, passing through stands of red fir, lodgepole pine, and aspen alternating with sagebrush-covered slopes and pockets of verdant foliage. The steady ascent continues well above the creek, leading across a stream draining a pair of unnamed tarns below King Spur and across exposed, rocky terrain to a boggy meadow. Beyond the meadow, pass through a gap in a drift fence, climb over a rocky ridge, and come to a pair of campsites near the crossing of the willow- and wildflower-lined stream draining Sixty Lakes Basin. A

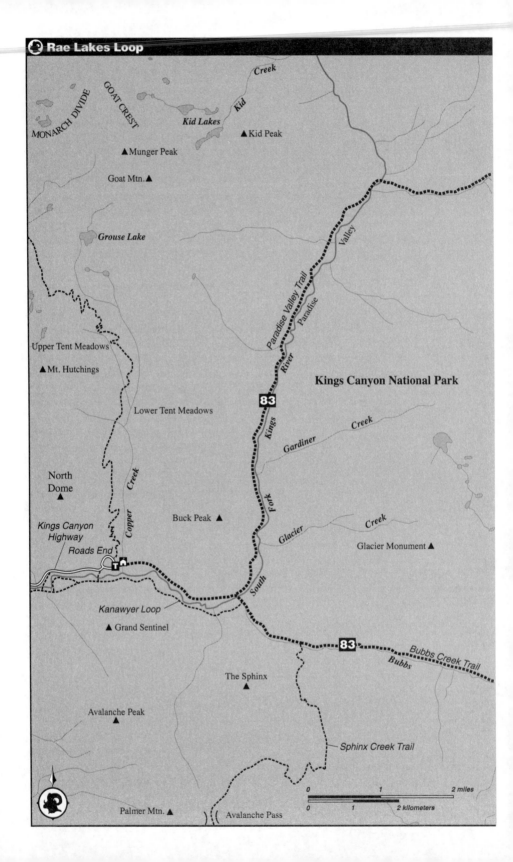

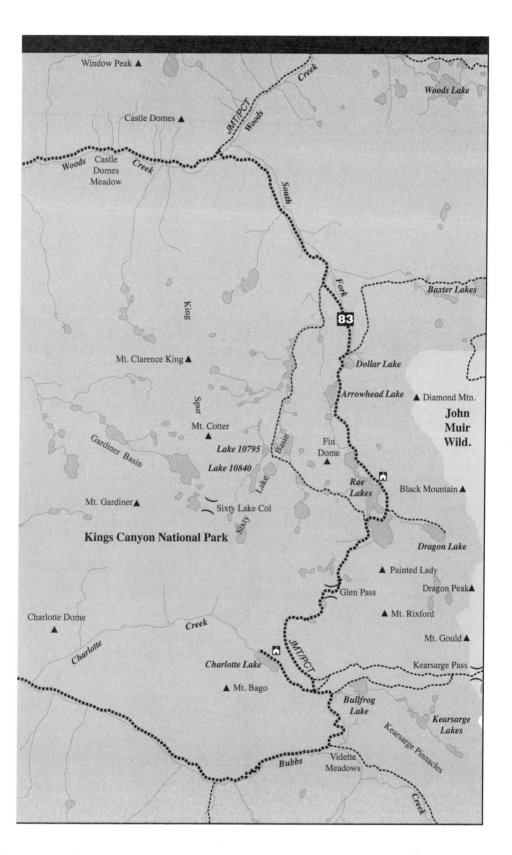

mile-long ascent through diminishing forest cover leads to a junction with the Baxter Pass Trail, just north of Dollar Lake, 17.25 miles from the trailhead, where an old post marks the junction. Solitude seekers, perhaps weary of the heavy traffic on the JMT, should find the 2.25-mile climb to decent campsites on the shore of the largest Baxter Lake a worthy diversion.

Although Dollar Lake has a few passable campsites, there are better sites a short distance ahead at Arrowhead Lake. Leaving Dollar Lake, continue the ascent on the JMT with improving scenery, including views of King Spur and Fine Dome, on the way past a small waterfall and to a crossing of the creek. Just beyond the crossing, a use trail veers around the north end of Arrowhead Lake to campsites (with a bear box).

Away from Arrowhead Lake, a short climb through widely scattered lodgepole pines and past a small, unnamed lake leads over the lip of Rae Lakes Basin and to the first of the three Rae Lakes. There are campsites (with bear boxes) along the shore of the first lake and also at the middle lake, where a ranger cabin is tucked into the pines above the northeast shore. Gently ascending tread leads across the basin around the east side of the first two lakes to Upper Rae Lake, where a trail heads east to more secluded campsites near Dragon Lake. The trail then bends around the north shore or the upper lake and fords a short stretch of creek between the two uppermost lakes.

The Rae Lakes Basin is one of the most scenic areas of the Sierra Nevada, with great views of monolithic Fin Dome, rugged King Spur, multihued Painted Lady, and rugged peaks along the Sierra Crest a fine complement to the sparkling, island-dotted lakes, bordered by glistening granite slabs and pockets of verdant, flower-carpeted meadows. Fishing for brook and rainbow trout is reported to be fair, despite the obvious pressure the area receives. Although the stunning scenery is more than worthy of a multiday visit, park regulations limit camping to two nights.

Just past the ford between the two uppermost lakes, reach a junction with the Sixty Lakes Basin Trail, 20.25 miles from the trailhead.

SIDE TRIP TO SIXTY LAKES BASIN: Any trip to Rae Lakes without a visit to Sixty Lakes Basin would be incomplete. Although the trail is unmaintained, the route through the basin has been so well used over the years that the defined tread is easy to follow. Once you are in the mostly open basin, cross-country travel between the lakes is fairly straightforward with plenty of nooks and crannies awaiting exploration.

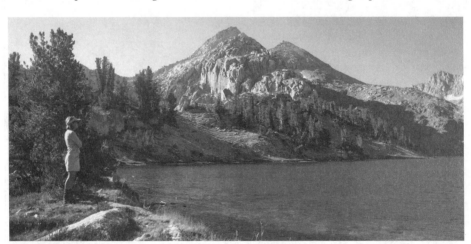

Sixty Lakes Basin

From the junction at the northwest shore of Upper Rae Lake, head south along the southwest shore of the middle lake, traverse a marshy clearing, and climb northwest to the lip of a small basin overlooking a tarn below. The view of Rae Lakes during this ascent is superb. Drop around the north side of the tarn, and climb shortly up to a saddle in the ridge dividing the Rae Lakes and Sixty Lakes Basins, where Mt. Clarence King and Mt. Cotter dominate the impressive view to the northwest. A winding, rocky descent leads to the shore of an irregularly shaped lake (approximately 10,925 feet), with campsites near the outlet.

Continuing northwest, round a ridge and enter the heart of Sixty Lakes Basin, approaching a sizable, island-dotted lake (approximately 10,795 feet), 1.9 miles from the junction. The trail continues north from here, eventually deteriorating to a cross-country route following the basin's outlet stream to a junction with the JMT, just south of Baxter Creek. You also have the option of returning to the JMT over Basin Notch, via a straightforward route through a gap in a ridge about 1 mile north of Fin Dome. From the notch, descend to the west shore of Arrowhead Lake, and work around the lake to the JMT above the east shore.

END OF SIDE TRIP

From the Sixty Lakes Basin junction, pass above the west shore of Upper Rae Lake, and then begin a 2-mile climb to Glen Pass, switchbacking through diminishing vegetation on the way to a tarn-dotted, rock-filled bench. From there, a winding ascent leads to the crest of a ridge, which you follow for a short distance to 11,978-foot Glen Pass, 22 miles from the trailhead. Hemmed in by the topography, the view is rather scanty compared to other High Sierra passes, but you do have a fine farewell vista of Rae Lakes.

From Glen Pass, the trail makes a rocky, switchbacking descent, passes a pair of greenish, rockbound tarns, and then crosses a seasonal stream with a pair of poor campsites nearby. The descent continues beside more rocks and boulders to more hospitable

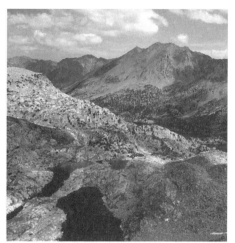

Rae Lakes Basin from Glen Pass

terrain farther down the slope, where the trail veers southeast. The grade eases on a descending traverse across a lodgepole pine–covered hillside above Charlotte Lake, where brief gaps in the forest allow views of the lake and Charlotte Dome farther down Charlotte Creek canyon.

At 2.3 miles from the pass, reach a junction with a connector to the Kearsarge Pass Trail. Continue south on the JMT, breaking out of the trees to a good view of Mt. Bago, and then stroll across a sandy flat to a four-way junction, 0.2 mile from the previous one. Here, the Kearsarge Pass Trail heads northeast, and the Charlotte Lake Trail heads northwest 0.8 mile to excellent campsites (with bear boxes) around the lake (which has a two-night camping limit).

Remaining on the JMT, head away from the junction, and climb east over a low rise. From there, short-legged switchbacks lead downhill through dense forest to a junction with the Bullfrog Lake Trail, which climbs northeast to the picturesque lake (where camping is prohibited) and continues east to Kearsarge Lakes (which have a two-night camping limit).

From the junction, continue descending, crossing Bullfrog Lake's outlet twice on the way to Lower Vidette Meadow and a junction with the Bubbs Creek Trail, 4.8 miles from Glen Pass.

Turn away from the JMT, and head west on Bubbs Creek Trail on a short descent to the north edge of expansive Lower Vidette Meadow. Overnighters will find excellent, but heavily used, campsites (with a bear box) nestled beneath lodgepole pines along the meadow's fringe.

Leaving the gently graded trail along the meadow behind, follow a more pronounced descent as the now tumbling creek plunges down the gorge. Momentarily break out into the open, where a large hump of granite provides an excellent vantage from which to survey the surrounding terrain. Head back into forest cover, and continue down the canyon, stepping over a number of lushly lined freshets along the way. The forest breaks enough on occasion to allow views of the dramatic topography above East Creek canyon, including Mt. Brewer, North Guard, and Mt. Farquhar. Farther down Bubbs Creek, picturesque waterfalls and cascades provide additional visual treats. The stiff descent eventually eases near the edge of grassy, fern-filled, and wildflower-covered Junction Meadow. Stroll across the meadow to a signed, three-way junction of the East Creek Trail, 2.3 miles from the JMT junction. Campsites can be found shortly down this trail on either side of a ford of Bubbs Creek and farther west on the Bubbs Creek Trail, past the horse camp.

Head away from Junction Meadow, as the moderate descent down the canyon resumes alongside turbulent Bubbs Creek through the moderate cover of a white fir forest. After nearly 2 miles of steady descent, the creek mellows and the grade eases through an aspen grove with a floor of ferns on the way to a log crossing of Charlotte Creek. Nearby, a short lateral leads to campsites near Bubbs Creek, where fishing for rainbow, brook, and brown trout is reportedly good.

Gently graded trail continues for a while beyond Charlotte Creek, as you hop across a trio of side streams and stroll through shoulder-high ferns, before Bubbs Creek returns to its tumultuous course down the gorge. A steady, moderate descent follows

the course of the creek for the next several miles. Farther down the canyon, moderate forest gives way to a light covering of trees, composed mainly of Jeffrey pines, with fewer firs, incense cedars, and black oaks. Reach Sphinx Creek Camp and a junction with the Sphinx Creek Trail, 8.25 miles from the JMT.

Away from Sphinx Creek, the trail descends moderately through coniferous forest and then mixed forest on the way to switchbacks that zigzag down the east wall of Kings Canyon. Reach the floor of the canyon, cross a few short, wood bridges across multiple channels of Bubbs Creek, and reach a junction with the Kanawyer Loop Trail on the left. Continue ahead from the junction, cross South Fork Kings River on a bridge, and immediately reach a junction with the Paradise Valley Trail, closing the loop. From there, retrace your steps 1.9 miles to Roads End.

An extra day in Sixty Lakes Basin allows hikers time for off-trail exploration of neighboring Gardiner Basin. From Lake 10795, head along the west shore of Lake 10840 to the inlet, climb southwest over talus and slabs to Sixty Lakes Col (approximately 11,680 feet), a saddle approximately 1 mile south of Mt. Cotter. A Class 2 descent of the west side of the col leads into remote Gardiner Basin. The old Gardiner Pass Trail, shown on the *Mt. Clarence King* quad map, has long been abandoned and is now a difficult cross-country route.

Mountaineers can attempt a Class 2 route up Painted Lady from the vicinity of the tarn-dotted bench just north of Glen Pass on the JMT. The west face of Fin Dome is Class 3–4 from Sixty Lakes Basin, and Mt. Cotter is Class 2–3.

A wilderness permit is required for overnight stays. Camping is limited to two nights in Paradise Valley, Rae Lakes Basin (including Dollar and Arrowhead Lakes), and at Charlotte Lake. Bear canisters are required. Campfires are prohibited above 10,000 feet.

TRIP 84

Copper Creek Trail to Granite Basin

S / **BP**

DISTANCE: 19 miles, out-and-back

ELEVATION: 5,045'/10,347'/10,093', +5,735'/-685'/±12,840'

SEASON: July to mid-October

USE: Light to moderate

MAP: *The Sphinx*

TRAIL LOG

4.0   Lower Tent Meadow
9.0   Granite Lake junction

INTRODUCTION: Granite Basin is a gently sloping bowl filled with scenic tarns and flower-bedecked meadows, accessed by a steep and usually scorching ascent from the floor of Kings Canyon. Successful backpackers can recuperate along the pine-dotted shore of Granite Lake or beside a bevy of tarns scattered across the picturesque basin. Anglers will find fishing in the basin's streams and lakes a fitting challenge.

Backpackers who choose not to make the full 9.5-mile climb to Granite Lake in one day will have to be satisfied with the passable campsites at Lower Tent Meadow; there are no other camping opportunities between there and the basin. Don't expect a typical meadow at Lower or Upper Tent Meadows. Neither offers anything close to the flat, grassy clearing typically associated with the term. Both "meadows" are moderately sloped and choked with brush.

DIRECTIONS TO TRAILHEAD: Follow Kings Canyon Highway into Kings Canyon and to the overnight parking areas at Roads End, 5 miles past the Cedar Grove turnoff.

DESCRIPTION: From the north side of the parking lot, follow switchbacks on a steady climb up a mostly open hillside dotted with Jeffrey pines and canyon live oaks. While granting insufficient shade, the sparse vegetation does allow fine views of the Grand Sentinel. More switchbacks lead high up the Copper Creek drainage and into partial shade from a light forest of sugar pines, incense cedars, Jeffrey pines, and white firs. Hop over tiny brooks and a tributary of Copper Creek, and then cross a sloping, manzanita-covered clearing. Soon cross a larger, aspen- and brush-filled clearing with a cramped campsite, step over a couple of rivulets, and head back into forest cover on a climb to the next creek crossing. Reach Lower Tent Meadow, immediately past the creek, 4 miles from the trailhead, where conifers shade five designated campsites (which have a bear box).

Climb moderately away from Lower Tent Meadow Camp, ascending brush-choked slopes and an avalanche swath. A long, steady, switchbacking climb leads back into a light covering of red firs, joined later on by western white pines and then lodgepole pines. Near the 7-mile mark, cross a moraine at the edge of Granite Basin, with fine views through the trees of 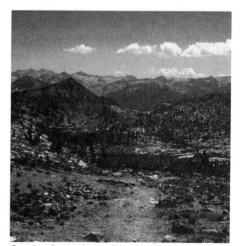 the basin below and Mt. Clarence King and Mt. Gardiner.

After 7 miles of climbing, a short, winding descent toward the basin is a welcome

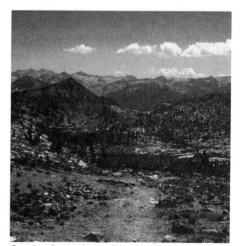

Granite Basin from Granite Pass

☉ Copper Creek Trail to Granite Basin

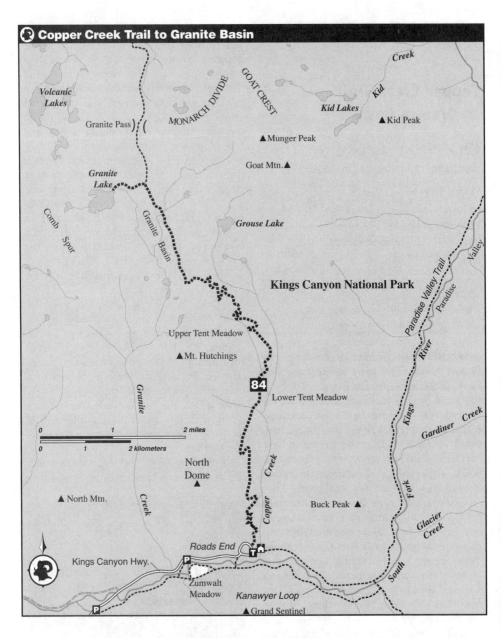

change; you pass through a drift fence along the way. The basin is filled with delightful tarns and irregularly shaped meadows. The trail avoids the basin in favor of an undulating traverse of the lodgepole pine–dotted hillside above. Parties interested in camping near the tarns must leave the trail and journey cross-country into the basin. In a pocket

of willows, just beyond the large meadow at the north end of Granite Basin, reach a signed junction on the left with a lateral to Granite Lake, 9 miles from the trailhead.

Turn left (west) at the junction, and follow the lateral over a stream and past a couple of seldom-used campsites on a mild ascent toward the lake. Step across the seasonal inlet, and reach some campsites along the north shore of Granite Lake, 0.5 mile from the junction. The island-dotted lake sits in a rocky basin below cliffs of the Monarch Divide. Sparsely distributed pines offer little shelter for the smattering of campsites scattered around the shore, but the scenery is marvelous. Anglers can test their skill on fair-size brook trout.

Cross-country enthusiasts can access Granite Lake from the Copper Creek Trail by following part of Steve Roper's classic Sierra High Route. Leave the trail near the crest of the moraine above Granite Basin, and traverse north for a half mile to the meadow bordering the outlet. From there, make the easy climb to the lake.

A wilderness permit is required for overnight stays. Campfires are prohibited above 10,000 feet.

ROADS END TRAILHEADS

TRIP 85

State and Horseshoe Lakes

Ⓢ ✎ BP

DISTANCE: 36 miles, out-and-back

ELEVATION: 5,045'/10,515', +7,735'/-2,275'/±20,020'

SEASON: Mid-July to mid-October

USE: Light

MAPS: *The Sphinx* and *Marion Peak*

TRAIL LOG

5.0	Lower Tent Meadow
9.0	Granite Lake junction
9.6	Granite Pass
12.25	Kennedy Pass Trail junction
15.9	Lower State Lake
18.0	Horseshoe Lakes

INTRODUCTION: The trip to Granite Basin and Granite Lake as described in Trip 82 (see page 262) is a worthy weekend goal for backpackers searching for great scenery. The extension to State and Horseshoe Lakes offers those with more time the opportunity to add a pair of pleasant lake basins that see few visitors.

After the initial protracted climb from Roads End to Granite Basin, the terrain mellows considerably on the way to the lakes. Anglers should enjoy fishing in a variety of lakes that see little pressure. Cross-country enthusiasts have numerous possibilities for further wanderings to the alpine terrain northeast of Horseshoe Lakes.

DIRECTIONS TO TRAILHEAD: Follow Kings Canyon Highway into Kings Canyon and to the overnight parking areas at Roads End, 5 miles past the Cedar Grove turnoff.

DESCRIPTION: From the north side of the parking lot, follow switchbacks on a steady climb up a mostly open hillside dotted with Jeffrey pines and canyon live oaks. While

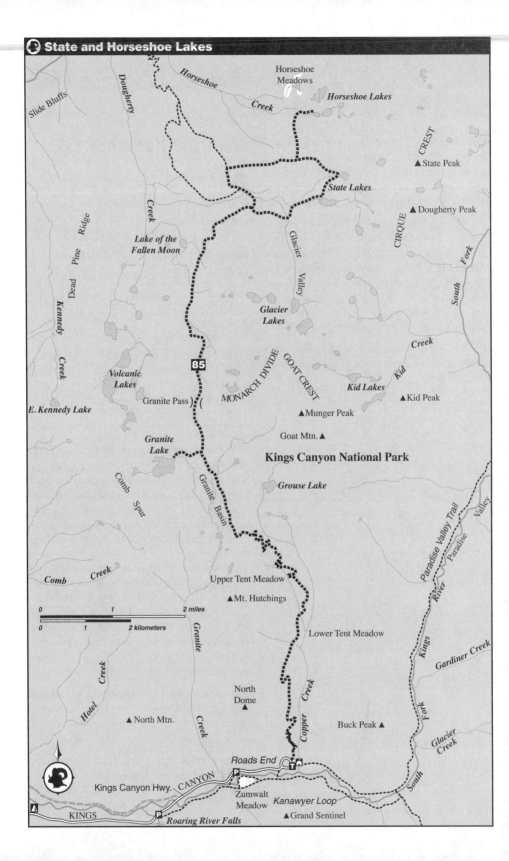

Slide Bluffs

Dougherty

Horseshoe

Horseshoe Meadows

Horseshoe Lakes

Creek

CREST

▲ State Peak

Creek

State Lakes

▲ Dougherty Peak

Lake of the Fallen Moon

Glacier Valley

CIRQUE

South Fork

Dead Pine Ridge

Kennedy Creek

Glacier Lakes

Creek

Volcanic Lakes

85

MONARCH DIVIDE

GOAT CREST

Kid Lakes

Kid

▲Kid Peak

E. Kennedy Lake

Granite Pass)(

▲Munger Peak

Granite Lake

Goat Mtn. ▲

Kings Canyon National Park

Comb Spur

Granite Basin

Grouse Lake

Paradise Valley Trail

Valley

Paradise

River

Comb   Creek

Upper Tent Meadow

Kings

Comb

▲Mt. Hutchings

Lower Tent Meadow

Gardiner Creek

0   1   2 miles

0   1   2 kilometers

Granite

Fork

Hotel   Creek

North Dome ▲

Glacier Creek

▲ North Mtn.

Creek

Copper Creek

Buck Peak ▲

South

Roads End

Kings Canyon Hwy.   CANYON

Zumwalt Meadow   *Kanawyer Loop*

▲Grand Sentinel

KINGS   *Roaring River Falls*

granting insufficient shade, the sparse vegetation does allow fine views of the Grand Sentinel. More switchbacks lead high up the Copper Creek drainage and into partial shade from a light forest of sugar pines, incense cedars, Jeffrey pines, and white firs. Hop over tiny brooks and a tributary of Copper Creek, and then cross a sloping, manzanita-covered clearing. Soon cross a larger, aspen- and brush-filled clearing with a cramped campsite, step over a couple of rivulets, and head back into forest cover on a climb to the next creek crossing. Reach Lower Tent Meadow, immediately past the creek, 4 miles from the trailhead, where conifers shade five designated campsites (which have a bear box).

Climb moderately away from Lower Tent Meadow Camp, ascending brush-choked slopes and an avalanche swath. A long, steady, switchbacking climb leads back into a light covering of red firs, joined later on by western white pines and then lodgepole pines. Near the 7-mile mark, cross a moraine at the edge of Granite Basin, with fine views through the trees of the basin below and Mt. Clarence King and Mt. Gardiner.

After 7 miles of climbing, a short, winding descent toward the basin is a welcome change; you pass through a drift fence along the way. The basin is filled with delightful tarns and irregularly shaped meadows. The trail avoids the basin in favor of an undulating traverse of the lodgepole pine–dotted hillside above. Parties interested in camping near the tarns must leave the trail and journey cross-country into the basin. In a pocket of willows, just beyond the large meadow at the north end of Granite Basin, reach a signed junction on the left with a lateral to Granite Lake, 9 miles from the trailhead.

SIDE TRIP TO GRANITE LAKE: Turn left (west) at the junction, and follow the lateral over a stream and past a couple of seldom-used campsites on a mild ascent toward the lake. Step across the seasonal inlet, and reach some campsites along the north shore of Granite Lake, 0.5 mile from the junction. The island-dotted lake sits in a rocky

basin below cliffs of the Monarch Divide. Sparsely distributed pines offer little shelter for the smattering of campsites scattered around the shore, but the scenery is marvelous. Anglers can test their skill on fair-size brook trout. **END OF SIDE TRIP**

Proceed straight ahead at the Granite Lake junction, breaking out of light forest and climbing steeply on rocky tread toward Granite Pass. After a 0.6-mile ascent, you stand atop Granite Pass on the Monarch Divide (10,673 feet), with good views of the surrounding terrain.

A zigzagging path leads down from the pass to a series of meadow-covered benches rimmed by granite walls. The trail nears Middle Fork Dougherty Creek several times during the descent. After passing through a pair of drift fences, continue winding downstream through scattered lodgepole pines, step over the creek three times, and climb a ridge with a fine view down the Middle Fork's canyon. Soon, gently graded trail leads to a junction with a connector on the left to the Lewis Creek and Kennedy Pass Trail, 12.25 miles from the trailhead.

Proceed straight ahead from the junction for 0.3 mile to the stream flowing northwest toward Lake of the Fallen Moon; about a quarter mile beyond the creek, an obscure, unmarked trail heads west toward the lake. A short, moderate climb leads to a traverse across a forested hillside, followed by a brief descent to a pocket meadow and a junction with the southern trail to State Lakes, 4 miles from Granite Pass.

From the junction, the Dougherty Creek Trail continues northeast to Dougherty Meadows before veering northwest and descending toward Simpson Meadow along Middle Fork Kings River. Your route turns right (east) at the junction and proceeds through lodgepole pine forest and past a fair-size meadow carpeted with wildflowers, including tiger lily, aster, and shooting star. From the meadow, climb to the crest of a rise, and then drop down the far side to the crossing of a stream draining lovely Glacier Valley and Glacier Lakes. From there, a short traverse north leads to the crossing of a vigorous stream plummeting from Lower State Lake, followed by a moderately steep climb up a hillside and over the lip of the basin. Stroll across gently rising, flower-dotted terrain to the northwest shore of Lower State Lake.

Backdropped by the impressive cliffs of Cirque Crest, Lower State Lake offers a few lodgepole pine–shaded campsites along the north shore. Fishing should be decent for good-size rainbow and golden trout since the lake receives little pressure.

A lightly used trail heads north from the lower lake on a mild to moderate 0.5-mile ascent through lodgepole pines, currant, and gooseberry to Upper State Lake. This seldom-visited lake is less desirable than its lower counterpart; it offers a limited view of State Peak and has only a couple of primitive campsites around its forest- and meadow-rimmed shore. Also, the shallow lake appears to be devoid of fish.

Step across the upper lake's outlet, and head through boulder-strewn, lightly forested terrain on moderately ascending trail past a small meadow to the crest of a hill and a Y-junction, 16.6 miles from the trailhead, where the faint tread heads west to a connection with the Dougherty Creek Trail.

From the junction, bend right (north) and make a short descent to a meadow and

a crossing of a flower-lined stream (neither the trail or the stream appear on the *Marion Peak* quad map). A mildly rising traverse follows, leading across a dry, sand slope dotted with lodgepole and western white pines. Approximately 0.75 mile from the junction, the trail rounds the nose of a moraine and veers northeast up the canyon of Horseshoe Creek, revealing impressive views of Windy Ridge and cliffs rimming the cirque basin ahead. Approach the creek through willows and wildflowers, boulder hop across, and then continue upstream to Horseshoe Lakes.

The first lake is rather small and shallow, but a short walk on a use trail leads to the second larger, deeper lake rimmed by cliffs and green hills dotted with pines and boulders. From the northwest shore of the second lake, a short, off-trail jaunt leads northwest across gently rising terrain to the third lake, a large, deep lake surrounded by pines and boulders. Seldom-used campsites are plentiful between the second and third lakes. Good-size rainbow trout will tempt the angler. Once your visit to Horseshoe Lakes is complete, retrace your steps back to the junction.

From the Horseshoe Lakes junction, follow faint tread west on a gently graded, 1.3-mile descent to a junction with the Dougherty Creek Trail. Turn left (south) at the junction, and descend for 0.3 mile to where the trail turns east and traverses to a ford of East Fork Dougherty Creek. From there, a short climb leads to the top of a ridge, followed by a gradual descent to the junction with the trail to Lower State Lake at the close of the loop.

From the junction, retrace your steps 13.6 miles to the trailhead.

Backpackers can access the remote Middle Fork Kings River at Simpson Meadow by continuing northbound on the Dougherty Creek Trail. However, such a journey necessitates a steep, 2,300-foot descent and subsequent ascent for a return to Roads End.

Experienced cross-country hikers can access the exquisite Marion Lake and Lake Basin region by continuing roughly north-

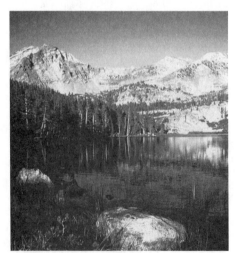

Early evening at State Lake

east from Horseshoe Lakes on the Sierra High Route over Grey, White, and Red Passes (consult *Sierra High Route* by Steve Roper for more information).

Both Dougherty and State Peaks on Cirque Crest are Class 2 climbs from State Lakes.

R A wilderness permit is required for overnight stays. Campfires are prohibited above 10,000 feet.

Introduction to John Muir Wilderness: West Side

The John Muir Wilderness forms a sizeable buffer on the west side of Kings Canyon National Park, positioned between the end of access roads from the foothills and the park's backcountry. Most of this section of the wilderness is heavily forested, interrupted occasionally by meadows and lakes, and reaching the high country only along the divides that form the west boundary of the park. The longer-than-weekend trips necessary to reach the heart of the backcountry, paired with the long drives to trailheads, ensure that backpackers who do visit this region will do so with a modicum of solitude.

Trail users who invest the time necessary to penetrate the forested wilderness will find magnificent scenery in the western realm of Kings Canyon National Park. High, lake-dotted basins beneath the shadow of the craggy Le Conte Divide, White Divide, and Kettle Ridge provide a suitable reward for hiking mile after mile of tree-lined trail. The few trails crossing into the park lead to impressive canyons, none more renowned than Middle Fork Kings River canyon.

ACCESS: Highway 168 from Fresno is the principal access to Sierra National Forest lands west of Kings Canyon National Park. Along the way, motorists pass through recreation areas at a series of artificial reservoirs—Shaver, Huntington, Courtright, and Wishon. The drives to trailheads are characteristically long, sometimes over narrow and winding secondary roads. Highway 168 is open year-round to Huntington Lake and usually beyond from late May to October, depending on conditions.

AMENITIES: A declining economy has recently reduced the range of services available in the resort communities of both Shaver Lake and Huntington Lake. Wishon Village has a general store. Florence Lake has a very small general store. Courtright Reservoir

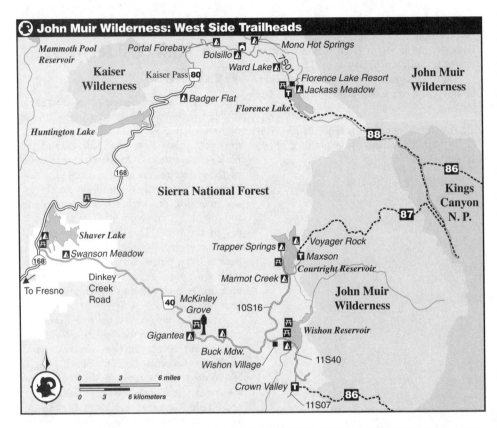

John Muir Wilderness: West Side Trailheads

Mammoth Pool Reservoir

Portal Forebay

Bolsillo

Mono Hot Springs

Ward Lake

7S01

Kaiser Wilderness

Kaiser Pass 80

Florence Lake Resort

Jackass Meadow

John Muir Wilderness

Badger Flat

Florence Lake

Huntington Lake

88

168

Sierra National Forest

86

Kings Canyon N. P.

87

Shaver Lake

Swanson Meadow

Trapper Springs

Voyager Rock

Maxson

Courtright Reservoir

168

Dinkey Creek Road

Marmot Creek

To Fresno

40

McKinley Grove

10S16

John Muir Wilderness

Gigantea

Wishon Reservoir

Buck Mdw.

Wishon Village

11S40

Crown Valley

11S07

86

0   3   6 miles

0   3   6 kilometers

Campgrounds

Campground	Fee	Elevation	Season	Restrooms	Water	Bear Boxes	Phone
Sawmill Flat (southwest of Wishon Reservoir)	Free	6,700 feet	May to October	Vault	No	No	No
Lily Pad (Wishon Reservoir)	$16	6,500 feet	May to October	Vault	Yes	No	No
Buck Meadow (west of Wishon Reservoir)	$16	6,800 feet	May to October	Vault	No	No	No
Marmot Rock (Courtright Reservoir)	$24	8,200 feet	May to October	Vault	Yes	No	No
Trapper Springs (Courtright Reservoir)	$24	8,300 feet	May to October	Vault	No	No	No
Voyager Rock (Courtright Reservoir)	Free	8,200 feet	May to October	Vault	No	No	No
Jackass Meadow (Florence Lake)	$18	7,200 feet	June to October	Vault	No	No	No
Ward Lake (north of Florence Lake)	$16	7,400 feet	June to October	Vault	No	No	No
Mono Hot Springs (north of Florence Lake)	$18	6,560 feet	June to October	Vault	No	No	No

has no services. Prather is perhaps the most reliable town for getting gas or a meal on the way to the trailhead.

Muir Trail Ranch (MTR), 4 miles by trail from Florence Lake and inside John Muir Wilderness, is a backcountry resort that offers rustic accommodations by reservation only (209-966-3195, **www.muirtrail ranch.com**). Backpacker services include accepting resupply packages for JMT thru-hikers, and a small store selling such items as batteries and matches. Recently, MTR has offered short stay packages to back-packers, which includes an overnight stay in a tent, or two-night stay in a cabin, meals, a sack lunch for the trail, and access to the hot springs (reservations necessary). Also, for a fee MTR will arrange to have your backpack hauled by pack horse to Heart Lake or Evolution Meadow (subject to availability). MTR also operates a ferry service ($11 one-way) across Florence Lake from late May to late September, which saves 4 miles of unremarkable hiking along the shoreline.

RANGER STATION: Wilderness permits are available at the High Sierra Ranger District office on Highway 168 in Prather. Back-packers headed for Florence Lake could pick up a permit at the High Sierra Visitor Information Station on Kaiser Pass Road, 0.75 mile prior to the Florence Lake and Edison Lake junction.

GOOD TO KNOW BEFORE YOU GO: Some-times narrow and curvy roads make for slow going on the way to trailheads, so plan on extra driving time. Lightly used and infrequently maintained trails on the west side of the wilderness may necessitate good navigational skills.

CROWN VALLEY TRAILHEAD

TRIP 86

Middle Fork Kings River

S / **BP**

DISTANCE: 82.6 miles, point-to-point

ELEVATION: 6,725'/4,120'/11,980'/8,485'/ 11,320'/7,990', +15,950'/-14,025'/±29,975'

SEASON: Mid-July to early October

USE: Light

MAPS: *Rough Spur, Tehipite Dome, Slide Bluffs, Marion Peak, North Palisade, Mt. Goddard, Mt. Darwin, Mt. Henry, Blackcap Mountain, Ward Mountain,* and *Courtright Reservoir*

TRAIL LOG

3.75	Statham Meadow junction
8.0	Crown Valley and Tehipite Trail junction
14.5	Tehipite Valley
25.5	Simpson Meadow and Middle Fork ford
32.0	Devils Washbowl
35.0	John Muir Trail junction
38.3	Bishop Pass Trail junction
45.3	Muir Pass
50.2	North shore of Evolution Lake
54.8	McClure Meadow Ranger Station
58.3	Goddard Canyon Trail junction
63.3	Hell-for-Sure Pass Trail junction
67.3	Hell-for-Sure Pass
70.8	Rae Lakes and Indian Lakes Trail junction
75.6	Post Corral Creek
82.6	Maxson Trailhead

INTRODUCTION: While the stunning scen-ery is unparalleled, much of the High Sierra has lost some of the sense of wildness and mystery the range once enjoyed during the bygone era of Frank Dusy's pioneer wander-ings and the Whitney Survey's discoveries.

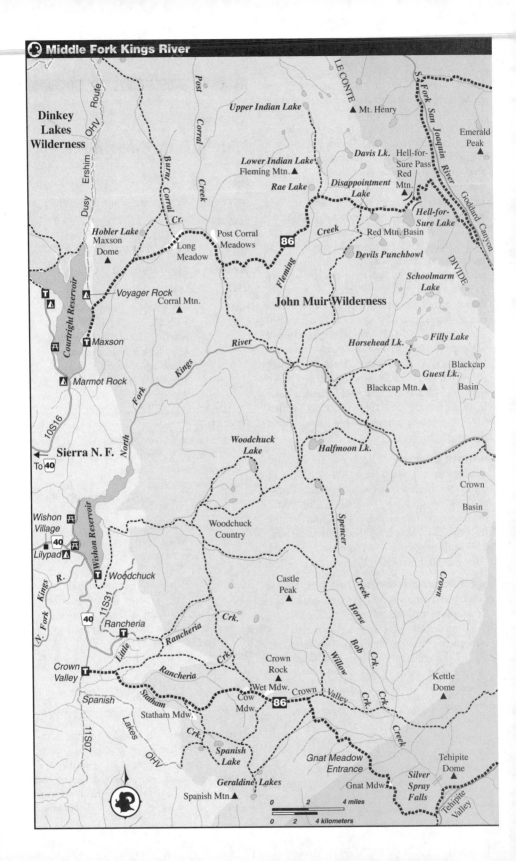

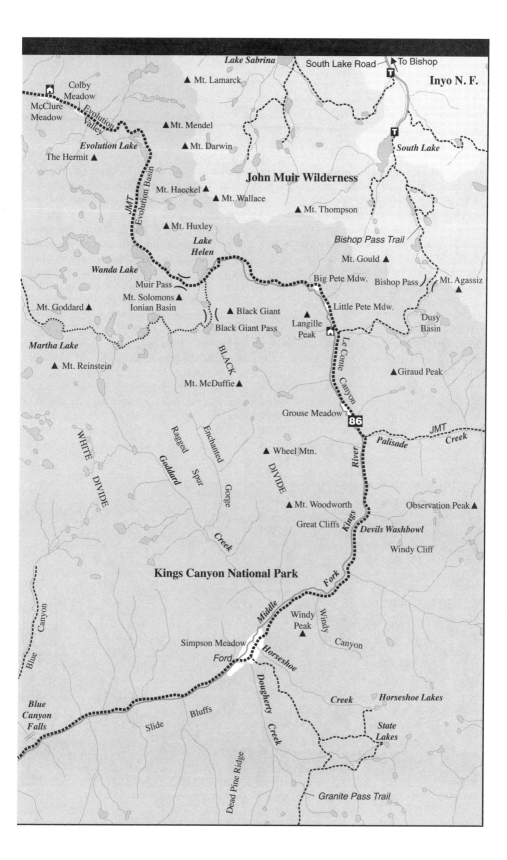

Today, parts of the more popular areas of the High Sierra seem anything but wild, with the John Muir Trail (JMT) often denigrated as a freeway, and backpackers routinely battling one another for a limited number of wilderness permits. However, all is not lost. A few places exist in the range where it's still possible to feel a sense of remoteness, where even though the mind will know you're not the first person to see such majestic terrain, the soul will revel in that feeling. Wild, remote, and infrequently traveled, the Middle Fork Kings River is just such a place. Plus it's one of the most stunningly scenic canyons in the entire range.

The remoteness of the Middle Fork results in large part from its extremely long approach. Although a highway and a dam were once proposed by competing water-grabbing interests from Los Angeles and the San Joaquin Valley, these proposals were fortunately defeated over time. The absence of a road into the canyon requires either a 15-mile hike from Courtright Reservoir (the route described here) or a 25-mile hike from Cedar Grove. The distance is not the only contributor to the area's isolation. Both routes are physically taxing; the shorter route requires a knee-wrenching, unrelenting, 3,000-foot descent from the canyon rim straight down to Tehipite Valley; the longer route is no picnic either, with a strenuous climb to 10,673-foot Granite Pass on Monarch Divide, followed by an equally unpleasant descent to 5,950-foot Simpson Meadow. If these deterrents are not enough, the relatively low elevations of the lower canyon create prime rattlesnake habitat and usually mean hot afternoon temperatures during the summer. Also, because of ongoing cattle grazing, indistinct sections of trail in Sierra National Forest may be difficult to follow and require some route-finding skills.

So, why would anyone want to overcome such a daunting set of obstacles to reach Middle Fork Kings River? For one, Tehipite Valley is a scenic rival to Yosemite Valley but without the hordes of tourists. In fact, odds are you may be the only one craning your neck to fully absorb the 3,500-foot view of the striking south face of Tehipite Dome, largest of the many note-

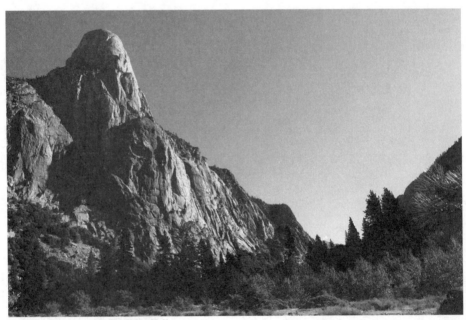

Tehipite Dome from Tehipite Valley

worthy domes in the Sierra. The dramatic cascade of Silver Spray Falls tumbling down Crown Creek canyon to the left of Tehipite Dome might be your own private domain and, while camped next to the spectacular Middle Fork Kings River, the evening howl of coyotes may be your only companion. If you can imagine Yosemite Valley without any people, you'll have a fairly good image of Tehipite Valley.

Tehipite Valley is not the only reward on this trip; the rest of Middle Fork Kings River canyon is quite scenic as well. The river courses through a magnificent gorge of granite, where picturesque waterfalls, such as Blue Canyon Falls, spill down high and steep canyon walls, and where dramatic cascades, such as Devils Punchbowl, tumble down rock steps and swirl into pools along the rolling river. The lush foliage of Simpson Meadow creates a pastoral ambiance near the midpoint of the Middle Fork Trail, well worth a layover day or two. The trail beyond the meadow passes through mostly open terrain through a narrow section of the canyon, with fine views of the soaring granite walls and the tumbling river. Hiking the 20-mile stretch of the Middle Fork Trail between Tehipite Valley and the JMT junction is a classic Sierra adventure.

While the contrast between the lonely Middle Fork Trail and the heavily traveled JMT can be a shock to your system after multiple days of encountering few, if any, people, the scenery along this stretch of the JMT is magnificent. Continuing up the Middle Fork Kings River, the trail passes through beautiful Le Conte Canyon and then climbs to the river's headwaters at Helen Lake below Muir Pass. Beyond the pass are two of the most precious gems along the JMT, dramatic Evolution Basin, with a string of alpine lakes, and lovely Evolution Valley, sprinkled with a trio of large, beautiful meadows.

Below Evolution Valley, this route leaves the JMT and follows a 5-mile stretch of South Fork San Joaquin River on the seldom-traveled Goddard Canyon Trail through another magnificent High Sierra gorge. From there, a climb up and over Hell-for-Sure Pass leads to a cluster of lovely lakes nestled in a sea of granite in Red Mountain Basin, followed by a lengthy forested journey to the ending trailhead at Courtright Reservoir.

DIRECTIONS TO TRAILHEAD:

START: From Fresno, follow State Highway 168 through Prather (ranger station), and continue toward the community of Shaver Lake. Just as you come into town, turn right onto Dinkey Creek Road, and proceed 11.5 miles to a right-hand turn onto McKinley Grove Road. Continue 13.6 more miles to the Courtright-Wishon junction.

Bear right at the Courtright-Wishon junction, pass through Wishon Village RV Park (general store), and continue past a junction near the west side of Wishon Reservoir with FS Road 10S64, which provides access to a campground and two picnic areas. Cross the one-way road over the dam, and head south for about 3 miles to a junction with FS Road 11S07 on the right. Following a sign for Crown Valley Trailhead, proceed another mile to the dirt parking area on the right (which has bear boxes).

END: To reach the ending trailhead, bear left at the Courtright-Wishon junction, and drive 7 miles to a junction near the south end of Courtright Reservoir. Following a sign for the Maxson Trailhead, veer right, cross the one-way road over the dam, and head above the southeast shore to the parking area (with a vault toilet). Courtright Reservoir has three developed campgrounds.

DESCRIPTION: Walk through the parking area and across the road to the start of the Crown Valley Trail, which climbs steeply up a forested hillside before mellowing out to a more moderate ascent. Hop over Little Rancheria Creek, and follow moderately rising tread to a junction with a trail to Three Springs, 0.75 mile from the trailhead.

Veer right (southeast) from the junction, and continue the climb. Drop briefly to a crossing of Rancheria Creek, and then resume the ascent along the south bank to the John Muir Wilderness boundary. Leaving

Rancheria Creek, the trail crosses Statham Creek, moves away, and then draws back alongside the creek on the way to Statham Meadow, a large clearing with a horse camp on a private inholding. Reach an indistinct junction at the west fringe of the meadow, 3.75 miles from the trailhead, where an old sign marks the obscure tread of the Crown Valley Trail angling uphill to the east (avoid the desire to proceed ahead into the meadow on the more distinct path toward the old structures of the horse camp).

From the junction, bear left and climb steeply up an open hillside to the north of Statham Meadow, where the tread becomes better defined, to the top of a rise immediately east of point 8516. Heading back into the trees, follow gently graded trail across the rise, cross a tributary, and then start a moderate descent toward Rancheria Creek. At the bottom, turn upstream and head toward a boggy clearing known appropriately as Cow Meadow, where the unfortunate effect of ongoing cattle grazing has been the destruction of the main trail and the creation of multiple stock paths that come and go randomly. Route-finding through this maze will be challenging, but the actual route passes around the southern fringe of the meadow, crosses the creek near the east edge, reaches an indistinct junction with a trail heading north to Round Corral Meadow, and then heads southeast across a spring-fed rivulet toward the south edge of Wet Meadow.

The tread becomes more defined again beyond Wet Meadow on a mild to moderate descent through mixed forest toward Crown Valley. Pass the Crown Valley ranger cabin, and soon reach the gravesite of Ike Smit. Continue the descent to a crossing of Crown Valley Creek at the west edge of the long, namesake valley. Curve around the south edge of the valley to a three-way junction with the Tehipite Valley Trail, 8 miles from the trailhead, just up from the old, worn-out cabins of the Crown Valley Ranch, a former guest ranch. An old sign indicates that backpackers should look elsewhere for a camp, but the notion of anyone caring about whether or not anyone camps here nowadays is hard to fathom.

At the junction, turn right (south) and follow the Tehipite Valley Trail on gently rising tread. Past a junction of a trail up Rogers Creek to Geraldine Lakes, the trail begins a lengthy descent toward the lip of the Middle Fork Kings River canyon, crossing the densely forested upper slopes of the Crown Creek drainage. Along the way, the route follows the folds and creases of the canyon and its tributaries, crossing numerous side streams along the way. A lightning-caused fire swept through this area in 2008, evidence of which you can see from here all the way to the Middle Fork canyon. The fire blackened more than 4,000 acres in the park, the unintended benefit of which was that firefighters bushwhacked this infrequently used trail, leaving behind a very distinct path.

At 3 miles from the Crown Valley junction, cross the signed park boundary at the Gnat Valley Entrance and continue the extended descent, now in Kings Canyon National Park. Proceed through featureless forest across some tributaries and around the nose of a ridge to Hay Meadow, a verdant, sloping clearing bisected by a rivulet. The trail arcs around the meadow and passes above the first decent campsite since Crown Valley, about 13 miles from the trailhead. The extended descent is interrupted by a steep but short climb over a ridge to the east of Hay Meadow. From there, resume the downward march to the lip of Middle Fork Kings River canyon above Tehipite Valley.

After the lengthy trip through dense forest, the canyon seems even more stupendous, as you stand at the very edge of the deep gorge and gaze straight down its sheer granite walls to the tumbling river 3,000 feet below. Just upstream is the beautiful plain of Tehipite Valley, a scenic rival to the much more famous Yosemite Valley. Standing guard over the deep cleft of the canyon is the strikingly dramatic profile of Tehipite Dome, at 7,708 feet the largest of the many noteworthy domes in the Sierra. Under the pen name of Montero, one of the first Euro-Americans to experience this stunning vista wrote:

> . . . at 4 o'clock p.m. of Sunday, July 13th, we stood on the brink of the cliff and gazed with wonder and awe upon one of the grandest views to be found in the Sierras. A grassy slope reaches to the very edge of the chasm, the bottom of which is more than a vertical mile below, and as one looks shudderingly down the giddy abyss he sees the majestic stream of the Middle Fork, appearing no larger than a brook, as it glistened in the sun. To the east we beheld mountains of solid rock, capped with snow, and increasing in grandeur and height as they near the summit, which was dimly outlined by the sky in the far distance. Lingering with enraptured visions we were loth [loathe] to withdraw our eyes from a scene at once sublime and awe-inspiring.

Without embellishment, this vista is truly one of the supreme classics of the Sierra.

The high price for such a marvelous view soon becomes obvious, as the trail starts a brutally steep, unrelenting, 3,000-foot descent that zigzags repeatedly down the west wall of the canyon on short, tight switchbacks. The notorious descent has earned the nickname "the son of a bitch," and any survivor would be hard-pressed to come up with a more appropriate moniker. Beginning in conifers on the canyon rim, the vegetation transitions to a mixture of conifers and broadleaf trees by the time the trail reaches the canyon floor. Despite sporadic maintenance, imagining a trail in worse shape is hard, as leaf litter from the previous autumn routinely piles up on the trail, creating plenty of opportunities for losing your footing. Even hikers who don't routinely use trekking poles may want to consider bringing them along for this knee-wrenching descent. With nary a level spot suitable for a moment's rest, the inexorable decline will tax the most highly conditioned backpackers before they reach the relatively level floor of Tehipite Valley. Complicating matters even more, watch for poison oak on the lower third of the descent, which grows profusely alongside the trail in some loca-

tions. After losing 3,000 feet of elevation in fewer than 3 miles, backpackers should feel an overwhelming sense of gratitude upon reaching the gentle terrain of Tehipite Valley at the bottom of the canyon.

Turning upstream, follow gently graded trail across the sandy floor of the valley, with towering Tehipite Dome continually looming above. Infrequently used camp- sites near the Middle Fork Kings River will issue a strong pull after the knee-wrenching descent. A lack of campers combined with plenty of driftwood should produce enough fuel for an evening campfire. Since the river is designated a National Wild and Scenic River, anglers can fish for wild trout with little pressure from fellow anglers.

The scenery of Tehipite Valley is outstanding, similar in grandeur to Yosemite but without the crowds. In fact, odds are you may have the entire valley to yourself. Trees, primarily oaks, may obscure views of Silver Spray Falls, requiring you to move about the valley in order to get a good look at Crown Valley Creek spilling down a wall of granite. After midsummer, you might consider a worthy side trip from the valley floor up the narrow gorge to the base of the 75-foot falls and the possibility of a chilly swim in the pool at the bottom. Before then, the incessant spray will quickly drench anyone bold enough to try to approach the falls. On the opposite side, the Gorge of Despair slices through the wall of the canyon in dramatic fashion and is topped by a series of stunningly scenic turrets that provide some of the finest technical rock climbing in the Sierra. The gorge, blocked by steep cliffs and waterfalls is virtually impenetrable from Tehipite Valley, although a few parties have descended the gorge with the aid of climbing gear and wetsuits. (More often hikers access the Gorge of Despair from Kings Canyon over Monarch Divide via a pass northeast of Mt. Harrington.) Tehipite Valley is truly one of the most majestic and wild locations in the Sierra.

At some point, you must leave the beauty of Tehipite Valley behind. The ford of Crown Creek may be difficult, if not impossible, early in the season but should not be any higher than mid-calf by mid-July. Simpson Meadow, the next logical stopping point, is 11 miles away from and 1,700 feet higher than Tehipite Valley. Such numbers would normally indicate a fairly easy stretch of trail, but the Middle Fork Kings River Trail defies convention by continuously gaining and then losing elevation along the way. The topography didn't allow the original trail builders to construct a steadily graded path. Instead the cliffs and walls of the canyon force the trail up and over numerous obstacles. Most of the journey to Simpson Meadow is under the cover of mixed forest and is usually a good distance away from the riverbank. However, the trail crosses several unnamed tributaries and three named creeks, Blue Canyon, Rattlesnake, and Alpine, on the way to the meadow, which provide plenty of places to get water. If you leave the trail at the crossing of Blue Canyon Creek and head upstream approximately 200 feet, you can enjoy a view of Blue Canyon Falls.

On the way to Simpson Meadow infrequent gaps in the trees allow excellent views of Slide Bluffs across Middle Fork Kings River and the occasional cascade plummeting down the canyon walls. Patches of lush vegetation offer intermittent breaks in the typical mixed forest, composed of ponderosa pines, incense cedars, black oaks, canyon oaks, cottonwoods, and laurels.

Across from Simpson Meadow, the previously undulating trail proceeds through the trees on the north side of the river and then reaches an obscure junction marked by a small cairn. If you miss this junction, the trail will eventually lead into a tangle of thick and lush vegetation where the tread completely disappears. From the cairn, turn right and follow a short path to the riverbank and a knee- to waist-deep ford of the river, which shouldn't present any difficulties after midsummer. Back downstream, near the south end of the meadow, there are reports of a high log that might be used to cross the river. Long ago, a bridge used to span the Middle Fork, but the structure was never rebuilt after repeated washouts. The Park Service is reluctant to design and

build a new bridge that so few backpackers would use; most of the limited traffic the Middle Fork receives is via the Granite Pass Trail from Kings Canyon over Monarch Divide and down to Simpson Meadow.

Reach the lush grassland of upper Simpson Meadow on the far side of the river. There are campsites in small groves of trees near the bank and also back down the Granite Pass Trail near Horseshoe Creek and farther still via a use trail leading to Dougherty Creek.

On the now-distinct tread of the Middle Fork Trail, proceed upstream from Simpson Meadow around the base of Windy Peak to a crossing of the stream draining Windy Canyon. Along the way, the mostly open topography allows for fine views across the river and up the enchanting canyon of Goddard Creek. From the stream crossing, follow the canyon as it bends to the north to a bridge over Cartridge Creek, about 2.5 miles from Simpson Meadow. Long ago, the JMT came over Cartridge Pass, went through lovely Lake Basin, and then descended Cartridge Creek to Middle Fork Kings River. Although traces of the path still exist, the former trail is now considered a tough cross-country route, especially through the brush-filled lower canyon. The route, as described in Secor's *The High Sierra: Peaks, Passes, and Trails*, begins about a quarter mile farther up the Middle Fork Trail.

Beyond the Cartridge Creek bridge, follow the trail through oak woodland, and then drop suddenly to a gravel bar along the river. From there, a steady climb leads through the narrowing canyon, sandwiched between Windy Cliff to the east and Great Cliffs at the end of the Black Divide to the west. Rocky tread ascends stiffly to one of the premier features of the Middle Fork, Devils Washbowl, where the river tumbles dramatically into a scenic pool, 1.5 miles from Cartridge Creek.

After taking in the sights of Devils Washbowl, resume the steady ascent through rock-filled, open terrain, with excellent views of the tumbling river and the high canyon walls. In the shadow of Rambaud Peak, hop across a side stream and continue up the narrow canyon. Nearing Palisade Creek, the grade eases on the way into the cover of Jeffrey pines. Walk across this flat to a ford of the creek, which shouldn't be difficult other than early in the season, when it could be potentially dangerous. A bridge used to span the creek farther upstream, but was not rebuilt after it washed out in the 1980s. On the far side is a well-used, tree-shaded 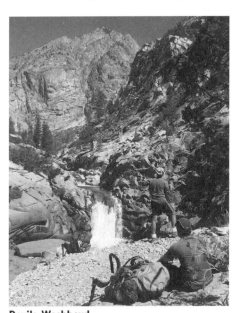 camping area just before a junction with the JMT, 3 miles from Devils Washbowl. Do not expect two things here: solitude, which will be particularly noticeable after the nearly guaranteed solitude of the Middle Fork, and easily available firewood, which will more than likely be picked over by midsummer.

Now on the JMT, a stiff climb away from the junction soon moderates under light forest along the course of the Middle Fork. Hop across a stream draining a trio of unnamed tarns below the southeast face of Giraud Peak, and then cross an open, sagebrush-covered hillside to Grouse Meadow, 1 mile from the junction. The meadow is quite scenic, as the river sedately meanders through an expanse of grassland,

Devils Washbowl

backdropped by the nearly vertical walls of Le Conte Canyon. View-filled campsites around the fringe are heavily used but quite scenic. Mosquitoes are quite bothersome in midsummer.

Beyond serene Grouse Meadow, the previously placid river picks up steam again, and the trail climbs mildly through scattered to light forest. The effects of an avalanche and a forest fire, combined with natural breaks in the forest, provide occasional views of the towering walls of Le Conte Canyon, along with the mighty ramparts of The Citadel accented by a cascading stream from Ladder Lake. Where the trail draws nearer to the river, shooting cascades of white water catapult across granite slabs. Farther up the trail, ribbons of water on the Dusy Branch slide gracefully down the sloping face of an extensive granite slab on the deep canyon's east wall. Pass campsites on either side of a bridge over Dusy Branch and reach a junction with the Bishop Pass Trail, 3.3 miles from the Middle Fork Trail junction. The Le Conte Canyon ranger cabin is nearby, and there are more campsites spread along the riverbank.

From the junction, head northbound on the JMT on gently graded tread through light forest. The grade increases and the forest cover diminishes, which allows views of 12,108-foot Langille Peak looming over the canyon. A prolific display of wildflowers lines the trail on the way into Lower Pete Meadow, where a mellow stretch of river meanders through a sloping, grass-covered clearing bordered by sagebrush and scattered groves of lodgepole pines and mountain hemlocks. The trees shelter several campsites sprinkled around the fringe of the meadow. Fishing for rainbow, brook, and golden trout is reported to be good here.

The climb resumes above the meadow, passing through open terrain with more views of the canyon and now cascading river. After crossing a couple of side streams, drop into a lush wildflower garden intermixed with young aspens. Pass through a drift fence, and climb to Big Pete Meadow, 1.75 miles from the Bishop Pass junction, with plenty of well-used campsites.

At Big Pete Meadow, the JMT turns west, hops over streams, and crosses an avalanche swath, where massive Langille Peak continues to dominate the view. About a quarter mile from the meadow, pass more campsites and closely follow the river in and out of the shade from a light forest. The trail starts climbing moderately to moderately steeply between steep granite walls, which may feel like an oven during the typically hot afternoons. Above a talus slope, skirt the side of the canyon and climb above granite slabs to a fine view of a waterfall on the turbulent Middle Fork. Follow the trail across a luxuriant, seep-watered hillside amid a bounty of colorful wildflowers to a series of rocky switchbacks leading above the falls and into a small basin filled with verdant meadows and delightful tarns. The grade eases on a stroll through this picturesque basin, passing through intermittent stands of mountain hemlocks and lodgepole, western white, and whitebark pines.

After crossing a small stream, a short climb leads to campsites nestled beneath the trees. Another set of switchbacks leads up to views of a pond-filled basin, where primitive campsites can be found scattered around the shorelines. After crossing the dwindling Middle Fork, wander around a tangle of rock humps to a large tarn. Overnighters could set up camp on the rock shelf at the south shore or on a hillside to the southwest amid widely scattered conifers.

Amid diminishing whitebark pines, climb above the tarn, cross back over the nascent Middle Fork, follow the diminishing river for a spell, veer away, and then rejoin it farther up the slope. Ascend past another tarn and up the narrowing, rocky cleft of the river to the east shore of sprawling, majestic, and austere Helen Lake, set into an expansive, rock-filled basin just below the Goddard Divide. The lake, named for one of John Muir's daughters, is the headwaters of Middle Fork Kings River. Exposed campsites are spread around the treeless shoreline in small patches of sand, the ground-hugging vegetation offering little protection from the elements. The stark beauty of Helen Lake and the rust-colored

surroundings provide compelling scenery. Anglers can accept the challenge of fishing for fair-size golden trout.

Bidding a final farewell to the Middle Fork, follow the south side of Helen Lake, weaving around some tarns across rock-filled terrain to the base of the final climb leading up a set of switchbacks to Muir Pass on the Goddard Divide. About 7,800 feet higher than Tehipite Valley, the reward for the previous 30-mile climb along Middle Fork Kings River is a sweeping view from the pass in both directions. Directly ahead, the shimmering waters of Lake McDermand and Wanda Lake lie at the head of enchanting Evolution Basin. Nearby, is the iconic landmark of Muir Hut.

> **MUIR HUT**
>
> The beehive-shaped stone hut was built by the Sierra Club in 1933 to honor the organization's most prestigious member, cofounder, and original president. The hut was also constructed to "offer protection and safety to storm-bound travelers." In keeping with this spirit, backpackers can use the hut temporarily during inclement weather, but camping in or near the hut is prohibited because of human waste concerns.

The descent from Muir Pass begins moderately and then eases to a gently descending grade across the upper slope of Evolution Basin. Less than a mile from the pass, skirt the west shore of lonely Lake McDermand, and proceed to the much larger Wanda Lake, named for Muir's other daughter. Spartan campsites near the outlet and widely scattered around the shoreline are bordered by low-growing alpine vegetation creating an austere vibe to the rocky surroundings, but the expansive scenery more than compensates for the lack of shrubs and trees. Glacier-clad Mt. Goddard and the north face of multihued Goddard

Divide provide a fine backdrop to the southwest, while the string of summits of Mounts Huxley, Spencer, Darwin, and Mendel line the northeast horizon.

Away from sprawling Wanda Lake, the JMT fords Evolution Creek and then gently descends along the course of the creek before dropping more moderately but shortly toward scenic Sapphire Lake. Sapphire is perhaps the prettiest of the Evolution Lakes, the glacier-polished canyon sandwiched between towering summits on both sides of the trail. Campsites seem to be even less prevalent here than at Wanda Lake. The trailless mini-basin to the east of the lake offers more remote campsites around smaller, 11,000-foot lakes and tarns sitting in scenic wonderland below a horseshoe of soaring peaks, including Mounts Huxley, Warlow, Fiske, Wallace, Haeckel, and Spencer.

Proceed downstream through the deep cleft of the canyon toward the most hospitable lake in the basin, Evolution Lake. Cross the inlet and proceed around the east side of the long and narrow lake to a short climb over a low rise separating two lobes of the lake. Arc around to the north shore to a small, elevated peninsula dotted with stunted whitebark pines. There are view-packed, well-used campsites on the peninsula, near the outlet, and on small flats on the hillside north of the lake.

Before leaving Evolution Lake, take one last look at the majesty of the surroundings. The slender basin, graced with a string of jeweled lakes and a procession of magnificent peaks, provides one of the most glorious sights in the High Sierra.

From Evolution Lake, follow sandy tread past some tarns and over granite slabs to the top of a set of switchbacks dropping into Evolution Valley. From the top of the switchbacks, several cross-country routes embark on crossings of the Glacier Divide and the Sierra Crest, including the popular Lamarck Col route (see Trip 121, page 431). A thickening forest of lodgepole pines coincides with the drop in elevation, with periodic gaps in the trees allowing fine views of the valley. The trail zigzags down the wall of the canyon and crosses a couple of flower-lined streams on the way. From early to midsummer the thunderous roar from a waterfall on the creek draining Darwin Bench and the canyons above usually heralds the approach to the floor of the canyon.

At the bottom of the switchbacks, the trail heads down Evolution Valley through stands of scattered pines, across small pocket meadows, and beside granite slabs and boulders to eventually reach Colby Meadow, 9.25 miles from Muir Pass. The verdant clearing of the meadow offers fine scenery of the valley, serpentine creek, and surrounding peaks. Overnighters will find good campsites scattered around the fringe of the meadow beneath lodgepole pines. Despite the heavy traffic on the JMT, fishing in nearby Evolution Creek is good for golden trout.

Continuing on the JMT, follow gently graded trail over a pair of streams and through light forest cover for 0.75 mile to the edge of McClure Meadow, the largest of the main meadows in Evolution Valley, with numerous campsites spread around fringe, some with excellent views of the lazy creek flowing sinuously through the verdant clearing. On a low rise just north of the trail sits a ranger cabin, the summer home for seasonal rangers who patrol this section of the park. Continue the gentle stroll to the end of the meadow, where the creek returns to its tumbling ways.

For the next couple of miles, the JMT travels in and out of lodgepole pine forest, crossing a trio of streams draining the south side of Glacier Divide. Breaks in the forest allow occasional views of the canyon, including a major avalanche swath and a picturesque waterfall below Emerald Peak. Reach the east edge of Evolution Meadow near the crossing of a twin-channeled creek.

Gently graded trail leads along the lodgepole pine–shaded fringe of Evolution Meadow, passing numerous campsites along the way. Beyond the meadow, the trail bends south toward a ford of Evolution Creek. Except during the height of snowmelt, the ford should not present any difficulties, although you should plan on getting your feet and lower legs wet.

After fording Evolution Creek, briefly follow gently graded trail along the south bank to where the creek suddenly begins a raucous plunge toward a union with South Fork San Joaquin River, tumbling over slabs and careening wildly around boulders. The trail seemingly attempts to match the fall of the creek with a zigzagging descent down the exposed, west-facing wall of the canyon, providing fine views along the way of the canyon and river below. Near the bottom of the descent, enter the welcome shade from a forest of aspens, lodgepole pines, and incense cedars, and stroll across the floor to a wood bridge spanning the river. On the far side of the bridge, reach a junction with the Goddard Canyon Trail, 4.25 miles from McClure Meadow. There are good campsites on both sides of the bridge and a short way up the Goddard Canyon Trail.

Leaving the JMT behind, turn south and follow the Goddard Canyon Trail on a moderate climb through light lodgepole pine forest, following the course of South Fork San Joaquin River. A half mile of climbing leads to Franklin Meadow, where a picturesque, wildflower-laden meadowland is dotted with tall aspens and occasional lodgepoles. Step across streams draining unnamed tarns below Le Conte Divide near the middle and far end of the meadow, where there are primitive campsites just above the river.

Beyond Franklin Meadow, follow the trail away from the riverbank for a while on a mild to moderate climb through more scattered lodgepole pines. Soon the canyon narrows, forcing the path up the hillside farther above the river. In the midst of this ascending traverse, you pass above some campsites occupying a narrow bench overlooking the South Fork. Soon, encounter a lush hillside carpeted with willows, aspens, and wildflowers, including paintbrush, clover, coneflower, columbine, and heather, well watered by a series of rivulets. On the far side of the river is Pig Chute, where a seasonal stream pours down a narrow cleft of rock beside a rocky, knife-edged protrusion. Farther up the trail, a spectacular waterfall spilling dramatically into an emerald pool further enhances the beautiful scenery.

For the next 1.5 miles, proceed upstream with splendid views of the cascading river plunging down the narrow, deep, and rocky cleft of Goddard Canyon. Pass two more waterfalls as scenic as any in the High Sierra, and jump across many flower-lined side streams along the way.

Near the confluence of North Goddard Creek, the canyon widens temporarily, allowing the river to adopt a more leisurely pace. Stroll through meadowlands with fine views of the two canyons, separated by a low rock dome. A short, moderate climb leads to an obscure, unsigned junction (approximately 9,900 feet) with the barely distinct Hell-for-Sure Pass Trail, 5 miles from the JMT junction. A small cairn may mark the junction, but the path is easy to miss. There are a couple of passable campsites just up the trail a short way, near the crossing of a stream draining a small, unnamed tarn (approximately 11,390 feet) below Le Conte Divide.

Turn right (southwest) and climb moderately on a series of switchbacks up the lightly forested hillside. Fortunately, the tread becomes more distinct above the junction and should provide few route-finding problems for the duration of the climb to Hell-for-Sure Pass. After the switchbacks, the trail begins an undulating, 2.5-mile traverse across the southwest wall of Goddard Canyon, roughly paralleling the section of trail you just followed up the canyon. You can't help but wonder if there could have been a more direct route from Goddard Canyon to Hell-for-Sure Pass. Nonetheless, follow the trail to the top of a bench, about 0.6 mile from the junction, which, oddly enough, is the high point of the traverse. From there, drop into a small bowl holding a tiny pond, and proceed to the crossing of a stream draining a tarn (approximately 10,400 feet) above. Shortly beyond the crossing, the trail descends more steeply for a half mile to the low point of the traverse before a short climb, followed by an even shorter descent to the next stream crossing, 2 miles from the junction. A moderate ascent ensues, from there leading past point 10191 to the brink of a small side drainage. Drop briefly into the drainage, cross the stream, and then climb up to a switchback at the end of the traverse. After the 2.5-mile traverse, you find yourself less than 500 feet above the junction, about even with the top of the initial switchbacks, but having lost and gained 1,400 feet of elevation in the process. At least the traverse offered a few good views of Goddard Canyon along the way.

Now the trail attacks the slopes below the pass with a vengeance, zigzagging steeply up a lightly forested hillside before arcing back toward the north bank of the creek that the trail previously crossed. Now out of the trees, the trail follows the creek for a while before angling away on a stiff climb to the top of a rocky rise. From there, the trail begins a long diagonal ascent across the upper slopes of the drainage and then doubles back before curving around over rocky terrain to 11,297-foot Hell-for-Sure Pass, 4 miles from the Goddard Canyon Trail junction. The view ahead of Red Mountain Basin and its bevy of sparkling lakes and out to the Sierra foothills beyond is quite pleasant, although you shouldn't forget to turn around for one final view of the deep cleft of Goddard Canyon crowned by the summits of Emerald Peak, Peter Peak, and Mt. McGee.

From Hell-for-Sure Pass, the path plummets steeply down the west face of Le Conte Divide on tightly winding, sandy tread amid large boulders before the grade eases immediately north of Hell-for-Sure Lake. Small pockets of meadow attempt to soften the extensive amount of glacier-polished granite slabs making up the open bowl holding the lake. Along with acres and acres of glistening white granite, the steep wall of the Le Conte Divide and the craggy cliffs on the north face of Mt. Hutton cast a decidedly alpine ambiance. Developed campsites, while few in number, are seemingly adequate for the low number of backpackers making the 15-mile journey from Courtright Reservoir. Anglers should enjoy fishing for medium-size brook trout. J. N. Le Conte, who first used the name in print, must have had some sort of difficulty negotiating the pass above since beautiful Hell-for-Sure Lake seems deserving of a less demonic name.

A short, moderately steep, winding descent leads away from the environs of Hell-for-Sure Lake and down into a long, nearly level bench holding a series of small tarns. Cross the outlet at the far end of the bench, and drop through open, rocky terrain to pass to the north of Disappointment Lake. Reach a junction with a lateral to the northwest shore of the lake, 1.5 mile from the pass. Backdropped by Mt. Hutton and Le Conte Divide, Disappointment Lake is as attractive as any of the High Sierra lakes with pockets of meadow alternating with rolling granite slabs and a strip of sandy beach on the near shore. There are tree-shaded, view-packed campsites just above the beach. While campfires are permitted, you probably won't be able to find enough firewood.

DISAPPOINTMENT LAKE

Hardly a disappointment to modern-day travelers, the lake received its name from some early anglers unhappy with their poor catch. Today, a healthy population of good-size brook trout should satisfy most anglers.

From the lateral to Disappointment Lake, continue ahead over granite slabs, following a series of cairns down a hillside through widely scattered dwarf pines to a junction with the Meadow Brook Trail on the left, which leads 1.5 miles to lovely Devils Punchbowl.

Continue straight ahead from the junction, cross a stream, and gently ascend through thickening forest to the crest of a rise. A moderate descent leads away from the crest and down to a shallow ford of meadow-lined Fleming Creek. A short distance beyond the ford is a signed junction with a trail heading north to Rae Lake and Indian Lakes, 3.5 miles from the pass. A short distance from the junction, Rae Lake offers fine campsites and good fishing.

Turn left (southwest) at the junction and follow gently graded tread past oval-shaped Fleming Lake. Heading into forest cover for the duration of the journey, the gentle stroll continues for a while beyond the lake, and then a moderate, occasionally switchbacking descent leads across the side of the canyon above Fleming Creek, crossing a number of small, lushly lined seasonal tributaries along the way. Following more gently graded tread for a mile or so, reach a saddle on a ridge dividing the drainages of Fleming and Post Corral Creeks.

A 2-mile descent from the saddle leads to Post Corral Creek. Initially, the descent is quite stiff, winding down the hillside to a series of granite slabs near the midpoint, from where there are limited views to the west. Beyond the slabs, the grade eases a bit, and the trail proceeds through viewless forest to a small meadow on the floor of the canyon and a junction with a trail on the left that eventually leads to Blackcap Basin, 4.75 miles from the Rae Lake junction. Turn right and proceed a short distance beyond the junction to a ford of Post Corral Creek. The crossing of the broad channel usually presents few problems, but until late summer plan on getting your feet wet. Campsites may be available on either side of the ford.

Seven miles is all that remains on the journey to Maxson Trailhead near Courtright Reservoir. Gently graded trail soon leads to Post Corral Meadows, where a series of posts line the trail and a use trail branches northeast across the creek to the heart of the meadow and a leaseholder's cabin. As part of the multiuse approach, the Forest Service has continued to allow grazing within the wilderness area, an effective deterrent to anyone searching for campsites near the meadow.

Away from Post Corral Meadows, the trail arcs around the nose of a hill on a gentle climb through the forest to the edge of Long Meadow and a junction with the Burnt Corral Meadow Trail, 2 miles from the ford of Post Corral Creek.

Continue the gentle stroll through Long Meadow, and then climb moderately back into the cover of lodgepole pine and red fir forest. At the top of the climb in a forested saddle, reach a junction with a trail to Hobler Lake, 1.5 miles from the previous junction.

Drop away from the saddle on a moderate, 0.75-mile descent, following the narrow cleft of a seasonal drainage before the grade eases near Chamberlains Camp. Nearby Maxson Dome, which cuts a dramatic profile when seen from the west above the waters of Courtright Reservoir, is completely obscured by the dense forest (as is the reservoir). Skirt a series of meadows alternating with dense stands of lodgepole pine forest for the next couple of miles to a junction with a jeep road, southwest of Maxson Meadows. Turn left (south) and walk along the road on a gentle descent through the trees for about 0.75 mile to where the road begins a steep uphill climb. Poorly marked, single-track trail veers slightly away to the left of the road and climbs up to the Maxson Traihead parking area, which occupies a saddle.

🅾 Enough options exist along this route to fill an entire guidebook; they are limited only by your imagination. One option is highly recommended for parties possessing the requisite skills: Cross-country enthusiasts could take advantage of a shortcut from Helen Lake through enchanted Ionian Basin to Martha Lake and then down Goddard Canyon to the Hell-for-Sure Pass Trail junction. However, doing so means missing the fine scenery of Evolution Basin, Evolution Valley, and lower Goddard Canyon.

🆁 A wilderness permit is required for overnight stays. Campfires are prohibited above 10,000 feet.

COURTRIGHT RESERVOIR TRAILHEAD

TRIP 87

Red Mountain Basin

Ⓜ ↗ BP

DISTANCE: 30.5 miles, out-and-back

ELEVATION: 7,990'/10,765',
+4,035'/-1,375'/±10,820'

SEASON: July to mid-October

USE: Light

MAPS: *Courtright Reservoir, Ward Mountain, Blackcap Mountain, and Mt. Henry*

TRAIL LOG

3.5	Hobler Lake junction
6.0	Post Corral Creek ford and Blackcap Basin Trail junction
11.75	Rae Lake and Indian Lakes junction
13.5	Meadow Brook Trail junction
13.75	Disappointment Lake
15.0	Hell-for-Sure Lake
15.25	Hell-for-Sure Pass

INTRODUCTION: Red Mountain Basin offers some of the scenery for which the High Sierra is famous. However, a fairly long journey through montane forest is necessary before you reach the classic granite terrain below rugged Le Conte Divide. Aside from 3 miles of moderate ascent, most of the 15-mile journey is over gently graded trail on the way to a bounty of picturesque lakes, some near the trail and others requiring straightforward cross-country travel. A remote trailhead, lightly used trail, and assortment of lakes from which to choose for campsites combine to ensure a reasonable expectation of solitude. Crossing Le Conte Divide at Hell-for-Sure Pass opens the gates to further adventures in Kings Canyon National Park.

DIRECTIONS TO TRAILHEAD: From Fresno, follow State Highway 168 through Prather (which has a ranger station), and continue toward the community of Shaver Lake. As you come into town, turn right onto Dinkey Creek Road, and proceed 11.5 miles to a right-hand turn onto McKinley Grove Road. Continue 13.6 more miles to the Courtright-Wishon junction. Bear left at the junction, and drive 7 miles to another junction near the south end of Courtright Reservoir. Following a sign for the Maxson Trailhead, veer right, cross the one-way road over the dam, and head above the southeast shore to the parking area (which has a vault toilet).

DESCRIPTION: From the Maxson Trailhead parking area, follow single-track trail on a short, winding descent through light lodgepole pine forest, past the equestrian trail, and down to a jeep road at the bottom of the hill. Head generally north on the gently graded road for a mile to a signed junction near Maxson Meadow. Leaving the road, bear right (northeast) and follow a trail across the meadow and back under forest cover. Gently climbing, the path follows and then crosses a stream near the 2-mile mark just before entering John Muir Wilderness. Ascend a forested hillside to the crest of a rise, and meet a junction with a trail to Hobler Lake, 3.5 miles from the trailhead.

🄾 **SIDE TRIP TO HOBLER LAKE:** A short descent leads to the crossing of a small stream, followed by a gentle, forested ascent to Hobler Lake, 0.75 mile from the junction. The placid lake is nearly surrounded by a forest of lodgepole pines and red firs, which shelters a smattering of campsites. Grassy meadows border the lakeshore in areas too wet for the conifers. Brook trout will entice anglers, and swimmers should find the temperate waters to be reasonably pleasant.

Rather than retrace your steps, follow the trail past the lake another mile to a junction, turn right (southeast) and follow the Burnt Corral Meadow Trail on a nearly mile-long descent to rejoin the Blackcap Basin Trail at Long Meadow and continue your journey to Red Mountain Basin. **END OF SIDE TRIP**

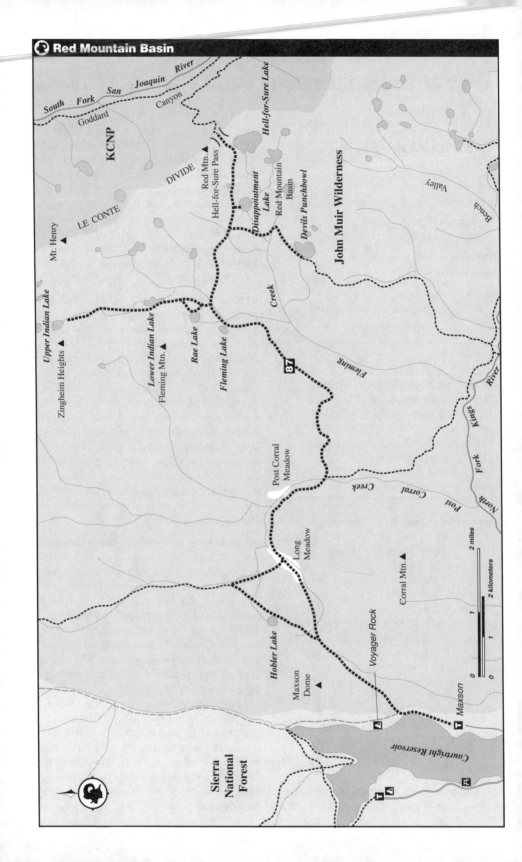

From the Hobler Lake junction, continue roughly northeast on gently descending tread to the fringe of Long Meadow. A pleasant walk through the meadow along Post Corral Creek provides enticing glimpses of the distant peaks and ridges to the east. In the midst of the meadow, reach a signed junction with the Burnt Corral Meadow Trail, 5 miles from the trailhead.

Just beyond the junction, ford the creek and continue a gentle descent around the nose of a hillside for 1.3 miles to the vicinity of Post Corral Meadow, where short posts line the trail. A use trail branches northeast across the creek and into the heart of the meadow to a leaseholder's cabin. As part of the Forest Service's multiuse approach, cattle grazing is still allowed in this part of the wilderness, which should effectively deter backpackers who want to camp near the meadow—there are better campsites a quarter mile farther down the trail near a crossing of Post Corral Creek.

Proceed downstream on nearly level trail to the ford, 7 miles from the trailhead, usually easy, although you should plan to get your feet wet. There are campsites on either side of the creek. A short distance beyond, reach a signed, three-way junction with Hell-for-Sure Pass Trail, where the Blackcap Trail continues east.

Continue straight ahead from the junction on the Hell-for-Sure Pass Trail. The gentle grade of the previous 7 miles is left behind, as a moderate climb leads up a ridge separating the Post Corral Creek and Fleming Creek drainages. Midway up the hillside, the grade increases on an ascent over granite slabs, where the Forest Service dynamited the route to provide easier stock travel. The 2-mile, moderately steep, sometimes winding climb ends at a saddle, with limited views of the mountainous terrain ahead.

A brief descent from the saddle leads to a gentle, mile-plus climb through lodgepole pine forest across the side of the canyon above Fleming Creek. Along the way, the trail crosses a number of small, lushly lined streams. A short, switchbacking climb is followed by gently graded trail alongside meadows dotted with scattered conifers.

Just beyond a low hummock, oval-shaped Fleming Lake springs into view, 11.5 miles from the trailhead.

After so many miles of forest, broken only by a handful of meadows, the lake offers a welcome change in scenery. Views of the craggy Le Conte Divide complement an exposed shoreline of boggy meadows. Widely scattered pines shelter a few good campsites on the hummock. Anglers can test their skill on a sizable population of brook trout. Halfway around the lakeshore, the trail crosses the outlet and passes an old campsite closed for restoration. Following the course of Fleming Creek, head northeast to impressive views of Le Conte Divide across a broad meadow, in the middle of which is a signed junction with the Rae Lake and Indian Lakes Trail, 11.75 miles from the trailhead.

SIDE TRIP TO RAE LAKE AND INDIAN LAKES: From the Rae Lake and Indian Lakes Trail junction, continue straight ahead, skirt the meadow, and reach an indistinct junction in a grove of conifers. Follow the left-hand trail over a forested rise, and then drop down to the northeast shore of meadow-rimmed Rae Lake. Fine campsites beneath scattered pines will appeal to overnighters, with the best sites on the west and north sides of the lake. Brook trout provide opportunities for anglers. Now named for a packer, the lake was originally called Wolverine Lake, but the appellation disappeared about the same time as its namesake mammal, which while not extinct, is no longer a resident of the southern Sierra.

From the indistinct junction with the lateral to Rae Lake, a moderate climb leads up a forested hillside. Where the grade eases, the trees start to thin, allowing improving views of Le Conte Divide across the expansive meadow encircling Lower Indian Lake. About 0.75 mile from the Hell-for-Sure Trail junction, draw alongside the narrow south finger of the lake. Although developed campsites are nonexistent, plenty of primitive camping is available in this secluded setting. Fishing pressure on the resident brook trout should be quite low.

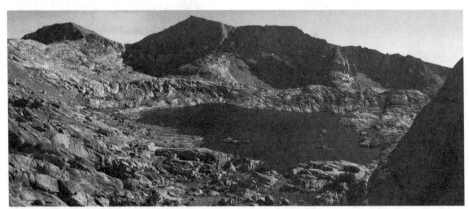

Hell-for-Sure Lake below Hell-for-Sure Pass on Le Conte Divide

Beyond the lower lake, discernible tread disappears in the lush vegetation, but the wide open basin, sprinkled with boulders and compact granite slabs, is easily traversed in the absence of a bona fide trail. At the far end of the meadow, hop over a seasonal stream and make a short, moderately steep climb alongside a creek pouring down a narrow cleft in the hillside above. A final, half-mile ascent leads to the south shore of pristine Upper Indian Lake, perched at the very head of the canyon. Steep slopes virtually surround the lake, culminating in the 11,318-foot Zingheim Heights above the west shore. Mosquito Pass, just above the far shore, offers a glance north down a canyon of South Fork San Joaquin River.

NOTE: The *Mt. Henry* quad indicates a shortcut from the northeast shore of Rae Lake to a connection with the trail to Lower Indian Lake. Although the faint path exists, finding it is difficult since insignificant cairns mark the indistinct path. The path ascends the hillside above the lake and then connects with the trail about a quarter mile south of Lower Indian Lake. **END OF SIDE TRIP**

From the Rae Lake and Indian Lakes junction, turn right (east) and follow the Hell-for-Sure Pass Trail across Fleming Creek and around the lower edge of a meadow. A moderate, lightly forested climb heads past a junction with a lateral to seldom-visited Dale Lake. Continue climbing through dwindling trees, boulder fields, and

pocket meadows to the crest of a ridge. As you enter Red Mountain Basin, a fine view unfolds of Le Conte Divide and the east ridge of Mt. Hutton. Beyond the crossing of a stream, reach a junction with the Meadow Brook Trail, 13.5 miles from the trailhead.

[O] SIDE TRIP TO DEVILS PUNCHBOWL: Turn away from the Hell-for-Sure Pass Trail, and head south on a gentle descent through light pine forest, passing a small, meadow-rimmed pond. Eventually the descent becomes more pronounced as the trail rounds a hill and winds down to lush meadowlands at the crossing of a picturesque stream. Beyond the creek, stroll past more meadows until a moderately steep climb regains most of the lost elevation. At the top of the climb, reach the beautiful lake dubbed Devils Punchbowl, 1.5 miles from the junction.

Devils Punchbowl sits in a scenic basin carved out of a rocky cleft at the very edge of steep cliffs overlooking Fleming Creek canyon. The outlet pours from the lake and immediately plummets dramatically down the cliff face, bound for the diminutive Jigger Lakes before adopting a less riotous path toward Fleming Creek. A trip to the lake would be incomplete without taking in the view from the edge of the cliffs near the outlet, particularly early in the season when the water flows at full force. An expansive and unobstructed view to the west provides a splendid opportunity to enjoy some magnificent sunsets. The lake is quite scenic as well, backdropped by rugged peaks and lined with a smattering of graceful pines. There are excellent campsites spread around the shoreline, and a sandy beach offers an excellent spot for sunbathing and swimming. Anglers can test their luck on rainbow and brook trout.

By visiting Devils Punchbowl on the way back through upper Red Mountain Basin, you could return via the Blackcap Basin Trail by continuing southwest from the lake for 6.5 miles to North Fork Kings River, turning northwest, and proceeding 4 miles to a junction with the Hell-for-Sure Pass Trail near the ford of Post Corral Creek. Such a detour offers picturesque meadows, views along the upper part of the Meadow Brook Trail, and a scenic mile-long stretch along the river. **END OF SIDE TRIP**

From the Meadow Brook Trail junction, head southeast, following cairns over granite slabs and past dwarf pines to an unmarked lateral to Disappointment Lake. A short stroll down this trail accesses the north shore of this scenic lake, which is backdropped by Mt. Hutton and Le Conte Divide. As attractive as any other High Sierra lake, the shore is bordered by alternating pockets of meadow, a strip of sandy beach on the near shore, and rolling granite slabs on the far shore. There are view-packed campsites shaded by pines just above the beach.

Continuing on the main trail, stroll along on sandy tread with good views of the surrounding terrain. Cross a stream and pass some delightful tarns before starting a moderate, winding climb up a hillside

DISAPPOINTMENT LAKE

Hardly a disappointment to modern-day travelers, the lake received its name from some early anglers unhappy with the size of their catch. Today, a healthy population of good-size brook trout should satisfy most anglers.

composed of granite slabs. At the top of the climb, you pass above Hell-for-Sure Lake, another spectacularly beautiful lake surrounded by polished granite slabs, with tiny pockets of meadow feebly attempting to soften the rock-filled basin. The lake is backdropped by the immediate presence of steep rock walls rising up toward the crest of Le Conte Divide and by the craggy cliffs on the north face of Mt. Hutton. Developed campsites are few but seem plentiful enough to provide for the hearty souls who venture this far from the trailhead. Fishing is reportedly good for medium-size brook trout. The name given to this gorgeous lake seems as uninspired and misguided as Disappointment Lake.

Beyond Hell-for-Sure Lake, the trail begins a steady climb along the banks of a lushly vegetated creek, heading toward a cleft in the divide above. Wind around, over, and beside large boulders all the way to 11,297-foot Hell-for-Sure Pass. A dramatic view down into Goddard Canyon is a worthy reward for the extra bit of climbing from the lake.

The Hell-for-Sure Pass Trail drops nearly 1,500 feet in 4 miles to a connection with the Goddard Canyon Trail, 2.75 miles north of Martha Lake (see Trip 88, page 298).

Red Mountain Basin provides excellent opportunities for further wanderings to many scenic lakes without maintained trails. Cross-country enthusiasts with a modicum of off-trail experience should be able to easily navigate the open terrain. The Two Passes cross-country route provides a Class 2 connection between Red Mountain Basin and Bench Valley.

Mountaineering is somewhat limited in and around the basin. From Hell-for-Sure Pass, Red Mountain, just northwest, is a short, Class 1 ascent. From the vicinity of Indian Lakes, both Zingheim Heights and Fleming Mountain are straightforward climbs.

R A wilderness permit is required for overnight stays. Campfires are permitted west of the park boundary.

TRIP 88

Blayney Hot Springs, Goddard Canyon, and Martha Lake

 BP

DISTANCE: 46 miles, out-and-back
38 miles, out-and-back via ferry

ELEVATION: 7,350'/11,005', +4,830'/-1,175'/±12,010'

SEASON: Mid-July to late September

USE: Moderate to the hot springs, and light beyond

MAPS: *Florence Lake, Ward Mountain, Blackcap Mountain, Mt. Henry,* and *Mount Goddard*

TRAIL LOG

3.5	South Fork San Joaquin River
4.0	Ferry landing junction
6.25	Lower Blayney Campground
7.0	Blayney Hot Springs junction
9.5	John Muir Trail junction
11.75	Piute Pass Trail junction
13.25	Aspen Meadow
15.25	Goddard Canyon Trail junction
16.0	Franklin Meadow
20.25	Hell-for-Sure Pass Trail junction
23.0	Martha Lake

INTRODUCTION: This multiday trip visits the remote northwestern corner of Kings Canyon National Park. Although you may see a number of people on their way to Muir Trail Ranch, you can expect a healthy dose of solitude once you reach Goddard Canyon. Solitude is not the only benefit—the scenery along South Fork San Joaquin River, including thrilling cataracts, cascades, and waterfalls from Florence Lake all the way to the headwaters, is superb. The

river offers anglers excellent fishing as well. The journey up the river reaches a splendid crescendo at beautiful Martha Lake, a large alpine lake cradled in a rocky basin and backdropped by craggy peaks and ridges. Along the way, gorgeous meadows, peaceful forests, and the opportunity to soak in a natural hot spring are added bonuses. A number of shady, riverside campsites provide pleasant overnight havens.

The first obstacle is the drive to the trailhead. The route over Kaiser Pass on narrow, twisting, single-lane road is quite time consuming—plan on an hour for the 21-mile drive from Huntington Lake. Once at Florence Lake, you must decide whether to hike 4 miles around the reservoir or to accept the favored alternative of paying to ride the ferry across.

The 4 miles of trail beyond Florence Lake parallel and sometimes share the route of a jeep road used regularly by Muir Trail Ranch (MTR) to transport guests to and from their backcountry resort. The ranch is a hubbub of activity at times, providing anglers, equestrians, and hikers a base camp from which to explore the nearby trails. Backpackers thru-hiking the John Muir and Pacific Crest Trails often use the ranch as a mail drop.

Blayney Hot Springs, just past MTR, is a popular spot with backpackers, a soothing place to soak weary bodies. However, you must ford the South Fork San Joaquin River, which can be dangerous early in the season, to reach the springs. Do *not* attempt this ford when the river is high and fast. Once you leave the ranch and hot springs behind, the activity along the trail diminishes considerably.

DIRECTIONS TO TRAILHEAD: From Fresno, follow State Highway 168 through Prather (which has a ranger station) and the community of Shaver Lake toward Huntington Lake. Just before Huntington Lake, turn right at a sign marked FLORENCE LAKE, and continue for 5.5 miles on a two-lane paved road to where it abruptly narrows. From this point, expect slow going on a narrow, winding road climbing steeply to

⊙ Blayney Hot Springs, Goddard Canyon, and Martha Lake

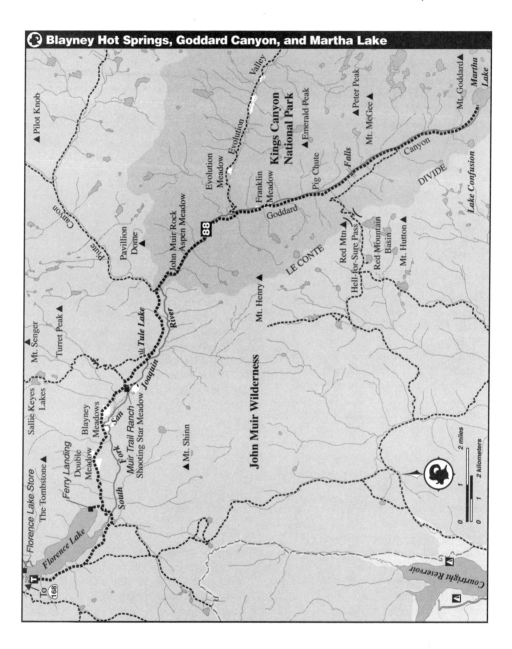

Kaiser Pass and then down to the High Sierra Ranger Station (which issues wilderness permits), 15 miles from Highway 168. Continue 0.75 mile to the Florence Lake and Lake Edison Y-junction, and proceed straight ahead. Pass the entrance to Ward Lake Campground, and continue to the trailhead parking area at Florence Lake, 21 miles from 168.

DESCRIPTION:

TRAIL AROUND FLORENCE LAKE: From the parking lot, follow paved road on an arcing descent through the picnic area and down to the lakeshore. From there, follow the road along the west shore to the start of single-track trail, where a set of stairs leads into John Muir Wilderness. Proceed on gently graded tread across a rolling hillside through a light, mixed forest of Jeffrey pines, ponderosa pines, white firs, western junipers, and aspens. The forest cover thins enough on occasion to allow views across Florence Lake of the dam and the granite walls above the far shore, as well as more distant Mt. Shinn and Ward Mountain to the southeast. Reach a junction with the Burnt Corral Meadow Trail heading south toward Thompson and Lost Lakes, 2 miles from the trailhead.

Continue straight ahead at the junction and travel above the southwest arm of Florence Lake for a mile to a junction with a connector to the Burnt Corral Meadow Trail. Head downhill to a bridge over a tributary, and stroll shortly over to a more substantial bridge spanning South Fork San Joaquin River, 3.5 miles from the trailhead. Fine campsites shaded by lodgepole pines line both banks of the river, and there is a pit toilet up the hillside above the far bank. Turn upstream and briefly follow the course of the river until embarking on a half-mile, moderate climb over sloping granite slabs to a junction with the ferry dock lateral, 4 miles from the trailhead.

FERRY SERVICE OPTION: Rather than backpack the 4 miles around Florence Lake, you can rest your legs while enjoying a $12 one-way or $23 round-trip (as of 2012) boat ride across the lake from late May to late September, subject to weather conditions. The ferry typically runs five times per day, more on weekends if necessary. Children 12 and under ride for $6 one-way ($10 round-trip); dogs can ride for $1 each way. Tickets are purchased at the Florence Lake Store. For more information, check out the website at **www.florence-lake.com**.

From the ferry dock at the far end of the lake, climb uphill over bare granite slopes for a half mile, following cairns and short patches of trail to a junction with the trail around the lake.

MUIR TRAIL RANCH

Keen eyes may notice a primitive jeep road beyond Florence Lake, which Muir Trail Ranch (MTR) uses to transport guests and supplies. The road parallels and sometimes coincides with sections of the hiking trail. Such activity would seem incompatible with the wilderness concept, but this longstanding family business was grandfathered into the original 1964 Wilderness Act. Despite the apparent intrusion of a resort in the backcountry, MTR is hiker-friendly, offers inexpensive ferry rides across Florence Lake, holds packages for John Muir Trail (JMT) and Pacific Crest Trail (PCT) thru-hikers, offers pack carrying services, and allows a limited number of short stay packages at the resort. However, individual meals are not available. For more information, consult the website at **www. muirtrailranch.com**.

NOTE: Mileages listed are from the trailhead at Florence Lake. If you are starting from the ferry dock on the far side of the lake, subtract 4 miles. From the junction of the ferry dock lateral and the trail around Florence Lake, climb over granite slabs and up dry gullies for a mile to the edge of pastoral Double Meadow. The trail soon veers away to skirt the meadow through light forest. Nearing the far end, step across a seasonal stream lined with grasses and wildflowers, and catch a glimpse of the meadow through the trees before a gentle, forested descent leads to a crossing of Alder Creek, 6 miles from the trailhead. Sheltered campsites can be found near the far bank. A short way beyond the creek, a lateral leads to fine campsites at Lower Blayney Campground along South Fork San Joaquin River.

Past the campground lateral is a splendid view across the broad expanse of Blayney Meadow, but the trail soon veers away from the lovely clearing in favor of a less scenic route through the forest. Approximately a half mile from Alder Creek, pass through a gate at the fenced boundary of privately owned MTR. Beyond the gate the backpacker route around the ranch may be difficult to discern among the maze of dusty stock trails and the churned-up jeep road. At a signed junction farther along the road, veer away from the dusty road, which continues toward MTR, onto single-track trail on the left.

Proceed through open terrain and light forest on gently graded trail to the crossings of Sallie Keyes and Senger Creeks. From there, a moderate climb leads up a hillside to a lightly forested traverse that passes through a gate. Continue across the open hillside within earshot of the rhythmic sound from a pelton wheel generating electricity for MTR. Reach an open knoll with a fine view of the surrounding terrain, before dropping to a signed Y-junction with a lateral to MTR and Blayney Hot Springs.

◻ SIDE TRIP TO BLAYNEY HOT SPRINGS: Just 50 feet from the Y-junction, reach another junction, where the left-hand path heads to MTR. Continue ahead from the second junction, and proceed down the hillside through lush vegetation and past numerous overused campsites to the north bank of South Fork San Joaquin River. A very short path travels upstream to a ford of the wide river. Proceed across the river with caution; early in the season the ford may be too dangerous to attempt. The riverbed can be quite slippery—wearing appropriate footwear might help. Once on the far bank, pass more campsites and head across Shooting Star Meadow to the hot springs. Beyond a patch of willow is Warm Lake, well suited for a refreshing swim after a lengthy soak in the springs. The vegetation around the lake and springs is quite fragile, so tread lightly.
END OF SIDE TRIP

From the hot springs junction, head southeast on a gentle climb through light forest, soon reaching a junction with a connector to the JMT on the left. Veer right at the junction, and proceed upstream, paralleling the river. Continue on gently graded tread through a scattered forest of aspens, lodgepole pines, and Jeffrey pines, passing a stagnant pond along the way. Soon, the trail passes above an extensive camping area on a bench above the river, just prior to a junction with the JMT, 9.5 miles from the trailhead.

Proceed straight ahead onto the JMT, following the course of the river through a mixture of granite and conifers. You have fine views of South Fork Canyon as the trail curves around for the next couple of miles, headed toward the confluence of Piute Creek. At 11.75 miles from the trailhead, just before a steel bridge spanning the tumultuous creek, reach a junction with the Piute Pass Trail.

Cross the bridge into Kings Canyon National Park and stroll through chaparral and widely scattered Jeffrey pines past several fine campsites spread across a flat. Proceed upstream on a gentle, exposed climb, rounding John Muir Rock and drawing near the tumbling river flowing through a narrow channel of rock. About 1.5 miles from the Piute Pass Trail junction, enter the cool, forested glade of aspens and pines misnamed Aspen Meadow. While a meadow no longer exists here, there are a few sheltered campsites.

Beyond Aspen Meadow, leave the shade behind, and follow the river on a gently graded, mile-long climb up another narrow, exposed part of the canyon. Cross a steel bridge over the river to a small forested flat, 14.25 miles from the trailhead, where a use trail leads shortly downstream to campsites.

Now on the south bank, pass through a gate near more campsites and then through lush wildflower gardens to a boulder hop of a vigorous stream draining several tarns below Le Conte Divide. Beneath the shade of aspens, lodgepole pines, and western junipers, pass more campsites on the way to a junction of the Goddard Canyon Trail, 15.25 miles from the trailhead. There are fine campsites a short way up Goddard Canyon and also across the river.

From the junction, continue ahead on the Goddard Canyon Trail, passing beneath the cover of a light lodgepole pine forest, within earshot of the churning South Fork on the left. A half mile of climbing leads to Franklin Meadow, where a picturesque, ❀ wildflower-laden meadowland is dotted with tall aspens and occasional lodgepoles. Step across streams draining unnamed tarns below Le Conte Divide near the middle and far end of the meadow, where there are primitive campsites just above the river.

Beyond Franklin Meadow, follow the trail away from the riverbank for a while on a mild to moderate climb through more scattered lodgepole pines. Soon the canyon narrows, forcing the path up the hillside farther above the river. In the midst of this ascending traverse, you pass above some campsites occupying a narrow bench overlooking the South Fork. Soon, encounter a lush hillside carpeted with willows, aspens, ❀ and wildflowers, including paintbrush, clover, coneflower, columbine, and heather, well watered by a series of rivulets. On the far side of the river is Pig Chute, where a seasonal stream pours down a narrow cleft of rock beside a knife-edged protrusion. Farther up the trail, a spectacular waterfall spilling dramatically into an emerald pool further enhances the beautiful scenery.

For the next 1.5 miles, proceed upstream with splendid views of the cascading river plunging down the narrow, deep, and rocky cleft of Goddard Canyon. Pass two more waterfalls as scenic as any in the High Sierra, and jump across a number of flower-lined side streams along the way.

Near the confluence of North Goddard Creek, the canyon widens temporarily, allowing the river to adopt a more leisurely pace. Stroll through meadowlands with fine views of the two canyons, separated by a low rock dome. A short, moderate climb leads to an obscure, unsigned junction (approximately 9,900 feet) with the barely distinct Hell-for-Sure Pass Trail, 5 miles from the JMT junction. There are a couple of passable campsites just up the trail a short way, near the crossing of a stream drain-

ing a small, unnamed tarn (approximately 11,390 feet) below Le Conte Divide.

Upper Goddard Canyon spreads out in subalpine splendor, as the trail ascends lush meadowlands, unbroken except for an occasional stunted pine or a small clump of willows. Patches of lupine and heather gracefully accent the deep green vegetation of the meadows, towered over by the mighty hulks of Mt. Goddard and Mt. Reinstein. The tread becomes indistinct in the upper canyon, but the route is clearly evident—follow the South Fork upstream to the headwaters beneath the Le Conte and Goddard Divides. Wildflowers, including daisy, shoot- ❀ ing star, and paintbrush, carpet the upper canyon. After crossing the outlet from Lake Confusion, begin a moderately steep, cross-country ascent over grassy benches and granite slabs to the lip of the basin, and then stroll easily to the west shore of Martha Lake, 23 miles from the trailhead.

Martha Lake is an austere, rockbound lake, where only a few small meadows soften the otherwise barren shoreline. Situated above timberline, near the convergence of three divides—Goddard, Le Conte, and White—the lake is truly alpine in nature. The dark, rugged flanks of 13,368-foot Mt. Goddard tower 2,500 feet over the lake to the northeast, while 12,604-foot Mt.

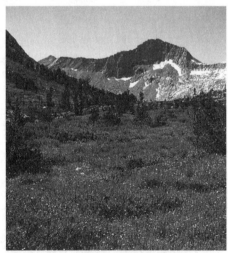

A tranquil meadow in Goddard Canyon

Reinstein provides a fine backdrop to the south. Developed campsites are virtually nonexistent, but resourceful backpackers should be able to locate suitable spots for pitching a tent. Anglers can ply the waters in search of rainbow and golden trout.

O Cross-country enthusiasts can use Martha Lake as the western gateway into one of the High Sierra's most spectacular trail-less areas, the mysterious realm of Ionian Basin. Traversing it is a classic High Sierra adventure. By connecting with the JMT near Lake Helen, you can follow a fine loop through Evolution Basin and Valley back to the Goddard Canyon Trail junction.

Southwest of Martha Lake, 11,760-foot Valor Pass offers a Class 2–3 route across Le Conte Divide to Blackcap Basin. Southeast of Martha Lake and 0.2 mile northeast of Mt. Reinstein, a Class 2 route over 11,880-foot Reinstein Pass leads to the Goddard Creek drainage.

Two moderately difficult cross-country routes cross Le Conte Divide from Goddard Canyon, approximately 1 mile below Martha Lake. The first, a Class 2 route, climbs tediously up talus to 11,370-foot Confusion Pass and Lake Confusion before dropping into Blackcap Basin. The second route, also Class 2, climbs west over talus-covered slopes to 11,635-foot Gunsight Pass, northwest of Lake Confusion, before descending the canyon of Bullet Lake into Bench Valley.

From Martha Lake, the southeast ridge of Mt. Goddard is Class 2–3. The northeast ridge of Mt. Reinstein is Class 3.

R A wilderness permit is required for overnight stays. Campfires are prohibited above 10,000 feet.

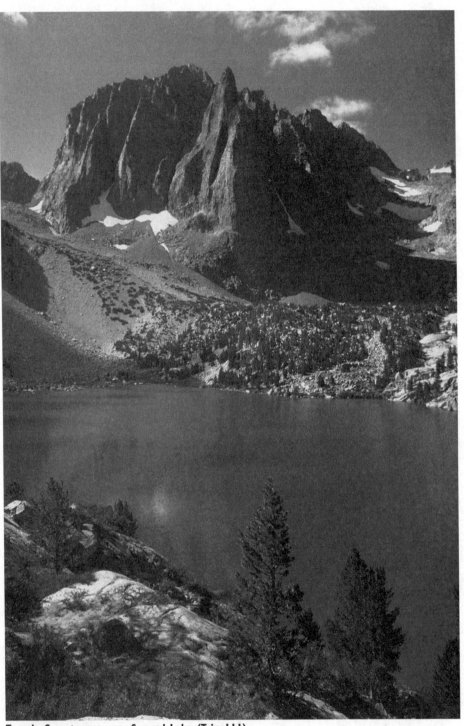

Temple Crag towers over Second Lake (Trip 111)

East Side Trips

In sharp contrast to the gradually rising terrain on the west side of the Sierra, the east side catapults from the floor of Owens Valley sharply upward to the crest of the range. This massive wall of mountains appears to be an impenetrable barrier to a wee, small individual peering upward thousands of feet from the western edge of the Great Basin to the Sierra spine. East side trails assume one of two approaches, either abandoning any possibility of crossing the range by following raucous streams to the heads of dead-end canyons or by steeply attacking the towering eastern escarpment on protracted climbs to a handful of high passes where the crest dips to around 11,000 or 12,000 feet. There is no easy approach to the backcountry on the east side; the principal reward of an eastern approach is the shorter distances required to access the alpine heights of the High Sierra.

The high and rugged terrain on the east boundary of Sequoia and Kings Canyon National Parks has limited the trailheads to ten (including Piute Pass to the north of Kings Canyon). Consequently, quotas for wilderness permits tend to fill up rapidly. Individuals or groups without reservations should plan to begin their trip on a weekday instead of on busy summer weekends.

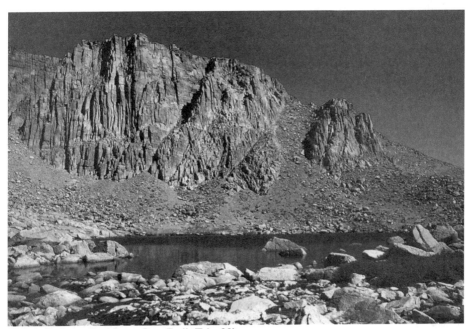

High Lake from New Army Pass Trail (Trip 90)

Introduction to the Mount Whitney Ranger District

The eastern escarpment of the Sierra spans the Mt. Whitney Ranger District, containing some of the area's most noteworthy topography. The majestic east face of the Mt. Whitney massif towers more than 10,000 feet above the community of Lone Pine. The Alabama Hills near the base have provided the scenery for numerous Hollywood movies. While this terrain is quite impressive when viewed from the windshield of a passing car or on the big screen, the area's real splendor is only available to those willing to venture into the backcountry on foot or horseback. Certainly the majority of trail users focus on the summit of Mt. Whitney, with hundreds of dayhikers and backpackers embarking each day on attempts of the Lower 48's highest peak. However, by concentrating on Whitney and ignoring the surrounding terrain, these travelers miss some of the most impressive scenery in the High Sierra.

The nearly impenetrable wall of the southern Sierra within the Whitney district remains untarnished by any road and is only successfully surmounted by five trails. These high peaks lure not only backpackers but also mountaineers, technical climbers, and cross-country enthusiasts from around the globe.

West of the Whitney spine, a horseshoe-shaped ring of peaks, incorporating the Sierra Crest, Kings-Kern Divide, Great Western Divide, and Kaweah Peaks Ridge, define some of the most remote and expansive backcountry in the range. A deep gorge cleaves the midsection of this arc, where the Kern River flows down a long, glacier-carved, Yosemite-like cleft before ultimately reaching the San Joaquin Valley. Between the top of Mt. Whitney and the bottom of Kern Trench, the terrain plunges 7,500 vertical feet in a mere 6 miles. This scenic backcountry is filled with craggy peaks, majestic canyons, wildflower-filled meadows, beautiful subalpine and alpine lakes, rushing streams, and gorgeous vistas.

ACCESS: The north-south thoroughfare of US 395 provides access for all eastside trips to secondary roads branching toward trailheads.

AMENITIES: The small towns of Lone Pine and Independence offer basic services to motorists on US 395, including motels, general stores, gas stations, and restaurants. Retailers sell a very limited selection of outdoor equipment, principally fishing and camping gear.

The Whitney Portal Store & Café has been serving outdoor recreationists for many years. The cafe serves burgers and hot cakes sure to satisfy the hungry hiker. Showers, souvenirs, and backcountry supplies are also available. They also run a hiker-friendly hostel in Lone Pine.

SHUTTLE SERVICE: A number of companies provide shuttle service to trailheads on the east side of the Sierra. Consult **www.climber. org** for a current list. *Note that Greyhound no longer services towns along US 395.*

OUTFITTERS: The following pack stations operate trips in this area:

> **Cottonwood Pack Station**
> c/o Dennis Y Tommi Winchester
> 910 Gibson Ranch Road
> Independence, CA 93526
> 760-878-2015

> **Rock Creek Pack Station**
> Craig London
> P.O. Box 248
> Bishop, CA 93515
> 760-935-4493

> **Sequoia Kings Pack Trains**
> P.O. Box 209
> Independence, CA 93526
> 800-962-0775

RANGER STATIONS: The Eastern Sierra Interagency Visitor Center is located 1 mile south of Lone Pine at the junction of US 395 and Highway 136 and is open daily from 8 a.m. to 4:30 p.m. Reserved and

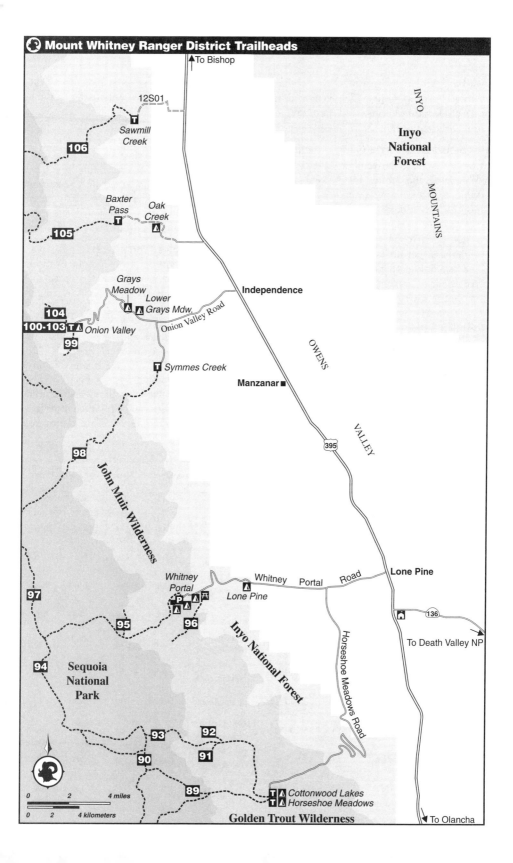

Mount Whitney Ranger District Trailheads

To Bishop

12S01

T Sawmill Creek

106

105

Baxter Pass **T**

Oak Creek **A**

Grays Meadow **A**

Lower Grays Mdw. **A**

104

100-103 **T** **A** Onion Valley

Onion Valley Road

99

T Symmes Creek

Independence

Manzanar ■

INYO

Inyo National Forest

MOUNTAINS

OWENS

VALLEY

395

98

John Muir Wilderness

97

Whitney Portal **A** Lone Pine

Whitney Portal Road

Lone Pine

P **A** **A** **A**

95

96

Inyo National Forest

136

A

To Death Valley NP

Horseshoe Meadows Road

94

Sequoia National Park

93

92

90

91

89

T **A** Cottonwood Lakes
T **A** Horseshoe Meadows

Golden Trout Wilderness

To Olancha

0   2   4 miles

0   2   4 kilometers

walk-in wilderness permits are available during business hours. The visitor center sells a selection of books and maps and also rents bear canisters.

WILDERNESS PERMITS: Quotas are in effect from May 1 to November 1. Except for Whitney Zone trails, 60 percent of the quota is available by reservation from six months to two days prior to the start of the trip ($5 per person). Inyo National Forest is scheduled to have an online system for wilderness permit applications by 2012. The remaining 40 percent is available for free walk-in permits, available one day before the start of the trip on a first-come, first-served basis. For more information call 760-873-2483.

WHITNEY ZONE DAY PERMITS: Dayhikers must secure a permit to enter the Whitney Zone. Reservations for day-use permits can be made through the Mt. Whitney Lottery at a cost of $15 per person. The entire quota can be reserved. Applications for reservations begin on February 1. The Inyo National Forest anticipates having an online reservation system up and running for 2012. Available dates not secured through the lottery can be reserved after late April and up to two days before departure. Unreserved spaces are available for free, on a first-come, first-served basis one day before departure. The Eastern Sierra Inter Agency Visitor Center south of Lone Pine issues all permits for the zone.

WHITNEY ZONE OVERNIGHT PERMITS: Backpackers planning to spend one or more nights must secure a permit to enter the Whitney Zone. Reservations for overnight permits can be made through the Mt. Whitney Lottery at a cost of $15 per person. The entire quota can be reserved. Applications for reservations begin on February 1. The Inyo National Forest anticipates having an online reservation system up and running for 2012. Available dates not secured through the lottery can be reserved after late April and up to two days before departure.

Campgrounds

Campground	Fee	Elevation	Season	Restrooms	Water	Bear Boxes	Phone
Cottonwood Lakes Trailhead (walk-in)	$6	9,900 feet	Late May to October	Vault	Yes	Yes	No
Horseshoe Meadows (walk-in)	$6	9,900 feet	Late May to October	Vault	Yes	Yes	No
Tuttle Creek (BLM)	Free	4,000 feet	March to November	Vault	No	No	No
Portagee Joe (Inyo County)	$10	8,200 feet	May to October	Vault	Yes	No	No
Lone Pine	$17	6,000 feet	Late April to mid-October	Vault	Yes	Yes	No
Whitney Portal	$17–$19	8,300 feet	Late May to mid-October	Flush	Yes	Yes	Yes
Mt. Whitney Trailhead (walk-in)	$10	8,300 feet	Late May to mid-October	Vault	Yes	Yes	Yes
Independence Creek (Inyo County)	$10	3,800 feet	Open all year	Flush	Yes	No	No
Lower Grays Meadow	$16	5,200 feet	Mid-March to mid-October	Flush	Yes	Yes	No
Upper Grays Meadow	$16	5,900 feet	Late May to November	Flush	Yes	Yes	No
Onion Valley	$16	9,200 feet	Early June to early October	Vault	Yes	Yes	No

Unreserved spaces are available free on a first-come, first-served basis one day before departure. The Eastern Sierra Inter Agency Visitor Center south of Lone Pine issues all permits for the zone.

Consult the Inyo National Forest website, **www.fs.usda.gov/inyo**, for current information on the Mt. Whitney Lottery, or call the Wilderness Permit Office at 760-873-2483.

GOOD TO KNOW BEFORE YOU GO: Both dayhikers and backpackers need a wilderness permit to enter the Mt. Whitney Zone, which includes both the Mt. Whitney and North Fork Lone Pine Creek Trails. Permits for this area are in extremely high demand.

The Onion Valley and Whitney Portal areas are notorious for bear activity, and space in the bear lockers near the trailhead is often at a premium. Backpackers must use bear canisters in the Cottonwood Lakes, Mt. Whitney, and Kearsarge Pass areas.

HORSESHOE MEADOW TRAILHEAD

TRIP 89

Chicken Spring Lake

Ⓜ ✗ **DH** or **BP**

DISTANCE: 8.2 miles, out-and-back

ELEVATION: 9,935'/11,245', +1,400'/-90'/±2,980'

SEASON: Mid-July to mid-October

USE: Moderate

MAPS: USGS's *Cirque Peak* or Tom Harrison Maps' *Golden Trout Wilderness Trail Map*

TRAIL LOG

3.4   Cottonwood Pass

4.1   Chicken Spring Lake

INTRODUCTION: Aside from the 0.75-mile climb to Cottonwood Pass, the grade to Chicken Spring Lake is mild, providing a relatively easy 4-plus-mile trip to a scenic destination. Solitude is usually in short supply at picturesque lakes along the Pacific Crest Trail (PCT), especially those so close to a trailhead, but Chicken Spring Lake offers more peace and quiet than the ever popular Cottonwood Lakes.

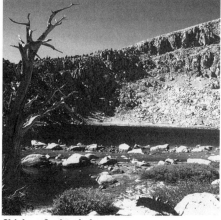

Chicken Spring Lake

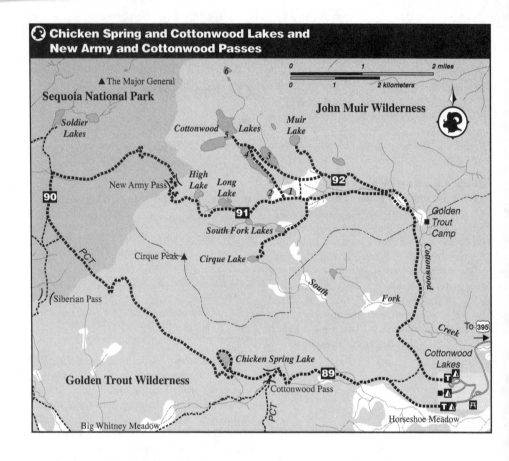

Chicken Spring and Cottonwood Lakes and New Army and Cottonwood Passes

DIRECTIONS TO TRAILHEAD: Turn west from US 395 in Lone Pine onto Whitney Portal Road, and proceed 3 miles to a left-hand turn onto Horseshoe Meadow Road. Continue south for 18.5 miles, past the turnoff for Cottonwood Lakes Trailhead, to the parking area. Nearby are bathrooms, running water, and a walk-in campground (which has a one-night limit).

DESCRIPTION: The well-signed trail begins at an interpretive display board near the restrooms. Follow gently graded, sandy tread across a slope dotted with lodgepole and foxtail pines and very little ground cover. Shortly, cross into Golden Trout Wilderness and reach a junction with trails heading south to Trail Pass and north to the pack station. Continue ahead (west) from the junction, skirting the north fringe of expansive Horseshoe Meadow. Although the grade is virtually level, hiking on the well-used, horse-trod soil is akin to trudging through beach sand.

Where the forest thickens, come alongside and then cross a stream, where a use trail leads to a dilapidated old cabin (where camping is prohibited). The trail soon crosses back over the stream, leaves the meadow behind, and begins a moderate ascent. Switchbacks lead up a rock-strewn hillside adjacent to a willow-lined drainage and ultimately to Cottonwood Pass (approximately 11,200 feet), 3.4 miles from the trailhead. You have excellent views of Horseshoe Meadow below, backdropped by the distant Panamint and Inyo Mountains to the east, as well as the southern extremity of the Great Western Divide to the west.

A short distance from the pass is a junction with the PCT and the trail to Big

Whitney Meadow. Following a sign marked ROCK CREEK, turn right and follow the PCT on an easy half-mile traverse to the seasonal outlet from Chicken Spring Lake. Turning away from the PCT, head upstream to the south shore.

Tucked into a cirque, Chicken Spring Lake is nearly surrounded by rugged granite cliffs. The shore is dotted with foxtail pines, with a number of weather-beaten old snags adding some character to the picture-postcard scene. There are several good campsites in patches of sand around a bay on the south side close to the outlet and amid scattered pines above the west shore. A use trail encircling the lake provides easy access for both anglers and swimmers.

From the lake, you can take side trips to Stokes Stringer Creek, Big Whitney Meadow, and Rocky Basin Lakes. A straightforward loop heads over Siberian Pass from the west side of Big Whitney Meadow to a connection with the PCT and then heads east back to Chicken Spring Lake.

A wilderness permit is required for overnight stays. Campfires are prohibited at Chicken Spring Lake.

HORSESHOE MEADOW TRAILHEAD

TRIP 90

Cottonwood Pass and New Army Pass Loop

M **Q** **BP**

DISTANCE: 19 miles, loop

ELEVATION: 9,935'/12,315'/9,935', +4,115'/-4,115'/±8,230'

SEASON: Mid-July to mid-October

USE: Moderate to heavy

MAPS: *Cirque Peak, Johnson Peak,* and *Mt. Whitney*

see map on p.310

TRAIL LOG

4.1	Chicken Spring Lake
9.0	Rock Creek Trail junction
11.5	New Army Pass
12.5	High Lake
15.8	Cottonwood Lakes Trail junction

INTRODUCTION: Strong backpackers may be able to complete this loop in a weekend, but the sublime High Sierra terrain invites those with more time to enjoy the vistas, lakes, canyons, and meadows along the southeastern fringe of Sequoia. Anglers should enjoy fishing for golden trout in many of the lakes and streams along the way.

DIRECTIONS TO TRAILHEAD: Turn west from US 395 in Lone Pine onto Whitney Portal Road, and proceed 3 miles to a left-hand turn onto Horseshoe Meadow Road. Continue south for 18.5 miles, past the turnoff for Cottonwood Pass Trailhead, to the parking area. Nearby are bathrooms, running water, and a walk-in campground (which has a one-night limit).

DESCRIPTION: The well-signed trail begins at an interpretive display board near the restrooms. Follow gently graded, sandy tread across a slope dotted with lodgepole and foxtail pines and very little ground cover. Shortly, cross into Golden Trout Wilderness, and reach a junction with trails heading south to Trail Pass and north to the pack station. Continue ahead (west) from the junction, skirting the north fringe of expansive Horseshoe Meadow. Although the grade is virtually level, hiking on the well-used, horse-trod soil is akin to trudging through beach sand.

Where the forest thickens, come alongside and then cross a stream, where a use trail leads to a dilapidated old cabin (where camping is prohibited). The trail soon crosses back over the stream, leaves the meadow behind, and begins a moderate ascent. Switchbacks lead up a rock-strewn hillside adjacent to a willow-lined drainage and ultimately to Cottonwood Pass (approximately 11,200 feet), 3.4 miles from the trailhead. You have excellent views of Horseshoe Meadow below, backdropped by the distant Panamint and Inyo Mountains to the east, as well as the southern extremity of the Great Western Divide to the west.

A short distance from the pass is a junction with the PCT and the trail to Big Whitney Meadow. Following a sign marked ROCK CREEK, turn right and follow the PCT on an easy half-mile traverse to the seasonal outlet from Chicken Spring Lake.

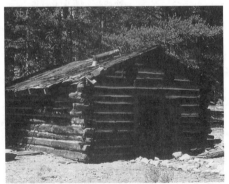

Historic cabin at Horseshoe Meadow, Cottonwood Lakes Trail

Turning away from the PCT, head upstream to the south shore.

Tucked into a cirque, Chicken Spring Lake is nearly surrounded by rugged granite cliffs. The shore is dotted with foxtail pines, with a number of weather-beaten old snags adding some character to the picture-postcard scene. There are several good campsites in patches of sand around a bay on the south side close to the outlet and amid scattered pines above the west shore. A use trail encircling the lake provides easy access for both anglers and swimmers.

From Chicken Spring Lake, retrace your steps to the PCT, and proceed northbound on a moderate ascent to the crest of a ridge above the west side of the lake, from where there are fine views of Big Whitney Meadow and the Great Western Divide. A mildly descending traverse on sandy tread amid scattered foxtail pines from the ridge skirts a verdant meadow with a seasonal tarn and then proceeds around the base of some cliffs. A short climb leads to a vista of Siberian Outpost, Mt. Kaweah, and the Great Western Divide, as well as some craggy peaks along the Sierra Crest above Rock Creek. A short distance farther, 7.5 miles from the trailhead, is the Sequoia National Park boundary. Traverse across a lightly forested hillside to a junction with the lightly used Siberian Pass Trail heading south and the PCT continuing west.

At the junction, turn right and head uphill toward Rock Creek. Proceed northwest, as the trail descends gently and then more steeply. Near the 9-mile mark, ford a meadow-lined tributary, and soon arrive at a junction with the New Army Pass Trail.

□ SIDE TRIP TO SOLDIER LAKES: Rather than immediately heading east toward the pass, continue northbound toward Soldier Lakes, passing a thin strip of meadow and a junction with a signed lateral to pine-shaded campsites (with a bear box) on a low rise above the lake's outlet. Boulder hop the outlet, and reach a junction with the trail to the lakes a short distance farther.

Turn right and follow the fringe of a thin band of flower-filled meadow through scattered pines to the south tip of Lower Soldier Lake, 0.75 mile from the New Army Pass Trail. A boot-beaten path continues along the west shore. To reach some pine-shaded campsites, cross the outlet just below the lake via some well-placed boulders, and continue on a faint path to the east shore. Dramatically framed by the towering walls of The Major General, Lower Soldier Lake reposes serenely in a scenic cirque. Anglers should enjoy fishing for golden trout.

A short, steep, cross-country jaunt from the north shore leads up the east side of the cirque to Upper Soldier Lake. **END OF SIDE TRIP**

From the Siberian Pass Trail and PCT junction, head east on the New Army Pass Trail on a moderate climb through scattered lodgepole pines, along the edge of a verdant, flower-bedecked meadow. Farther upstream, the trees thin on the way to an open, boulder-studded basin rimmed by rocky cliffs and ridges. A steady, lengthy climb leads to New Army Pass (approximately 12,315 feet), 11.5 miles from the trailhead, which is not at the low point (Army Pass) but is 0.4 mile south and 700 feet higher. The new trail was built to avoid the old pass, which typically harbored a large snowfield well into summer and was prone to rockfall. Fine views of Cottonwood Lakes and the Cottonwood Creek drainage invite you to linger at the pass while catching your breath.

From the pass, descend rocky switchbacks to High Lake, proceed down more rocky switchbacks past timberline, and continue through widely scattered dwarf pines, low-growing alpine plants, and grasses and sedges to Long Lake (approximately 11,135 feet). The best campsites are beneath a stand of pines along the southeast shore, with some less protected sites above the north shore.

A moderate descent from Long Lake brings you to a lateral to additional campsites, followed by a stretch of trail cutting across a sea of rock. Beyond this desolate area the trail passes across meadowlands below Cottonwood Lakes 2 and 1 on the way to a Y-junction. Continue ahead a short distance to another Y-junction, this one with the South Fork Lakes Trail on the right.

From the junction, follow Cottonwood Creek downstream for a mile to where the trail crosses the creek and reaches a junction with the Cottonwood Lakes Trail angling in from the left. Proceed downstream, soon crossing a side stream and then following the main creek as it curves south. After crossing Cottonwood Creek on a beveled log, cross the boundary between the John Muir and Golden Trout Wildernesses. Then pass below some steep cliffs on the right and the wood buildings of Golden Trout Camp across a meadow to the left. As the canyon widens, the grade eases to a gentle descent, which eventually leads to a crossing of South Fork Cottonwood Creek.

Gently graded trail continues to a junction with a lateral to the pack station just prior to the wilderness boundary. Turn left and follow this lateral through the pack station, and continue south toward a junction with the New Army Pass Trail. From there, head east a short distance to the Horseshoe Meadow Trailhead.

O Off-trail enthusiasts will find plenty of stunningly scenic terrain by following Rock Creek to Miter Basin (see options in Trip 93, page 318).

Mountaineers may enjoy a straightforward Class 1 ascent of Cirque Peak from New Army Pass.

R A wilderness permit is required for overnight stays. Campfires are prohibited at Chicken Spring Lake. Bear canisters are required in Cottonwood Lakes Basin.

COTTONWOOD LAKES TRAILHEAD

TRIP 91

New Army Pass Trail

E ✗ **DH or BP**

DISTANCE: 13 miles, out-and-back

ELEVATION: 10,040'/11,483',
+1,650'/-215'/±3,730'

SEASON: Mid-July to early October

USE: Moderate to heavy

MAP: *Cirque Peak*

see map on p.310

TRAIL LOG

3.25 New Army Pass Trail junction
4.3 South Fork Lakes junction
5.75 Long Lake
6.5 High Lake

INTRODUCTION: Weekend backpackers enjoy a reasonably easy trip to a handful of scenic lakes along the New Army Pass and South Fork Trails. Open, rock-strewn basins and sprawling, grassy meadows allow fine views of the rugged Sierra Crest. Although the general area is quite popular, Cirque Lake and South Fork Lakes receive relatively light use. If you have more time, the neighboring Cottonwood Lakes present a fine trip addition.

DIRECTIONS TO TRAILHEAD: Turn west from US 395 in Lone Pine onto Whitney Portal Road, and proceed 3 miles to a left-hand turn onto Horseshoe Meadow Road. Continue south for 18 miles to a junction, and turn right, following a sign for NEW ARMY PASS, COTTONWOOD LAKES. Pass the Cottonwood Lakes Walk-In Campground, and continue to the parking area, 0.5 mile from Horseshoe Meadow Road.

DESCRIPTION: The trail begins auspiciously as a brick-lined path near a restroom and trailhead signboard. From there, follow gently graded, sandy tread slightly uphill through widely scattered foxtail and lodgepole pines, where virtually no ground cover has taken root in the sandy soil. Soon you cross the Golden Trout Wilderness boundary and pass a spur on the left to the Cottonwood Lakes Pack Station. On an equally gentle descent, reach South Fork Cottonwood Creek, 1 mile from the trailhead, where a couple of campsites appear on the far bank. The vegetation lining the creek seems quite vibrant after the previous lack of ground cover.

From the crossing, climb gently through scattered pines, soon meeting the main branch of Cottonwood Creek to head upstream through a broad valley for the next 1.5 miles. Simultaneously leaving the Golden Trout Wilderness and entering the John Muir Wilderness, you pass beneath steep cliffs on the left and pass the wood structures of Golden Trout Camp across a meadow to the right. Where the trail bends west, the canyon narrows and the grade increases on the way to a crossing of the creek on a beveled log, 2.5 miles from the trailhead. A pair of campsites near the crossing may tempt backpackers who got a late start.

Continue climbing through light forest past meadows lining the creek. Just after crossing a side stream, reach a Y-junction between the Cottonwood Lakes Trail on the right and the New Army Trail on the left, 3.25 miles from the trailhead.

From the junction, veer left and soon cross Cottonwood Creek. Climb moderately along the creek for a little more than a mile to the junction of the South Fork Lakes Trail beside a large meadow, 4.3 miles from the trailhead.

SIDE TRIP TO SOUTH FORK AND CIRQUE LAKES: From the South Fork Lakes and New Army Pass junction, head south along the edge of a sloping meadow lined with willows. Soon the trail bends southwest and climbs gently through scattered foxtail pines, followed by a brief descent to a crossing of South Fork Cottonwood Creek. The trail then cuts across a large meadow on the way to the easternmost South Fork Lake (approximately 11,200 feet). The roughly oval-shaped lake has a splendid backdrop of rocky ridges and craggy peaks. A few 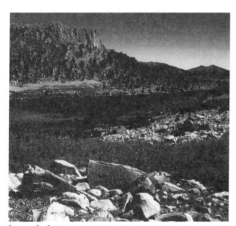 campsites on a hill above the south shore may lure overnighters.

Cirque Lake is reached by following a moderate climb through scattered foxtail pines to the top of a ridge and then dropping down shortly to the northeast shore, 1.3 miles from the junction. Cradled in a bowl at the base of steep cliffs forming the west flank of Cirque Peak, the lake feels decidedly alpine. A few campsites scattered around the sparsely forested shore seem adequate for the few adventurous souls who make the trip. **END OF SIDE TRIP**

From the junction of the South Fork Lakes and New Army Pass Trails, continue westbound, climbing a low hillside to another Y-junction, this one with a lateral to Cottonwood Lakes. Keep heading west, skirting the edge of an expansive meadow encircling Cottonwood Lake 1. Near the far end of the meadow, you pass Lake 2 before leaving the verdant grassland behind. A short climb leads to a desolate area covered with large boulders, where a few pockets of pines are the only vegetation capable of gaining a foothold in this sea of rock.

Eventually, you leave the desolate area behind, as gently graded tread arcs across a lightly forested hillside. Below, a meadow-lined stream rushes toward the westernmost South Fork Lake. A faint path heads across the stream to forested campsites between the lake and Long Lake above. A moderate climb through thinning forest leads to the south shore of Long Lake (approximately 11,135 feet), 5.75 miles from the trailhead. The best campsites are beneath a stand of pines near the southeast shore, with less protected sites above the north shore.

From the east side of Long Lake, the trail climbs more steeply on an ascending traverse toward High Lake. Through grasses, low-growing alpine vegetation, and widely scattered dwarf pines, you ascend past timberline and then wind up rocky switchbacks to High Lake (approximately 11,510 feet), 6.5 miles from the trailhead. The lake reposes in a rocky, open bowl rimmed by steep cliffs. Campsites around the exposed lakeshore are extremely limited. Following the trail toward New Army Pass offers wide-ranging views.

Thanks to a network of trails and open terrain easily navigable with a modicum of cross-country skill, a number of side trips are possible to the nearby Cottonwood Lakes (see Trip 92, page 316).

Hopeful mountaineers can follow the strenuous but straightforward route from New Army Pass to the summit of Mt. Langley, the southernmost 14,000-high peak in the range. Cirque Peak is also a nontechnical climb from either the pass or from Cirque Lake.

A wilderness permit is required for overnight stays. Campfires are prohibited. Bear canisters are required in Cottonwood Lakes Basin.

SPECIAL FISHING REGULATIONS: Catch-and-release fishing is allowed at Cottonwood Lakes 1, 2, 3, and 4 and their tributaries. All other lakes in the basin are restricted to artificial lures or flies with barbless hooks; the daily limit is five fish. Fishing season runs from July 1 to October 1.

Long Lake

COTTONWOOD LAKES TRAILHEAD

TRIP 92

Cottonwood Lakes

E ↗ **DH** or **BP**

DISTANCE: 11.8 miles, out-and-back

ELEVATION: 10,040'/11,160', +1,450'/-295'/±3,490'

SEASON: Mid-July to early October

USE: Moderate to heavy

MAPS: *Cirque Peak* and *Mt. Langley*

see map on p.310

TRAIL LOG

3.25　New Army Pass Trail junction
4.5　　Muir Lake junction
5.25　Lake 3
5.5　　Lake 4
5.75　Lake 5

INTRODUCTION: Most of the journey to Cottonwood Lakes is on gently graded tread, with only 1.75 miles of moderate climbing. The relatively easy route's outstanding scenery and notable golden trout fishery make it a popular destination for recreationists. Solitude seekers should not despair though; the high number of lakes tends to effectively disperse visitors around the basin. An expansive network of trails and cross-country routes provides straightforward travel between the lakes.

DIRECTIONS TO TRAILHEAD: Turn west from US 395 in Lone Pine onto Whitney Portal Road, and proceed 3 miles to a left-hand turn onto Horseshoe Meadow Road. Continue south for 18 miles to a junction, and turn right, following a sign for NEW ARMY PASS, COTTONWOOD LAKES. Pass the Cottonwood Lakes Walk-In Campground, and continue to the parking area, 0.5 mile from Horseshoe Meadow Road.

DESCRIPTION: The trail begins auspiciously as a brick-lined path near a restroom and trailhead signboard. From there, follow gently graded, sandy tread slightly uphill through widely scattered foxtail and lodgepole pines, where virtually no ground cover has taken root in the sandy soil. Soon you cross the Golden Trout Wilderness boundary and pass a spur on the left to the Cottonwood Lakes Pack Station. On an equally gentle descent, reach South Fork Cottonwood Creek, 1 mile from the trailhead, where a couple of campsites appear on the far bank. The vegetation lining the creek seems quite vibrant after the previous lack of ground cover.

From the crossing, climb gently through scattered pines, soon meeting the main branch of Cottonwood Creek and following it up a broad valley for the next 1.5 miles. Simultaneously leaving the Golden Trout Wilderness and entering the John Muir Wilderness, you pass beneath steep cliffs on the left and pass the wood structures of Golden Trout Camp across a meadow to the right. Where the trail bends west, the canyon narrows and the grade increases on the way to a crossing of the creek on a beveled log, 2.5 miles from the trailhead. A pair of campsites near the crossing may tempt backpackers who got a late start.

Continue climbing through light forest past meadows lining the creek. Just after crossing a side stream, reach a Y-junction between the Cottonwood Lakes Trail on the right and the New Army Trail on the left, 3.25 miles from the trailhead.

From the junction, veer right and proceed on a moderate climb through lodgepole and foxtail pine forest. The ascent leads well above the creek to a set of switchbacks. Along the way are periodic views through gaps in the trees of Cirque Peak and the Sierra Crest. Near the east edge of a large meadow at the lip of Cottonwood Lakes Basin, you reach a junction with the Muir Lake Trail, 4.5 miles from the trailhead.

SIDE TRIP TO MUIR LAKE: Initially, the correct route to Muir Lake is a bit difficult to determine. The faint path skirts the northeast edge of a meadow before bending north toward the lake. Complicating matters, a boot-beaten path heads northeast up a low hillside to the right, which is the beginning of a cross-country route to Hidden Lake. After following the correct path around the meadow, ascend north through pines and scattered boulders. Hop over a flower-lined rivulet, and proceed to the south shore of Muir Lake.

While the trail may be hard to follow in places, the location of the lake is hard to miss—tucked into a horseshoe basin at the base of an unnamed peak. Muir Lake (approximately 11,010 feet) is quite scenic, with rugged cliffs encircling the lakeshore and Mt. Langley rising to the northwest. Judging by the trail's condition, the lake receives light use, in spite of its pleasant surroundings and the several fine campsites nestled beneath scattered pines. **END OF SIDE TRIP**

From the Muir Lake junction, continue west on level trail across a meadow, well north of Cottonwood Lake 1. The path soon bends northwest up a low, forested rise (which has campsites), crosses a stream, and then passes through grassy meadows dotted with boulders, clumps of willow, and widely scattered pines. The massive east Sierra wall dominates the surroundings, as you pass

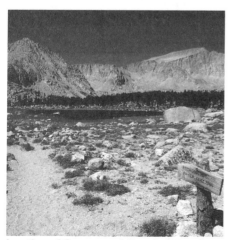

Junction of Cottonwood Pass and New Army Pass Trails

a corrugated metal shed on the left and a small tarn to the right on the way to willow-rimmed Lake 3 (approximately 11,075 feet), 5.25 miles from the trailhead. There are additional campsites on the forested rise between Lake 3 and Lake 4.

At the far end of Lake 3, briefly skirt a meadow and then wind around on an easy course through mostly open terrain to the northeast shore of Lake 4 (approximately 11,110 feet), a quarter mile from Lake 3. At an indistinct junction, a faint path follows the east shore for a mile to a junction with the New Army Pass Trail near Lake 1.

To reach Lake 5 you must travel another quarter mile, first around the north shore of Lake 4 and then up a steep hillside to the south shore. A short stretch of the creek flows between two large lakes in the basin, both designated as Lake 5. Nestled in a rocky basin just below the crest, these two lakes are rimmed by cliffs and talus. Meadows surround the lakeshore, with clumps of willow here and there, but very few trees have taken hold. There are a few campsites around the lake, but better, more protected sites pepper the low rise between Lakes 3 and 4. While there are golden trout in all of the Cottonwood Lakes, Lake 5 is the only one that is not catch and release.

A good network of trails connects just about every lake in the basin, and short cross-country routes easily access the rest. A straightforward, 1-mile cross-country route along the creek flowing into Lake 5 provides a route to diminutive Lake 6.

A wilderness permit is required for overnight stays. Campfires are prohibited. Bear canisters are required in Cottonwood Lakes Basin.

SPECIAL FISHING REGULATIONS: Catch-and-release fishing is permitted at Cottonwood Lakes 1, 2, 3, and 4 and their tributaries. All other lakes in the basin are restricted to artificial lures or flies with barbless hooks; the daily limit is five fish. Fishing season runs from July 1 to October 1.

TRIP 93

Soldier Lakes and Rock Creek

Ⓜ ↗ BP

DISTANCE: 29.2 miles, out-and-back

ELEVATION: 10,040'/12,315',
+2,555'/-445'/±6,000'

SEASON: Mid-July to mid-October

USE: Moderate

MAPS: *Cirque Peak, Johnson Peak,* and *Mount Whitney*

TRAIL LOG

6.5	High Lake
7.5	New Army Pass
10.5	Soldier Lake junction
14.6	Rock Creek crossing

INTRODUCTION: Easy access and stunning scenery in Cottonwood Lakes Basin make the area one of the more popular weekend destinations on the east side of the southern Sierra. However, most weekenders don't possess the extra time or energy to continue over the divide at New Army Pass and down to the exquisite backcountry in the Rock Creek drainage. The Rock Creek Trail leads to wildflower-laden meadows, quiet forests, and lovely subalpine lakes. This trip also provides the option of an off-trail journey into Miter Basin, one of the most dramatic alpine basins in the High Sierra, where a bevy of pristine lakes reflect towering peaks.

DIRECTIONS TO TRAILHEAD: Turn west from US 395 in Lone Pine onto Whitney Portal Road, and proceed 3 miles to a left-hand turn onto Horseshoe Meadow Road. Continue south for 18 miles to a junction, and turn right, following a sign for NEW ARMY PASS, COTTONWOOD LAKES. Pass the Cottonwood Lakes Walk-In Camp-

ground, and continue to the parking area, 0.5 mile from Horseshoe Meadow Road.

DESCRIPTION: The trail begins auspiciously as a brick-lined path near a restroom and trailhead signboard. From there, follow gently graded, sandy tread slightly uphill through widely scattered foxtail and lodgepole pines, where virtually no ground cover has taken root in the sandy soil. Soon you cross the Golden Trout Wilderness boundary and pass a spur on the left to the Cottonwood Lakes Pack Station. On an equally gentle descent, reach South Fork Cottonwood Creek, 1 mile from the trailhead, where a couple of campsites appear on the far bank. The vegetation lining the creek seems quite vibrant after the previous lack of ground cover.

From the crossing, climb gently through scattered pines, soon meeting the main branch of Cottonwood Creek and following it up a broad valley for the next 1.5 miles. Simultaneously leaving the Golden Trout Wilderness and entering the John Muir Wilderness, you pass beneath steep cliffs on the left and pass the wood structures of Golden Trout Camp across a meadow to the right. Where the trail bends west, the canyon narrows and the grade increases on the way to a crossing of the creek on a beveled log, 2.5 miles from the trailhead. A pair of campsites near the crossing may tempt backpackers who got a late start.

Continue climbing through light forest past meadows lining the creek. Just after crossing a side stream, reach a Y-junction between the Cottonwood Lakes Trail on the right and the New Army Trail on the left, 3.25 miles from the trailhead.

From the junction, veer left and soon cross Cottonwood Creek. Climb moderately along the creek for a little more than a mile to the junction of the South Fork Lakes Trail beside a large meadow, 4.3 miles from the trailhead.

From the junction of the South Fork Lakes and New Army Pass Trails, continue westbound, climbing a low hillside to another Y-junction with a lateral to Cottonwood Lakes. Keep heading west,

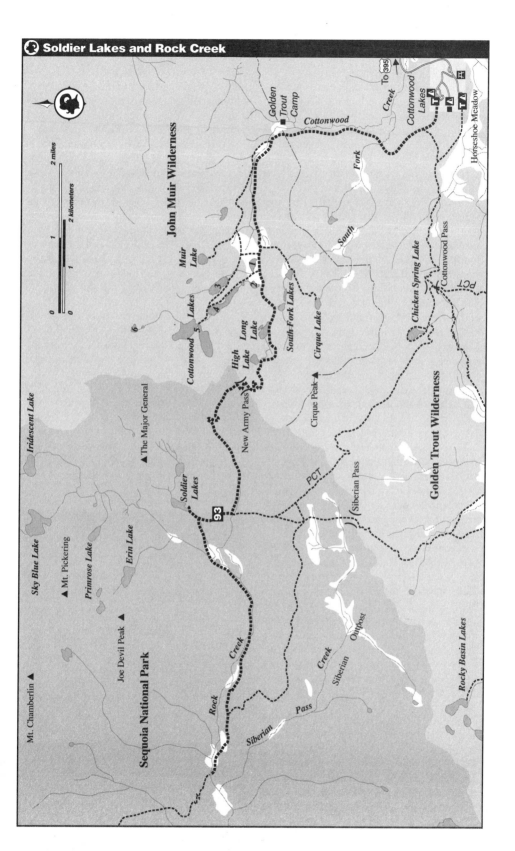

skirting the edge of an expansive meadow encircling Cottonwood Lake 1. Near the far end of the meadow, you pass Lake 2 before leaving the verdant grassland behind. A short climb leads to a desolate area covered with large boulders, where a few pockets of pines are the only vegetation capable of gaining a foothold in this sea of rock.

Eventually, you leave the desolate area behind, as gently graded tread arcs across a lightly forested hillside. Below, a meadow-lined stream rushes toward the westernmost South Fork Lake. A faint path heads across the stream to forested campsites between the lake and Long Lake above. A moderate climb through thinning forest leads to the south shore of Long Lake (approximately 11,135 feet), 5.75 miles from the trailhead. The best campsites are beneath a stand of pines near the southeast shore, with less protected sites above the north shore.

From the east side of Long Lake, the trail climbs more steeply on an ascending traverse toward High Lake. Through grasses, low-growing alpine vegetation, and widely scattered, dwarf pines, you ascend past timberline and then wind up rocky switchbacks to High Lake (approximately 11,510 feet), 6.5 miles from the trailhead. The lake reposes in a rocky, open bowl rimmed by steep cliffs. Campsites around the exposed lakeshore are extremely limited.

From High Lake, ascend a mile of rocky switchbacks to New Army Pass (approximately 12,315 feet), 7.5 miles from the trailhead, which is not at the low point (Army Pass) but is 0.4 mile south and 700 feet higher. The new trail was built to avoid the old pass, which typically harbored a large snowfield well into summer and was prone to rockfall. Fine views of Cottonwood Lakes and the Cottonwood Creek drainage invite you to linger at the pass while catching your breath.

A moderate descent across barren slopes leads to more hospitable terrain, eventually meeting and following a tributary of Rock Creek. Continue downstream through boulder-sprinkled meadows rimmed by rocky cliffs and ridges to where stunted pines reappear. Soon you're skirting flower-filled

meadows through a scattered to light forest of lodgepole and foxtail pines on the way to a junction with a lateral to the Pacific Crest Trail (PCT), 9.9 miles from the trailhead.

Veer right at the junction, and travel past a thin strip of meadow to a signed lateral leading to pine-shaded campsites (with a bear box) on a low rise above the outlet from Soldier Lakes. A short distance farther boulder hop the outlet, and reach a junction with a spur to the lakes at 10.5 miles.

Veer right (northeast), and follow the spur along the edge of a narrow, flower-filled meadow through scattered pines to the south tip of Lower Soldier Lake (approximately 10,805 feet). A boot-beaten path continues along the west side of the lake, but to reach the pine-shaded campsites you'll have to cross the outlet just below the lake via some well-placed boulders and logs to a faint path along the east shore.

Dramatically framed by the towering walls of The Major General, Lower Soldier Lake reposes serenely in a scenic cirque, where anglers should enjoy fishing for golden trout. A short, steep, cross-country jaunt from the north shore leads up the east side of the cirque to Upper Soldier Lake.

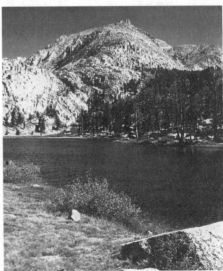

Soldier Lake and The Major General from the Pacific Crest Trail

After a stay at Soldier Lakes, retrace your steps to the junction with the Rock Creek Trail, and then continue downstream alongside the tumbling creek through a thickening forest of lodgepole pines. A short, steep descent down a narrow gully alongside a riotous section of the creek heads past a campsite just before the edge of a broad meadow. An obscure use trail begins near this campsite and leads along the east side of Rock Creek toward Miter Basin. The path is fairly well defined to where the creek exits the lower basin but evaporates into a bona fide cross-country route above (see options below).

Gently graded tread leads around the fringe of the meadow to ford the branch of Rock Creek draining Sky Blue Lake. Pass a large pond, beyond which are more campsites (with a bear box) in a grove of pines. Head back into the trees at the far edge of the meadow, and pass through a drift fence, as the moderate descent resumes and the trail veers away from the creek for a while. Return to the creek, which dances over slabs and cascades over boulders between meadow- and willow-lined banks. At 2 miles from Lower Soldier Lake, the trail crosses Rock Creek on a pair of logs and continues downstream for a half mile to another picturesque meadow, with a number of lodgepole-shaded campsites along the fringe. Beyond the meadow, a short, forested descent leads to a junction of the PCT, 3.25 miles from Lower Soldier Lake.

From the junction, a winding, moderate descent along the PCT heads through alternating sections of forest and flower- and fern-filled meadows, where the summit of massive Mt. Guyot looms to the west. As the descent continues, pass a signed spur leading to the Rock Creek Ranger Station, and then stroll by some shady campsites.

After yet another verdant meadow, additional campsites (with a bear box) line the trail on the way to the Rock Creek crossing, 4.1 miles from Lower Soldier Lake.

By using a section of the PCT, backpackers can create a loop over Cottonwood Pass and back to the Cottonwood Lakes Trailhead (see Trip 91, page 314), as well as a number of fine dayhikes.

The cross-country route to Miter Basin is a classic High Sierra adventure. From Lower Soldier Lake, a faint use trail steeply ascends the westernmost inlet to open slopes below The Major General. From there, follow the west bank of upper Rock Creek into the stunning amphitheater of Miter Basin, where iridescent lakes and a semicircle of craggy peaks create alpine scenery as dramatic as any in the range. A moderate, off-trail route continues past the east and north shores of Sky Blue Lake along the inlet to the west side of the unnamed lake (3697) above and then climbs north to Crabtree Pass (Class 2 and approximately 12,560 feet).

From the pass, descend steep talus, or traverse north toward Whitney Pass to avoid the talus, and drop to the north shore of the tarn below (approximately 12,100 feet). At the tarn, a use trail leads down the canyon to Crabtree Lakes, where maintained trail continues to a junction with the PCT near Crabtree Meadow. To return to the trailhead, head southbound on the PCT to the Rock Creek crossing and cross New Army Pass, or continue southbound on the PCT to Cottonwood Pass.

A wilderness permit is required for overnight stays. Campfires are prohibited. Bear canisters are required in Cottonwood Lakes Basin.

COTTONWOOD LAKES TRAILHEAD

TRIP 94

Cottonwood Lakes to Whitney Portal

MS / BP

DISTANCE: 35 miles, point-to-point

ELEVATION: 10,040'/12,315'/9,595'/
13,580'/8,360',
+8,070'/-9,805'/±17,875'

SEASON: Mid-July to mid-October

USE: Moderate

MAPS: USGS's *Cirque Peak, Johnson Peak, Mount Whitney,* and *Mt. Langley* or Tom Harrison Maps' *Mt. Whitney High Country Trail Map*

TRAIL LOG

6.5	High Lake
7.5	New Army Pass
10.5	Soldier Lake junction
14.6	Rock Creek crossing
20.25	Lower Crabtree Meadow
21.5	John Muir Trail junction
25.75	Mt. Whitney Trail junction

INTRODUCTION: A multitude of peak baggers set their sights on the summit of Mt. Whitney each season, which places a high demand on the limited number of wilderness permits available for both dayhikers and backpackers wishing to depart from Whitney Portal. For groups with extra days and the capacity to arrange for the 29-mile shuttle between trailheads, the longer approach to the peak from Cottonwood Lakes Trailhead passes through some sublime mountain scenery. Beautiful lakes, stunning vistas, tumbling creeks, flower-filled meadows, and serene forests are all here in abundance. Although the Whitney and Cottonwood Lakes areas are typically crammed with people, solitude seekers should find doses of peace and quiet along

the lightly used Rock Creek Trail and a somewhat neglected stretch of the Pacific Crest Trail (PCT).

DIRECTIONS TO TRAILHEAD:
START: Turn west from US 395 in Lone Pine onto Whitney Portal Road, and proceed 3 miles to a left-hand turn onto Horseshoe Meadow Road. Continue south for 18 miles to a junction, and turn right, following a sign for NEW ARMY PASS, COTTONWOOD LAKES. Pass the Cottonwood Lakes Walk-In Campground, and continue to the parking area, 0.5 mile from Horseshoe Meadow Road.

END: Turn west from US 395 in Lone Pine onto Whitney Portal Road, and proceed 13 miles to the overnight parking lot at Whitney Portal. Campgrounds, restrooms, and a small store with a cafe are nearby.

DESCRIPTION: The trail begins auspiciously as a brick-lined path near a restroom and trailhead signboard. From there, follow gently graded, sandy tread slightly uphill through widely scattered foxtail and lodgepole pines, where virtually no ground cover has taken root in the sandy soil. Soon you cross the Golden Trout Wilderness boundary, and pass a spur on the left to the Cottonwood Lakes Pack Station. On an equally gentle descent, reach South Fork Cottonwood Creek, 1 mile from the trailhead, where a couple of campsites appear on the far bank. The vegetation lining the creek seems quite vibrant after the previous lack of ground cover.

From the crossing, climb gently through scattered pines, soon meeting the main branch of Cottonwood Creek and following it up a broad valley for the next 1.5 miles. Simultaneously leaving the Golden Trout Wilderness and entering the John Muir Wilderness, you pass beneath steep cliffs on the left and pass the wood structures of Golden Trout Camp across a meadow to the right. Where the trail bends west, the canyon narrows and the grade increases on the way to a crossing of the creek on a beveled log, 2.5 miles from the trailhead. A pair

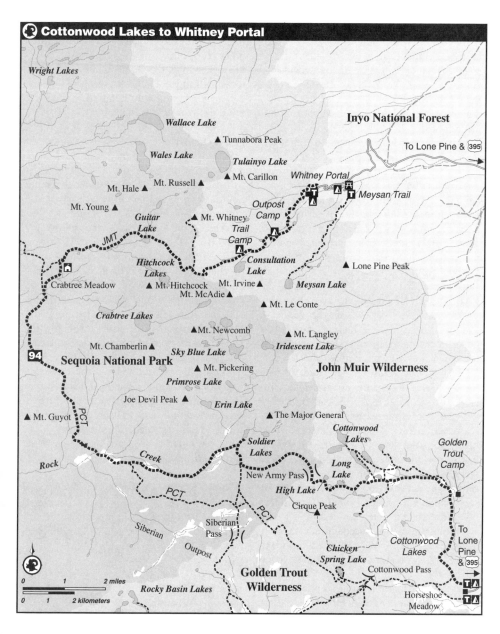

Cottonwood Lakes to Whitney Portal

of campsites near the crossing may tempt backpackers who got a late start.

Continue climbing through light forest past meadows lining the creek. Just after crossing a side stream, reach a Y-junction between the Cottonwood Lakes Trail on the right and the New Army Trail on the left, 3.25 miles from the trailhead.

From the junction, veer left and soon cross Cottonwood Creek. Climb moderately along the creek for a little more than a mile to the junction of the South Fork Lakes Trail beside a large meadow, 4.3 miles from the trailhead.

From the junction of the South Fork Lakes and New Army Pass Trails, continue westbound, climbing a low hillside to another Y-junction with a lateral to Cottonwood Lakes. Keep heading west, skirting the edge of an expansive meadow encircling Cottonwood Lake 1. Near the far end of the meadow, you pass Lake 2 before leaving the verdant grassland behind. A short climb leads to a desolate area covered with large boulders, where a few pockets of pines are the only vegetation capable of gaining a foothold in this sea of rock.

Eventually, you leave the desolate area behind, as gently graded tread arcs across a lightly forested hillside. Below, a meadow-lined stream rushes toward the westernmost South Fork Lake. A faint path heads across the stream to forested campsites between the lake and Long Lake above. A moderate climb through thinning forest leads to the south shore of Long Lake (approximately 11,135 feet), 5.75 miles from the trailhead. The best campsites are beneath a stand of pines near the southeast shore, with less protected sites above the north shore.

From the east side of Long Lake, the trail climbs more steeply on an ascending traverse toward High Lake. Through grasses, low-growing alpine vegetation, and widely scattered, dwarf pines, you ascend past timberline and then wind up rocky switchbacks to High Lake (approximately 11,510 feet), 6.5 miles from the trailhead. The lake reposes in a rocky, open bowl rimmed by steep cliffs. Campsites around the exposed lakeshore are extremely limited.

From High Lake, ascend a mile of rocky switchbacks to New Army Pass (approximately 12,315 feet), 7.5 miles from the trailhead, which is not at the low point (Army Pass) but is 0.4 mile south and 700 feet higher. The new trail was built to avoid the old pass, which typically harbored a large snowfield well into summer and was prone to rockfall. Fine views of Cottonwood Lakes and the Cottonwood Creek drainage invite you to linger at the pass while catching your breath.

A moderate descent across barren slopes leads to more hospitable terrain, eventually meeting and following a tributary of Rock Creek. Continue downstream through

boulder-sprinkled meadows rimmed by rocky cliffs and ridges to where stunted pines reappear. Soon you're skirting flower-filled meadows through a scattered to light forest of lodgepole and foxtail pines on the way to a junction with a lateral to the PCT, 9.9 miles from the trailhead.

Veer right at the junction, and travel past a thin strip of meadow to a signed lateral leading to pine-shaded campsites (with a bear box) on a low rise above the outlet from Soldier Lakes. A short distance farther boulder hop the outlet, and reach a junction with a spur to the lakes at 10.5 miles.

Veer right (northeast), and follow the spur along the edge of a narrow, flower-filled meadow through scattered pines to the south tip of Lower Soldier Lake (approximately 10,805 feet). A boot-beaten path continues along the west side of the lake, but to reach the pine-shaded campsites you'll have to cross the outlet just below the lake via some well-placed boulders and logs to a faint path along the east shore.

Dramatically framed by the towering walls of The Major General, Lower Soldier Lake reposes serenely in a scenic cirque. Anglers should enjoy fishing for golden trout. A short, steep, cross-country jaunt from the north shore leads up the east side of the cirque to Upper Soldier Lake.

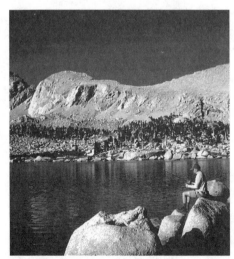

Angler in Cottonwood Lakes Basin

After a stay at Soldier Lakes, retrace your steps to the junction with the Rock Creek Trail and then continue downstream alongside the tumbling creek through a thickening forest of lodgepole pines. A short, steep descent down a narrow gully alongside a riotous section of the creek heads past a campsite just before the edge of a broad meadow. An obscure use trail begins near this campsite and leads along the east side of Rock Creek toward Miter Basin. The path is fairly well defined to where the creek exits the lower basin but evaporates into a bona fide cross-country route above (see options, page 326).

Gently graded tread leads around the fringe of the meadow to ford the branch of Rock Creek draining Sky Blue Lake. Pass a large pond, beyond which are more campsites (with a bear box) in a grove of pines. Head back into the trees at the far edge of the meadow, and pass through a drift fence, as the moderate descent resumes and the trail veers away from the creek for a while. Return to the creek, which dances over slabs and cascades over boulders between meadow- and willow-lined banks. At 2 miles from Lower Soldier Lake, the trail crosses Rock Creek on a pair of logs and continues downstream for a half mile to another picturesque meadow, with a number of lodgepole-shaded campsites along the fringe. Beyond the meadow, a short, forested descent leads to a junction of the PCT, 3.25 miles from Lower Soldier Lake.

From the junction, a winding, moderate descent along the PCT heads through alternating sections of forest and flower- and fern-filled meadows, where the summit of massive Mt. Guyot looms to the west. As the descent continues, pass a signed spur leading to the Rock Creek Ranger Station, and then stroll by some shady campsites. After yet another verdant meadow, additional campsites (with a bear box) line the trail on the way to Rock Creek crossing, 4.1 miles from Lower Soldier Lake.

Upon fording Rock Creek, begin a moderately steep, switchbacking climb along the PCT up the north wall of the canyon through a light forest of lodgepole pines.

After about 0.75 mile, the grade eases and climbs more gently toward a crossing of Guyot Creek (with campsites nearby). Before departing, make sure your water supply is sufficient for the next 4.5 miles of dry trail. Fine views of Mt. Guyot and Joe Devil Peak grace the next section of gently graded tread on the way to a steeper, boulder-filled climb through young pines to Guyot Pass (approximately 10,920 feet), directly northeast of Mt. Guyot.

Beyond the pass, a moderate descent ensues with excellent views of the Great Western Divide, Kern Canyon, Red Spur, and Kaweah Peaks. Soon, easy tread leads across the wide expanse of a sandy basin known as Guyot Flat, where few plants are capable of taking root. The fine views continue until you enter a light forest of foxtail pines at the far end of the flat. For the next couple of miles, the trail follows an undulating traverse to the south lip of Whitney Creek canyon, where steep switchbacks descend to the floor. A gentle stroll over rocky terrain leads to Lower Crabtree Meadow (approximately 10,320 feet) and campsites (with a bear box) near a ford of the creek. Just past the creek is a junction with your route toward Mt. Whitney, 20.3 miles from the trailhead.

With the west face of Mt. Whitney in constant view, leave the PCT and make a gentle, half-mile ascent along the north bank of Whitney Creek to the lush environs of Upper Crabtree Meadow. Near the far end, just prior to where the trail crosses the creek, the Crabtree Lakes Trail branches east. Beyond the ford, a lateral heads to campsites (with a bear box) and the Crabtree Ranger Station before crossing back over the creek to the north bank. Shortly beyond this crossing, the lateral intersects the John Muir Trail (JMT), where there are campsites, 1.2 miles from the previous junction of the PCT.

Now on the JMT, ascend along the north bank of Whitney Creek through a smattering of lodgepole and foxtail pines. About a half mile from the junction, pass some campsites on the way to picturesque Timberline Lake. Although closed to camping, the lake is worthy of an extended visit, especially a vantage point on the south shore, where the bulk of Mt. Whitney is reflected in the placid surface.

Beyond Timberline Lake, the steady ascent continues through an open basin laden with granite slabs and benches. You climb over a flat-topped ridge to Guitar Lake (approximately 11,460 feet), 3.5 miles from the PCT junction, where camping is still allowed in sandy pockets away from the meadow grass. Away from the lake, a pair of tarns offers additional campsites and the last reliable water source before the stiff climb to Trail Crest.

As the grade increases, Hitchcock Lakes appear to the south, luring knapsackers to a remote location beneath the precipitous north face of Mt. Hitchcock. Long-legged switchbacks lead up the steep west face of the Sierra Crest on a steady, 1,500-foot climb to a junction with the Mt. Whitney Trail, 5.5 miles from the PCT junction. A typical summer day will see a plethora of backpacks reposing against a steep wall of rock nearby, as backpackers jettison their fully loaded backpacks for the final 2-mile climb to Whitney's summit.

Ⓞ **SIDE TRIP TO MOUNT WHITNEY:** Unless the weather is threatening, to come all this way and not proceed the additional 2 miles to the summit would be a lapse in judgment. Climb steadily along the west side of the crest, where the trail periodically enters airy notches that provide acrophobic vistas straight down the east face. Proceed along rocky tread to the final slope below the summit, where the grade increases and several paths angle toward the top. Cairns may aid you, but the route is obvious—head for the highest point! The top of the peak is a broad, sloping plateau of jumbled slabs and large boulders, with an indescribable view. **END OF SIDE TRIP**

From the Mt. Whitney junction, a short climb leads to Trail Crest (approximately 13,650 feet), 8.2 miles from Whitney Portal. Now you must descend the 100 switchbacks to Trail Camp. Zigzag down the rocky slope, which may have snow patches through midseason. A seep about halfway down, which is oftentimes in the shade, may have icy conditions as well. Unless you are longing for human contact, you'll most likely want to breeze past Trail Camp, as the last legal camping area below Mt. Whitney is usually a hubbub of frenetic activity. If you must camp for the night, sites near Consultation Lake may be slightly less crowded.

Continue the descent through a sea of rock to lovely Trailside Meadow (where camping is prohibited), a verdant strip of meadowlands contrasting starkly with the otherwise rocky terrain. Beyond the meadow, the trail crosses Lone Pine Creek and proceeds downstream. Switchbacks lead down to Mirror Lake (where camping is also prohibited) and onward to a crossing of Mirror Creek just before reaching Outpost Camp .

With 4.6 miles to go, cross Lone Pine Creek, and stroll through the willow-lined meadows of Bighorn Park. From there, switchbacks descend a rocky slope and down a rock-filled wash to a junction with the lateral to Lone Pine Lake. A short way beyond the junction the trail fords Lone Pine Creek and begins a steady, mostly shadeless descent with occasional switchbacks out of the wilderness, across North Fork Lone Pine Creek, and back into forest on the way to the Whitney Portal Trailhead.

Ⓡ A wilderness permit is required for overnight stay. Campfires are prohibited in Cottonwood Lakes Basin, above 10,400 feet, or within the Whitney Zone. Bear canisters are required. Camping is prohibited at Timberline Lake, in Trailside Meadow, and at Mirror Lake.

Within the Whitney Zone the Forest Service has instituted mandatory use of WAG (waste alleviation and gelling) bags for disposal of all human waste. Hikers should pick up bags at the Crabtree Meadow junction and then dispose of them at Whitney Portal.

TRIP 95

Mount Whitney

S ↗ **DH** or **BP**

DISTANCE: 21.4 miles, out-and-back

ELEVATION: 8,361'/14,494',
+7,830'/-1,875'/±19,410'

SEASON: Mid-July to early October

USE: Extremely heavy

MAPS: USGS's *Mount Whitney* or
Tom Harrison Maps' *Mt.
Whitney Zone Trail Map*

TRAIL LOG

2.5   Lone Pine Lake junction
3.6   Outpost Camp
4.0   Mirror Lake
5.75 Trailside Meadow
5.9   Trail Camp
8.2   Trail Crest
8.4   John Muir Trail junction
10.7 Mt. Whitney summit

INTRODUCTION: Mt. Whitney is one of the most impressive mountains in North America with a classic east face presenting a towering and dramatic alpine profile to rival any peak in the West. Not only is the view of the mountain exceptional, but the vista from the summit is even more extraordinary, a commensurate reward for the diligence required to reach the climax of the Sierra. Standing atop the 14,494-foot summit remains a crowning achievement for many recreationists.

To say that Mt. Whitney is a coveted ascent would be quite an understatement; so many people desire to climb the highest US summit outside of Alaska that the Forest Service long ago implemented a lottery system to dole out a limited number of permits well short of the exceedingly high demand. The $15 per person fee for reservations has done little, if anything, to temper these desires. (See the introduction to the

Mt. Whitney Ranger District, page 306, for Whitney Zone permit information.)

Before submitting an application, prospective climbers must decide whether to make their attempt as a dayhike or overnight (or longer) backpack. The main advantage of the single-day option is not having to lug a heavy backpack to a campsite at either Outpost Camp or Trail Camp. However, to complete the trip in one day, hikers must be in top condition and well acclimated, as well as prepared for a long and strenuous day. In addition to being similarly prepared, backpackers must trudge up the steep trail like beasts of burden laden with all the necessary gear for setting up camp. In so doing, they have the advantage of a more leisurely ascent (if any climb of Whitney could be considered so) and more time to acclimatize along the way. Either approach makes for an arduous ascent.

Even with your permit in hand, the actual climb raises several concerns. The high altitude (14,494 feet), elevation gain (7,830 feet), and total distance (21.4 miles) all require excellent fitness and proper acclimatization. Spending a night at the backpackers' walk-in campground at Whitney Portal at 8,350 feet is a good way to begin the acclimatization process. If the campground is full, the regular Whitney Portal (8,000 feet) or Lone Pine (6,000 feet) campgrounds are alternatives. The 4.5-mile Meysan Trail nearby provides an excellent conditioning hike the day before a Whitney climb (see Trip 96, page 332). Once you are on the trail, stay well hydrated, eat plenty of high-energy foods, and monitor your condition and that of your companions for any signs of altitude sickness or other malady.

Not only does a climb of Whitney require excellent physical fitness and acclimatization, but proper equipment as well. The sun's intensity at these elevations necessitates the use of sunglasses, and the regular application of sunblock to unprotected areas of skin. A wide-brimmed hat helps too. Pack clothing suitable for a wide range of temperatures, which can fluctuate dramatically from trailhead to summit. Weather conditions can change rapidly—

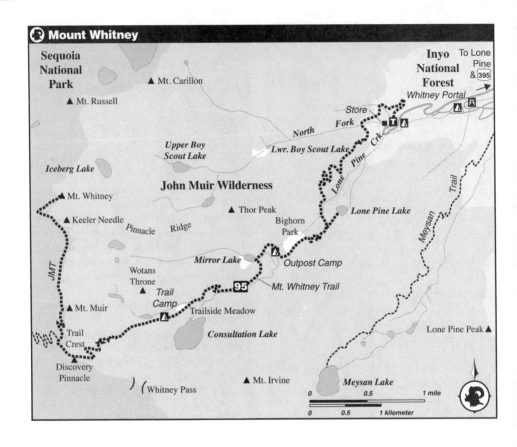

Mount Whitney

high winds, heavy rain, hail, and even snow are possible during any month of the year. Afternoon thunderstorms are not uncommon; beat a hasty retreat at the first signs of developing thunderclouds. There is no place high on the mountain, particularly between Trail Crest and the summit, to hide from lightning strikes.

Finally, be aware of the special regulations put in place by the Forest Service in an attempt to minimize the impact of so many humans on a sensitive mountain environment. Above Lone Pine Lake, camping is restricted to Outpost Camp and Trail Camp, and campfires are prohibited. WAG (waste alleviation and gelling) bags are mandatory for removal of all human waste within the Whitney Zone. Hikers can pick up the bags at the Whitney Portal Trailhead and bring their used bags back out with them.

MOUNT WILLIAMSON

What is the second highest peak in California? The correct answer is 14,375-foot Mt. Williamson, 5.5 miles north of Mt. Whitney. While almost everyone recognizes Whitney as the tallest mountain in the Lower 48, Williamson languishes in relative obscurity. While hundreds of pilgrims toil up toward Whitney's summit every day of the season, far fewer set their sights on number two. If a mere 120 feet could be added to Mt. Williamson, no doubt a trail would lead to the summit and hundreds of devotees would make that climb.

Warnings about overcrowding, permits, strenuous climbing, potential health problems, adverse weather conditions, and regulations might lead hikers to consider avoiding this area altogether. However, the reward of standing on top of Mt. Whitney still outweighs any potential drawbacks.

DIRECTIONS TO TRAILHEAD: Turn west from US 395 in Lone Pine onto Whitney Portal Road, and proceed 13 miles to the day-use or overnight parking lots at Whitney Portal. Campgrounds, restrooms, and a small store with a cafe are nearby.

DESCRIPTION: Abundant signs, placards, and display boards create quite a fanfare at the start of the Mt. Whitney Trail, which seems perversely suited to the most heavily regulated and popular backcountry thoroughfare in the High Sierra. After the bombardment of multiple regulations and warnings, you pass a human waste receptacle, perhaps the most vivid reminder of the limitations of an alpine environment to handle such a high level of human impact.

Away from the trailhead hoopla, a well-beaten path winds through a light forest of red firs, Jeffrey pines, and mountain mahogany before curving up the slope to the first major switchback. Now heading roughly east across a chaparral-covered slope, you have a fine view up the canyon of a waterfall on Lone Pine Creek. Soon the trail crosses an unnamed tributary lined with lush foliage, followed by a rising quarter-mile traverse to a crossing of North Fork Lone Pine Creek, where a steep mountaineer's route ascends this drainage to alpine lakes below Whitney's east face (see options, page 331). Beyond, the trail crosses the John Muir Wilderness boundary.

A mostly shadeless, steady climb, incorporating numerous switchbacks, ensues. If the forecast is for hot weather, try to avoid this section during the heat of the day. After 1.5 miles, relief comes in the shade of lodgepole pine forest on the way to a ford of Lone Pine Creek. Shortly beyond the ford, reach a junction with the short spur to Lone Pine Lake, 2.5 miles from the trailhead.

 SIDE TRIP TO LONE PINE LAKE: From the junction, follow the spur 200 yards through light forest to the shore of the lake. Perched at the edge of a steep cliff, the roughly oval lake is blessed with fine views down the cleft of Lone Pine Creek's canyon across the mostly open, boulder-strewn shore. With no permanent inlet, the lake depends on snowmelt. Angers can test their luck on rainbow and brook trout. There are a small number of foxtail pine–shaded campsites by the trail above the southwest shore. **END OF SIDE TRIP**

From the Lone Pine Lake junction, stroll through a rocky wash on gently graded tread through a light covering of pine and cross the boundary into the Whitney Zone. Soon, steeper climbing resumes, as switchbacks lead up and over a rocky slope to Bighorn Park, a large, willow-lined meadow carpeted with wildflowers in season. Follow a gently graded path along the meadow to the far end, and then turn northwest to a crossing of the creek. Just beyond the creek, near a vigorous waterfall, is Outpost Camp (10,335 feet), 3.6 miles from the trailhead.

In olden days, Outpost Camp bustled with even more activity when a packer's wife rented tents and sold meals to travelers, while tending stock grazing in the lush grasses of Bighorn Park nearby (named for the native sheep that once inhabited the area). Although camping is legal at Lone Pine Lake, the sloping campsites at Outpost Camp, bordered by rock and gravel and sheltered below widely scattered pines, represents the first practical alternative for Whitney bound backpackers. Using the required bear canisters protects your food from the resident rodents as well.

Leave the peaceful surroundings of Outpost Camp, cross Mirror Creek, and then make a steep, switchbacking climb alongside a tumbling stream lined with flowers. At the top of the climb, boulder hop back over the creek, and pass through head-high willows on the way to the southeast shore of Mirror Lake (10,460 feet), 4 miles from the trailhead.

Mirror Lake is quite attractive, set in a deep cirque below the steep cliffs of Thor Peak. Anglers can test their skill on the brook trout rumored to live here, but backpackers will have to continue to Trail Camp for legal camping. The Forest Service banned overnight stays at the lake in 1972 to protect it from overuse. However, the lake is a fine haven for a rest stop or lunch break.

More switchbacks climb steeply out of Mirror Lake's cirque to the top of a ridge near timberline. As the trail resumes a more southwesterly direction, the east face of Mt. Whitney pops into view over Pinnacle Ridge. Climb moderately through boulders and rocks, the otherwise rugged landscape occasionally broken by scattered wildflowers and small shrubs. Rock steps lead closer to the banks of Lone Pine Creek and eventually across a stone bridge spanning the stream. Beyond, you reach lovely Trailside Meadow (11,855 feet) carpeted in season by shooting stars, paintbrush, and columbine, 5.75 miles from Whitney Portal.

Beyond this lovely oasis is an interminable climb amid a nearly endless sea of rock. After crossing Lone Pine Creek again, Consultation Lake comes into view, flanked dramatically by Mts. Irvine and McAdie. Continue climbing steadily around boulders and over rock steps. Just past a short, nearly level stretch, a final climb leads to Trail Camp (12,035 feet), 5.9 miles from the trailhead, where every possible semi-flat campsite has been scratched out of the sand between here and Consultation Lake. Ample amounts of water should be available from streams and tarns nearby.

Although Trail Camp's atmosphere is circuslike, its setting below the rugged east face of the Whitney massif is spectacular. To the north lies Wotan's Throne, with Pinnacle Ridge behind; to the south, 13,680-foot Mt. McAdie and 13,770-foot Mt. Irvine form an impressive amphitheater for the icy waters of Consultation Lake. Directly above the camp loom the 100 switchbacks to the low gap in the Sierra Crest known as Trail Crest. Many a Whitney climber has experienced a restless night in their foreboding shadow.

TRAIL CAMP

On just about any summer day, Trail Camp assumes the aura of an expedition base camp. While colorful nylon tents flap in the breeze, expectant summiteers sort and check equipment, while others gaze upward at the route, or check the skies for hints of the weather. Still others make inquiries of returning climbers about their experiences on the mountain.

Trail Camp is definitely not the place for isolationists in search of a solitary wilderness experience. *Don't expect any privacy.* With 100 dayhikers and 60 overnighters allowed to depart every day, along with 25 backpackers starting from alternate trailheads allowed to exit at Whitney Portal, up to 250 people pass through Trail Camp on a given day.

Away from Trail Camp, the trail has a fairly mellow grade initially but soon increases on the way to the first of the switchbacks leading to Trail Crest. Zigzag up the rocky slope, enjoying the ever expanding views (Mt. Whitney becomes hidden behind the Needles). Near the midpoint, climb the side of a rock wall, where a seep oozing across the tread may create icy conditions and old iron railings may add a feeling of apprehensive safety. The interminable switchbacks continue, eventually leading to Trail Crest (13,580 feet), 8.2 miles from Whitney Portal, where staggering views to the west of the Great Western Divide and of a large portion of Sequoia National Park greet you. Directly below, in the barren basin, lie the shimmering Hitchcock Lakes.

A short descent from Trail Crest takes you to the junction of the John Muir Trail (JMT), where the final 2.5-mile climb to the summit begins. A steady ascent leads along the west side of the ridge, where the trail periodically dips into notches with acrophobic views straight down the east face. Farther on, sharp eyes will pick out the hut on the summit plateau, built in 1909 by the Smithsonian Institute for research purposes. Below the final slope, the grade increases and multiple paths head toward the summit. Cairns may aid you here, but the way forward is unmistakable—simply head toward the highest point!

Soon the hut's metal roof pops into view above the horizon, and you shortly reach the highest piece of terra firma in the continental United States. The top of the mountain is a broad, sloping plateau, made up of jumbled slabs and boulders. Make sure you mark your accomplishment by signing the summit register. Any adjective will seem inadequate to describe the view. Suffice it to say, the scene encompasses a 360-degree vista, with each bearing of the compass holding something extraordinary

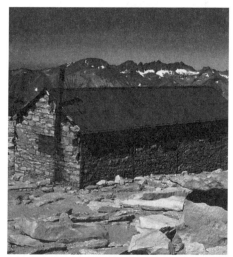

The Smithsonian's stone hut on top of Mt. Whitney

to discover—a just reward for the toil necessary to achieve such a lofty aerie.

○ The nearby Meysan Trail provides a good way to acclimatize for the ascent of Whitney (see Trip 96, page 332). Approximately 1 mile up the Mt. Whitney Trail, an interesting but strenuous trip follows the mountaineers' trail up North Fork Lone Pine Creek to Boy Scout and Iceberg Lakes, nestled in a scenic alpine basin below the impressive north face of Mt. Whitney. From Iceberg Lake, skilled climbers can attempt the Class 3 Mountaineers Route on Mt. Whitney, although by climbing standards the popular route can feel crowded at times.

From Iceberg Lake, a Class 2 cross-country route proceeds over the crest at Whitney-Russell Pass (13,040 feet) and then descends west to Arctic Lake, from where you can continue to connect with the JMT near Guitar Lake. Whitney hikers with the requisite off-trail skills could alter their return from the summit by descending the north slope of Whitney to Whitney-Russell Pass and then descending the North Fork route back to the Mt. Whitney Trail.

R A wilderness permit is required for overnight stay. Campfires are prohibited within the Whitney Zone. Bear canisters are required. Camping is prohibited at Mirror Lake and in Trailside Meadow. Stock is prohibited.

Within the Whitney Zone the Forest Service has instituted mandatory use of WAG (waste alleviation and gelling) bags for disposal of all human waste. Hikers should pick up bags and dispose of them at the Whitney Portal Trailhead.

TRIP 96

Meysan Trail

MS ↗ **DH** or **BP**

DISTANCE: 10.2 miles, out-and-back

ELEVATION: 7,890'/11,625',
+3,860'/-310'/±8,340'

SEASON: Mid-July to early-October

USE: Light

MAPS: USGS's *Mt. Langley* or Tom
Harrison Maps' *Mt. Whitney
Zone Trail Map*

INTRODUCTION: What a difference a mile
makes! Each summer day hundreds trudge
up the Mt. Whitney Trail toward the high-

est point in the continental United States,
but in a canyon just a mile away only a few
people hike the Meysan Trail. Although the
rewards may not be as prestigious as those
of scaling Whitney, the scenery and relative
solitude in the canyon of Meysan Creek
have their own appeal. As an added bonus,
since the trail lies outside the Whitney Zone,
dayhikers are *not* required to get a permit,
and backpackers face far less competition
for permits and campsites. However, upon
reaching Meysan Lake, visitors may feel like
they completed the equivalent of a Whitney
climb, as the trail grinds steadily uphill,
gaining nearly 4,000 feet in 4.5 miles.

DIRECTIONS TO TRAILHEAD: Turn west
from US 395 in Lone Pine onto Whitney
Portal Road and proceed 13 miles to the
day-use or overnight parking lots at Whitney Portal. Campgrounds, restrooms, and a
small store with a cafe are nearby.

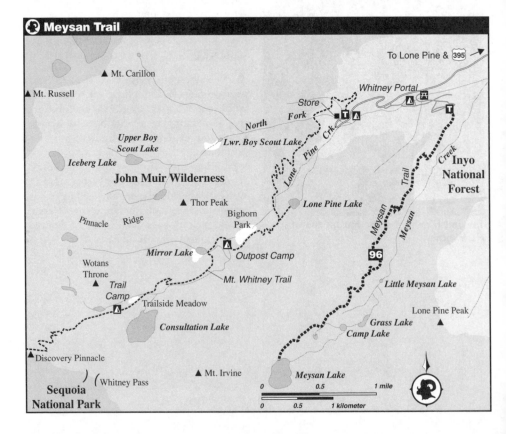

Meysan Trail

DESCRIPTION: The first leg of the journey requires you to descend the old service road from the Whitney Portal Road to the Whitney Portal Campground. Following signs, go left on the campground loop road, and cross the bridge over Lone Pine Creek to an intersection. Turn left again, passing some cabins on the way to the official trailhead.

From the trailhead, make a steep climb up a hillside on single-track tread. The stiff ascent may give you second thoughts about the wisdom of doing this hike, but the grade fortunately eases on the approach to another road. Follow the road past more cabins to the resumption of trail.

Having now left the last vestiges of civilization behind, you make a moderate climb across a dry hillside dotted with red firs, pinyon pines, Jeffrey pines, and mountain mahogany. Soon the trail reaches the canyon of Meysan Creek and curves southwest, climbing moderately up a steep hillside, well above the level of the creek. Reach the first of many switchbacks to come, where views open up to the northeast of the Alabama Hills and Owens Valley. Cross the wilderness boundary near the 1.5-mile mark.

Where the trail draws slightly closer to the creek, you may catch glimpses of a pretty cascade gliding down a rock slab into a delightful pool. More switchbacks lead to even better views of the canyon and another cascade dropping down the headwall of the lake-filled basin above. Scattered foxtail pines appear just prior to a grassy meadow, about 3.5 miles from the parking area, where a sign at a junction provides directions to Grass Lake straight ahead and Camp and Meysan Lakes to the right.

Beyond the junction, cairns periodically mark the faint tread on the final climb to Meysan Lake. Proceed around a large meadow bordering Camp Lake, and then ascend a grassy draw. Where the slope becomes steeper, veer southwest and climb over rock slabs to a gap above the lake, where a short descent leads to the northeast shore. Small pockets of flower-filled meadow dot the otherwise rocky shore, which is backdropped by a dramatic headwall formed by Mts. Irvine and Mallory. While there are places to camp around Meysan Lake, Camp Lake has better sites.

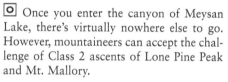 Once you enter the canyon of Meysan Lake, there's virtually nowhere else to go. However, mountaineers can accept the challenge of Class 2 ascents of Lone Pine Peak and Mt. Mallory.

A wilderness permit is required for overnight stays. Campfires and stock are prohibited.

WHITNEY PORTAL TRAILHEAD

TRIP 97

John Muir Trail: Whitney Portal to Onion Valley

MS / BP

DISTANCE: 44.5 miles, point-to-point

ELEVATION: 8,361'/13,650'/10,405'/ 13,070'/9,535'/11,823'/9,185', +15,250'/-13,250'/±28,500'

SEASON: Mid- or late July to early October

USE: High

MAPS: USGS's *Mount Whitney, Mt. Kaweah, Mt. Brewer, Mt. Williamson, Mt.Clarence King,* and *Kearsarge Peak* or Tom Harrison Maps' *John Muir Trail Map-Pack*

TRAIL LOG

2.5	Lone Pine Lake junction
3.6	Outpost Camp
4.0	Mirror Lake
5.75	Trailside Meadow
5.9	Trail Camp
8.2	Trail Crest
8.4	Mt. Whitney Trail and John Muir Trail junction
14.8	Pacific Crest Trail junction
18.3	High Sierra Trail junction and Wallace Creek
21.8	Tyndall Frog Ponds
22.6	Tyndall Creek Trail junction
22.9	Shepherd Pass Trail junction and Tyndall Creek ford
27.6	Forester Pass
32.0	Center Basin Trail junction
35.5	Vidette Meadow and Bubbs Creek Trail junction
36.6	Bullfrog Lake junction
37.1	Kearsarge Pass and Charlotte Lake junction
41.6	Kearsarge Pass

INTRODUCTION: Without a doubt, you will see some of the most impressive High Sierra scenery around on this stretch of the 200-plus-mile John Muir Trail (JMT). Access from the east side is via the very popular 8.4-mile Mt. Whitney Trail from Whitney Portal, with wilderness permits at a premium (see Trip 95, page 327). Those fortunate enough to score a permit have the opportunity to scale Mt. Whitney along the way and continue their journey along the JMT, exiting at Onion Valley via the Kearsarge Pass Trail.

DIRECTIONS TO TRAILHEAD:
START: Turn west from US 395 in Lone Pine onto Whitney Portal Road, and proceed 13 miles to the day-use or overnight parking lots at Whitney Portal. Campgrounds, restrooms, and a small store with a cafe are nearby.
END: From US 395 in Independence, turn west onto Market Street, and proceed out of town for 12.5 miles on steep and winding Onion Valley Road to the parking area. A campground, vault toilets, and running water are near the trailhead.

DESCRIPTION: Follow the description in Trip 95 for 8.4 miles to the junction between the Mt. Whitney Trail and the JMT just below Trail Crest. Those with an interest in scaling the highest peak in the continental United States should drop their backpacks and make the 4-mile round-trip to Mt. Whitney's summit and back.

From the JMT and Mt. Whitney Trail junction, descend a series of switchbacks, with constant views of the shimmering Hitchcock Lakes below, backdropped regally by the northeast wall of Mt. Hitchcock. Beyond the switchbacks, a moderate descent leads to a bench holding a pair of tarns and some overused, exposed campsites (there are better spots off-trail around Hitchcock Lakes). Continue descending to Guitar Lake (approximately 11,480 feet), where the grade eases momentarily and there are more overused campsites. Once again, there are superior campsites away from the lake, on

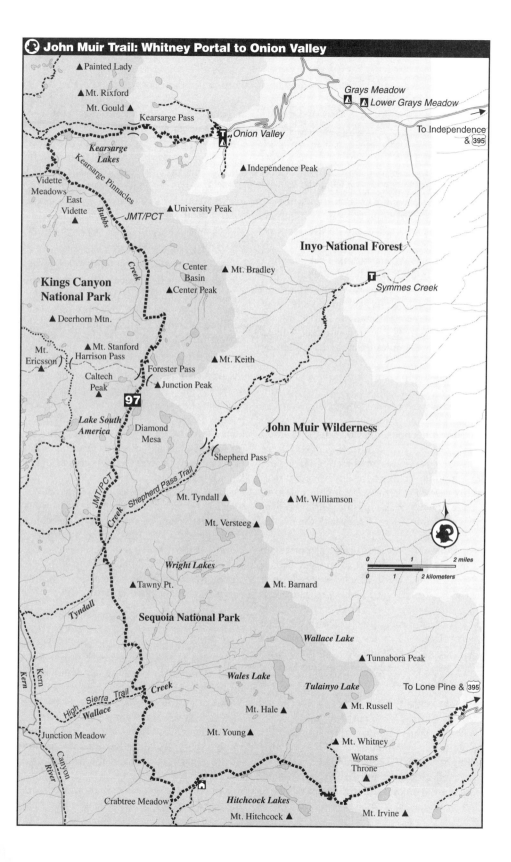

rises above the south shore and along the outlet from Arctic Lake.

After crossing Arctic Lake's outlet, follow a mile-long, moderately steep descent on rocky tread through a sparse cover of lodgepole pines to Timberline Lake, which is closed to camping but offers a fine reflection of Mt. Whitney from its southwest shore. Beyond the lake, pass a lovely meadow and drop into the vale of Whitney Creek, meeting a junction with the Crabtree Meadow lateral, from which a spur leads to the Crabtree Ranger Station. There are fine campsites (with a bear box) along the spur on either side of a ford of Whitney Creek.

From the junction, continue west away from the creek through a smattering of foxtail pines to a junction with the Pacific Crest Trail, 6.4 miles from the Mt. Whitney Trail junction.

Turn north at the junction, and climb over a rise to a ford of a seasonal stream. Skirt Sandy Meadow, stepping across many small brooks, and then make a steady climb through lodgepole pines to a saddle (10,963 feet). Beyond this saddle, a gentle descent leads across the west shoulder of Mt. Young to a boulder field, where the grade momentarily eases. From there, a moderate descent heads down a rocky hillside, with excellent views of the Sierra Crest and the Kings-Kern Divide. Stepping across several rivulets along the way, you drop into a stream canyon and reach the broad ford of Wallace Creek (10,403 feet), which can be difficult early in the season. There are numerous campsites (with a bear box) on the far side of the creek, near a junction with the High Sierra Trail, 3.7 miles from the JMT and PCT junction. From here, an unmaintained path heads east upstream to scenic Wallace and Wales Lakes.

◉ SIDE TRIP TO WALLACE AND WALES LAKES: Although the path to Wallace Lake is unmaintained and indistinct in places, by cross-country standards the route is fairly straightforward. From the JMT, follow a use trail along the north bank of Wallace Creek on a gentle ascent through a light to moderate cover of lodgepole pines. Near a

meadow at the confluence with the outlet from Wales Lake, cross to the south bank of Wallace Creek, ford the outlet, and then continue upstream to a cluster of timberline campsites about a half mile below Wallace Lake. From there, proceed along the south bank of the main branch to Wallace Lake (11,473 feet), 3.6 miles from the JMT. Anglers can ply the waters for good-size golden trout. Less-visited Wales Lake is just a short, off-trail jaunt away. **END OF SIDE TRIP**

Away from the junction, ascend a boulder-strewn hillside through light forest on a sustained climb out of Wallace Creek canyon. Before reaching Wrights Creek, you will pass a few shady campsites. A moderate climb follows the creek briefly before bending away.

◉ SIDE TRIP TO WRIGHT LAKES: The wide-open Wright Lakes basin provides easy off-trail travel to spectacular scenery and good fishing. Leave the JMT where it bends away from Wright Creek, and continue upstream through lodgepole pines. The trail soon breaks out of the trees and enters the open, lake-dotted basin.

In early to midseason the meadows, which are fed by a plethora of springs and rivulets, can be quite boggy. Reaching the highest lake requires a short but steep climb up the brush- and rock-filled slope, but it rewards the diligent hiker with fine views. More ambitious souls can continue to Tulainyo Lake. **END OF SIDE TRIP**

A steeper climb leads across open slopes with excellent views of Wright Lakes basin backdropped by Mts. Tyndall, Versteeg, and Barnard. Soon you're back into a scattered forest of lodgepole and foxtail pines on the way to the broad, barren expanse of Bighorn Plateau. Across this sandy flat are more good views, this time a sweeping vista of the Great Western Divide, from Red Spur in the south to Kings-Kern Divide in the north. A tarn just west of the trail offers a nice touch for photographs.

At the far edge of Bighorn Plateau, scattered foxtails greet you once more on a mild descent across the west slope of Tawny Point. At 3.8 miles from the High Sierra Trail junction, hop across a tributary of Tyndall Creek, which is the outlet from a trio of tarns known as Tyndall Frog Ponds. Just off the trail are good campsites (with a bear box), with more secluded sites closer to the ponds. The shallow tarns offer pleasant swimming by midsummer. A winding, 0.75-mile descent through lodgepole pine cover leads to a junction with the Tyndall Creek Trail. A short distance down this trail there is a seasonal ranger station and some campsites along the creek.

A quarter-mile climb from the junction leads to a junction with the Shepherd Pass Trail, 4.6 miles from the High Sierra Trail junction, and the potentially daunting ford of Tyndall Creek just beyond. Campsites (with a bear box) on the far bank may tempt overnighters. Beyond the ford, the ascent continues, leading 0.3 mile to a junction with a trail toward Lake South America, a worthy diversion for those with extra time and energy. A tarn west of the trail offers secluded campsites.

A mild to moderate ascent leads above timberline, where there are fine views of the upper Tyndall Creek basin. Pass lovely tarns and hop across rollicking streams along the way to the base of a headwall below Forester Pass. As with many of the High Sierra passes, a viable route over the headwall seems unlikely, at least until you can see the switchbacking trail zigzagging up the slope. This section is something of an engineering marvel, literally blasted and cut out of a vertical rock wall—portions of it are definitely not for acrophobes. Reach the narrow gap of Forester Pass (13,180 feet) on the Kings-Kern Divide at the boundary between Sequoia and Kings Canyon National Parks, 4.7 miles from the Shepherd Pass Trail junction. Expansive vistas include myriad peaks to both the north and south.

After you have scaled the precipitous terrain on the south side of the pass, the descent of the north side on smooth, sandy tread that switchbacks down to the top of a rock rib above a tarn in the head of the canyon seems straightforward. Follow the trail to the end of the rib, enjoying excellent views along the way. An angling descent from there leads to a crossing of Bubbs Creek and a grand alpine view of the tarn backdropped by Junction Peak.

Continue the winding, rocky descent, fording the stream a couple more times, as it bends west and drops into more hospitable terrain. Pass a pair of poor campsites in a grove of pines tiered down the steep slope and follow more switchbacks into a light forest of scattered lodgepole and whitebark pines and past small pockets of verdant, wildflower-dotted meadows and clumps of willow. Ford Center Basin Creek and reach campsites (with a bear box) near a junction with the old Center Basin Trail, 4.4 miles from Forester Pass, from where a side trip to Golden Bear Lake is a worthy diversion.

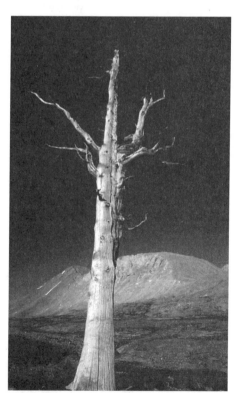

Old snag and Mt. Tyndall from the John Muir Trail

Continue the descent along tumbling Bubbs Creek, which is sandwiched between the towering pinnacle of East Vidette to the west and the rugged spine of the Kearsarge Pinnacles to the east. Along the way, you travel in and out of scattered to light lodgepole forest and hop across a number of tributaries. Eventually, after passing through a wire fence, the trail reaches Upper Vidette Meadow, where a number of over-used campsites repose under pines along the creek. Beyond the campsites, an unmarked lateral leads down to a large packer's camp near the creek. Farther on is the ever popular Vidette Meadows Camp (with bear boxes) catering to JMT thru-hikers and backpackers on the Rae Lakes Loop. After a pair of stream crossings, reach a junction with the Bubbs Creek Trail to Cedar Grove, 7.7 miles from Forester Pass.

From the Bubbs Creek junction, follow a moderate, switchbacking climb up the north wall of the canyon. Views to the right of the Kearsarge Pinnacles are dramatic, but don't neglect the view of the Videttes and Deerhorn Mountain behind you. After a couple of stream crossings, reach the Bullfrog Lake Trail junction (the old Kearsarge Pass Trail and the shortest route to Kearsarge Pass), 1.3 miles from the Bubbs Creek Trail junction. Picturesque Bullfrog Lake, 0.4 mile east of the JMT, has been closed to camping for several decades to allow it to recover from overuse, but it provides an excellent spot for a break. Farther on, Kearsarge Lakes have a two-night camping limit.

Short switchbacks climb a half mile over a lightly forested rise to a broad sandy flat and a multi-signed junction, 1.8 miles from the Bubbs Creek Trail junction. Here a 0.75-mile lateral heads toward campsites around

lovely Charlotte Lake (with a bear box and a two-night limit), and the Kearsarge Pass Trail heads east 7 miles to the Onion Valley Trailhead.

To exit at Onion Valley, either reverse the description in Trip 101 (page 348) for the Bullfrog Lake Trail, or Trip 102 (page 352) for the Kearsarge Pass Trail.

O Options abound for further wanderings away from the JMT. Center Basin is a worthy goal (see Trip 98, page 339). Mountaineers also have a number of potential peaks to climb. From Wallace Creek, the southwest slope of Mt. Barnard is Class 1. From Upper Wright Lake, the southwest slope of both Mt. Versteeg and Mt. Tyndall are Class 2. Below Forester Pass, a Class 2 route up Caltech Peak follows the southwest slope. From the pass, a moderate Class 3 climb of Junction Peak is possible via the west ridge. North of the pass, the east ridge of East Vidette is a fine Class 3 ascent.

R A wilderness permit is required for overnight stays (see Trip 95, page 327, for information on the Whitney Zone lottery). Campfires are prohibited within the Whitney Zone, Lower Crabtree Meadow, and above 10,400 feet. Bear canisters are required. Camping is prohibited at Mirror Lake, in Trailside Meadow, and at Timberline and Bullfrog Lakes. Camping at Charlotte and Kearsarge Lakes is limited to two nights. Stock is prohibited on Mt. Whitney Trail.

Within the Whitney Zone the Forest Service has instituted mandatory use of WAG (waste alleviation and gelling) bags for disposal of all human waste. Hikers should pick up bags at the Whitney Portal Trailhead and carry the used bags out with them. Near Crabtree Meadows hikers may dispose of their waste in the sandy soil.

TRIP 98

Shepherd Pass Trail

S ↗ BP

DISTANCE: 25 miles, out-and-back to the John Muir Trail

ELEVATION: 6,310'/12,050'/10,890', +6,785'/-2,205'/±17,960'

SEASON: Mid-July to mid-October

USE: Light

MAPS: *Mt. Williamson* and *Mt. Brewer*

TRAIL LOG

7.0 Anvil Camp
9.0 Shepherd Pass
12.5 John Muir Trail junction

INTRODUCTION: The Shepherd Pass Trail is not for the weak or timid. But for those who don't mind low-elevation starts, exposed climbs, and hauling extra water, the trail is a gateway to some incredible backcountry. Its rugged nature also keeps fellow travelers to a minimum.

Beginning almost on the floor of Owens Valley, the trail is steep and usually hot, with little shade or water within the first 7 miles. However, diligent hikers in excellent condition will be rewarded for their efforts. Unlike sister trails over Baxter, Sawmill, and Taboose Passes, this route is much better maintained.

The initial ascent follows two typical Sierra canyons slicing into the rugged eastside escarpment. Beyond the pinyon-sagebrush zone, hikers climb into subalpine and alpine terrain on the way to the 12,050-foot pass at the boundary of Sequoia National Park. In these higher elevations, visitors are treated to dramatic mountain scenery, lush meadowlands, and the potential for extended wanderings to lake-dotted basins. Cross-country enthusi-

asts and mountaineers will enjoy the numerous routes possible from this trail.

DIRECTIONS TO TRAILHEAD: From US 395 in Independence, turn west onto Market Street, following signed directions for the Onion Valley Trailhead. At 4.4 miles, leave the Onion Valley Road, and turn left onto Foothill Road, heading south on well-graded dirt road (FS 13S08). Continue 2.6 miles to a junction, and turn left onto FS 13S07 toward the signed hiker trailhead (equestrian parking is a short distance up the right-hand road). Immediately cross Symmes Creek, and continue for a half mile to another signed junction. Turn right and head southwest, taking the right-hand forks at two junctions. After 1.6 miles you reach the Symmes Creek Trailhead, which has a screened pit toilet and parking for about a dozen cars.

DESCRIPTION: Through flora typical of the eastside pinyon-sagebrush zone, you follow sandy tread along the edge of a riparian zone lining the south bank of Symmes Creek into a narrowing canyon. Just past a junction with the stock trail and before the first ford of the creek, signs offer information about the Bighorn Sheep Zoological Area and Sequoia National Park. After a trio of fords, cross the John Muir Wilderness boundary, and proceed upstream through the deep cleft of the canyon to the beginning of a long, switchbacking climb up the south wall. Fill up on water before leaving the creek; the upcoming climb is steep and hot, and most of the water sources between here and Shepherd Creek are usually dry by midsummer.

The nearly 2-mile, winding climb gains 2,000 feet from the floor of the canyon to the crest of a ridge. Initially, scattered pinyon pines and mountain mahogany offer little shade, and there is not much more amid a sprinkling of red firs and western white pines higher up the slope. In the midst of the interminable climb, reach a small, pinyon-shaded flat with a campsite near a seasonal stream, which usually dries up shortly after snowmelt. The switchbacks continue away from the flat to the crest of

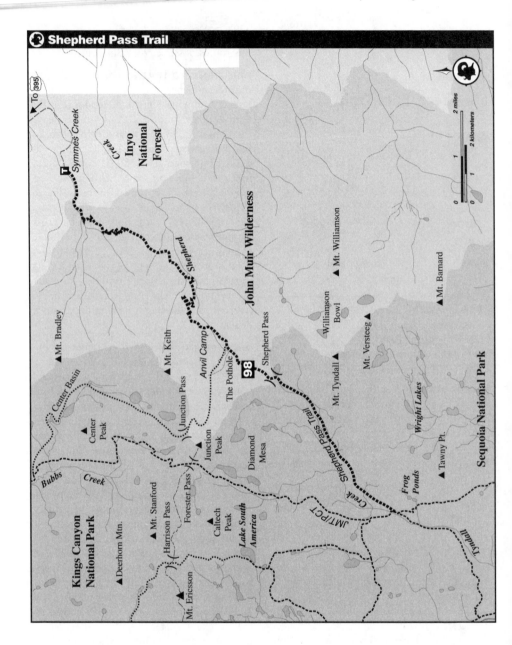

Shepherd Pass Trail

a ridge, from where you have fine views of Mt. Williamson and the deep cleft of Shepherd Creek.

A welcome stretch of gentler tread leads across a couple of low ridges and then on a generally descending traverse across a steep hillside above the deep gash formed by Shepherd Creek. Although you will likely welcome the easier hiking, losing some of that hard-won elevation is a tad discouraging when you contemplate the upcoming climb. The brief respite ends at a seasonal stream, where a moderate half-mile climb ensues to a perennial tributary draining the slopes below Mt. Keith, 4.6 miles from the trailhead.

Continue up and around the hillside to a switchback with a fine view of a waterfall. From there, pass marginal campsites at Mahogany Flat (which isn't much of a flat), well above Shepherd Creek, and then follow long-legged switchbacks up manzanita- and mahogany-covered slopes across the north wall of the canyon into a talus field. Eventually, a light forest of pines heralds the approach to Anvil Camp (shown incorrectly on the *Mt. Williamson* quad).

A short distance beyond the crossing of a tiny brook and past a NO FIRES sign, a bounty of campsites appear just prior to a crossing of Shepherd Creek, heralding your arrival at Anvil Camp (approximately 10,300 feet), 7 miles and nearly 4,000 vertical feet from the trailhead. Since the camp has the only campsites of any acceptable quality within the first 7 miles, it receives a fair amount of use, despite the trail's generally low use. A number of level campsites nestle beneath young foxtail pines near the willow-lined creek.

After a well-earned rest at Anvil Camp, cross Shepherd Creek and resume the ascent, leaving the pines behind to climb around a boulder-covered hillside to the Pothole, a willow-carpeted depression at the convergence of several watercourses. Beyond the crossing of a rivulet, a short and steep climb leads up a hillside dotted with stunted whitebark pines and past a couple of poor campsites on the way to the crossing of a more substantial stream. The trail then passes through treeless, boulder-strewn, morainal debris, with diminishing patches of alpine flora.

Proceeding up a deep, rocky gorge, you reach the base of a headwall below the Sierra Crest and begin the final climb up a slope often holding snow patches well into summer. Follow switchbacks that zigzag across the headwall to Shepherd Pass (approximately 12,050 feet), 9 miles from the trailhead. Here at the boundary of Sequoia National Park, a fine view of the Kaweah Peaks unfolds.

Just over the pass, a large tarn provides an exposed alpine base camp for a possible climb of Mt. Tyndall, with good views

into the Williamson Bowl. On sandy tread, you make a gentle descent through boulder-strewn meadows heading downstream along Tyndall Creek, with additional views of the Great Western Divide. Hop across numerous tributaries toward clumps of lodgepole pines, as the trail curves toward a junction with the John Muir Trail (JMT), 12.5 miles from the trailhead. There are campsites are near the junction, as well as farther south along a spur to the Tyndall Creek Ranger Station and along the JMT near the crossing of a stream draining some small, unnamed tarns.

CENTER BASIN TRAIL

Before the JMT was completed over Forester Pass in 1932, the Center Basin Trail over Junction Pass was the maintained route. Nowadays, with only traces remaining, this old trail is a bona fide cross-country route between Golden Bear Lake and the Shepherd Pass Trail.

CENTER BASIN AND JUNCTION PASS LOOP: A multiday, semiloop follows the JMT northbound over Forester Pass to the Center Basin Trail and then heads cross-country over Junction Pass, returning to the Shepherd Pass Trail near The Pothole. Head north on the JMT to a junction with the Center Basin Trail, 4.5 miles north of Forester Pass (there are campsites with a bear box just beyond the ford of Center Basin Creek). Turn east at the junction, and climb moderately up a hillside, crossing a flower-lined tributary and passing marshy stretches on the way to Golden Bear Lake (which has campsites).

Above the lake, gently ascending tread passes through nearly idyllic flower gardens before a more pronounced climb through talus-covered terrain leads to the first of a pair of alpine tarns (which has campsites). Pass the tarn on the west side, and climb

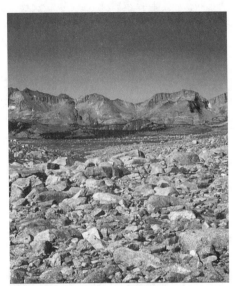

View west from Shepherd Pass

toward a ridge to the west above the second tarn. From there, follow an ascending arc to the east over to the flat saddle of Junction Pass (approximately 13,085 feet), 0.4 mile northeast of Junction Peak (the pass is shown incorrectly shown on the *Mt. Williamson* quad).

Beyond the pass, few traces of the old trail remain, as you follow a steep, rocky descent toward a reunion with the Shepherd Pass Trail. Initially, the route heads south down steep talus, before veering east to follow a stream down the valley. After about a mile, where the stream bends sharply toward The Pothole, descend a steep slope to the west of a beautiful subalpine meadow to the trail.

O Wright Lakes offer a pleasant trip extension, where a bevy of remote lakes repose in a broad, meadow-covered basin. The highest lake is particularly stunning, backdropped by the rugged Sierra Crest between Mt. Tyndall and Mt. Versteeg. The fishing here is reported to be quite good. About 1.5 miles west of Shepherd Pass, leave the trail and head south toward a prominent saddle. From there, a straightforward descent leads into the Wright Lakes basin.

A view into barren Williamson Bowl coupled with the opportunity to spy some bighorn sheep is worth the minor effort involved. From Shepherd Pass, head southeast about a mile to a broad gap in the crest above the westernmost lake in Williamson Bowl. Here you have an excellent view nearly straight down into an austere, lake-dotted basin. Drop from the crest down 300 feet of rough talus to the head of the bowl.

Mountaineers have plenty of ascents to choose from. From Shepherd Pass, the northwest ridge of Mt. Tyndall and the south face of Mt. Keith are Class 2. A moderate Class 3 route follows the southeast ridge of Junction Peak from the pass. A stay in Center Basin offers Class 2 climbs of the east face of Center Peak and the west face of Mt. Bradley; more technical routes on the five Center Basin Crags provide more technical climbing.

R A wilderness permit is required for overnight stays. Campfires are prohibited within 1,000 feet of Anvil Camp and above 10,400 feet. Dogs and domestic sheep are prohibited in the bighorn sheep zone.

TRIP 99

Robinson Lake

Ⓜ ✗ **DH** or **BP**

DISTANCE: 3 miles, out-and-back

ELEVATION: 9,185'/10,535', +1,335'/negligible/±2,670'

SEASON: Mid-July to early-October

USE: Light

MAPS: USGS's *Kearsarge Peak* or Tom Harrison Maps' *Kearsarge Pass-Rae Lakes Loop Trail Map*

INTRODUCTION: A short hike leading to splendid alpine scenery is generally a recipe for severe overuse. However, such is not the case with the trail to Robinson Lake. Perhaps the majority of hikers dismiss the area, which lies outside of the John Muir Wilderness, as unworthy, but nothing could be further from the truth; the lake, cradled in a dramatic glacial cirque topped with craggy pinnacles, is quite scenic. Sections of the 1.5-mile climb are steep, but it is short enough for a pleasant hike or overnight backpack.

DIRECTIONS TO TRAILHEAD: From US 395 in Independence, turn west onto Market Street, and proceed out of town for 12.5 miles on steep and winding Onion Valley Road to the parking area. A campground, △ vault toilets, and running water are near the trailhead.

DESCRIPTION: A small sign directs hikers from the parking area to the Onion Valley Campground and the signed trailhead near campsite 8. Follow a stone-filled path, which sometimes doubles as the course of a seasonal stream, to sandy tread above.

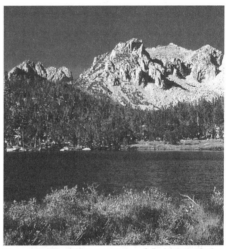

The sparkling blue waters of Robinson Lake

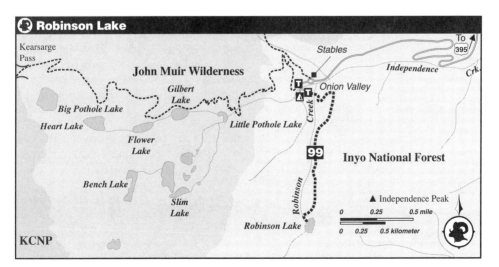

Through aspens, whitebark pines, and foxtail pines, follow switchbacks up a steep hillside to a small, sloping basin, where scattered timber provides evidence of previous avalanches. A more moderate climb eventually leads near the east bank of Robinson Creek. As you proceed upstream, the grade increases again where a large swath of willows carpets the drainage. Above the willows, climb beside and then across a small tributary, wind through a boulder field, and then crest the lip of Robinson Lake's basin. From there, gentler tread leads across an open area of rock, sand, and dwarf pines to the north shore.

Nestled in a steep, horseshoe-shaped basin, sapphire Robinson Lake radiates a bold alpine presence. Steep granite walls and talus rise up from the surface toward the summits of University and Independence Peaks. Foxtail pines above the west shore shade a number of pleasant campsites. Rainbow and brook trout will tempt anglers.

[O] Robinson Lake is the end of the line for most hikers, but mountaineers can accept the challenge of a difficult, Class 2 cross-country route over University Pass to Center Basin, or a similarly rated climb of 13,632-foot University Peak.

[R] Campfires are prohibited at the lake.

ONION VALLEY TRAILHEAD

TRIP 100

Kearsarge and Bullfrog Lakes

(M) ∕ DH or BP

DISTANCE: 14.4 miles, out-and-back

ELEVATION: 9,185'/11,823'/10,895', +2,685'/-1,415'/±8,380'

SEASON: Mid-July to early October

USE: Heavy

MAPS: USGS's *Kearsarge Peak* and *Mt. Clarence King* or Tom Harrison Maps' *Kearsarge Pass-Rae Lakes Loop Trail Map*

TRAIL LOG

2.2   Gilbert Lake
2.5   Flower Lake
5.0   Kearsarge Pass
5.7   Bullfrog Lake Trail junction
6.3   Use trail to Kearsarge Lakes
7.2   Bullfrog Lake

INTRODUCTION: Kearsarge Pass provides one of the least difficult eastern gateways across the Sierra Crest. Consequently, the trail is heavily used. The climb to the pass still requires an elevation gain of more than 2,500 feet in 5 miles at high altitude, but the ascent is short by eastern Sierra standards and rarely climbs at more than a moderate grade.

Relative ease alone is not what makes this trail so popular; its stunning scenery composed of serrated peaks, glistening subalpine lakes, flower-filled meadows, and rushing streams are the real lures. In addition, short connections to the John Muir Trail (JMT) and Bubbs Creek Trail offer a bounty of options for trip extensions, including the ever popular Rae Lakes. Unfortunately, severe overuse has resulted in a camping ban at Bullfrog Lake and a two-night limit at Kearsarge Lakes.

DIRECTIONS TO TRAILHEAD: From US 395 in Independence, turn west onto Market Street, and proceed out of town for 12.5 miles on steep and winding Onion Valley Road to the parking area. A campground, vault toilets, and running water are near the trailhead.

DESCRIPTION: Locate the signed trailhead near the restroom building (running water is usually available), and climb moderately across a sagebrush-covered slope, soon reaching the first of several switchbacks. Nearing Golden Trout Creek, a short spur to the Golden Trout Lakes Trail comes in from the right. Proceed through manzanita, mountain mahogany, and widely scattered red fir and limber pine into the Independence Creek drainage. After the wilderness

boundary, more switchbacks zigzag across a steep hillside, as the trail plays hide-and-seek with the creek. At one point, the wildflower-lined stream is handy enough for a thirst-slaking break.

Along the ascent, you have fine views down the canyon and across Owens Valley to the Inyo Mountains. To the south, University Peak looms above. More gently graded switchbacks lead to Little Pothole Lake at 1.5 miles from the trailhead. The willow-lined lake is attractively set in a compact, half moon–shaped basin, where waterfalls pour down cliffs and flow briefly through willow patches into the lake. There are a few overused campsites scattered around the shore beneath foxtail pines.

More switchbacks lead away from the lake and up the canyon to a long talus slope. Beyond, you return to the banks of Independence Creek and soon reach Gilbert Lake, 2.2 miles from the trailhead. Gilbert

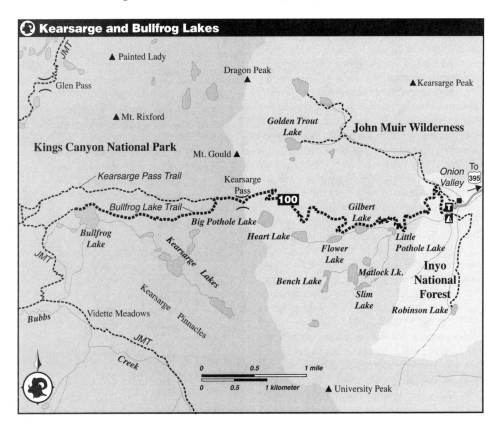

Kearsarge and Bullfrog Lakes

Painted Lady

Dragon Peak

Kearsarge Peak

Glen Pass

Mt. Rixford

Golden Trout Lake

John Muir Wilderness

Kings Canyon National Park

Mt. Gould

Kearsarge Pass Trail

Kearsarge Pass

Onion Valley

To 395

Bullfrog Lake Trail

100

Gilbert Lake

Big Pothole Lake

Little Pothole Lake

Bullfrog Lake

Heart Lake

Flower Lake

Inyo National Forest

Kearsarge Lakes

Bench Lake

Matlock Lk.

Slim Lake

Robinson Lake

Bubbs

Vidette Meadows

Kearsarge Pinnacles

JMT

Creek

0   0.5   1 mile

0   0.5   1 kilometer

University Peak

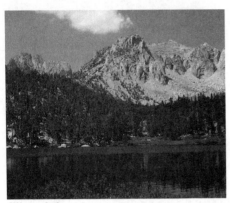

Gilbert Lake

is an oval lake with a pleasant backdrop of craggy spires. Grassy meadows dotted with clumps of willow ring the shore and provide straightforward access for anglers plying the waters for brook and brown trout, although the lake's proximity to the trailhead usually means that it is fished out by midseason; however, swimming should be quite refreshing by then. There are plenty of overused campsites here as well.

The trail follows a gentle course around the north side of the lake before resuming the ascent along Independence Creek. Shortly, you reach the vicinity of Flower Lake, where a short spur heads down to a forest-rimmed shore harboring good campsites. Anglers can fish for brook trout.

Near the north side of Flower Lake, switchbacks veer northeast to attack a headwall, zigzagging through scattered whitebark and foxtail pines on the way to an overlook of Heart Lake. Additional switchbacks climb through diminishing timber and rockier terrain to another overlook, where photogenic Big Pothole Lake pops into view. Despite its name, given by Joseph N. Le Conte, the deep-blue lake, set in a horseshoe-shaped cirque below the Sierra Crest is quite scenic and worth the short cross-country ramble necessary to visit it. Although it has no permanent inlet or outlet, the lake is reported to harbor a small population of brook trout. There are a smattering of exposed campsites around its austere shoreline.

Now the trail crosses stark, shalelike terrain via some long-legged switchbacks on the way toward the pass. A smattering of gnarled, dwarfed whitebark pines defy the elements at this altitude and cling desperately to small pockets of soil, appearing more like wind-blasted shrubs than actual trees. A moderate, upward traverse culminates in a sweeping vista at 11,823-foot Kearsarge Pass, from where Kearsarge and Bullfrog Lakes shimmer beneath the Sierra sun. Above the lakes rest the Kearsarge Pinnacles, and farther out is the crenellated crest of the Kings-Kern Divide. The impressive peak directly west is 11,868-foot Mt. Bago. The pass marks the boundary between the John Muir Wilderness behind you and the backcountry of Kings Canyon National Park ahead.

A moderately steep descent leads toward more hospitable terrain below. Near timberline, 0.7 mile from the pass, you reach a junction with the Bullfrog Lake Trail heading south toward Kearsarge Lakes.

TREAD LIGHTLY

Originally, the main trail from Kearsarge Pass followed the older route now known as the Bullfrog Lake Trail. The new alignment minimizes the tremendously destructive impact continuous overuse had created at Bullfrog and Kearsarge Lakes. The relocation of the trail away from the lake basin, along with a ban on camping at Bullfrog Lake and a two-night limit at Kearsarge Lakes, has sufficiently dissuaded the hordes of backpackers who previously visited the area. While traveling in this area, please be ultrasensitive to the environment by observing all minimum-impact practices and regulations.

Now on the Bullfrog Lake Trail, follow switchbacks down the slope, crossing several seasonal streams on the way toward Kearsarge Lakes. Approximately 0.3 mile from the junction, a faint use trail branches south from the main trail toward the northernmost lakes. You head across a granite-filled basin through widely scattered clumps of whitebark pines and past a pair of delightful tarns to the largest of the Kearsarge Lakes (10,895 feet). Tucked beneath the impressive wall of the serrated Kearsarge Pinnacles, the lakes are quite picturesque. Use trails lead to plentiful campsites and bear boxes. Anglers should find that the rainbow trout sufficiently test their skills.

Back on the main Bullfrog Lake Trail, head west on a moderate descent through stunted pines and pockets of meadow, hopping across numerous rivulets along the way. Soon the trail approaches the main branch of the creek and proceeds through delightful meadowlands to the north shore of scenic Bullfrog Lake.

Near the edge of the blue-green waters of Bullfrog Lake, you realize why this area was so popular with backpackers—the meadow-rimmed lake rivals any other Sierra lake for picturesque scenery. Across the deep trench of Bubbs Creek, the pyramidal summit of East Vidette rises sharply into the sky, providing a dramatic counterpoint to the usually placid waters of Bullfrog Lake. Above the shore, clumps of pine shelter former campsites graced with stunning views.

OPTIONAL RETURN VIA JMT: Rather than simply return the way you came, continue west to the JMT and head northbound to a junction with the Kearsarge Pass Trail for a slightly longer semiloop back to Kearsarge Pass. Follow gently graded tread along the north shore of Bullfrog Lake followed by a moderate descent. The grade eases momentarily near a pair of meadow-rimmed ponds before the moderate descent resumes, passing through scattered lodgepole pines on the way to the JMT junction.

Turn right and climb for 0.3 mile to a sandy flat and a four-way junction with the Charlotte Lake and Kearsarge Pass Trails. The 0.75-mile Charlotte Lake Trail leads to campsites (with a bear box) and a seasonal ranger station. Follow the Kearsarge Pass Trail northeast, soon encountering a Y-junction with a spur providing a shortcut

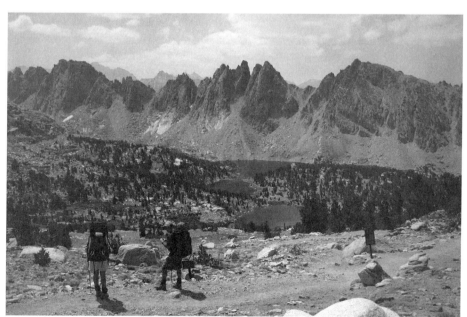

Kearsarge Lakes backdropped by Kearsarge Pinnacles

to the JMT for northbound hikers from Kearsarge Pass. Bear right (east) at the junction, and travel 2 miles on a steady climb to the Bullfrog Lake Trail junction. From there, retrace your steps to the Onion Valley Trailhead.

◯ A straightforward cross-country route from Gilbert Lake and a faint use trail from Flower Lake both lead across a low ridge into the forested cirque of Slim (10,545 feet) and Matlock (10,558 feet) Lakes. Hidden in the shadow of University Peak, these lakes provide anglers with a better opportunity to fish for brook and rainbow trout than the more popular lakes along the Kearsarge Pass Trail do; backpackers should appreciate the lesser-used campsites as well. Even less visited is Bench Lake (10,889 feet), a short but steep jaunt from the lower lakes.

To visit Heart Lake, follow a faint path west from Flower Lake upstream along a creek to the east shore. The lake is seldom visited, even though it lies just 0.1 mile from the Kearsarge Pass Trail. There are fine campsites beneath whitebark pines at the east end. Fishing for rainbow and brook trout is reported to be fair.

An ascent of 13,005-foot Mt. Gould is relatively straightforward from Kearsarge Pass.

R A wilderness permit is required for overnight stays. Camping is prohibited at Bullfrog Lake, and there's a two-night limit at Kearsarge and Charlotte Lakes. Bear canisters are required. Campfires are prohibited.

ONION VALLEY TRAILHEAD

TRIP 101

Charlotte Lake and Rae Lakes Basin

Ⓜ ╱ BP

DISTANCE: 28.6 miles, out-and-back

ELEVATION: 9,185'/11,823'/10,790'/ 11,978'/10,540', +4,050'/-2,685'/±13,470'

SEASON: Mid-July to early October

USE: Heavy

MAPS: USGS's *Kearsarge Peak* and *Mt. Clarence King* or Tom Harrison Maps' *Kearsarge Pass-Rae Lakes Loop Trail Map*

TRAIL LOG

2.3	Gilbert Lake
2.6	Flower Lake
6.0	Kearsarge Pass
7.5	John Muir Trail junction
9.5	Glen Pass
11.4	Sixty Lakes Basin Trail junction
14.3	Rae Lakes Ranger Station

INTRODUCTION: The Rae Lakes Basin is arguably one of the prettiest alpine basins in the Sierra Nevada. Large numbers of backpackers certainly think so—this is one of most heavily used and regulated backcountry areas outside of the Whitney Zone (bear canisters are required, and there's a two-night camping limit). Restrictions aside, a trip to the Rae Lakes may be the quintessential High Sierra outing. Along the way you encounter a wide range of environments, including the arid eastern Sierra approach, the above timberline moonscape at Kearsarge Pass, the serene forest around Charlotte Lake, and the splendid alpine and subalpine scenery around Rae Lakes. Toss in some wildflower-laden meadows, sparkling streams, and splendid views, and

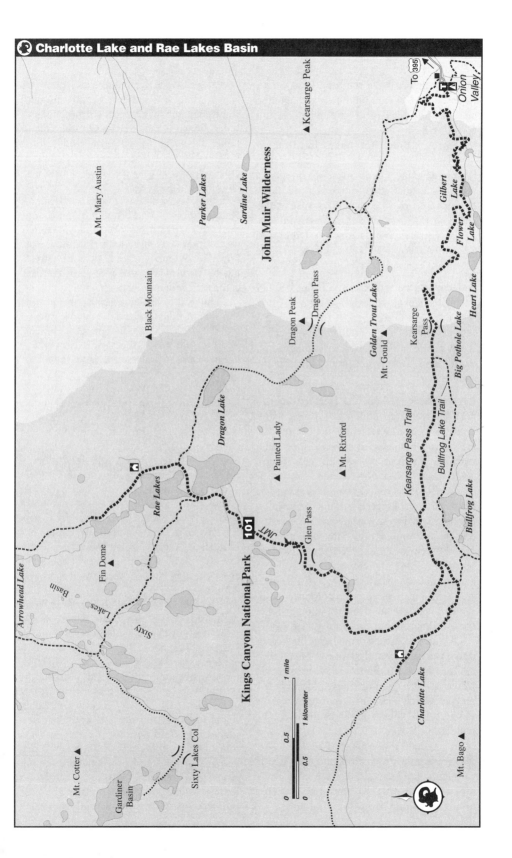

Kearsarge Peak ▲

To 395

Onion Valley

Mt. Mary Austin ▲

Parker Lakes

Sardine Lake

Black Mountain ▲

John Muir Wilderness

Gilbert Lake

Flower Lake

Heart Lake

Dragon Peak

Dragon Pass

Golden Trout Lake

Mt. Gould ▲

Kearsarge Pass

Big Pothole Lake

Dragon Lake

Rae Lakes

Painted Lady ▲

Mt. Rixford ▲

Kearsarge Pass Trail

Bullfrog Lake Trail

Bullfrog Lake

Arrowhead Lake

Fin Dome ▲

Sixty Lakes Basin

Kings Canyon National Park

101

JMT

Glen Pass

Charlotte Lake

Mt. Bago ▲

Mt. Cotter ▲

Gardiner Basin

Sixty Lakes Col

1 mile

1 kilometer

0.5

0.5

0

you may indeed have the total High Sierra experience. Off-trail enthusiasts have the added bonus of side trips to Sixty Lakes and Gardiner Basins.

Since reaching Rae Lakes from Onion Valley involves crossing two high passes, Kearsarge and Glen, most backpackers should consider the journey a multiday outing. Besides, the terrain is spectacular enough to warrant any extra time you have to devote to it. Both Kearsarge Lakes and Charlotte Lake offer excellent spots for a first night's camp.

DIRECTIONS TO TRAILHEAD: From US 395 in Independence, turn west onto Market Street, and proceed out of town for 12.5 miles on steep and winding Onion Valley Road to the parking area. A campground, vault toilets, and running water are near the trailhead.

DESCRIPTION: Locate the signed trailhead near the restroom building (running water is usually available), and climb moderately across a sagebrush-covered slope, soon reaching the first of several switchbacks. Nearing Golden Trout Creek, a short spur to the Golden Trout Lakes Trail comes in from the right. Proceed through manzanita, mountain mahogany, and widely scattered red fir and limber pine into the Independence Creek drainage. After the wilderness boundary, more switchbacks zigzag across a steep hillside, as the trail plays hide-and-seek with the creek. At one point, the wildflower-lined stream is handy enough for a thirst-slaking break.

Along the ascent, you have fine views down the canyon and across Owens Valley to the Inyo Mountains. To the south, University Peak looms above. More gently graded switchbacks lead to Little Pothole Lake at 1.5 miles from the trailhead. The willow-lined lake is attractively set in a compact, half moon–shaped basin, where waterfalls pour down cliffs and flow briefly through willow patches into the lake. There are a few overused campsites scattered around the shore beneath foxtail pines.

More switchbacks lead away from the lake and up the canyon to a long talus slope. Beyond, you return to the banks of Independence Creek and soon reach Gilbert Lake, 2.2 miles from the trailhead. Gilbert is an oval lake with a pleasant backdrop of craggy spires. Grassy meadows dotted with clumps of willow ring the shore and provide straightforward access for anglers plying the waters for brook and brown trout, although the lake's proximity to the trailhead usually means that it is fished out by midseason; however, swimming should be quite refreshing by then. There are plenty of overused campsites here as well.

The trail follows a gentle course around the north side of the lake before resuming the ascent along Independence Creek. Shortly, you reach the vicinity of Flower Lake, where a short spur heads down to a forest-rimmed shore harboring good campsites. Anglers can fish for brook trout.

Near the north side of Flower Lake, switchbacks veer northeast to attack a headwall, zigzagging through scattered whitebark and foxtail pines on the way to an overlook of Heart Lake. Additional switchbacks climb through diminishing timber and rockier terrain to another overlook, where photogenic Big Pothole Lake pops into view. Despite its name, given by Joseph N. Le Conte, the deep-blue lake, set in a horseshoe-shaped cirque below the Sierra Crest, is quite scenic and worth the short cross-country ramble necessary to visit it. Although it has no permanent inlet or outlet, the lake is reported to harbor a small population of brook trout. There are a smattering of exposed campsites around its austere shoreline.

Now the trail crosses stark, shalelike terrain via some long-legged switchbacks on the way toward the pass. A smattering of gnarled, dwarfed whitebark pines defy the elements at this altitude and cling desperately to small pockets of soil, appearing more like wind-blasted shrubs than actual trees. A moderate, upward traverse culminates in a sweeping vista at 11,823-foot Kearsarge Pass, from where Kearsarge and Bullfrog Lakes shimmer beneath the Sierra sun. Above the lakes rest the Kearsarge Pinnacles and farther out is the crenellated crest of the Kings-Kern Divide. The impressive peak directly west is 11,868-foot Mt. Bago. The pass marks the boundary between the John Muir Wilderness behind you and the backcountry of Kings Canyon National Park ahead.

A moderately steep descent leads toward more hospitable terrain below. Near timberline, 0.7 mile from the pass, you reach a junction with the Bullfrog Lake Trail heading south toward Kearsarge Lakes. Unless you're planning to camp at one of the Kearsarge Lakes, continue west on the Kearsarge Pass Trail, entering more hospitable terrain, where meadow grasses, clumps of willow, and scattered wildflowers watered by seasonal streams soften the rocky slopes. Fine view of Kearsarge Pinnacles and Lakes are your constant companions along the moderate descent. Farther on, scenic Bullfrog Lake pops into view, framed by the spiked summits of East and West Vidette across the deep chasm of Bubbs Creek canyon, joined by Junction and Center Peaks to the south. Eventually, the expansive views diminish, obscured by a scattered to light forest of whitebark and foxtail pines. Continue to a Y-junction with a spur that offers a shortcut for hikers northbound on the John Muir Trail (JMT).

SIDE TRIP TO CHARLOTTE LAKE: To visit Charlotte Lake, go straight at the spur junction, heading south and then southwest through forest until breaking out into the open at a sandy flat with a four-way junction with the JMT and Charlotte Lake Trail, 0.3 mile from the previous junction. Head west and then northwest on a 0.75-mile, winding, forested descent to the lake (10,370 feet).

Charlotte is a delightful lake, rimmed by pines and nearly surrounded by high hills. At the outlet on the northwest end, a splayed, V-shaped notch frames the sunset. As the only lake with decent campsites close to the JMT between Forester and Glen Passes, Charlotte receives a fair amount of use, which has resulted in a two-night limit.

Campsites (with a bear box) and a patrol cabin occupy the northeast shore. Solitude seekers may find a few more secluded campsites scattered around the south and southwest shores. Anglers will be tempted by rainbow and brook trout. **END OF SIDE TRIP**

Unless you're bound for a campsite at Charlotte Lake, veer right at the junction, and follow the spur trail 0.2 mile to a junction with the JMT. Turn right and head northbound on a gently graded section of the JMT, with periodic views of Charlotte Lake through the trees. Where the grade increases, granite Charlotte Dome springs briefly into view down the Charlotte Creek drainage. Proceed into rock- and boulder-filled terrain, which will accompany you all the way over Glen Pass until more hospitable terrain appears just above Rae Lakes. As the trail bends east, make a short descent before the climbing resumes and you bend back around to the north. A pair of marginal campsites appears near a seasonal stream, which are even less desirable after the stream quits running.

Beyond, steeper switchbacks lead past a couple of greenish tarns. Gazing toward the vicinity of Glen Pass, your mind should remain steadfast in the knowledge that a trail as significant as the JMT must somehow cross the formidable crest ahead. More switchbacks and more climbing eventually lead up the rocky headwall to Glen Pass (11,978 feet), 2 miles from the junction. Because of the cirque headwall's angle, the view from the pass is not as remarkable as some of the other high passes on the JMT, but the Rae Lakes Basin below is certainly a welcome sight.

Follow the crest of the ridge momentarily before beginning a rocky, winding descent that may seem a bit tedious. The grade eases a bit where you cross a tarn-dotted bench, until another series of switchbacks lead down the slope. Eventually, signs of life become more evident along the banks of rollicking rivulets, where wildflowers, sedges, grasses, and small shrubs tenuously hold onto small pockets of soil. Farther down, scattered pines give further evidence of the more temperate surroundings.

Still more switchbacks lead across additional watercourses and finally down to the uppermost Rae Lake (10,541 feet). The JMT continues along the northwest side of the upper lake toward an isthmus separating it from the middle lake. Just before the isthmus, reach a junction with the trail to Sixty Lakes Basin, 1.9 miles from Glen Pass.

SIDE TRIP TO SIXTY LAKES BASIN: Any trip to Rae Lakes without a visit to Sixty Lakes Basin would be incomplete. Although the trail is unmaintained, the route through the basin has been so well used over the years that defined tread is easy to follow. Once you are in the mostly open basin, cross-country travel between the lakes is fairly straightforward, with plenty of nooks and crannies awaiting exploration.

From the junction at the northwest shore of Upper Rae Lake, head south along the southwest shore of the middle lake, traverse a marshy clearing, and climb northwest to the lip of a small basin overlooking a tarn below. The view of Rae Lakes during this ascent is superb. Drop around the north side of the tarn, and climb shortly up to a saddle in the ridge dividing Rae Lakes and Sixty Lakes Basins, where Mt. Clarence King and Mt. Cotter dominate the impressive view to the northwest. A winding, rocky descent leads to the shore of an irregularly shaped lake (approximately 10,925 feet), with campsites near its outlet.

Continuing northwest, round a ridge and enter the heart of Sixty Lakes Basin, approaching a sizable, island-dotted lake (approximately 10,795 feet), 1.9 miles from the junction. The trail continues north from here, eventually deteriorating to a cross-country route following the basin's outlet stream to a junction with the JMT, just south of Baxter Creek. You also have the option of returning to the JMT over Basin Notch, via a straightforward route through a gap in a ridge about 1 mile north of Fin Dome. From the notch, descend to the west shore of Arrowhead Lake, and work around the lake to the JMT above the east shore.
END OF SIDE TRIP

Beyond the Sixty Lakes Basin junction, follow the JMT to a ford of the short stretch of creek between the upper and middle lakes, and then continue around the east shorelines of the middle and lower lakes. A patrol cabin sits just up the hill above the northeast shore.

The Rae Lakes Basin is characterized by beautiful aquamarine lakes dotted with tiny islands, by shorelines of rolling granite humps interspersed with pockets of verdant meadow and scattered pines, and by a border of steep cliffs and picturesque peaks. Fine views of exfoliated Fin Dome, multicolored Painted Lady, and King Spur are common throughout the basin. There are campsites (with bear boxes) around the middle and lower lakes. Despite the area's popularity, fishing for rainbow and brook trout is reported to be quite good. The sublime beauty of the basin and the plentiful options for further wanderings are attractive enough to easily pass whatever time you spend here.

In addition to the must-do trip into Sixty Lakes Basin, Dragon Lake, a half mile east of the JMT, is worth a visit. There are decent campsites scattered around the lake.

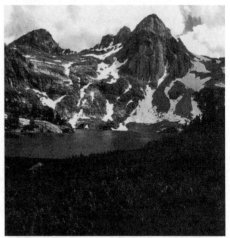

The multicolored Painted Lady above the Rae Lakes

Experienced cross-country enthusiasts can alter their return to the Onion Valley Trailhead by crossing the Sierra Crest at Dragon Pass (12,800 feet), also known as Gould Pass, which lies halfway between Dragon Peak and Mt. Gould. This Class 2 route involves a seemingly interminable scramble over loose talus south of Dragon Lake to the easternmost of three unnamed tarns, which then climbs more talus to the steep chute leading up to the pass. More talus awaits on the far side of the pass until you reach the tread of an unmaintained trail from Golden Trout Lake. Beyond the lake, the more defined tread of the Golden Trout Lakes Trail (see Trip 105, page 372) leads back to the trailhead.

Peakbaggers are at a disadvantage in the basin, since most of the routes on the nearby mountains are technical climbs. Painted Lady is perhaps the easiest ascent; rated Class 2, the route leaves the JMT from the granite bench below Glen Pass and ascends the west face to the summit.

R A wilderness permit is required for overnight stays. Rae Lakes Basin has a two-night camping limit. Campfires are prohibited. Bear canisters required.

ONION VALLEY TRAILHEAD

TRIP 102

Trans-Sierra Trek: Onion Valley to Cedar Grove

Ⓜ / DH or BP

DISTANCE: 22.3 miles, point-to-point

ELEVATION: 9,185'/11,823'/5,045', +2,845'/-4,140'/±13,970'

SEASON: Mid-July to mid-October

USE: Heavy

MAPS: USGS's *Kearsarge Peak, Mt. Clarence King,* and *The Sphinx* or Tom Harrison Maps' *Kearsarge Pass-Rae Lakes Loop Trail Map*

TRAIL LOG

2.4	Gilbert Lake
2.7	Flower Lake
6.0	Kearsarge Pass
6.7	Bullfrog Lake Trail junction
8.9	John Muir Trail junction
10.2	Bubbs Creek Trail junction
12.5	Junction Meadow
18.8	Sphinx Creek Camp
22.3	Roads End Trailhead

INTRODUCTION: This route provides the least difficult east-west traverse across the High Sierra. However, the trip is not easy: the long drive between Onion Valley and Roads End Trailheads, which requires almost as much time as the hike itself, is enough to deter most hikers. You have to decide whether to attempt this trip as a dayhike or as an overnight backpack. The main advantage to a one-day trip is not having to carry a full backpack, but the 21-mile distance requires an early start and excellent conditioning. Additionally, dayhikers do not have to compete for the limited number of wilderness permits. Backpackers will need more time to complete the journey,

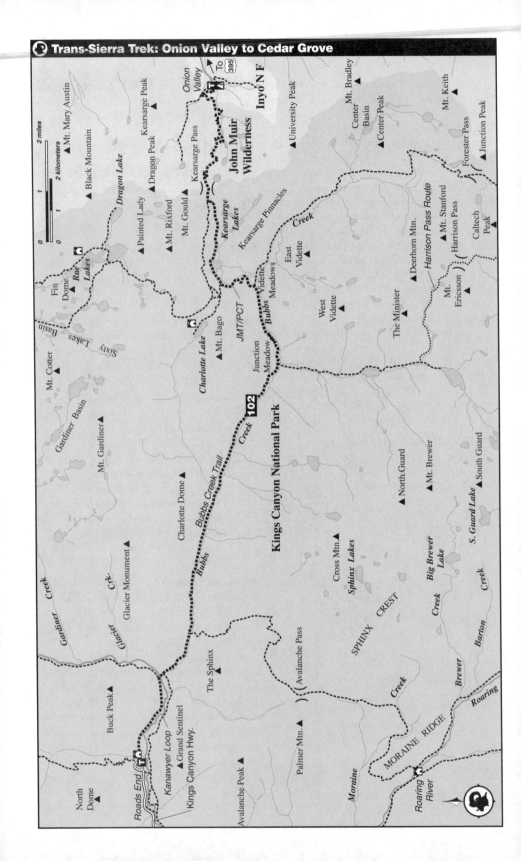

but they can appreciate the scenery at a slower pace.

Whatever time frame you chose, you will be treated to some great scenery and diverse flora. Starting in Onion Valley, in a typical eastside environment, you climb through subalpine and alpine zones to Kearsarge Pass, passing a lovely set of lakes in the Independence Creek drainage along the way. Beyond the pass, a nearly 6,800-foot descent leads through dramatic alpine and subalpine realms of Kearsarge and Bullfrog Lakes and then down into mixed-coniferous forests along Bubbs Creek, intermixed with pockets of lovely, flower-filled meadows. The trip ends in stunningly beautiful Kings Canyon, a fitting climax for this classic High Sierra traverse.

DIRECTIONS TO TRAILHEAD:

START: From US 395 in Independence, turn west onto Market Street, and proceed out of town for 12.5 miles on steep and winding Onion Valley Road to the parking area. A campground, vault toilets, and running water are near the trailhead.

END: Follow Highway 180 east from Fresno into Kings Canyon, and continue to the parking lot at Roads End, 5 miles from the Cedar Grove turnoff.

DESCRIPTION: Locate the signed trailhead near the restroom building (running water is usually available), and climb moderately across a sagebrush-covered slope, soon reaching the first of several switchbacks. Nearing Golden Trout Creek, a short spur to the Golden Trout Lakes Trail comes in from the right. Proceed through manzanita, mountain mahogany, and widely scattered red fir and limber pine into the Independence Creek drainage. After the wilderness boundary, more switchbacks zigzag across a steep hillside, as the trail plays hide-and-seek with the creek. At one point, the wildflower-lined stream is handy enough for a thirst-slaking break.

Along the ascent, you have fine views down the canyon and across Owens Valley to the Inyo Mountains. To the south, University Peak looms above. More gently graded switchbacks lead to Little Pothole Lake at 1.5 miles from the trailhead. The willow-lined lake is attractively set in a compact, half moon–shaped basin, where waterfalls pour down cliffs and flow briefly through willow patches into the lake. There are a few overused campsites scattered around the shore beneath foxtail pines.

More switchbacks lead away from the lake and up the canyon to a long talus slope. Beyond, you return to the banks of Independence Creek and soon reach Gilbert Lake, 2.2 miles from the trailhead. Gilbert is an oval lake with a pleasant backdrop of craggy spires. Grassy meadows dotted with clumps of willow ring the shore and provide straightforward access for anglers plying the waters for brook and brown trout, although the lake's proximity to the trailhead usually means that it is fished out by midseason; however, swimming should be quite refreshing by then. There are plenty of overused campsites here as well.

The trail follows a gentle course around the north side of the lake before resuming the ascent along Independence Creek. Shortly, you reach the vicinity of Flower Lake, where a short spur heads down to a forest-rimmed shore harboring good campsites. Anglers can fish for brook trout.

Near the north side of Flower Lake, switchbacks veer northeast to attack a headwall, zigzagging through scattered whitebark and foxtail pines on the way to an overlook of Heart Lake. Additional switchbacks climb through diminishing timber and rockier terrain to another overlook, where photogenic Big Pothole Lake pops into view. Despite its name, given by Joseph N. Le Conte, the deep-blue lake, set in a horseshoe-shaped cirque below the Sierra Crest, is quite scenic and worth the short cross-country ramble. Without a permanent inlet or outlet, the lake is reported to harbor a small population of brook trout. There are a smattering of exposed campsites around its austere shoreline.

Now the trail crosses stark, shalelike terrain via some long-legged switchbacks on the way toward the pass. A smattering of gnarled, dwarfed whitebark pines defy the elements at this altitude and cling desperately to small pockets of soil, appearing more like wind-blasted shrubs than actual trees. A moderate, upward traverse culminates in a sweeping vista at 11,823-foot Kearsarge Pass, from where Kearsarge and Bullfrog Lakes shimmer beneath the Sierra sun. Above the lakes rest the Kearsarge Pinnacles and farther out is the crenellated crest of the Kings-Kern Divide. The impressive peak directly west is 11,868-foot Mt. Bago. The pass marks the boundary between the John Muir Wilderness behind you and the backcountry of Kings Canyon National Park ahead.

A moderately steep descent leads toward more hospitable terrain below. Near timberline, 0.7 mile from the pass, you reach a junction with the Bullfrog Lake Trail heading south toward Kearsarge Lakes.

Turn left and follow the Bullfrog Lake Trail down some switchbacks and across seasonal streams toward Kearsarge Lakes. About 0.3 mile from the junction, a faint use trail branches south across a granite basin through scattered whitebark pines and past a pair of delightful tarns to the largest of the Kearsarge Lakes (10,895 feet). From there, paths lead to the other lakes and campsites (with bear boxes) scattered about the basin.

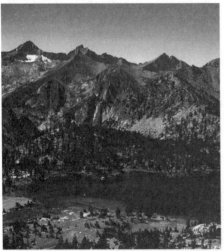
Bullfrog Lakes from the Kearsarge Pass Trail

From the junction of the use trail to the lakes, continue on the Bullfrog Lake Trail, heading west through stunted pines and pocket meadows on a moderate descent, hopping across seasonal streams along the way. Soon, the trail draws near to the main branch of the creek and proceeds through open meadowlands to Bullfrog Lake (10,895 feet). Near the edge of the blue-green waters of the lake, you realize why this area was so popular with backpackers—the meadow-rimmed lake rivals any other Sierra lake for picturesque scenery. Across the deep trench of Bubbs Creek, the pyramidal summit of East Vidette rises sharply into the sky and provides a dramatic counterpoint to the usually placid waters of Bullfrog Lake. Above the shore, clumps of pine shelter former campsites graced with stunning views.

Beyond the lake, the trail continues a mostly moderate descent through scattered lodgepole pines to a junction with the John Muir Trail (JMT), 2.2 miles from the previous junction between the Kearsarge Pass and Bullfrog Lakes Trails.

Turn left (south) on the JMT, and descend toward Bubbs Creek. After a pair of crossings over Bullfrog Lake's outlet, follow steep switchbacks down the wall of the canyon to Lower Vidette Meadow and a junction with the Bubbs Creek Trail, 1.3 miles from the previous junction.

Following a sign toward Cedar Grove, leave the JMT, and head west on the Bubbs Creek Trail, making a short descent to the north edge of expansive Lower Vidette Meadow. Overnighters will find excellent campsites (with a bear box) nestled beneath lodgepole pines along the meadow's fringe. Leaving the gently graded trail along the meadows behind, begin a pronounced descent, following the now tumbling creek plunging down the gorge. Momentarily break out into the open, where a large hump of granite offers an excellent vantage from which to survey the surrounding landscape.

Head back into the trees, and continue downstream, stepping over numerous lushly lined freshets along the way. Switchbacking periodically, you have occasional views of the dramatic topography above East Creek gorge, including rugged Mt. Brewer, North Guard, and Mt. Farquhar. Farther down the canyon, picturesque waterfalls and cascades on Bubbs Creek provide additional visual treats.

The stiff descent eventually eases nearing the grassy, fern-filled, and wildflower-covered clearing of Junction Meadow (approximately 8,190 feet), as you stroll over to a three-way junction with the East Creek Trail toward East Lake and Lake Reflection, 2.3 miles from the JMT junction. Overnights may find campsites down this trail on either side of the ford of Bubbs Creek. There are additional campsites farther west on the Bubbs Creek Trail, at the west edge of the meadow past the horse packer camp.

The moderate descent down the canyon resumes away from Junction Meadow, following the turbulent creek through a moderate forest of mainly white firs. After nearly 2 miles of steady descent, the creek mellows; you hike on gently graded tread through a grove of aspens and ferns on the way to a log crossing of Charlotte Creek. Nearby, a short spur leads to fair campsites near Bubbs Creek, where fishing for rainbow, brook, and brown trout is reported to be good.

Gently graded trail continues for a bit beyond Charlotte Creek. You hop across a trio of rills, and walk through shoulder-high ferns, and then Bubbs Creek returns to a tumultuous course down the gorge. The trail follows a steady, moderate descent for the next several miles. As you head farther down the canyon, the moderate fir forest gives way to a light cover of mostly Jeffrey pines, with a smattering of firs, incense cedars, and black oaks. At 8.3 miles from

the JMT junction, reach Sphinx Creek Camp and a three-way junction with the Sphinx Creek Trail. Excellent, heavily used campsites (with bear boxes) on either side of the log-and-plank bridge spanning Bubbs Creek will appeal to overnighters seeking one final night under the stars.

Away from Sphinx Creek Camp, the descent resumes across the east side of the canyon well above the creek, passing through thickening conifers. Soon, numerous switchbacks descend the steep wall of the canyon of South Fork Kings River. During the descent, gaps in the scrubby forest allow fine views into Kings Canyon below and The Sphinx above. Early in the season hikers have the added bonus of a spectacular cascade plunging across the steep granite wall of the canyon. The switchbacks eventually end at the floor of the canyon, near the first junction of the Kanawyer Loop Trail. Continue northwest and walk across a series of short, wood bridges over braided Bubbs Creek to a junction with the Kanawyer Loop and Paradise Valley Trails.

At the junction, turn west and follow gently descending tread along South Fork Kings River through a mixed forest of ponderosa pines, incense cedars, black oaks, sugar pines, and white firs. Just past a short bridge over Copper Creek, you pass the wilderness permit station and shortly reach Roads End Trailhead, 3.5 miles from Sphinx Creek Camp.

R A wilderness permit is required for overnight stays. Camping is limited to two nights at Kearsarge Lakes and prohibited at Bullfrog Lake. Campfires are allowed only along Bubbs Creek. Bear canisters are required.

TRIP 103

John Muir Trail:
Onion Valley to South Lake

(MS) / BP

DISTANCE: 61.2 miles, point-to-point

ELEVATION: 9,185'/11,823'/10,865'/
11,978'/8,547'/12,130'/
10,098'/12,100'/8,020'/
8,745'/11,972'/9,845',
+17,260'/-14,535'/±31,795'

SEASON: Late July to early October

USE: Heavy

MAPS: USGS's *Kearsarge Peak, Mt.
Clarence King, Mt. Pinchot,
Split Mountain, North
Palisade,* and *Mt. Thompson*
or Tom Harrison Maps' *John
Muir Trail Map-Pack*

TRAIL LOG

2.5	Gilbert Lake
2.8	Flower Lake
7.0	Kearsarge Pass
7.6	John Muir Trail junction
9.6	Glen Pass
11.5	Rae Lakes and Sixty Lakes Basin Trail junction
14.6	Baxter Pass Trail junction
18.3	Woods Creek crossing
19.1	Explorer Pass cross-country route
21.8	Sawmill Pass Trail junction
25.5	Pinchot Pass
28.5	Bench Lake junction
28.6	Taboose Pass Trail junction
30.1	South Fork Kings River crossing
32.8	Vennacher Col route
33.1	Mather Pass
36.7	Lower Palisade Lake and Cirque Pass route
40.2	Deer Meadow and Cataract Creek route
43.6	Middle Fork Trail junction
46.2	Grouse Meadow
47.0	Bishop Pass Trail junction
54.0	Bishop Pass
61.2	South Lake Trailhead

INTRODUCTION: This stretch of the John Muir Trail (JMT) between the Kearsarge Pass and Bishop Pass Trails is one of the most scenic along the 210-mile route. Backpackers must cross three 12,000-foot passes en route—Glen, Pinchot, and Mather—all of which provide fine vantages from which to observe the length and breadth of the High Sierra. Additionally, hikers will encounter three "holes"—Woods Creek, South Fork Kings River, and Le Conte Canyon. The trail also follows a lengthy romp up a portion of Middle Fork Kings River.

A number of picturesque basins provide rich scenery and a plethora of enticing campsites. Striking alpine peaks, exquisite lakes, rushing rivers, tumbling creeks, wildflower-covered meadows, and magnificent forests will delight wilderness lovers throughout the journey. Encompassing a wide range of elevation, the trip also exposes travelers to an equally diverse range of flora, including montane, subalpine, and alpine zones.

Aside from the usual concerns of a long-distance High Sierra backpacking trip, hikers should consider a few additional matters. Winters of average to above average snowfall may drape the high passes with snow, which can persist throughout much of the summer. When such conditions exist, you may need to use an ice axe to safely navigate the crossings. Additionally, the unbridged river and creek crossings may be unsafe during high water periods. Check with the Park Service about current conditions.

DIRECTIONS TO TRAILHEAD:
START: From US 395 in Independence, turn west onto Market Street, and proceed out of town for 12.5 miles on steep and winding Onion Valley Road to the parking area. A campground, vault toilets, and running water are near the trailhead.

END: From Bishop, leave US 395 and turn west onto Line Drive (which is known as South Lake Road and Highway 168 outside of town). Proceed southwest 15 miles to a junction with Lake Sabrina Road, and turn left, remaining on South Lake Road. Continue 6.75 miles to the end of the road near South Lake. Backpackers must park in the overnight lot (when full, additional parking may be available 1.3 miles back down the road—a footpath connects to the trailhead). Restrooms and water are available at the trailhead.

DESCRIPTION: From Onion Valley, locate the signed trailhead near the restroom building (running water is usually available), and climb moderately across a sagebrush-covered slope, soon reaching the first of several switchbacks. Nearing Golden Trout Creek, a short spur to the Golden Trout Lakes Trail comes in from the right. Proceed through manzanita, mountain mahogany, and widely scattered red fir and limber pine into the Independence Creek drainage. After the wilderness boundary, more switchbacks zigzag across a steep hillside, as the trail plays hide-and-seek with the creek. At one point, the wildflower-lined stream is handy enough for a thirst-slaking break.

Along the ascent, you have fine views down the canyon and across Owens Valley to the Inyo Mountains. To the south, University Peak looms above. More gently graded switchbacks lead to Little Pothole Lake at 1.5 miles from the trailhead. The willow-lined lake is attractively set in a compact, half moon–shaped basin, where waterfalls pour down cliffs and flow briefly through willow patches into the lake. There are a few overused campsites scattered around the shore beneath foxtail pines.

More switchbacks lead away from the lake and up the canyon to a long talus slope. Beyond, you return to the banks of Independence Creek and soon reach Gilbert Lake, 2.2 miles from the trailhead. Gilbert is an oval lake with a pleasant backdrop of craggy spires. Grassy meadows dotted with clumps of willow ring the shore and provide straightforward access for anglers plying the waters for brook and brown trout, although the lake's proximity to the trailhead usually means that it is fished out by midseason;

however, swimming should be quite refreshing by then. There are plenty of overused campsites here as well.

The trail follows a gentle course around the north side of the lake before resuming the ascent along Independence Creek. Shortly, you reach the vicinity of Flower Lake, where a short spur heads down to a forest-rimmed shore harboring good campsites. Anglers can fish for brook trout.

Near the north side of Flower Lake, switchbacks veer northeast to attack a headwall, zigzagging through scattered whitebark and foxtail pines on the way to an overlook of Heart Lake. Additional switchbacks climb through diminishing timber and rockier terrain to another overlook, where photogenic Big Pothole Lake pops into view. Despite its name, given by Joseph N. Le Conte, the deep-blue lake, set in a horseshoe-shaped cirque below the Sierra Crest, is quite scenic and worth the short cross-country ramble necessary to visit it. Although it has no permanent inlet or outlet, the lake is reported to harbor a small population of brook trout. There are a smattering of exposed campsites around its austere shoreline.

Now the trail crosses stark, shalelike terrain via some long-legged switchbacks on the way toward the pass. A smattering of gnarled, dwarf whitebark pines defy the elements at this altitude and cling desperately to small pockets of soil, appearing more like wind-blasted shrubs than actual trees. A moderate, upward traverse culminates in a sweeping vista at 11,823-foot Kearsarge Pass, from where Kearsarge and Bullfrog Lakes shimmer beneath the Sierra sun. Above the lakes rest the Kearsarge Pinnacles and farther out is the crenellated crest of the Kings-Kern Divide. The impressive peak directly west is 11,868-foot Mt. Bago. The pass marks the boundary between the John Muir Wilderness behind you and the backcountry of Kings Canyon National Park ahead.

A moderately steep descent leads toward more hospitable terrain below. Near timberline, 0.7 mile from the pass, you reach a junction with the Bullfrog Lake Trail

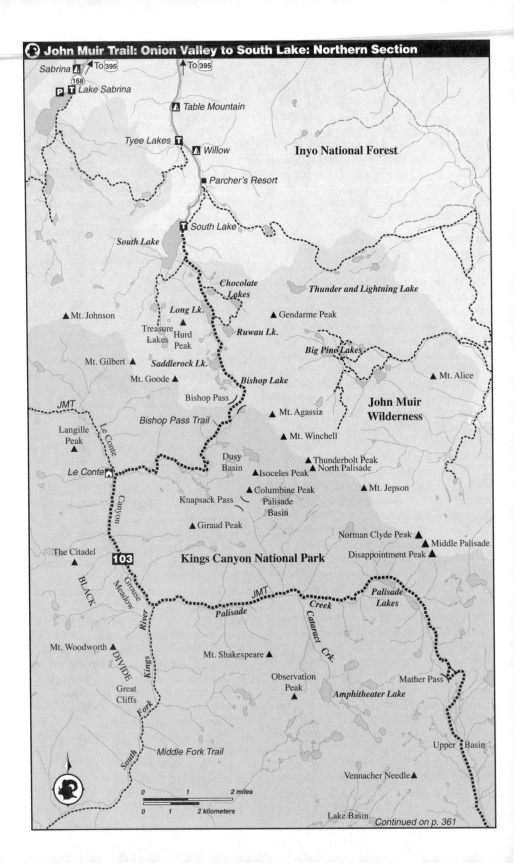

Sabrina △ ↑To 395 ↑To 395

(168)
P T Lake Sabrina

△ Table Mountain

Tyee Lakes T △ Willow **Inyo National Forest**

■ Parcher's Resort

T South Lake

South Lake

Chocolate Lakes

Thunder and Lightning Lake

▲ Mt. Johnson *Long Lk.* ▲ Gendarme Peak

Treasure Lakes Hurd Peak *Ruwau Lk.*

Mt. Gilbert ▲ *Saddlerock Lk.* *Big Pine Lakes* ▲ Mt. Alice

Mt. Goode ▲ *Bishop Lake*

Bishop Pass **John Muir Wilderness**

JMT *Bishop Pass Trail* ▲ Mt. Agassiz

Langille Peak ▲ ▲ Mt. Winchell

Le Conte Dusy Basin ▲ Thunderbolt Peak

Le Conte △ ▲ Isoceles Peak ▲ North Palisade

▲ Columbine Peak ▲ Mt. Jepson

Knapsack Pass Palisade Basin

Canyon ▲ Giraud Peak Norman Clyde Peak ▲

The Citadel ▲ Middle Palisade ▲

103 **Kings Canyon National Park** Disappointment Peak ▲

BLACK Grouse Meadow JMT *Creek* *Palisade Lakes*

Mt. Woodworth ▲ River *Palisade* Cataract Crk.

DIVIDE Kings

Great Cliffs Fork Mt. Shakespeare ▲

Observation Peak ▲ *Amphitheater Lake* Mather Pass

South

Middle Fork Trail Upper Basin

Vennacher Needle ▲

0   1   2 miles

0   1   2 kilometers

Lake Basin Continued on p. 361

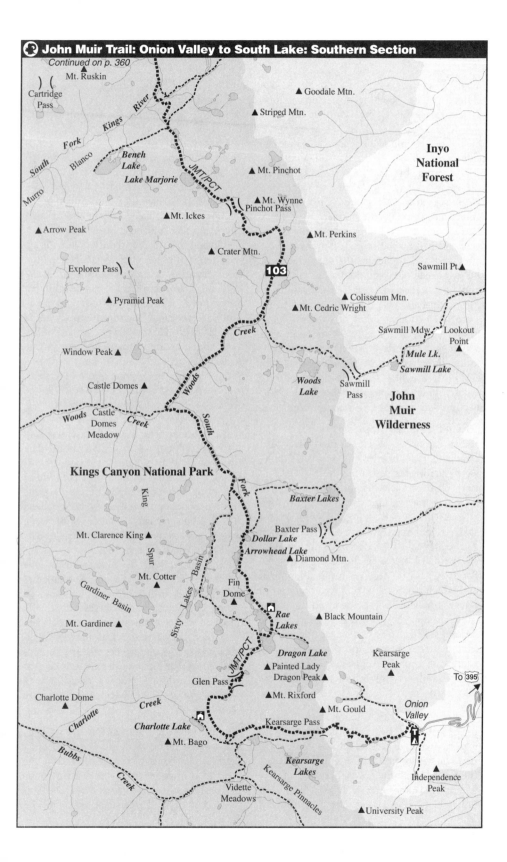

Continued on p. 360

▲ Mt. Ruskin

Cartridge
Pass

Kings   River

South   Fork   Blanco

Murro

**Bench
Lake**

Lake Marjorie

JMT/PCT

▲ Goodale Mtn.

▲ Striped Mtn.

**Inyo
National
Forest**

▲ Mt. Pinchot

▲ Mt. Wynne
Pinchot Pass

▲Mt. Ickes

▲ Arrow Peak

▲ Crater Mtn.

Explorer Pass)

▲ Pyramid Peak

▲Mt. Perkins

Sawmill Pt.▲

103

▲ Colisseum Mtn.

▲Mt. Cedric Wright

Sawmill Mdw. Lookout
Point

Mule Lk.

Window Peak ▲

Castle Domes ▲

Woods

Creek

**Woods
Lake**

Sawmill
Pass

Sawmill Lake

**John
Muir
Wilderness**

Woods   Castle   Creek
Domes
Meadow

Kings Canyon National Park

King

South   Fork

Baxter Lakes

Mt. Clarence King ▲

Spur

Baxter Pass)

Dollar Lake

Arrowhead Lake

▲ Diamond Mtn.

Mt. Cotter ▲

Gardiner Basin

Sixty   Lakes   Basin

Fin
Dome
▲

▲ Black Mountain

Mt. Gardiner ▲

**Rae
Lakes**

Dragon Lake

Kearsarge
Peak
▲

JMT/PCT

Glen Pass

▲ Painted Lady
Dragon Peak ▲

To 395

Charlotte Dome
▲

Creek

Charlotte

▲Mt. Rixford

Charlotte Lake

Kearsarge Pass

Onion
Valley

▲ Mt. Gould

▲Mt. Bago

Bubbs   Creek

**Kearsarge
Lakes**

Vidette
Meadows

Kearsarge Pinnacles

Independence
Peak
▲

▲University Peak

heading south toward Kearsarge Lakes. Unless you're planning to camp at one of the Kearsarge Lakes, continue west on the Kearsarge Pass Trail, entering more hospitable terrain, where meadow grasses, clumps of willow, and scattered wildflowers watered by seasonal streams soften the rocky slopes. Fine views of Kearsarge Pinnacles and Lakes are your constant companions along the moderate descent. Farther on, scenic Bullfrog Lake pops into view, framed by the spiked summits of East and West Vidette across the deep chasm of Bubbs Creek canyon, joined by Junction and Center Peaks to the south. Eventually, the expansive views diminish, obscured by a scattered to light forest of whitebark and foxtail pines. Continue to a Y-junction with a spur that offers a shortcut for hikers continuing northbound on the John Muir Trail (JMT). If you plan on bypassing Charlotte Lake, follow this spur for 0.2 mile to a connection with the JMT.

◻ SIDE TRIP TO CHARLOTTE LAKE: To access campsites at Charlotte Lake, head west and then northwest on a 0.75-mile, winding, forested descent to the lake (10,370 feet). Charlotte is a delightful lake, rimmed by pines and nearly surrounded by high hills. At the outlet on its northwest end, a splayed, V-shaped notch frames the sunset. As the only lake with decent campsites close to the JMT between Forester and Glen Passes, Charlotte receives a fair amount of use, which has resulted in a two-night limit. Campsites (with a bear box) and a patrol cabin occupy the northeast shore. Solitude seekers may find a few more secluded campsites scattered around the lake's south and southwest shores. Anglers will be tempted by rainbow and brook trout. **END OF SIDE TRIP**

At the four-way junction with the spur to Charlotte Lake, head northbound on a gently graded section of the JMT, with periodic views of Charlotte Lake through the trees. Where the grade increases, granite Charlotte Dome springs briefly into view down the Charlotte Creek drainage. Proceed into rock- and boulder-filled terrain, which will accompany you all the way over Glen Pass until more hospitable terrain appears just above Rae Lakes. As the trail bends east, make a short descent before the climbing resumes and you bend back around to the north. A pair of marginal campsites appears near a seasonal stream, which are even less desirable after the stream quits running. Beyond, steeper switchbacks lead past a couple of greenish tarns.

Gazing toward the vicinity of Glen Pass, your mind should remain steadfast in the knowledge that a trail as significant as the JMT must somehow cross the formidable crest ahead. More switchbacks and more climbing eventually lead up the rocky headwall to Glen Pass (11,978 feet), 2 miles from the junction. Because of the cirque headwall's angle, the view from the pass is not as remarkable as some of the other high passes on the JMT, but the Rae Lakes Basin below is certainly a welcome sight.

Follow the crest of the ridge momentarily before beginning a rocky, winding descent that may seem a bit tedious. The grade eases a bit where you cross a tarn-dotted bench, until another series of switchbacks lead down the slope. Eventually, signs of life become more evident along the banks of rollicking rivulets, where wildflowers, sedges, grasses, and small shrubs tenuously hold onto small pockets of soil.

Farther down, scattered pines give further evidence of the more temperate surroundings. Still more switchbacks lead across additional watercourses and finally down to the uppermost Rae Lake (10,541 feet). The JMT continues along the northwest side of the upper lake toward an isthmus separating it from the middle lake. Just before the isthmus, reach a junction with the trail to Sixty Lakes Basin, 1.9 miles from Glen Pass.

◻ SIDE TRIP TO SIXTY LAKES BASIN: Any trip to Rae Lakes without a visit to Sixty Lakes Basin would be incomplete. Although the trail is unmaintained, the route through the basin has been so well used over the years that defined tread is easy to follow.

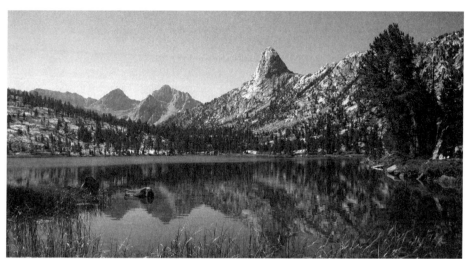

Arrowhead Lake

Once you are in the mostly open basin, cross-country travel between the lakes is fairly straightforward, with plenty of nooks and crannies awaiting exploration.

From the junction at the northwest shore of Upper Rae Lake, head south along the southwest shore of the middle lake, traverse a marshy clearing, and climb northwest to the lip of a small basin overlooking a tarn below. The view of Rae Lakes during this ascent is superb. Drop around the north side of the tarn, and climb shortly up to a saddle in the ridge dividing Rae Lakes and Sixty Lakes Basins, where Mt. Clarence King and Mt. Cotter dominate the impressive view to the northwest. A winding, rocky descent leads to the shore of an irregularly shaped lake (approximately 10,925 feet), with campsites near its outlet.

Continuing northwest, round a ridge and enter the heart of Sixty Lakes Basin, approaching a sizable, island-dotted lake (approximately 10,795 feet), 1.9 miles from the junction. The trail continues north from here, eventually deteriorating to a cross-country route following the basin's outlet stream to a junction with the JMT, just south of Baxter Creek. You also have the option of returning to the JMT over Basin Notch, via a straightforward route through a gap in a ridge about 1 mile north of Fin Dome. From the notch, descend to the west shore of Arrowhead Lake and work around the lake to the JMT above the east shore. **END OF SIDE TRIP**

Beyond the Sixty Lakes Basin junction, follow the JMT to a ford of the short stretch of creek between the upper and middle lakes and then continue around the east shorelines of the middle and lower lakes. A patrol cabin sits just up the hill above the northeast shore.

The Rae Lakes Basin is characterized by beautiful aquamarine lakes dotted with tiny islands, by shorelines of rolling granite humps interspersed with pockets of verdant meadow and scattered pines, and by a border of steep cliffs and picturesque peaks. Fine views of exfoliated Fin Dome, multicolored Painted Lady, and King Spur are common throughout the basin. There are campsites (with bear boxes) around the middle and lower lakes. Despite the area's popularity, fishing for rainbow and brook trout is reported to be quite good. The sublime beauty of the basin and the plentiful options for further wanderings are attractive enough to easily pass whatever time you spend here.

Beyond Lower Rae Lake, follow gently descending tread across a hillside dotted

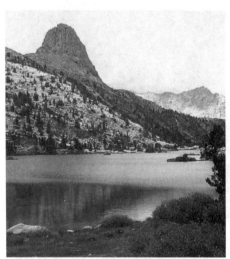

One of the Rae Lakes and Fin Dome

with widely scattered lodgepole pines, pass a pond, and then come above the east shore of meadow-rimmed Arrowhead Lake (10,292 feet), backdropped nicely by King Spur. The JMT reaches the level of the lake near the far shore, where a use trail branches away to potential campsites (with a bear box).

Cross Arrowhead Lake's outlet on a log just past a small waterfall, soon spying the next lake in the chain, Dollar Lake. A brief descent leads past steep cliffs and along the willow-choked creek to the north-west shore. Granite outcrops and groves of lodgepole pines share the west shore, and a large talus slope rises upward from the east shore toward Diamond Peak along the Sierra Crest. As from Rae Lakes above, fine views of Fin Dome and King Spur add a sublime sense of alpine beauty to the setting. Dollar Lake has a limited number of campsites—there are better sites back at Arrowhead Lake. Near the north shore is a junction with the little-used trail to Baxter Lakes and Pass, 3.1 miles from the Sixty Lakes junction. There are fair campsites around the largest Baxter Lake, 2.3 miles from Dollar Lake.

Leave the Rae Lakes area behind, and follow gently graded tread alongside South Fork Woods Creek through meadows, widely scattered lodgepole pines, and granite boulders. A mile-long descent leads through thickening forest to a crossing of the wildflower- and willow-lined stream draining Sixty Lakes Basin, with a pair of campsites nearby. Pass through a drift fence, descend a rocky ridge, and then come to a boggy meadow. Proceed across open, rocky terrain to the crossing of a small stream draining Lake 10315, and continue downstream, well above the South Fork, passing through stretches of lush vegetation, alternating with sagebrush-covered slopes and a light mixed forest of lodgepole pines, red firs, and aspens. The trail arcs around the end of King Spur and drops down to Woods Creek crossing, 1.7 miles from the Baxter Pass junction.

Numerous campsites nestle beneath red firs, lodgepole pines, aspens, and alders on either side of Woods Creek, which is a major stop for both thru-hikers on the JMT and backpackers on the Rae Lakes Loop—*don't expect solitude.* Although campfires are permitted, most of the firewood is already picked over early in the season. An impressive suspension bridge high above Woods Creek avoids the washouts that plague the previous bridges the Park Service had constructed.

On the north side of the bridge is a junction with the Paradise Valley Trail to Cedar Grove and Roads End Trailhead, which is 15 miles away. Heading northbound on the JMT, climb out of the deep cleft of Woods Creek through manzanita and scattered Jeffrey pines and junipers. Draw alongside Woods Creek cascading mightily down sloping slabs of granite in dramatic spouts, fountains, and swirling pools. Where the trail crosses a flower-lined tributary, the trees give way to a view up the canyon, including a lovely cascade on the stream draining Window Peak Lake. Continuing, you soon hop across this stream, 0.75 mile from Woods Crossing. The Explorer Pass cross-country route begins here (see options, page 369).

As you proceed up the canyon, take the time to turn around and enjoy the view into the deep cleft of Woods Creek, topped by the mighty ramparts of King Spur. Beyond a barbed wire fence, you ford White Fork Woods Creek; although potentially difficult early in the season, the creek should be a boulder hop later in the summer. The moderate climb continues through a lush area of wildflowers, ferns, willows, and aspens on the way to a set of switchbacks. After crossing a brook lined with flowers, enter lodgepole pine forest and pass a pair of campsites. In the midst of more switchbacks, break out into the open to a wonderful view of Mt. Cedric Wright. The winding trail crosses another creek and comes to the junction of the Sawmill Pass Trail, 3.5 miles from Woods Creek crossing. There are fine campsites along the creek or near Woods Lake (approximately 10,760 feet), 1.75 miles up this trail.

From the junction, follow gently graded tread west of Mt. Cedric Wright for a half mile to a junction with a short use trail on the right heading toward Twin Lakes. The lakes are set in an open, view-packed bowl below the rocky northwest slope of Mt. Cedric Wright. Scattered pines offer partial shade to fair campsites above the west shore of both lakes. Despite the lakes' location just off the JMT, overnight use seems to be light.

Back on the JMT, climb moderately through open terrain filled with grasses, sedges, and scattered clumps of whitebark pines, until the grade momentarily eases near a pond. There are a few fair campsites on a low hill east of the trail overlooking the pond. A moderate climb leads away from the pond through open terrain with expansive views of upper Woods Creek drainage, including the barren, rust-covered slopes of Mt. Wynne to the northwest. Unnamed tarns short distances off the trail offer secluded camping.

As you enter the above timberline realm, the trail curves west around a rocky hillside into a side canyon sprinkled with delightful tarns rimmed by small pockets of tundralike meadows. Beyond the meadows, a moderate climb leads across barren slopes filled with boulders and talus. A set of switchbacks leads you up to Pinchot Pass (12,110

feet), 3.7 miles from the Sawmill Pass junction. The splendid vista to the northwest reveals a string of sparkling tarns set in the stark canyon descending toward South Fork Kings River. In the distant northwest rise the dark, brooding summits of the Palisades. Behind, past the hulk of Mt. Cedric Wright, lies a seemingly endless sea of peaks.

From the pass, follow a rocky, zigzagging descent across barren slopes. Before reaching the first tarn below the pass, the grade mellows a bit, where patches of grass and a refreshing creek herald a welcome return to more hospitable terrain. Pass above the tarn on a winding, moderate descent across sandy slopes, broken by pockets of grassy meadow and scattered wildflowers. Proceed past a small pond and over a tiny stream to lovely Lake Marjorie (11,132 feet), 1.3 miles from the pass. The steep and dark gray cliffs of Mt. Ickes nicely frame the lake, which has a few spartan campsites among scattered whitebark pines.

Away from Lake Marjorie, the descent continues past lovely tarns, each with a few pleasant campsites nearby. Along the way, you cross a number of small rivulets successively bordered by increasing amounts of vegetation. Whitebark pines give way to lodgepole pines near the last tarn, where the inlet cascades over granite blocks before sinuously drifting across green meadows above the south shore. Passing along the tarn's west shore, reach an impressive view of Cirque Crest across the deep divide of the South Fork Canyon.

Beyond the tarn, a moderate descent leads through lush meadows and shrubs to a junction with the Bench Lake Trail on the left, 3 miles from Pinchot Pass. The 2-mile trail to Bench Lake is well worth the diversion for its excellent campsites and beautiful sunrises. Shortly after the junction, the JMT fords the creek, passes a lateral to a seasonal patrol cabin, and passes through light lodgepole pine forest on the way to a junction with the Taboose Pass Trail, 0.1 mile from the previous junction.

A moderate to steep descent from the junction winds down toward South Fork Kings River, as the roar of the water reverberates off the canyon walls. In the middle of the switchbacking descent, cross a tributary and proceed to the bottom of the forested canyon, reaching the riverbank at 4.6 miles from Pinchot Pass. You have to negotiate the churning waters using a combination of well-placed boulders and logs or else find a convenient place to ford. An islet just downstream divides the river into two channels, which may provide the safest crossing (but it still may be difficult early in the season). There are a limited number of campsites along the river, but you may find better sites a short way farther up the JMT.

After the long descent from Pinchot Pass, you now begin a 5.5-mile climb toward Mather Pass. A short way beyond the ford, a use trail heads downstream, providing access to off-trail routes down Murro Blanco or over Cartridge Pass. Remaining on the JMT, ascend the South Fork drainage to the north, crossing a couple of flower-lined side streams along the way. Near the second crossing, about 0.3 mile from the ford, an unsigned path veers right to fair campsites along the bank of the South Fork. Beyond these campsites, this path crosses the river and then climbs toward Taboose Pass.

Past the use trail junction, the ascent continues through wildflower-covered meadows and groves of lodgepole pines. About 0.75 mile from the South Fork crossing is a stream draining the slopes below Mt. Ruskin, where a cross-country route heads generally northwest toward Vennacher Col (see options, page 369). Farther on, ever expanding views of Upper Basin and distant Mather Pass drive you forward across numerous streams and rivulets and through sweeping terrain, composed of tranquil, wildflower-carpeted meadows, clumps of shrubs, scattered whitebark pines, and acres of granite boulders and slabs. The ever widening basin is encircled by steep, craggy ridges on three sides, culminating in the rugged Sierra Crest to the east. Cardinal Mountain (13,397 feet), Split Mountain (14,058 feet), and Mt. Prater (13,329 feet) stand guard along this spine, towering over the scenic basin.

Cross the nascent South Fork, and continue climbing through Upper Basin past timberline toward the seemingly impassable headwall below Mather Pass. Along the way, you hop across several rivulets and pass lovely tarns. Larger, more distant tarns issue a siren call, beckoning the unhurried traveler off the trail to explore the far reaches of the basin, which offers austere yet dramatically scenic locales for possible campsites. Approach the pass from the east, sweeping around the base of the headwall on a long, ascending traverse. With an incredible view as your companion, follow a series of switchbacks up to rockbound Mather Pass, 3 miles from the South Fork crossing.

Gazing north from the pass, you witness the dark-gray, 14,000-foot spires of the Palisades piercing the usually deep-blue Sierra sky. In a canyon to the northwest, dark tarns and the uppermost Palisade Lake contrast vividly with the surrounding granite basin. Final glimpses south of Upper Basin, east to Split Mountain, and northeast to Mt. Prater are stunning as well.

From Mather Pass, wind down rocky tread across a talus-covered slope. Signs of life—pockets of grasses, sedges, and wildflowers—start to appear between fields of boulders. Cross a number of flower-lined brooks along the descent, as widely scattered whitebark pines start to reappear. Along the way, you have fine views of Palisade Lakes and the surrounding peaks and ridges. About 2.25 miles from the pass, the trail passes well above the northeast shore of Upper Palisade Lake, crosses a picturesque stream cascading steeply down toward the lake through a willow- and flower-lined glade, and reaches a couple of small campsites just beyond the far bank (offering great views but little privacy). Pass across a hillside toward the far end of the upper lake to an area of lush vegetation near a pair of tiny rivulets.

Continue the descending traverse toward the lower lake on a series of granite benches interspersed with pockets of flora. After hopping across another charming rivulet that dances across the trail and tumbles down toward the lower lake, follow the trail around slabs and cliffs to a series of short-legged switchbacks, which drop you to the northwest shore of Lower Palisade Lake, 3.6 miles from the pass. If you're in need of a campsite, travel around the lake to its east end. Near the far (west) end of the lake, step across a stream below a picturesque waterfall pouring down a rock face.

Leaving Lower Palisade Lake, soon encounter a small, delightful side canyon, where yet another brook cascades down a hillside and then flows through clumps of willow and tiny pockets of wildflower-covered meadow before joining the main branch of Palisade Creek. Campers may find a cozy site somewhere around the floor of this petite basin. A cross-country route leaves the JMT here and climbs over Cirque Pass into Palisade Basin (see options, page 369). A short, pleasant stroll leads around the edge of this compact basin to the beginning of a major descent.

Ease into the descent, briefly following Palisade Creek before it plummets down short waterfalls, cataracts, and cascades toward the valley below. Soon, the trail makes a winding descent sandwiched between low humps of granite, with occasional glimpses of the plunging creek. Pass over a granite outcrop, from where there is an incredible view of the deep cleft 1,500 feet below, along with the towering peaks along the crest above; Mt. Shakespeare is southwest; Devils Crags, the Black Divide, and The Citadel rise sharply in the west; and 12,608-foot Giraud Peak dominates the skyline to the northwest.

Follow the trail around some cliffs to the start of a series of tight switchbacks, known as the Golden Staircase, carved straight out of the granite on the north wall of the canyon. The fact that this section of the 200-mile-plus trail was the last to be completed comes as no surprise to those who experience this section firsthand. Near the bottom, pass across a lushly vegetated hillside, well watered by a number of seeps, and continue down rocky tread to the floor of the canyon amid a forest of young aspens, lodgepole pines, and red firs.

The cool shade of the forest is quite welcome following the mostly exposed journey from Palisade Lakes, and your feet should appreciate the dirt trail carpeted with pine needles after the knee-wrenching descent along the rocky tread of the Golden Staircase. Pass campsites along the creek, cross braided Glacier Creek, and stroll above Deer Meadow, which, now covered with lodgepole pines, only faintly resembles a meadow anymore. Reach an unmarked junction, 3.5 miles from Lower Palisade Lake, with the old Cataract Creek Trail. There are some good campsites just beyond the junction.

On a moderate descent, cross the multibranched stream draining Palisade Basin to the north, and continue down the canyon. The forest here is composed primarily of lodgepole pines in the upper part of the canyon, with aspens, white firs, and Jeffrey pines mixed in farther downstream. Manzanita and snowbrush provide the principal ground cover. The first break in the timber occurs where a large avalanche tore through a stand of fair-size trees. About 2 miles from Deer Meadow, you enter a large clearing bordered by aspens and willows, known locally as Stillwater Meadow, where Palisade Creek glides lazily through the peaceful flat, reportedly offering good fishing for golden trout. There are fine campsites near the far end of the clearing.

Continue the descent away from Stillwater Meadow, as the gradient increases over the next mile. Wind down past the concrete supports for the former bridge spanning Palisade Creek, which provided access to the Middle Fork Trail. Flooding in the early 1980s destroyed the bridge, and the Park Service has no intentions of building a replacement. The descent concludes near the confluence of Palisade Creek with Middle Fork Kings River to a junction with the Middle Fork Trail, 3.4 miles from Deer Meadow. The small, forested flat nearby offers fair but overused campsites near the tumbling rapids on the Middle Fork. From the flat, a short path leads to a ford of the broad channel of Palisade Creek and the resumption of the Middle Fork Trail on the far side. This ford may be difficult early in the season.

A stiff climb away from the flat soon leads to a more moderate ascent, as you follow the course of the Middle Fork through light forest. Cross a stream draining a trio of unnamed lakes below the southeast face of Mt. Giraud, and then pass across an open hillside carpeted with sagebrush to Grouse Meadow (8,250 feet), 1 mile from the Middle Fork junction. Grouse Meadow is quite scenic, as the Middle Fork assumes a sedate, meandering course through expansive meadowlands, backdropped by the near-vertical, granite wall of Le Conte Canyon, a scene slightly reminiscent of Yosemite Valley. A number of heavily used campsites offer fine views of the meadow and river, although mosquitoes can be quite bothersome here early in the season.

Beyond the serene grassland of Grouse Meadow, the formerly placid river picks up speed again, as you climb gently through scattered to light forest. Farther on, the combined effects of another avalanche and a forest fire create openings in the forest cover, which offer good views of the canyon. Towering over Le Conte Canyon, the massive ramparts of The Citadel combine with a cascading stream from Ladder Lake to paint a dramatic mountain portrait on the west side of the canyon. Where the trail draws closer to the Middle Fork, shooting cascades of whitewater catapult across granite slabs, creating an equally exciting scene.

Farther up the trail, watery ribbons of the Dusy Branch slide gracefully down the sloping face of an extensive granite slab on the east canyon wall. As you approach the bridged crossing of the Dusy Branch, campsites are just off the trail and on either side of the Le Conte Canyon Ranger Station. At 3.4 miles from the Middle Fork junction is the junction with the Bishop Pass Trail heading east.

From the junction, turn right (east) and begin a moderate climb, initially through lodgepole pine forest, but soon across chaparral-covered slopes, which allow for fine views of Le Conte Canyon and mas-

sive Langille Peak. Numerous switchbacks follow the Dusy Branch upstream to where the grade eases momentarily on a bench with several good tree-shaded campsites away from the trail. Away from the bench the stiff climb resumes, switchbacking up the wall of the canyon to a bridge over Dusy Branch and then continuing to the west edge of lovely Dusy Basin. Verdant meadows carpeted with vibrant wildflowers encircle a seemingly innumerable number of sparkling tarns; the towering Palisades along the Sierra Crest and a southwest trending sub-ridge of peaks, including Isosceles and Columbine Peaks, borders this magnificent landscape. Dusy may be the finest alpine basin in all of the High Sierra, and well worth any time you may have to spend here.

Beyond Dusy Basin, the trail climbs for a mile and a half on sandy tread with occasional switchbacks to 11,972-foot Bishop Pass at the border between Kings Canyon National Park and John Muir Wilderness. Before you begin descending toward South Lake, take one last look at the view of Dusy Basin backdropped by the deep cleft of Le Conte Canyon and the rugged Black Divide.

A rocky, winding descent leads through rugged alpine terrain toward more hospitable surroundings below. Approaching timberline, you pass to the west of Bishop Lake, the first in a series of lovely lakes at the head of South Fork Bishop Creek, followed by Saddlerock Lake, Timberline Tarns, Spearhead Lake, and Long Lake. Reach the south junction with the Chocolate Lakes Trail to the right along the west shore of Long Lake. North of Long Lake, 0.8 mile from the previous junction, you reach the north junction of the Chocolate Lakes Trail and then follow a moderate, mostly forested descent with a couple of stream crossings to the Treasure Lakes junction. From there, exit the John Muir Wilderness and follow a descending traverse above the west shore of South Lake to the trailhead at the far end.

There are numerous options for further wanderings along the course of the JMT between the Kearsarge Pass and Bishop Pass Trails.

The Explorer Pass cross-country route leaves the JMT 0.75 mile north of Woods Creek crossing and heads up brush-filled slopes east of the outlet from Window Peak Lake and then south of a small, unnamed lake (approximately 10,360 feet) to Window Peak Lake. From there, follow the rock-filled drainage north along the east bank of a stream to Explorer Pass (approximately 12,250 feet). Descending a Class 3, often snow-filled chute (which will require an ice axe) down the northeast side of the pass is the crux of the route. Once you are past this difficult section, descend to the valley below, and traverse northeast to forest-rimmed Bench Lake. Return to the JMT via the 2-mile trail from the lake.

The Cartridge Pass route leaves the JMT from the north bank of South Fork Kings River and heads downstream along the river for 2 miles to a small brook draining a pair of good-size tarns below the pass. Follow an old trail on a climb along the east bank of this stream up to the tarns, and then ascend talus slopes to Cartridge Pass (approximately 11,680 feet, Class 1). A steep, rocky descent leads to easier talus slopes on the way into exquisite Lakes Basin.

Two possible routes exit Lakes Basin: The first follows a 4.5-mile off-trail descent along Cartridge Creek from Marion Lake northwest to the Middle Fork Kings River Trail. From there, follow the trail 4.5 miles north to the ford of Palisade Creek and the JMT junction just beyond. The second route heads north from the basin over Dumbbell

Lakes Pass (approximately 11,640 feet, Class 2), passes by Dumbbell Lakes, climbs to Cataract Creek Pass (approximately 11,520 feet, Class 2), and then drops to Amphitheater Lake. From there, follow an abandoned trail down Cataract Creek to a ford of Palisade Creek and the JMT beyond at Deer Meadow.

Cross-country enthusiasts can take a shortcut to the JMT to the Bishop Pass Trail by leaving the JMT just beyond the northwest shore of Lower Palisade Lake. Ascend northwest over a series of granite ledges to the west of a small tarn near the head of the cirque above. Climb to the broad saddle of Cirque Pass (approximately 12,000 feet, Class 3) and then descend to the Lake 11672 below (which has campsites). Cross Glacier Creek near the southwest shore, and climb over scree and granite ledges to Potluck Pass (approximately 12,120 feet, Class 2).

From the pass, follow a slightly descending traverse to a flat saddle directly northeast of Peak 12005, and then drop to the northeast shore of the largest Barrett Lake (11,523 feet). Pass south of Lake 11468, and traverse the south slope of Columbine Peak to Knapsack Pass (approximately 11,680 feet, Class 1). Descend the rocky gully west of the pass to the lower lakes in Dusy Basin, where an easy traverse northwest leads to the Bishop Pass Trail.

[R] A wilderness permit is required for overnight stays. Camping is limited to two nights at Kearsarge Lakes and Charlotte Lake and in Rae Lakes Basin. Bear canisters are required. Campfires are prohibited above 10,000 feet.

TRIP 104

Golden Trout Lakes

Ⓜ ∕ **DH** or **BP**

DISTANCE: 5 miles, out-and-back
to first lake

ELEVATION: 9,185'/11,390',
+2,295'/-80'/±4,750'

SEASON: Mid-July to mid-October

USE: Light

MAP: *Kearsarge Peak*

INTRODUCTION: The Golden Trout Lakes provide a fine destination for either a pleasant dayhike or an overnight backpack. The lakes are cradled in a talus-filled cirque just below the Sierra Crest in the shadow of Mt. Gould and Dragon Peak. Few trails allow hikers into such an austere alpine setting so quickly.

Although the Kearsarge Pass Trail in the next canyon south is one of the most popular eastern Sierra trails, relatively few hikers find their way up the Golden Trout Lakes Trail; a lack of maintenance helps deter some users from hiking it. Despite the trail conditions, the route is straightforward, and the impressive mountain scenery compensates for any rough sections.

DIRECTIONS TO TRAILHEAD: From US 395 in Independence, turn west onto Market Street, and proceed out of town for 12.5 miles on steep and winding Onion Valley Road to the parking area. A campground, vault toilets, and running water are near the trailhead.

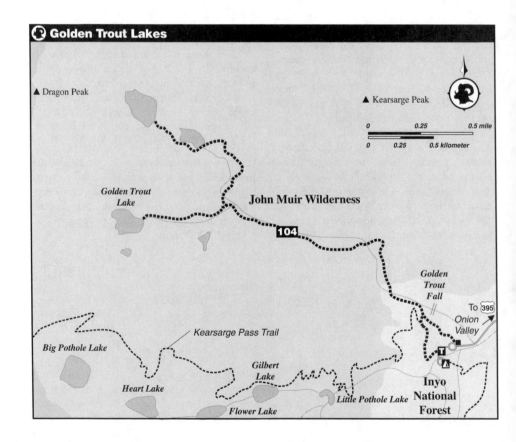

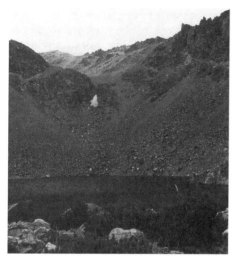

One of the Golden Trout Lakes above Onion Valley

DESCRIPTION: There are two options for the beginning of the hike to Golden Trout Lakes, and neither possesses much advantage over the other: Either follow the Kearsarge Pass Trail for a quarter mile to a junction with a short spur to the Golden Trout Lakes Trail, or hike up the access road near the pack station and branch left past a snow survey shelter and a couple of wood structures to the start of single-track trail, soon meeting the spur from the Kearsarge Pass Trail.

From the spur junction, proceed up the canyon through open pinyon pine and sagebrush scrub with views of Golden Trout Falls. Soon, riparian vegetation appears along a stretch of Golden Trout Creek, and you pass into John Muir Wilderness. Eventually, the trail crosses the creek and follows a winding climb through loose rock on the way above the falls. From there, pass through a flower-lined gully, and cross back over the creek. Above the crossing, the path becomes faint and hard to follow in places, particularly in areas of boulders and talus, but the way is obvious—simply head upstream through the narrow canyon. The established route fords the creek and soon crosses back again, but the trail is so faint that it's easy to miss these crossings. Eventually, you reach less steep terrain at a lush meadow near where the creek forks into two branches. A low rise nearby offers passable campsites.

To reach Golden Trout Lake, cross the left-hand branch, and head west along the north bank through gnarled whitebark pines and a few foxtail pines. Once again, the tread becomes sketchy, but the route is obvious—continue upstream to the lake. A few matted shrubs and widely scattered dwarf pines meet you at the east shore of Golden Trout Lake, where the boulders and talus from a glacier-carved cirque border the shore. The apex of this amphitheater is 13,005-foot Mt. Gould. Backpackers may be tempted by a couple of fine campsites near the outlet, while anglers can try their luck on brook and golden trout.

The quad map indicates a trail following the right-hand branch of the creek to a pair of unnamed lakes east of Dragon Peak. Although this path has mostly disappeared, the route is an easily managed cross-country jaunt. Both lakes are scenic and nicely backdropped by the multihued slopes of Dragon Peak. There are a few campsites around both lakes.

O If you want to explore further, you can take a shortcut to Rae Lakes via a cross-country route over Dragon Pass, just south of Dragon Peak.

R A wilderness permit is required for overnight stays. Campfires are prohibited.

OAK CREEK TRAILHEAD

TRIP 105

Baxter Pass Trail

S / **BP**

DISTANCE: 22 miles, out-and-back
to the John Muir Trail

ELEVATION: 5,990'/12,245'/10,210',
+6,650'/-2,430'/±18,160'

SEASON: Mid-July to mid-October

USE: Light

MAPS: USGS's *Kearsarge Peak* and
Mt. Clarence King or Tom
Harrison Maps' *Kings Canyon
High Country Trail Map*

TRAIL LOG

4.0 Summit Meadow
6.3 Baxter Pass
7.7 Upper Baxter Lake

INTRODUCTION: Only a very small percentage of the backpacking population will find this trip enjoyable—loners in incredible shape with a penchant for masochism. The trail—if the unmaintained, overgrown, washed-out, disappearing track can still be called a trail—is a long, steep, difficult, nasty route that begins practically on the floor of Owens Valley. The climb to Baxter Pass gains 6,300 feet in a little more than 6 miles, a 1,000-feet-per-mile ascent. But the trip is not entirely bad news. The Baxter Lakes are quite scenic and justifiably deserted. However, most hikers will prefer to access the lakes from the John Muir Trail (JMT) instead of from the Oak Creek Trailhead.

DIRECTIONS TO TRAILHEAD: Approximately 2.5 miles north of Independence, leave US 395 and turn west onto Fish Hatchery Road. Proceed on pavement 1.3 miles to a Y-junction, and turn right onto FS Road 13S04A, passing Oak Creek Campground on the way to the trailhead, 5.8 miles from the junction.

DESCRIPTION: From an oak-shaded campsite at the end of the road, follow an old roadbed up North Fork Oak Creek canyon through typical eastside terrain. Eventually the road narrows to single-track trail, although much of the path may be washed out, overgrown with brush, and generally indistinguishable. Ford a tributary and then the main channel of the creek near the 1-mile mark. A zigzagging path proceeds another 1.5 miles to the next ford, followed by a steady climb to Summit Meadow, about 4 miles from the trailhead.

Another mile beyond the meadow, the path becomes rockier and veers away from the creek to bend north toward the pass. Proceed over a scree field dotted with a smattering of pines to barren Baxter Pass (approximately 12,245 feet) at the Kings Canyon boundary, 6.3 miles from the trailhead. The fine view includes portions of the Sierra Crest, and Owens Valley and Independence to the east.

A steep, rocky descent from the pass leads to the gentler terrain of the Baxter Lakes basin, where wildflowers, grasses, and sedges give it a feeling of vibrant life after the mostly barren terrain around the pass. Seldomly used campsites are scattered around the shore of the upper lake (11,145 feet). Farther down, near the lower string of lakes, backpackers may find additional sites in small groves of whitebark pines.

Cross Baxter Creek, and continue the descent west until the path bends south and drops more steeply to Dollar Lake and South Fork Woods Creek. Along the descent, there are good views of King Spur, Fin Dome, and Dollar Lake. Reach an unsigned junction with the JMT, 11 miles from the trailhead.

|O| Although quite arduous, this route provides an alternative for accessing the Rae Lakes Basin if all of the permits for the Kearsarge Pass Trail have been gobbled up.

|R| A wilderness permit is required for overnight stays. Campfires are prohibited in the Kings Canyon National Park area of this trip. Dogs and sheep are prohibited.

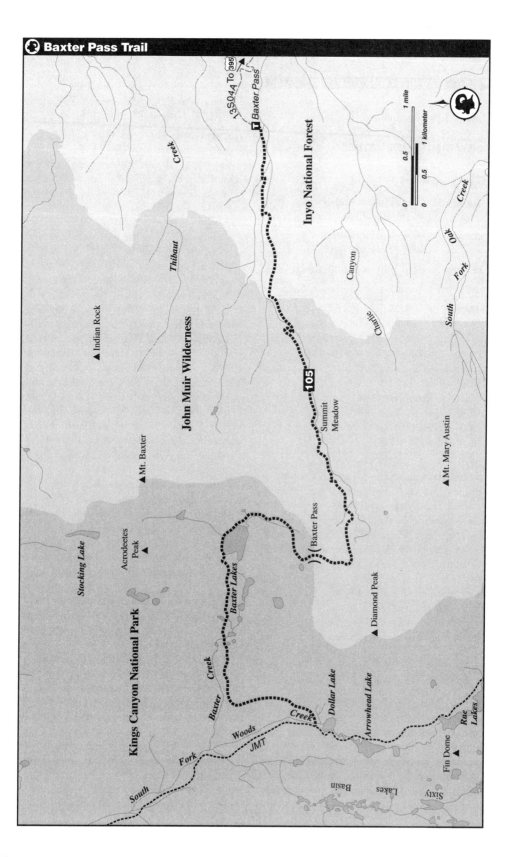

Stocking Lake

▲ Indian Rock

Thibaut

Creek

To 395

13S04A

Baxter Pass

Inyo National Forest

John Muir Wilderness

▲ Mt. Baxter

Acrodectes Peak ▲

Kings Canyon National Park

Baxter Creek

Baxter Lakes

Baxter Pass

105

Summit Meadow

▲ Diamond Peak

▲ Mt. Mary Austin

Canyon

Charlie

Oak

Creek

South Fork

South

Fork

Woods

JMT

Creek

Dollar Lake

Arrowhead Lake

Sixty Lakes Basin

Fin Dome ▲

Rae Lakes

0   0.5   1 kilometer

0   0.5   1 mile

SAWMILL CREEK TRAILHEAD

TRIP 106

Sawmill Pass Trail

S ⟋ **BP**

DISTANCE: 25 miles, out-and-back to the John Muir Trail

ELEVATION: 4,600'/11,300'/10,350', +7,325'/-1,550'/±17,750'

SEASON: Mid-July to mid-October

USE: Light

MAPS: USGS's *Aberdeen* and *Mt. Pinchot* or Tom Harrison Maps' *Kings Canyon High Country Trail Map*

TRAIL LOG

5.5	Sawmill Meadow
7.5	Sawmill Lake
9.3	Sawmill Pass
11.0	Woods Lake

INTRODUCTION: This is another of those grueling eastside approaches on unmaintained trail that will repel almost any clear-thinking backpacker; it starts near a sinkhole in Owens Valley at an elevation 1,300 feet lower than the Baxter Pass Trail (Trip 105, page 372). There is no shade for the first 4 miles, and little promise of much more beyond. Sections of tread have virtually disappeared.

For those who can overcome the hellish beginning, the terrain eventually becomes quite scenic, culminating in a splendid alpine basin on the west side of Sawmill Pass. However, similar to the Baxter Pass Trail, this area is more easily accessed from the JMT.

DIRECTIONS TO TRAILHEAD: About 17.5 miles south of Big Pine, leave US 395 and turn west onto Black Springs Road. Proceed 0.8 mile to a T-junction with Tinemaha Road, and turn right. After 1.2 miles, turn left onto Division Creek Road, proceed 1.5 miles to the end of pavement near a powerhouse, and then continue on dirt road another 0.4 mile to the trailhead.

DESCRIPTION: The trail begins seemingly in the middle of nowhere, heading across a vast ocean of sagebrush toward distant Sawmill Creek canyon; hikers must overcome the first 4 miles of trail—a shadeless, waterless, rising traverse across the east base of the Sierra—just to reach the mouth of the canyon. Along the way, you have fine views of the Big Pine Volcanic Field, where reddish cinder cones and black lava fields break up the sagebrush-covered slopes.

Staggering into the canyon, you encounter a smattering of Jeffrey pines, white firs, and oaks, which provide a mirage of shade on the way to The Hogsback. As the trail parallels this sloping ridge, ford the north tributary of Sawmill Creek three times before crossing over The Hogsback, veering south toward Sawmill Creek canyon, and then climbing to Sawmill Meadow (approximately 8,415 feet). A pine-covered bench just before the meadow offers a couple of marginal campsites, and there are a few more around the fringe of the meadow.

Away from the meadow, begin a moderate climb up the southwest-trending canyon. A steeper, zigzagging section of trail leads through Jeffrey pines and red firs to marshy Mule Lake, 6.9 miles from the trailhead. From there, a rocky climb with a pair of creek crossings leads to lovely Sawmill Lake (10,023 feet), 7.5 miles from the trailhead. Fine campsites beneath foxtail pines are quite appealing, especially after the long, stiff climb. A healthy population of rainbow trout will tempt anglers.

Leaving the lake behind, the winding trail heads for the pass through a diminishing forest of whitebark and foxtail pines and eventually passes above timberline, where a final climb leads to Sawmill Pass (11,347 feet) at the Kings Canyon National Park boundary, 9.3 miles from the trailhead.

Beyond the pass, stunning alpine scenery awaits, as a gently graded trail leads to a slightly more pronounced descent into a lovely basin filled with shimmering lakes

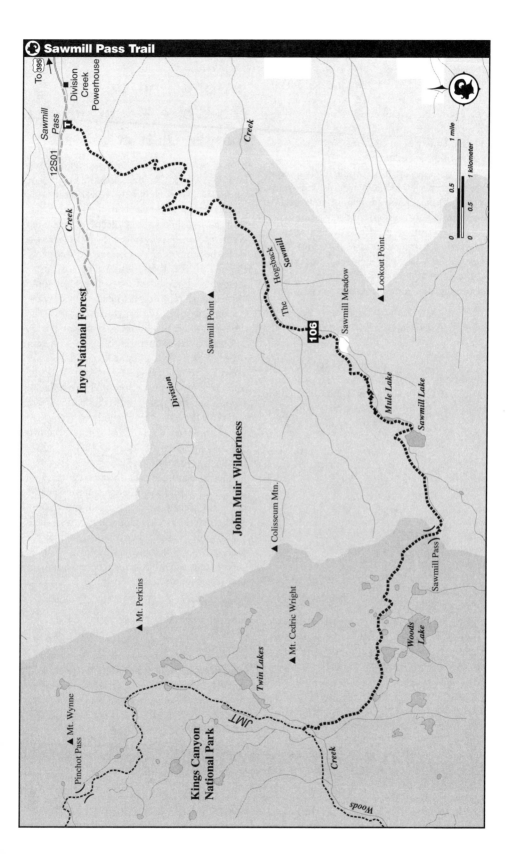

and ponds. A few whitebark pines dot verdant, wildflower-carpeted meadows around the lakes, almost beautiful enough to blot the previously tortuous, 9-mile ascent from your memory. The obscure path becomes a route-finding challenge, but if you've survived so far, you more than likely possess the wherewithal to navigate this convoluted basin. Woods Lake (approximately 10,710 feet) is a short cross-country jaunt south from the trail and offers decent camping and good fishing for rainbow trout. Faint tread continues west before arcing around the slopes of Mt. Cedric Wright and then dropping to a junction with the JMT.

O Both Mt. Cedric Wright and Colisseum Mountain provide Class 1 ascents from the trail.

R A wilderness permit is required for overnight stays. Campfires are prohibited in Kings Canyon National Park. Dogs and sheep are prohibited east of Sawmill Pass.

Introduction to the White Mountain Ranger District

Many outdoor recreationists have long known about the magnificent beauty of the eastern Sierra, where towering peaks, glacial cirques, flower-bedecked meadows, shimmering lakes, and deep-cut canyons create picture-postcard scenes. Whether you seek the airy summits of the Palisades or the depths of Evolution Valley, exquisite scenery is abundant in every direction. Some of the most remote and nearly inaccessible backcountry lies within this portion of the wilderness or neighboring national parks, offering cross-country enthusiasts a virtual off-trail mecca for extended trips into such areas as the Enchanted Gorge and Palisade and Ionian Basins. Bounded by Glacier Divide on the north and the main Sierra Crest on the east, this rugged terrain is also the birthplace of two of the region's mightiest rivers, the San Joaquin and Kings.

Such mountain splendor has attracted hordes of admirers over the decades, creating a high demand for wilderness permits, especially for areas within easy reach of weekend backpackers. Backpackers favor less difficult routes over the Sierra Crest, such as the Bishop Pass and Piute Pass Trails. Planning or creative scheduling may be essential for securing a wilderness permit.

ACCESS: The north-south thoroughfare of US 395 is the principal access for all eastside trips to secondary roads branching toward trailheads.

AMENITIES: Big Pine offers a few small motels, eateries, and gas stations. Bishop has a much more extensive list of these services, as well as a couple of outdoor suppliers and other retail stores.

West of Big Pine, Glacier Lodge (www.jewelofthsierra.com) is located near the end of Glacier Lodge Road. Although the main lodge building burned down many years ago, cabins and a trailer park are still open.

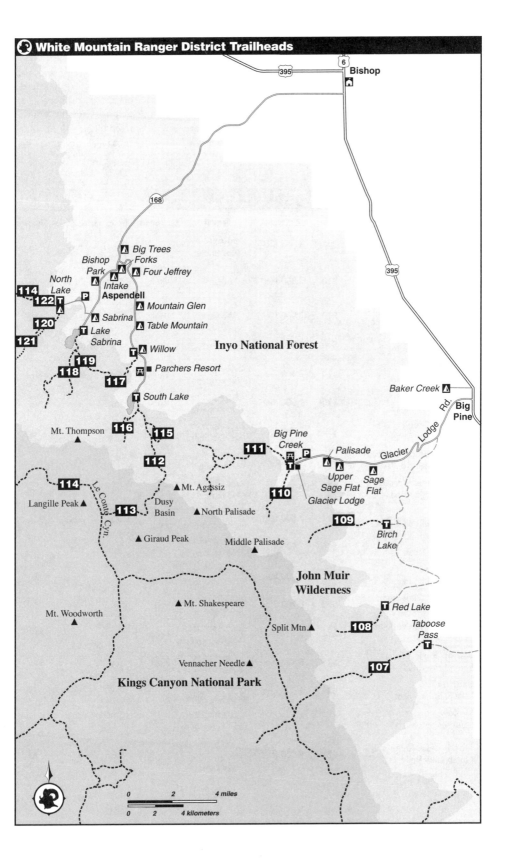

The resort also offers guided backcountry trips. Showers are available to the public.

Mountain lodges west of Bishop include Bishop Creek Lodge (www.bishopcreekresort.com), Cardinal Village Resort (www.cardinalvillageresort.com), and Parchers Resort (www.parchersresort.net).

SHUTTLE SERVICES: A number of companies provide shuttle service to trailheads on the east side of the Sierra. Consult www.climber.org for a current list. *Note that Greyhound no longer services towns along US 395.*

Campgrounds

Campground	Fee	Elevation	Season	Restrooms	Water	Bear Boxes	Phone
Goodale Creek (BLM) 14 miles south of Big Pine	$5	4,000 feet	Mid-April to November	Vault	No	No	No
Taboose Creek (Inyo County) 13 miles south of Big Pine	$10	3,900 feet	All year	Vault	Yes	No	No
Tinemaha (Inyo County) 9 miles south of Big Pine	$10	3,900 feet	All year	Vault	Yes	No	No
Baker Creek (Inyo County) 0.5 mile north of Big Pine	$10	8,200 feet	All year	Vault	Yes	No	No
Sage Flat Glacier Lodge Road	$20	7,400 feet	Late April to November	Vault	Yes	No	No
Upper Sage Flat Glacier Lodge Road	$20	7,600 feet	Late April to November	Vault	Yes	No	No
Big Pine Creek Glacier Lodge Road	$20	7,700 feet	Late April to late October	Flush	Yes	Yes	Yes
Palisade Glacier (group) Glacier Lodge Road	$60	8,300 feet	Late April to November	Flush	Yes	Yes	No
Clyde Glacier (group) Glacier Lodge Road	$60	8,300 feet	Late April to November	Flush	Yes	Yes	No
Big Trees South Lake Road	$21	7,500 feet	Late April to mid-September	Flush and vault	Yes	Yes	No
Forks South Lake Road	$16	5,900 feet	Late May to November	Flush	Yes	Yes	No
Four Jeffrey South Lake Road	$21	8,100 feet	Late April to late October	Flush	Yes	Yes	No
Mountain Glen (tents only) South Lake Road	$20	8,200 feet	Early May to October	Vault	No	Yes	No
Intake 2 and Walk-In Lake Sabrina Road	$21	8,200 feet	Late April to late October	Flush	Yes	Yes	No
Bishop Park (tents) South Lake Road	$21	8,400 feet	Late April to late October	Flush	Yes	Yes	No
Sabrina Lake Sabrina Road	$21	9,000 feet	Early May to late September	Flush	Yes	Yes	Yes
Willow South Lake Road	$20	9,000 feet	Early May to mid-September	Vault	No	Yes	No
North Lake (tents only) North Lake Road	$21	9,500 feet	Early to mid-June to October	Vault	Yes	Yes	No

OUTFITTERS: The following pack stations operate trips in this area:

Bishop Pack Outfitters
Morgan Livestock Company
247 Cataract Rd.
Aspendell, CA 93514
760-873-4785
www.bishoppackoutfitters.com

Glacier Pack Train
P.O. Box 321
Big Pine, CA 93513
760-938-2538

Pine Creek Pack Station
P.O. Box 968
Bishop, CA 93515
800-962-0775
bernerspack@yahoo.com

Rainbow Pack Outfitters
P.O. Box 1791
Bishop, CA 93515
760-873-8877
rainbowpackers@aol.com

Rock Creek Pack Station
Craig London
P.O. Box 248
Bishop, CA 93515
760-935-4493

Sequoia-Kings Pack Train
P.O. Box 209
Independence, CA 93526
800-962-2797

RANGER STATION: The White Mountain Ranger Station is located in the north part of Bishop on US 395 (798 Main Street). Wilderness permits, maps, guidebooks, and bear canister rentals are available during normal business hours. For more information call 760-873-2485.

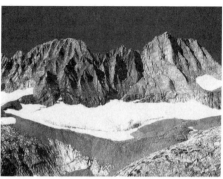

Middle Palisade and Disappointment Peak, South Fork Big Pine Creek Trail (Trip 110)

WILDERNESS PERMITS: Wilderness permits are required year-round. Quotas are in effect between May 1 and November 1, and 60 percent of the quota is available by reservation ($5 per person fee). Reservations can be made up to six months in advance to two days before the start of a trip. Download the application from the Inyo National Forest website, fill it out, and mail it to: Inyo National Forest, Wilderness Permit Reservation Office, 351 Pacu Lane, Suite 200, Bishop, CA 93514. You can also fax it to 760-873-2484. The Inyo National Forest is working on an online reservation system that should be operational in the near future.

The remaining 40 percent of the quota is available as free walk-in permits on a first-come, first-served basis. You can get a permit as late as the day before your departure. Consult the website or contact the Wilderness Permit Reservation Office at 760-873-2483 for more information.

GOOD TO KNOW BEFORE YOU GO: Even though gas is not inexpensive in Bishop, it is cheaper there than it is in the smaller towns of Big Pine, Independence, and Lone Pine.

TABOOSE CREEK TRAILHEAD

TRIP 107

Taboose Pass Trail

S ⭧ BP

DISTANCE: 23.5 miles, out-and-back to Bench Lake

ELEVATION: 5,425'/11,418'/10,560', +6,205'/-1,065'/±14,540'

SEASON: Mid-July to mid-October

USE: Light

MAPS: USGS's *Fish Springs, Aberdeen,* and *Mt. Pinchot* or Tom Harrison Maps' *Kings Canyon High Country Trail Map*

TRAIL LOG

7.4 Taboose Pass
10.0 John Muir Trail junction

INTRODUCTION: The Taboose Pass Trail is the northern entry in the "three not to see" category, along with its sister trails over Baxter and Sawmill Passes. A low-elevation start, lack of shade, and poorly maintained tread combine to make this a trip for backpackers in great shape who don't mind heat and poor conditions. However, for those who aren't vanquished by the grueling climb up to the pass, the sweeping view across a sloping, flower-splashed meadow is one of the more impressive vistas in the High Sierra. In addition, the easy stroll over to Bench Lake with its fine campsites is a very pleasant journey.

DIRECTIONS TO TRAILHEAD: From US 395, about 12 miles south of Big Pine, turn west onto paved Taboose Creek Road, and proceed 1.1 miles to a four-way intersection with Tinemaha Road. Continue straight ahead as the pavement turns to dirt, proceeding 3.5 miles to a Y-junction, and bear right onto rough FS Road 11S04. Reach a corral after 1.5 miles and park nearby. With a 4WD vehicle you could proceed another half mile on very rough road.

DESCRIPTION: The initial part of the journey involves a steadily rising ascent along Taboose Creek through an ocean of sagebrush toward the deep gash of the canyon. Once at the mouth of the canyon, follow the tumbling, willow-lined creek up a set of switchbacks and then traverse over to a ford, 4 miles from the corral.

The trail continues its zigzagging course up the canyon, passing a number of benches and fording the creek again on the way past timberline, where meadows, wildflow- ers, and tarns lend an alpine ambiance to the basin below the pass. At 8 miles, you reach the boulder field of Taboose Pass (11,487 feet) at the boundary of Kings Canyon National Park. The sweeping vista across flower-filled slopes down toward the deep cleft of South Fork Kings River, the shimmering surface of Bench Lake is backdropped by symmetrical Arrow Peak, and the towering summit of Mt. Ruskin is outstanding.

A gradual descent greets you on the west side of the pass on a stroll through gardens of green foliage and colorful wildflowers. After hopping over a rivulet, you reach an obscure junction. Take the left-hand fork, and continue the gentle descent, crossing more sprightly streams along the way, including one that drains a set of tarns to the east. Pass through a thickening forest of lodgepole pines, and then drop down to a junction with the JMT in a broad, sloping meadow, 11 miles from the corral.

Turn left (southbound) on the JMT, cross a small stream, pass the signed lateral to a patrol cabin, and come to a ford of the creek draining Lake Marjorie. Immediately beyond the creek is a junction with the faint tread of the Bench Lake Trail, 0.1 mile from the previous junction.

Head southwest away from the JMT across a flower-laden meadow, and then traverse a granite bench through scattered lodgepole pines. A little more than a mile from the junction, you ford a shallow stream and pass a pair of ponds on the

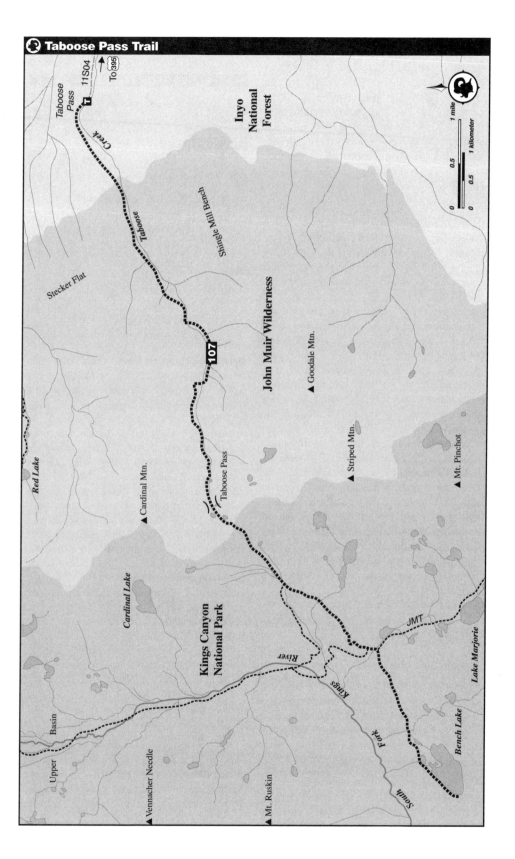

way to the northeast shore of Bench Lake (10,558 feet). The trail continues to the west end of the lake before fading out. Backpackers should find plenty of good campsites under pines along the northwest shore. Rainbow and brook trout will entice anglers. The sight of Arrow Peak from the lakeshore is one of the premier scenes in the High Sierra.

[O] Maintained trail may end at Bench Lake, but a couple of intriguing cross-country routes continue into the backcountry beyond. The first leaves the northwest shore, arcs around to Arrow Pass (approximately 11,600 feet, 0.7 mile southeast of Arrow Peak, Class 2), and then descends the drainage on the south side to the trail along Woods Creek at the north end of Paradise Valley.

The second route is more difficult and may require an ice axe. Initially it is the same until you reach the basin just northeast of Arrow Pass. Instead of crossing the pass, ascend southeast to the head of a canyon, and climb a steep chute (usually snow-covered) to Explorer Pass (12,160 feet, 0.9 mile northeast of Pyramid Peak, Class 3). Drop from the pass heading south and then southeast into a basin east of Pyramid Peak. Follow a stream past a trio of small tarns to the north shore of beautiful Window Peak Lake (approximately 10,600 feet), which has excellent, secluded campsites. From the lake, follow the outlet to an intersection with the JMT, approximately 1 mile northeast of Woods Creek crossing.

From Arrow Pass, both Arrow Peak and Pyramid Peak are Class 2 climbs. From Explorer Pass, a moderate Class 3 route ascends the northeast ridge of Pyramid Peak.

[R] A wilderness permit is required for overnight stays. Campfires are allowed along Taboose Creek but not in Kings Canyon.

RED CREEK TRAILHEAD

TRIP 108

Red Lake

(S) ↗ **DH or BP**

DISTANCE: 9 miles, out-and-back

ELEVATION: 6,575'/10,460', +4,200'/-1,065'/±10,530'

SEASON: Late June to mid-October

USE: Very light

MAPS: USGS's *Fish Springs* and *Split Mountain* or Tom Harrison Maps' *Kings Canyon High Country Trail Map*

INTRODUCTION: A long drive over dirt roads followed by a steep, sweltering climb on rough, poorly maintained, and sometimes indistinct trail—why would anyone bother with a trip to Red Lake? The rewards for such an arduous adventure are solitude and scenery. So few people are drawn to the area that the Forest Service didn't even have a quota for this trail until 2002, when all trails received one, whether they needed it or not. The few hardy souls who make the effort will be rewarded with a superbly picturesque lake backdropped by the impressive east face of Split Mountain (once known as South Palisade), where twin summits are separated by a narrow cleft. A high percentage of those on the trail are likely to be mountaineers bound for the easiest ascent of a fourteener in the Sierra outside of Mt. Whitney.

To make this trip more enjoyable make sure your vehicle is roadworthy. Second, get an early start to avoid the steep and exposed climb during the hottest part of the day. Finally, pack and drink plenty of water on the ascent. With these few precautions, you might enjoy going where few others dare to tread.

DIRECTIONS TO TRAILHEAD: Following the 12 miles of dirt road to the trailhead is a big part of the adventure of this trip—plan on an hour of travel time from Big Pine. In Big Pine, turn west from US 395 onto Crocker Street (which becomes Glacier Lodge Road outside of town), and follow paved road 2.75 miles to a left-hand turn onto McMurry Meadows Road (FS 9S03). Immediately after the turn, bear left, bypassing a 4WD road angling in from the right (south). After a very brief climb, veer right, pass under a powerline, and continue on well-traveled McMurry Meadows Road, ignoring lesser roads along the way.

At 5.75 miles from Glacier Lodge Road, a less-used road on the right heads north toward the Birch Creek Trailhead (see Trip 109, page 385). Cross Birch Creek immediately after the junction, and continue past McMurry Meadows to a Y-junction near the 7-mile mark. Bear left, where a crude sign marked RED LAKE offers some assurance that you're still on the right route. A quarter-mile descent leads to a crossing of

Fuller Creek and a T-junction just beyond. Turn left at the junction, and parallel the creek downstream on rougher road for 0.4 mile to another creek crossing. Continue down the creek along the north bank to a major intersection, 9 miles from Glacier Lodge Road, where a locked gate blocks forward progress.

Turn right (south) at the intersection, crossing Fuller and Tinemaha Creeks, to another T-junction, 0.75 mile from the previous junction. Turn right (west) and follow FS Road 9S03 another 2 miles to a fork. A small sign directs traffic to the left toward the trailhead parking area and right toward the start of the trail.

DESCRIPTION: Begin by following the north branch of the road uphill toward the start of single-track trail near a water diversion structure (although the south branch of the road heads directly toward Red

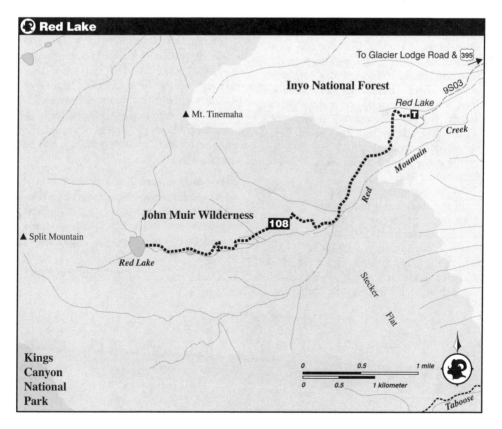

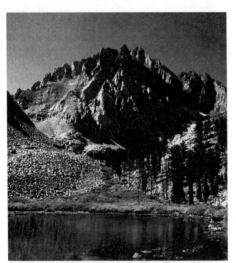

Split Mountain rises above an unnamed pond along the Red Lake Trail.

Mountain Creek, there is not a trail up the steep, brush-choked canyon). Climb moderately steeply up the hillside, paralleling a spring-fed tributary. Beyond a series of short-legged switchbacks, continue climbing steadily, soon bending south to cross a seasonal stream channel and a sagebrush-covered slope. Pass into the unmarked John Muir Wilderness, and make a curving ascent into Red Mountain Creek canyon, where the grade momentarily eases. Before the moderately steep climb resumes, you briefly come alongside the creek, 1.5 miles from the trailhead.

A steep, zigzagging climb leads away from the creek, up a gully, and then across a seasonal stream toward some cliffs. After a more moderate ascent, the steep climb resumes, as you cross a rocky wash and zigzag up the slope to a thicket of vegetation, where a cool, refreshing stream courses through a rock cleft. A few lonely pines

make an appearance, granting some hope that all of this climbing will eventually lead to more mountainlike terrain. Soon cross another stream lined by lush vegetation, step over a rocky wash, and then emerge onto a slope above the creek once more.

Just as you near the willow-lined stream, a switchback leads away on a lengthy diagonal ascent across a hillside. Views east of the Owens Valley and Inyo Mountains improve on the way up the slope. Another switchback leads back toward the canyon and a fine view of Split Mountain. After even more climbing, the trail levels near an unnamed pond. Here the view of Split Mountain is even more impressive. At the far end of the pond, a number of campsites will appeal to weary backpackers.

The trail passes halfway around the north shore of the pond, disappears in some talus, reappears briefly farther beyond the pond (campsites), and then vanishes for good beneath a talus slide. A quarter-mile scramble from there leads to Red Lake.

Surrounded by pockets of willow and widely scattered whitebark and foxtail pines, Red Lake (10,459 feet) rests dramatically below the steep talus slopes of 14,058-foot Split Mountain. Crude campsites suggest that camping is far better back down the trail along the creek or around the unnamed pond. Anglers may wish to ply the waters for golden trout.

[O] For most hikers, Red Lake will be the end of the line. However, competent cross-country travelers can cross the Sierra Crest via a Class 2 route over Red Lake Pass, 0.4 mile north of Split Mountain, into Upper Basin.

[R] A wilderness permit is required for overnight stays.

BIRCH CREEK TRAILHEAD

TRIP 109

Birch Lake

Ⓢ ↗ DH or BP

DISTANCE: 11 miles, out-and-back

ELEVATION: 6,485'/10,800',
+4,615'/-300'/±9,830'

SEASON: Late June to mid-October

USE: Very light

MAPS: USGS's *Fish Springs* and *Split Mountain* or Tom Harrison Maps' *Kings Canyon High Country Trail Map*

INTRODUCTION: Dirt road access, a low-elevation trailhead, and an infrequently maintained trail combine to dissuade most hikers from even considering this trip to Birch Lake. Despite the perceived drawbacks, Birch Lake is quite scenic, nestled beneath the Sierra Crest in the broad canyon of aspen-lined Birch Creek and sandwiched between The Thumb and Birch Mountain. The sketchy trail dead-ends below the lake, making this a trip suitable for a dayhike or overnight backpack.

DIRECTIONS TO TRAILHEAD: Following the 12 miles of dirt road to the trailhead is a big part of the adventure of this trip—plan on an hour of travel time from Big Pine. In Big Pine, turn west from US 395 onto Crocker Street (which becomes Glacier Lodge Road outside of town), and follow paved road 2.75 miles to a left-hand turn onto McMurry Meadows Road (FS 9S03).

Immediately after the turn, bear left, bypassing a 4WD road angling in from the right (south). After a very brief climb, veer right, pass under a powerline, and continue on well-traveled McMurry Meadows Road, ignoring lesser roads along the way. At 5.75 miles from Glacier Lodge Road, just before Birch Creek, turn right onto a less-used road heading north toward the Birch Creek Trailhead. Continue 0.6 mile to a T-junction, and bear right, proceeding another 0.1 mile to a small parking area near a closed gate.

DESCRIPTION: Initially, the route follows a closed 4WD road for about 100 yards to a trailhead sign and then continues through a field of tall grass and clumps of wild rose. Sagebrush-covered terrain alternates with meadows on the way to a Y-junction, 0.75 mile from the trailhead. Although the left-hand road heads toward Birch Creek, your route follows the right-hand branch up a seasonal drainage. Eventually, the road narrows to single-track trail heading directly up a sandy wash to a switchback leading onto more solid footing, where you have fine views of Owens Valley and the White Mountains to the east. On steady, winding tread, proceed over a hill, and then follow a more moderate ascent into the canyon of a seasonal tributary of Birch Creek. A moderately steep climb leads past a tiny, spring-fed stream and then up a grassy slope to an unsigned junction, 3.8 miles from the trailhead.

Bear left at the junction, and follow a horseshoe curve around a broad canyon, followed by a climb to the top of a rise with a spectacular view of Owens Valley. Drop 👁 off the rise into the next drainage, where the sketchy tread becomes hard to follow, splitting into two faint paths, each offering a slightly different approach to Birch Creek canyon. The route shown on the *Split Mountain* quad continues up the drainage

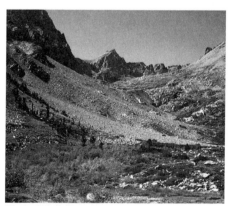

Birch Creek Canyon

and crosses the creek above a spring, before heading south on a 0.75-mile traverse into the main canyon just below Birch Lake. The other route crosses the drainage immediately and then heads directly over to the main canyon well below the lake. Both routes lead you into the beautiful vale of Birch Creek, where there are a number of primitive campsites below Birch Lake alongside the tumbling creek.

To reach the lake, head upstream through the open canyon and then across talus to a meadow just below the lake, which sits in a broad valley with excellent views up the canyon toward the Sierra Crest. Anglers can test their skill on good-size cutthroat trout.

There are few options for further wanderings in the Birch Creek drainage. A Class 3 cross-country route provides access to the upper Palisade Creek drainage over Birch Creek Pass (12,800 feet), 0.8 mile south of The Thumb.

Mountaineers can climb a Class 2 route up Birch Mountain by ascending the moraine south of Birch Lake to a saddle southwest of the peak and then along a ridge to the summit. Overall, a Class 2–3 ascent of The Thumb is straightforward once you surmount a cliff, 0.5 mile southwest of the lake.

R A wilderness permit is required for overnight stays.

BIG PINE CREEK TRAILHEAD

TRIP 110

Brainerd and Finger Lakes

⑤ ✗ DH or **BP**

DISTANCE: 10 miles, out-and-back to Brainerd Lake

ELEVATION: 7,750'/10,790', +3,740'/-700'/±8,880'

SEASON: Mid-July to early October

USE: Moderate

MAPS: USGS's *Coyote Flat* and *Split Mountain* or Tom Harrison Maps' *The Palisades Trail Map*

TRAIL LOG

3.8   Willow Lake junction
5.0   Brainerd Lake
5.5   Finger Lake

INTRODUCTION: Alpinists from all over the globe come to test their skills on the bevy of 13,000- to 14,000-foot peaks known as the Palisades. Splendid Sierra granite combined with dependably pleasant weather lure many mountaineers and technical climbers to the faces and ridges of these highly challenging and picturesque mountains. Hikers have the opportunity to enjoy the splendid alpine scenery of the Middle Palisades on the trail up South Fork Big Pine Creek to Brainerd Lake and then on a straightforward, off-trail route to Finger Lake and beyond. This is definitely a trip you'll want to capture with your camera.

Although the scenery is heavenly, parts of the steep climb seem to have less divine origins. The first half of the route is a reasonable climb on decent tread up the moderate angle of South Fork Big Pine Creek, but the second half requires hikers to surmount steep terrain on rough, poorly maintained trail. Those fortunate enough to complete the climb may find superb rooms with a view at campsites near either Brainerd or Finger Lakes.

DIRECTIONS TO TRAILHEAD: In Big Pine, turn west from US 395 onto Crocker Street (Glacier Lodge Road outside of town), and follow the two-lane, paved road past campgrounds to the overnight parking area, 9.2 miles from the highway. Dayhikers may continue another 0.75 mile to the day-use parking lot at the end of the road. There are vault toilets near both trailheads.

DESCRIPTION: Rather than starting the trip from the overnight parking lot and following the trail that traverses the hillside north of the road, backpackers should descend shortly to the Glacier Lodge Road and follow the pavement 0.75 mile to the dayhiker trailhead.

From the day-use parking lot, walk through forest along Big Pine Creek past a closed gate and up the road past some cabins. Soon the road narrows to single-track trail and climbs up rock steps to a bridge over the creek. From the bridge, continue 0.1 mile to a junction, and bear left, crossing an open, sagebrush-covered slope with striking views up the canyon of Norman Clyde Peak and Middle Palisade. Cross an old road, and follow cottonwood-lined South Fork Big Pine Creek through drought-tolerant vegetation on a moderate climb. Cross a seasonal stream, and proceed across boulder-strewn slopes to a ford of

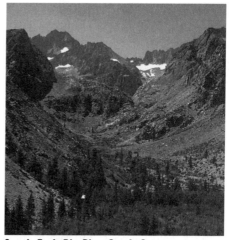

South Fork Big Pine Creek Canyon

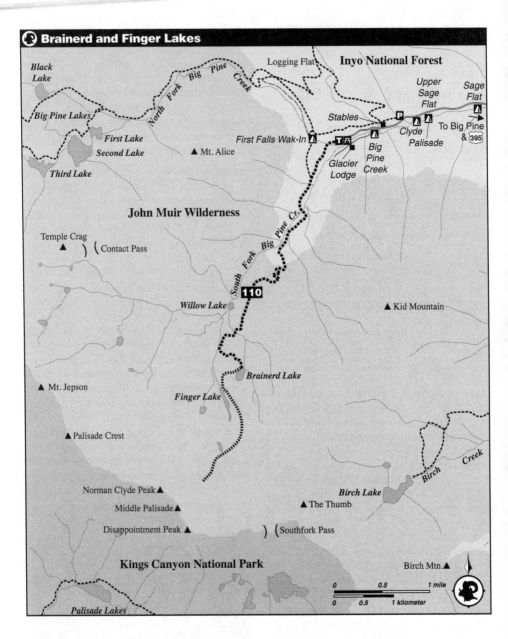

Brainerd and Finger Lakes

Black Lake

Big Pine Lakes

First Lake

Second Lake

Third Lake

North Fork Big Pine Creek

Logging Flat

Inyo National Forest

Upper Sage Flat

Sage Flat

Stables

Clyde Palisade

To Big Pine & 395

First Falls Wak-In

Big Pine Creek

Glacier Lodge

▲ Mt. Alice

John Muir Wilderness

Temple Crag ▲

) (Contact Pass

South Fork Big Pine Cr.

110

Willow Lake

▲ Kid Mountain

▲ Mt. Jepson

Finger Lake

Brainerd Lake

▲ Palisade Crest

Norman Clyde Peak ▲

Middle Palisade ▲

Disappointment Peak ▲

Birch Creek

Birch Lake

▲ The Thumb

) (Southfork Pass

Kings Canyon National Park

Birch Mtn. ▲

0   0.5   1 mile

0   0.5   1 kilometer

the willow- and birch-lined creek, 1.7 miles from the backpacker parking lot.

Beyond the ford, head upstream on gently graded tread toward a hillside. Soon the grade increases on a winding, steep ascent. Rocky switchbacks lead up through scattered limber pines to the base of some nearly vertical cliffs. Traverse across a hillside before bending left and climbing steeply up a narrow cleft of rock to a crest. A short distance ahead awaits a splendid panorama of the southern Palisades, stretching from Mt. Sill to The Thumb, a vista rivaling any in the High Sierra for stunning alpine scenery. From this viewpoint, drop briefly into the cover of lodgepole pines, pass a spring-fed rivulet, and then reach a T-junction with a lateral to Willow Lake, 3.9 miles from the backpacker parking lot.

⊡ SIDE TRIP TO WILLOW LAKE: Willow Lake (9,565 feet) is just 0.3 mile off the main trail. Sediments are steadily transforming this body of water into more of a marshy meadow than a lake, and in early summer the standing water creates a favorable environment for hordes of breeding mosquitoes. However, a couple of nice campsites beneath lodgepole pines will tempt those who got a late start or who are too pooped for the next stretch of climbing to Brainerd Lake. **END OF SIDE TRIP**

From the Willow Lake junction, descend to a crossing of the lushly lined outlet from Brainerd Lake, and then resume the climb on a winding ascent beneath lodgepole pines toward the stream draining Finger Lake. Head upstream for a while, and then turn east, passing a small pond and continuing up switchbacks to a granite hump, from where you can see Willow Lake below. Pass a second pond, make a short descent across a marshy meadow, and then swing around a granite ledge on a final climb to the lip of Brainerd Lake's basin.

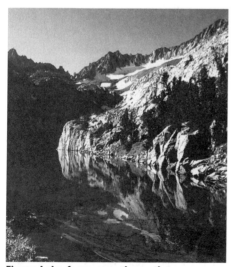

Finger Lake from near the outlet

The opal-tinted, icy waters of Brainerd Lake are tucked into a deep, glacier-carved bowl of granite, with steep cliffs nearly surrounding the lake. Snow oftentimes lingers in the narrow crevices of the bowl well into summer. The summits of the craggy, glacier-clad Palisades loom over the top of the cliffs thousands of feet above. There are a smattering of compact campsites sheltered by lodgepole and whitebark pines near the outlet. Anglers my wish to test their luck on brook trout, but don't expect any trophy-size fish at this elevation.

Without question, the setting of Brainerd Lake is absolutely stunning, but to come all this way and not go beyond would be missing out on some extraordinary scenery. With a modicum of cross-country skill, you can quite easily make the half-mile ascent to Finger Lake. Follow a use trail starting near the outlet of Brainerd Lake and continuing on an arcing climb above the cliffs around the northwest shore. Cairns mark the route, as you weave through a boulder field on the way to the lakeshore.

Finger Lake (10,787 feet) conjures up visions of a miniature Norwegian fjord, occupying a slim cleft of rock arcing toward the Palisade Crest. Scattered pines dot the shoreline, while tiny pockets of grasses, sedges, and wildflowers attempt to soften the otherwise rocky basin. There are a number of campsites between the outlet and the trail. From Finger Lake, you can continue easily cross-country to the base of the Middle Palisade Glacier and a stunning view of the Palisades (see options below).

⊡ A Class 2 cross-country route over Contact Pass affords a fine connection to the Big Pine Lakes. From Willow Lake, head across the meadow above, and follow the south bank of a stream draining the east slopes of Mt. Gayley for 0.6 mile to a meadow. Cross the stream, and continue up the north bank across talus slopes past the creek draining Elinore Lake. Continue west then northwest to a small tarn in the cirque between Mt. Gayley and Temple Crag. From there, climb north toward the notch of Contact Pass (11,760 feet). Descend slopes north of the pass along the contact zone of dark and light rock to a bench above Third Lake, and then continue the descent to the south shore of Second Lake, where you can pick up use trails to the North Fork Trail.

A difficult Class 3 route requiring mountaineering equipment crosses the Sierra Crest southwest of The Thumb at Southfork Pass (12,560 feet). However, for those who wish simply to see one of the larger Sierra glaciers, the cross-country route above Finger Lake to the base of Middle Palisade is straightforward and not technically challenging, but it can be physically taxing, especially for flatlanders at this altitude. The rewards of seeing such dramatic alpine scenery more than compensates for the strenuous effort the hike requires.

R A wilderness permit is required for overnight stays. Campfires are prohibited.

BIG PINE CREEK TRAILHEAD

TRIP 111

Big Pine Lakes

MS **𝄐 DH or BP**

DISTANCE: 12.5 miles, semiloop

ELEVATION: 7,750'/10,815', +3,170'/-3,170'/±6,340'

SEASON: Mid-July to early October

USE: Moderate to heavy

MAPS: USGS's *Coyote Flat, Split Mountain, Mt. Thompson,* and *North Palisade* or Tom Harrison Maps' *The Palisades Trail Map*

TRAIL LOG

4.3	Black Lake Trail junction
4.6	First Lake
5.5	Third Lake
6.3	Glacier Trail junction
6.6	Four-way trail junction
7.3	Black Lake
8.3	North Fork Trail junction

INTRODUCTION: The North Fork Big Pine Creek Trail offers some of the best mountain scenery in the entire High Sierra. Piercing the sky near the upper heights of the range, the Palisades comprise a craggy spine of tall peaks robed in scenic splendor as picturesque and dramatic as any in California, if not the entire West.

Clinging beneath the north faces of these rugged 13,000- to 14,000-foot peaks, glaciers, including the Palisade Glacier (the largest in the Sierra), lend the area a definite alpine ambiance. Even the lower peaks, such as the exceedingly stunning Temple Crag, which offers a classic challenge for technical climbers and a spectacular profile from various vantages around the basin, cast a bold and rugged presence. Nestled beneath the shadow of these giant peaks, glacier-scoured Big Pine Lakes, with their milky-turquoise waters, offer rewarding

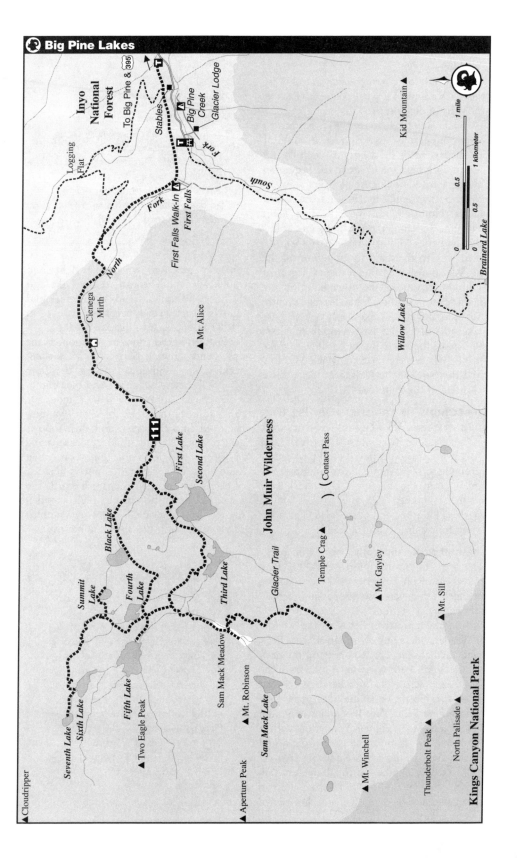

Big Pine Lakes

destinations for overnight stays. Many of the lakes are blessed with excellent vistas of the surrounding peaks.

Such awesome scenery is bound to inspire numerous visits by recreationists of all stripes. After the nearly 5-mile hike up North Fork Big Pine Creek to the beginning of Big Pine Lakes, most campers seem to congregate around First, Second, and Third Lakes. Not only are they the first lakes encountered after a stiff climb, mountaineers and rock climbers must pass them on their way to the majority of routes on the big peaks. You may find a higher degree of solitude at some of the other lakes off the main loop, including Fifth, Sixth, Seventh, Summit, and Black Lakes. Any one of these lakes provides a fine base camp from which to explore the basin. If time permits, dayhike up the Glacier Trail to Sam Mack Meadow and the base of the Palisade Glacier for a close-up of the Palisades.

DIRECTIONS TO TRAILHEAD: In Big Pine, turn west from US 395 onto Crocker Street (Glacier Lodge Road outside of town), and follow the two-lane, paved road past campgrounds to the overnight parking area, 9.2 miles from the highway. Dayhikers may continue another 0.75 mile to the day-use parking lot at the end of the road. There are vault toilets near both trailheads.

DESCRIPTION: From the overnight parking area, follow the North Fork Big Pine Creek Trail on an upward traverse across a sagebrush-covered slope, passing directly above a pack station.

Soon, impressive views of the Middle Palisades, including Norman Clyde Peak and the Palisade Crest, appear up the gash of the South Fork Canyon. A mile from the trailhead, where the trail bends northwest into the North Fork drainage, you pass above First Falls Walk-In Campground and soon come to a signed Y-junction with a trail angling through the campground and down-slope to the day-use parking area.

Continue climbing through open terrain with a fine view of Second Falls a mile up the canyon. Eventually, you reach a signed

GLACIER LODGE

Across the highway are Big Pine Campground, cabins, a general store, and the foundation of the historic Glacier Lodge. The cabins, general store, and trailer park remain open, but the main lodge building, which had been rebuilt following a 1969 avalanche, burned down in 1998.

four-way junction, where the right-hand trail heads uphill toward Baker Lake and the left-hand trail descends to the creek and follows a closed road, partially destroyed in a 1982 flood, back to the day-use lot.

Proceed ahead from the junction, as the trail bends toward Second Falls, switchbacking up a hillside, crossing the John Muir Wilderness boundary, and then climbing a chasm. Above the falls, a moderate climb follows the creek for a bit, wanders back out into the open, and then follows gently graded tread amid a dense stand of aspens and lodgepole pines on a flat known as Cienega Mirth (a combination of *cienega*, a misspelled Spanish word, and *mirth*, a Scottish word, which together mean "swampy place"). There are a number of pleasant campsites spread about the flat.

LON CHANEY CABIN

Currently used as a Forest Service wilderness cabin, this distinguished granite fieldstone cabin with a gabled roof and overhanging eaves was originally built in the 1920s at the direction of silent film star Lon Chaney, Sr., who used it as a summer retreat for fishing, hunting, and relaxing. Listed on the National Register of Historic Places, the cabin was designed by Paul Revere Williams (1894–1980), the first African-American granted a fellowship by the American Institute of Architects.

A short way up the trail, you may be surprised to see a renovated cabin in the midst of the wilderness.

Beyond the Lon Chaney cabin, you pass through an open area with a brief glimpse of the rugged peaks up the canyon and then resume climbing. The trail wanders to and from the creek numerous times through lush vegetation and light forest and then curves west, offering occasional views of the dramatic face of Temple Crag along the way. At 4 miles, cross willow-lined North Fork and then climb more steeply via switchbacks to another creek crossing. More climbing leads to a signed junction with the Black Lake Trail on the right, 4.3 miles from the parking lot.

Follow the left-hand trail across the North Fork and past a couple of campsites, continuing the climb through scattered trees, across granite slabs, and around boulders. Soon, you hear the sound of running water and catch a glimpse through the trees of milky-turquoise, glacier-fed First Lake (approximately 9,975 feet) below. There are slightly overused campsites above its west shore. A zigzagging ascent leads to a spectacular overlook of Second Lake with the ramparts of Temple Crag behind. Although Second Lake is the largest in the chain, the steep shoreline limits campsites on the trail side of the lake. Anglers can try their luck on rainbow, brook, and brown trout in both lakes.

Gently graded tread leads well above the north shore of Second Lake, where a sparse covering of trees permits fine views of the surrounding terrain, including dramatic, precipitous flying buttresses of Temple Crag looming high above the shimmering water. In stark contrast is the massive rockpile east of Second Lake known as Mt. Alice (Steve Roper expressed his disdain for the peak in *Climber's Guide to the High Sierra*, referring to it as "one of the ugliest peaks in the Sierra—a veritable pile of rubble"). Separating the two peaks is Contact Pass, where the distinction between darker and lighter shades of rock is quite evident. A cross-country route over the pass is a fine

way to access the South Fork (see options, Trip 110, page 389).

Beyond Second Lake, draw alongside the inlet, and climb through rocky terrain under a cover of lodgepole pines. Veer away from the creek and soon come to the north shore of Third Lake (10,249 feet), 5.5 miles from the parking lot. The lakeshore offers an even more impressive view of Temple Crag, which may account for the lake's popularity, or perhaps that's because of its abundance of campsites. Anglers may be tempted by rainbow and brook trout gliding through the water.

Leaving Third Lake behind, the trail switchbacks north up a hillside, where you have excellent views behind of Third Lake occupying a rocky bowl beneath the face of Temple Crag. To the south, the summits of the Palisades burst into view over a foreground ridge. The massive face of Mt. Robinson, with Aperture Peak poking out from behind, captures the view from the southwest. The grade eases a bit around a small meadow and the crossing of the tiny stream draining Fourth Lake. Just past the stream, reach a signed junction with the

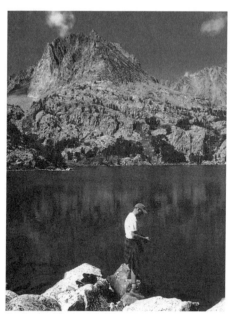

Angler at Second Lake

Glacier Trail near a grove of pines, 0.8 mile from Third Lake.

◎ **SIDE TRIP TO SAM MACK MEADOW AND PALISADE GLACIER:** From the junction with the Glacier Trail, head southwest through a willow-covered meadow and across a stream from Fifth Lake to a rocky slope, where a moderately steep, zigzagging ascent leads up a hillside through widely scattered whitebark pines. Pass a luxuriant, spring-fed grotto carpeted with wildflowers along the way. Farther up the slope, ascend alongside the main branch of the creek through more flowers, including paintbrush, buttercup, shooting star, daisy, aster, and columbine. The climb eases at the lip of a basin, as you stroll onto the verdant meadowlands of Sam Mack Meadow (approximately 11,035 feet).

The long, thin band of verdant Sam Mack Meadow is hemmed by steep walls of gray granite and bisected by the sinuous creek tinged with glacial milk. Snow patches cling to precipitous walls near the head of the vale, lingering throughout the short summers common at this elevation. There are a few campsites perched on the sloping, sandy bench adjacent to the meadow, surrounded by scattered clumps of dwarf pines. A footpath extends to the far end of the meadow, but those who wish to visit remote Sam Mack Lake will find the route up the west lip of the canyon wall easier than climbing up the headwall.

To reach the Palisade Glacier, ford the creek near the lower end of the meadow, where a small sign marked simply TRAIL points the way to a use trail on the far side. Ford the wide but shallow creek, and ascend the east slope on a winding course up a rocky hillside to a ridgecrest. From there, bend right (south), and continue winding around boulders and over slabs on the left-hand side of a ridge amid scattered whitebark pines. Excellent views of Big Pine Lakes basin are plentiful along the climb. Approximately a mile from the meadow, the route bends southeast on an ascending traverse over to a moraine. The path becomes faint, as you climb more steeply over talus,

boulders, and slabs, but cairns may help to keep you on route, until you reach an overlook of the Palisade Glacier with a stunning view of the Palisades. The semicircle vista includes, from right to left: Mt. Robinson, Aperture Peak, Mt. Agassiz, Mt. Winchell, Thunderbolt Peak, North Palisade, Mt. Sill, Mt. Gayley, and Temple Crag. **END OF SIDE TRIP**

From the Glacier Trail junction, head northwest on a moderate climb beside rocks, boulders, and scattered pines, with pleasant views of the Palisades above. At 6.6 miles, reach a prominent four-way junction, where the Black Lake Trail heads right and a lateral to Fifth Lake goes left, reaching the lake in a quarter mile. The middle route, a continuation of the North Fork Trail, provides access to Sixth, Seventh, and Summit Lakes. Directly ahead is Fourth Lake, a forest-rimmed body of water that lacks some of the views some of the other lakes offer but has plenty of campsites.

FOURTH LAKE LODGE

The amazing vista of the Palisades, spanning from Temple Crag to Mt. Winchell and including the Palisade Glacier, is the reason the Fourth Lake Lodge was built on this site in the 1920s. The Forest Service removed the lodge's stone house and eight wood cabins after the passage of the original Wilderness Act in 1964, leaving only a flat area and some scattered pieces of very small lumber.

◎ **SIDE TRIP TO FIFTH LAKE:** From the four-way junction, a short trail heads left (southwest) through light pine forest to the creek draining Fifth Lake. Follow alongside the willow-lined creek on a gentle climb to the east shore of the pretty lake. Rugged mountains, including Mt. Robinson, Two Eagle Peak, and Aperture Peak, form a scenic arc around the sapphire lake. As if these peaks failed to provide a stunning enough backdrop, the more distant summits of Temple Crag, Mt. Gayley, Mt. Sill, and the Inconsolable Range add even more picturesque alpine scenery. A smattering of pines dot the shoreline and lower slopes of the basin, while grasses, sedges, and shrubs take hold in small pockets of soil between rock cliffs and talus slopes. There are several pleasant campsites sprinkled around the inlet and farther around the shoreline. **END OF SIDE TRIP**

◉ **SIDE TRIP TO SIXTH AND SEVENTH LAKES:** From the four-way junction, follow the trail straight ahead (northwest) above the west shore of Fourth Lake, and then climb a hillside above the lake past some campsites. The grade increases where you cross a willow-lined stream flowing into the lake. Near the stream, an old, obscure path heads left toward Sixth Lake, which ends up being more of a cross-country route than a bona fide trail. In the opposite direction, a faint path soon leads to a level ridgetop camping area with incredible views.

From the junction with the obscure paths to Sixth Lake and the site of Fourth Lake Lodge, continue the ascent to a signed junction, 0.5 mile from the four-way junction. The left-hand trail heads to Sixth and Seventh Lakes, while the right-hand path goes to Summit Lake.

Turn left (north), and climb moderately steeply on rocky tread up some switchbacks to a pond surrounded by a small meadow. Resume the climb beyond the meadow, switchbacking to the top of a lightly forested rise, where a short stroll away from the trail leads to another incredible view of the Palisades. Drop off the rise into a meadow, hop across a creek, and then follow a short climb over a rock hump to a smaller meadow. After another stretch of climbing, the grade eases as Sixth Lake comes into view.

The atmosphere at Sixth Lake (11,088 feet) is more pastoral than that of most of the other lakes in the basin. Meadows surround the lake, and low rises dotted with whitebark pines present a softer background. The open terrain around the lake

affords good views of Mt. Robinson, Two Eagle Peak, and Cloudripper, as well as the more distant Temple Crag and Mt. Gayley. There are campsites scattered above the lake on top of the low rises.

Although a maintained trail does not connect Sixth and Seventh Lakes, the route is easy over open meadowlands dotted with clumps of willow. Simply travel northwest, paralleling the creek for less than a quarter mile to the east shore of Seventh Lake, which is quite pleasantly tucked into an open basin below the slopes of Cloudripper. There are few campsites, but they seem sufficient enough for the small number of campers who reach the lake. **END OF SIDE TRIP**

◉ **SIDE TRIP TO SUMMIT LAKE:** Follow the description above to the junction with the trail to Sixth Lake. Turn right (northeast) at the junction, and follow a moderate climb to the crest of a ridge. Soon, the lake appears through the trees, and a short descent delivers you to the shore, 0.5 mile from the junction. The roughly oval, forest-rimmed lake is perched on a bench above a steep drop plummeting toward Black Lake below. Campsites seem plentiful for the low numbers of backpackers seeking overnight shelter, and anglers can fish for brook trout. **END OF SIDE TRIP**

To continue the loop, turn right at the four-way junction, and head northeast on the Black Lake Trail, skirting the south shore of

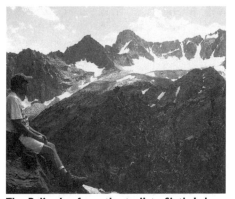

The Palisades from the trail to Sixth Lake

Fourth Lake on a mild decline through scattered to light forest. Soon, a gentle ascent leads over a forested rise before a moderate descent through a stand of lodgepole pines leads to Black Lake (approximately 10,690 feet), 7.3 miles from the overnight lot. A number of fine campsites around the lake will lure overnighters, and brook and rainbow trout will tempt anglers.

A steeper descent leads away from Black Lake, eventually leaving the forest behind to break out into the open to views of Temple Crag and Mt. Alice across the canyon and of Mt. Sill and North Palisade along the Sierra Crest. Farther along the trail, several of the Big Pine Lakes also come into view. Long-legged switchbacks lead across a sagebrush-covered sloped dotted with mountain mahogany, wild rose, and occasionally by whitebark and lodgepole pines. About 1 mile from Black Lake, you close the loop portion of the trip at the junction with the North Fork Trail. From there, turn left and retrace your steps 4.3 miles to the overnight parking lot.

Options abound for the backpacker blessed with plenty of time to explore the hinterlands beyond the lakes. A number of off-trail options, including the route over Contact Pass to South Fork Big Pine Creek and the Middle Palisade area (see options, Trip 110, page 389), may entice cross-country enthusiasts.

A Class 2–3 route over Jigsaw Pass in the Inconsolable Range links Fifth Lake with Bishop Pass Trail and Dusy Basin beyond. More technical routes over Agassiz Col and Glacier Notch may appeal to mountaineers.

The Palisades are a climber's paradise. No other area in the High Sierra provide as many challenging routes up so many classic peaks. Unfortunately, nontechnical climbers have few ascents to choose from other than the south ridge of Mt. Agassiz from Agassiz Col and the east ridge of Cloudripper.

R A wilderness permit is required for overnight stays. Campfires are prohibited.

SOUTH LAKE TRAILHEAD

TRIP 112

Long, Saddlerock, and Bishop Lakes

M / **DH or BP**

DISTANCE: 8.4 miles, out-and-back

ELEVATION: 9,845'/11,325', +1,740'/-260'/±4,000'

SEASON: Early July to early October

USE: Heavy

MAPS: USGS's *Mt. Thompson* and *North Palisade* or Tom Harrison Maps' *Bishop Pass North Lake-South Lake Loop Trail Map*

TRAIL LOG

0.75 Treasure Lakes Trail junction
1.9 Chocolate Lakes North Trail junction
2.3 Long Lake
2.7 Chocolate Lakes South Trail junction
3.8 Saddlerock Lake
4.3 Bishop Lake

INTRODUCTION: The Bishop Pass Trail is one of the least difficult ways over the Sierra Crest and into the backcountry of Kings Canyon National Park. The terrain south of Bishop Pass is highly popular with recreationists, which makes getting both a wilderness permit and a parking spot difficult on busy summer weekends.

Solitude is in short supply here, at least without stepping off maintained trail. However, if a little company isn't a problem, then picturesque lakes surrounded by stunning alpine peaks provide opportunities for either a dayhike or overnight backpack. Rushing streams, vibrant wildflowers, verdant meadows, and pine groves offer the finishing touches to a classic east Sierra journey.

DIRECTIONS TO TRAILHEAD: From Bishop, leave US 395, and turn west onto Line Drive, which is known as South Lake Road and Highway 168 outside of town. Proceed southwest 15 miles to a junction with Lake Sabrina Road, and turn left, remaining on South Lake Road. Continue 6.75 miles to the end of the road near South Lake. Backpackers must park in the overnight lot (when it is full, additional parking may be available 1.3 miles back down the road—a footpath connects to the trailhead). Dayhikers can park vehicles below the backpacker lot in spaces marked NO OVERNIGHT PARKING. Restrooms and water are available at the trailhead.

DESCRIPTION: Begin with a short, steep descent through lush vegetation, and then gently ascend above the east shore of South Lake through young aspens and lodgepole pines. Soon, break out into the open to fine

views up the canyon, as a steeper climb ensues. Cross the wilderness boundary, and continue climbing to a Y-junction with the Treasure Lakes Trail (see Trip 116, page 418), 0.75 mile from the trailhead.

Veer left (southeast), and continue through light lodgepole forest to a plank-bridge crossing of a small, flower-lined creek. A moderate climb leads to an unmarked, faint junction, 1.4 miles from the trailhead, with the partly cross-country route to Marie Lakes. Solitude seekers can follow this route northeast to a marshy meadow and then steeply southeast to the lakes.

Just beyond the junction, come alongside and then cross another small stream. Short-legged switchbacks lead over granite outcrops and boulders to the north junction of the Chocolate Lakes Trail, 1.9 miles from the trailhead.

From the junction, an easy quarter-mile stroll leads to the north shore of aptly

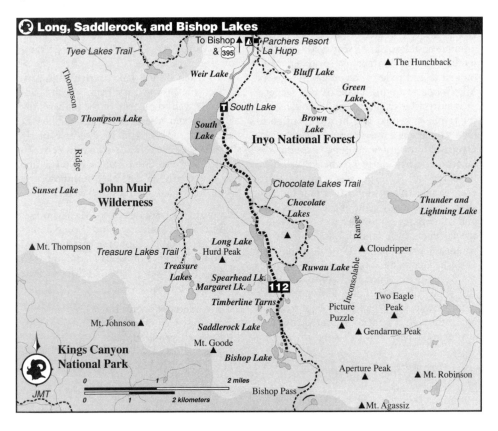

Long, Saddlerock, and Bishop Lakes

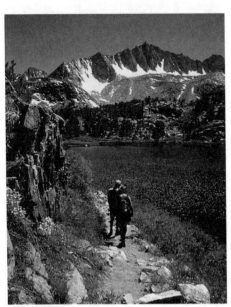

Long Lake and Mt. Goode

named Long Lake (10,753 feet). The elongated lake is bordered by green meadows, granite boulders, and scattered conifers. Its crystal-blue surface is sprinkled with tiny islets and reflects the craggy images of Mt. Goode and Hurd Peak. Its fine scenery, proximity to a trailhead, and good fishing for rainbow, brook, and brown trout combine to make it a very popular destination. Overused campsites abound around the lakeshore, particularly on the knoll above the south end. The lake seems to go on forever, as you follow the trail along the east shore, occasionally right at the water's edge and other times a good distance away. Near the far end of the lake, 2.7 miles from the trailhead, you come to the south junction with the Chocolate Lakes Trail.

Beyond the junction, continue along the shore of Long Lake, cross the inlet from Ruwau Lake, and then begin to climb again through a light to scattered forest of whitebark pines. Through small meadows,

boulder fields, and patches of wildflowers, climb across the slope east of Spearhead Lake (approximately 10,730 feet), which is quite picturesquely backdropped by the spine of the Inconsolable Range. There are limited campsites scattered around the lake, and fishing for rainbow and brook trout is reported to be fair. Easy cross-country travel leads west from the lake to isolated Margaret Lake.

A half-mile climb leads up a rocky slope to lovely Timberline Tarns, and sparkling waterfalls and tumbling cascades greet you along the way. Although most campers bypass this area, a handful of excellent, out-of-the-way campsites nearby are worthwhile spots for spending a night or two. A straightforward cross-country route from the east tarn leads north to Ruwau Lake.

From the tarns, a short climb leads up to island-dotted Saddlerock Lake (11,128 feet), 3.8 miles from the trailhead. Cradled in a glacier-scoured basin at the foot of the northeast buttress of towering Mt. Goode, the lake offers an austere haven for backpackers. Anglers can test their skill on rainbow and brook trout.

To reach Bishop Lake, rather than proceed on the Bishop Pass Trail, which skirts a hillside well to the east of the lake, follow an unmarked use trail from Saddlerock Lake over a low rise to the irregularly shaped shoreline (approximately 11,230 feet). There are good campsites on a low rise just north of the lake. Rainbow and brook trout also inhabit these waters.

O Short, off-trail forays to Marie Louise, Inconsolable, Margaret, and Ledge Lakes are quite possible. Mountaineers interested in nontechnical climbs can attempt Mt. Goode from Bishop Lake, or Mt. Agassiz from Bishop Pass.

R A wilderness permit is required for overnight stays. Campfires are prohibited. Bear canisters are required.

SOUTH LAKE TRAILHEAD

TRIP 113

Dusy Basin
and Le Conte Canyon

Ⓜ ⟋ BP

DISTANCE: 16 miles, out-and-back to Dusy Basin

26 miles, out-and-back to Le Conte Canyon

ELEVATION: 9,845'/11,972'/11,350', +2,500'/-1,550'/±6,100'

9,845'/11,972'/8,745', +2,585'/-3,680'/±12,530'

SEASON: Mid-July to early October

USE: Moderate to heavy

MAPS: USGS's *Mt. Thompson* and *North Palisade* or Tom Harrison Maps' *Bishop Pass North Lake-South Lake Loop Trail Map*

TRAIL LOG

0.75 Treasure Lakes Trail junction
1.9 Chocolate Lakes North Trail junction
2.3 Long Lake
2.7 Chocolate Lakes South Trail junction
3.8 Saddlerock Lake
4.3 Bishop Lake
6.0 Bishop Pass
8.0 Dusy Basin
10.5 Dusy Branch bridge
13.0 Le Conte Canyon and John Muir Trail junction

INTRODUCTION: Dusy Basin, where picturesque tarns encircled by lush meadows and sparkling granite slabs contrast vividly with a border of craggy peaks, is one of the prettiest alpine basins in the High Sierra. While the basin is a modest 8 miles from the trailhead, the moderately steep climb over a nearly 12,000-foot-high pass presents enough of a challenge that most backpackers use two days to reach it. With such stunning scenery, you should spend at least one additional day exploring the nooks and crannies of this exquisite parkland. Although there is no maintained trail through Dusy Basin, the terrain is uncomplicated, allowing for straightforward cross-country travel.

Extraordinary scenery coupled with relatively easy access makes Dusy Basin a popular destination. Such popularity creates pressure on the environment and increases competition for wilderness permits. Please observe all minimum impact guidelines while traveling or camping in Dusy Basin.

DIRECTIONS TO TRAILHEAD: From Bishop, leave US 395, and turn west onto Line Drive, which is known as South Lake Road and Highway 168 outside of town. Proceed southwest 15 miles to a junction with Lake Sabrina Road, and turn left, remaining on South Lake Road. Continue 6.75 miles to the end of the road near South Lake. Backpackers must park in the overnight lot (when full, additional parking may be available 1.3 miles back down the road—a footpath connects to the trailhead). Dayhikers can park vehicles below the backpacker lot in spaces marked NO OVERNIGHT PARKING. Restrooms and water are available at the trailhead.

DESCRIPTION: Begin with a short, steep descent through lush vegetation, and then gently ascend above the east shore of South Lake through young aspens and lodgepole pines. Soon, break out into the open to fine views up the canyon, as a steeper climb ensues. Cross the wilderness boundary, and continue climbing to a Y-junction with the Treasure Lakes Trail (see Trip 116, page 418), 0.75 mile from the trailhead.

Veer left (southeast), and continue through light lodgepole forest to a plank-bridge crossing of a small, flower-lined creek. A moderate climb leads to an unmarked, faint junction, 1.4 miles from the trailhead, with the partly cross-country route to Marie Lakes. Solitude seekers can follow this route

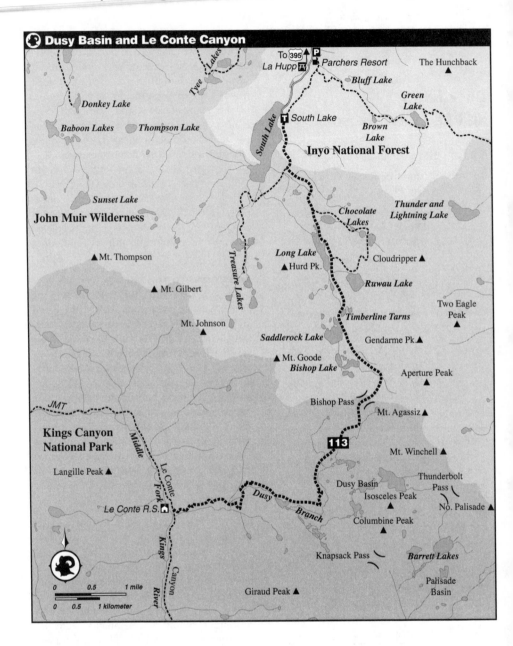

Dusy Basin and Le Conte Canyon

Tyee Lakes

To 395
La Hupp
Parchers Resort
The Hunchback ▲
Bluff Lake

Donkey Lake

Green Lake

Baboon Lakes   Thompson Lake   South Lake

Brown Lake

Inyo National Forest

South Lake

Sunset Lake

Chocolate Lakes

Thunder and Lightning Lake

John Muir Wilderness

Treasure Lakes

Long Lake
▲ Hurd Pk.

Cloudripper ▲

▲ Mt. Thompson

Ruwau Lake

▲ Mt. Gilbert

Two Eagle Peak ▲

Mt. Johnson ▲

Timberline Tarns

Saddlerock Lake

Gendarme Pk.▲

▲ Mt. Goode
Bishop Lake

Aperture Peak ▲

Bishop Pass

JMT

Mt. Agassiz ▲

Kings Canyon National Park

113

Mt. Winchell ▲

Langille Peak ▲

Middle

Thunderbolt Pass

Dusy Basin
Isosceles Peak ▲

No. Palisade ▲

Le Conte Fork

Dusy

Le Conte R.S.

Branch

Columbine Peak ▲

Kings Canyon River

Knapsack Pass

Barrett Lakes

0   0.5   1 mile

Palisade Basin

0   0.5   1 kilometer

Giraud Peak ▲

northeast to a marshy meadow and then steeply southeast to the lakes.

Just beyond the junction, come alongside and then cross another small stream. Short-legged switchbacks lead over granite outcrops and boulders to the north junction of the Chocolate Lakes Trail, 1.9 miles from the trailhead.

From the junction, an easy quarter-mile stroll leads to the north shore of aptly named Long Lake (10,753 feet). The elongated lake is bordered by green meadows, granite boulders, and scattered conifers. The crystal-blue surface is sprinkled with tiny islets and reflects the craggy images of Mt. Goode and Hurd Peak. Its fine scenery, proximity to a trailhead, and good fishing for rainbow, brook, and brown trout combine to make it a very popular destination. Overused campsites abound around the overused lakeshore, particularly on the knoll above the south end. The lake seems to go on forever, as you follow the trail along the east shore, occasionally right at the water's edge and other times a good distance away. Near the far end of the lake, 2.7 miles from the trailhead, you come to the south junction with the Chocolate Lakes Trail.

Beyond the junction, continue along the shore of Long Lake, cross the inlet from Ruwau Lake, and then begin to climb again through a light to scattered forest of whitebark pines. Through small meadows, boulder fields, and patches of wildflowers, climb across the slope east of Spearhead Lake (approximately 10,730 feet), which is quite picturesque backdropped by the spine of the Inconsolable Range. There are limited campsites scattered around the lake, and fishing for rainbow and brook trout is reported to be fair. Easy cross-country travel leads west from the lake to isolated Margaret Lake.

A half-mile climb leads up a rocky slope to lovely Timberline Tarns, and sparkling waterfalls and tumbling cascades greet you along the way. Although most campers bypass this area, a handful of excellent, out-of-the-way campsites nearby are worthwhile spots for spending a night or two. A straightforward cross-country route from the east tarn leads north to Ruwau Lake.

From the tarns, a short climb leads up to island-dotted Saddlerock Lake (11,128 feet), 3.8 miles from the trailhead. Cradled in a glacier-scoured basin at the foot of the northeast buttress of towering Mt. Goode, the lake offers an austere haven for backpackers. Anglers can test their skill on rainbow and brook trout.

If you're planning on camping at Bishop Lake, follow an unmarked use trail from Saddlerock Lake over a low rise to irregularly shaped Bishop Lake (approximately 11,230 feet), as the Bishop Pass Trail skirts a hillside well to the east of the lake. There are good campsites on a low rise just north

of the lake. Rainbow and brook trout also inhabit these waters.

Continuing on the Bishop Pass Trail, hike above timberline into the alpine zone on rocky tread composed of red metamorphosed rock. Soon the grade increases, where the winding trail passes through granite terrain on a climb of the dramatic cirque wall up to the pass. Through a seemingly endless sea of boulders and slabs, continue the laborious ascent, perhaps pausing occasionally to catch your breath while enjoying spectacular views of Mt. Goode and the spires of the Inconsolable Range.

Depending on the previous winter's snowpack, snow patches may cover the trail well into summer on the way to Bishop Pass (11,972 feet), 6 miles from the trailhead, where signs herald your arrival at the boundary of Kings Canyon National Park. The westward vista is quite striking, with the meadow-rimmed tarns of Dusy Basin directly below, backdropped nicely by Giraud and Columbine Peaks. To the southwest, beyond the deep chasm of Le Conte Canyon, the Black Divide casts a regal profile against the Sierra sky. Flanking the pass to the northeast, Mt. Agassiz beckons energetic climbers toward its summit.

After the taxing uphill climb, descend from the pass on sandy tread to some

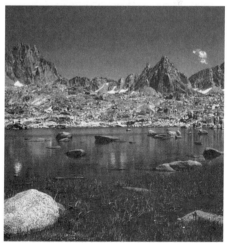

One of the many unnamed tarns in beautiful Dusy Basin

switchbacks, where a fairly defined use trail leads shortly to the top of a cliff, from where you have an excellent view of Dusy Basin and the surrounding peaks and ridges. Back on the main trail, continue the winding descent, encountering welcome patches of verdant meadow and an assortment of wildflowers, well watered through midseason by gurgling freshets. Along the descent, you will have plenty of fine views of Dusy Basin dramatically framed by the crags of the Palisades and Isosceles and Columbine Peaks.

Approximately 1.5 miles from the pass, a use trail branches left and leads to the uppermost tarn (approximately 11,350 feet) in the basin. You can follow this path to campsites around this tarn or continue to more secluded sites near Lake 11388 or Lake 11425. By continuing down the Bishop Pass Trail another 0.75 mile, you can access another use trail to campsites around the lower tarns.

FRANK DUSY

Dusy Basin's namesake was a Canadian-born shepherd who drove his flocks from the western foothills into the Kings River backcountry, exploring the Middle Fork all the way upstream to the Palisades. He was credited with the 1869 discovery of Tehipite Valley and for taking the first photos of the area 10 years later.

Wherever you stay, Dusy Basin is an exquisitely beautiful area, with small pockets of luxuriant meadow and acres of sparkling granite bordering azure tarns and tiny, crystalline rivulets. The neighboring peaks create a splendid alpine backdrop, with rugged spires piercing the rarified air and precipitous faces and knife-edge ridges providing plenty of challenges for the hardiest mountaineer. The delicate alpine vegetation is colorfully vibrant and quite fragile—camp only in pockets of sandy soil devoid of plant life.

While traveling across the basin, follow the least noxious routes to damage the vegetation as little as possible. There are plenty of campsites throughout the basin, but campers seem to congregate in areas closest to the Bishop Pass Trail. Possibilities for seclusion increase at campsites around tarns farthest from the main trail. From a base camp, you could spend days exploring the more remote corners of the basin on dayhikes. Anglers may test their skill on golden and brook trout. Along with recreationists, photographers are also drawn to the incredible scenery in Dusy Basin; alpenglow on the west faces of the Palisades can create a dreamlike climax to a spectacular sunset, an ideal conclusion to a day in Dusy Basin.

Those bound for Le Conte Canyon and a connection with the John Muir Trail (JMT) should continue the scenic descent from Dusy Basin down the Bishop Pass Trail. Widely scattered whitebark pines grace the upper end of the basin and become slightly less scattered as the elevation drops. Interspersed between granite slabs and boulders are pockets of verdant meadow, clumps of willow and heather, and colorful wildflowers, including shooting star, penstemon, aster, and buttercup. Such vegetation greets you along the trail, which follows the winding Dusy Branch dancing toward the Middle Fork Kings River below in Le Conte Canyon. Just beyond Lake 10742, the trail reaches the lip of Dusy Basin, from where you gaze into the deep declivity of the canyon.

More switchbacks follow as the stiff descent continues, offering periodic views of the Dusy Branch spilling down a nearly vertical wall of granite. Gazing down the hillside below reveals an avalanche swath, where a large stand of trees was swept away in years past. The trail plunges down the slope to a lightly forested bench and a pair of crossings over the multibranched creek. Among the nearby trees are a number of excellent campsites along the creek.

Beyond the crossings, proceed down the canyon wall through light to scattered lodgepole pine forest, interrupted briefly by an open chaparral-covered slope offering a dramatic view of the canyon and towering Langille Peak. As the descent ends, the open vegetation gives way to a light covering of forest shading the floor of the canyon. Reach a signed junction with the JMT, 13 miles from the trailhead. Campsites are spread around the area on either side of the Le Conte Canyon Ranger Station.

[O] An adventurous but straightforward cross-country loop leads from Dusy Basin over Knapsack Pass (approximately 11,680 feet) through stunning Palisade Basin, and then back to Dusy Basin over Thunderbolt Pass (approximately 12,360 feet). The route is not technically demanding, but ascending and descending the passes over slopes filled with talus can be tedious. From lower Dusy Basin, head east toward the saddle directly south of Columbine Peak, and ascend a gully, working your way through brush and then rocks. A use trail that once made the climb easier was partially destroyed in a rockslide years ago.

Traverse east from the saddle, and then drop to barren Barrett Lakes. From the uppermost lake, climb north over talus toward the distinct saddle immediately southeast of Thunderbolt Peak. Descend from the saddle over more talus to the uppermost lake in Dusy Basin.

Extended backpack routes are easy to create from Dusy Basin through neighboring Palisade Basin and over Potluck Pass (approximately 12,120 feet), connecting with the JMT near Lower Palisade Lake. From there, an uncomplicated loop back to Dusy Basin follows the JMT north through Le Conte Canyon and then east up the Bishop Pass Trail (37 miles round-trip with 6 miles off-trail).

If Dusy Basin seems too crowded, the narrow canyon holding Rainbow Lakes should provide more seclusion. These seldom-visited lakes are cradled in glacier-scoured bowls beneath the north face of Giraud Peak and quite scenic. To reach the lakes, leave the Bishop Pass Trail near the lower end of Dusy Basin, about 0.3 mile northwest of Lake 10742, and traverse cross-country a half mile to the first lake (approximately 10,720 feet). Brook trout are reported to inhabit the two larger lakes.

While all the impressive peaks of the Palisades require technical climbing in order to reach their summits, mountaineers will find less demanding challenges on Class 2 routes from Bishop Pass to either Mt. Agassiz or Mt. Goode. Columbine Peak, on the southeast edge of Dusy Basin, is Class 2 from Knapsack Pass. An ascent of the east ridge of Giraud Peak from the peak immediately northeast is also rated Class 2.

Once you are on the JMT, you have numerous options for further wanderings, especially if you can make shuttle arrangements for alternate trailheads. With a minimal distance between trailheads, a multiday trip northbound on the JMT to the Piute Pass Trail and then east over Piute Pass to North Lake is a popular near-loop journey. Cross-country enthusiasts can accomplish the same goal over a shorter distance by crossing the Glacier Divide at either Snow Tongue Pass (approximately 12,200 feet, 1.5 miles northwest of Mt. Goethe, Class 2–3), or Alpine Col (approximately 12,320 feet, Class 2) and then connecting to the Piute Pass Trail in Humphreys Basin. Heading southbound on the JMT, backpackers can connect with a variety of eastside trailheads.

[R] A wilderness permit is required for overnight stays. Campfires are prohibited. Bear canisters are required. Stock is prohibited in Dusy Basin.

SOUTH LAKE TRAILHEAD

TRIP 114

John Muir Trail: South Lake to North Lake

(MS) ✗ **BPx**

DISTANCE: 55.1 miles, point-to-point

ELEVATION: 9,845'/11,972'/8,745'/
11,955'/8,075'/11,423'/9,255',
+10,580'/-11,150'/±21,730'

SEASON: Mid-July to early October

USE: Moderate to heavy

MAPS: USGS's *Mt. Thompson,*
North Palisade, Mt. Goddard,
Mt. Darwin, Mt. Henry,
Mt. Hilgard, and *Mt. Tom* or
Tom Harrison Maps' *Bishop*
Pass North Lake-South Loop
Trail Map

TRAIL LOG

6.0 Bishop Pass
13.0 John Muir Trail junction
13.5 Little Pete Meadow
14.9 Big Pete Meadow
19.5 Helen Lake and Ionian Basin route
20.8 Muir Pass
23.0 Wanda Lake
24.8 Sapphire Lake and McGee Lakes route
25.5 Evolution Lake
26.5 Lamarck Col, The Keyhole, Alpine Col, and Snow Tongue Pass routes
29.9 Colby Meadow
30.7 McClure Meadow and McGee Lakes route
33.1 Evolution Creek ford
34.6 Goddard Canyon Trail junction
36.9 Aspen Meadow
38.1 Piute Pass Trail junction
43.2 Hutchinson Meadow and Piute Creek Pass Trail junction
50.5 Piute Pass
55.1 North Lake Trailhead

INTRODUCTION: This 25-mile stretch of the John Muir Trail (JMT) between the Bishop Pass and Piute Pass junctions passes through the remarkably scenic Evolution Basin, where a narrow rockbound canyon holds a string of jeweled alpine lakes in the shadow of towering peaks. Referred to as the Evolution Group, Mounts Huxley, Fiske, Wallace, Haeckel, Spencer, Darwin, and Mendel reign over the region in absolute mountain majesty. Six of these summits reach elevations of more than 13,000 feet, with 12,431-foot Mt. Spencer the lone exception. Although Theodore S. Solomons, explorer, charter member of the Sierra Club, and JMT visionary, named the peaks in 1895 for contemporary proponents of evolutionary theory, such appellations fall short of capturing the area's true grandeur.

Farther downstream, Evolution Valley is the picturesque subalpine equivalent to the alpine basin, where serene lodgepole pine forests separate the verdant meadowlands of Colby, McClure, and Evolution Meadows. The oftentimes sinuous course of Evolution Creek flowing gracefully through the namesake valley provides the ideal complement to the pastoral ambiance found in the meadows.

If Evolution Basin and Valley were the only treasures, the trip would be well worth the time and effort involved. However, additional gems await your discovery, including the parklands of Dusy Basin, the Middle Fork Kings River flowing through the deep granite cleft of Le Conte Canyon, the alpine wonderland around Muir Pass, and the beautiful canyon of South Fork San Joaquin River. If you consider wildflower-laden meadows, glacier-carved canyons, striking alpine peaks, and crystalline lakes to be essentials to a classic High Sierra adventure, then this trip will not disappoint you.

Since you follow well-maintained trails for the duration of this trip, you will face no major route-finding challenges. However, you will need to consider the usual factors involved with high-altitude journeys through the High Sierra, including the potential for snow-covered slopes below the high passes and potentially difficult fords at the crossings of major rivers and creeks.

DIRECTIONS TO TRAILHEAD:

START: From Bishop, leave US 395, and turn west onto Line Drive, which is known as South Lake Road and Highway 168 outside of town. Proceed southwest 15 miles to a junction with Lake Sabrina Road, and turn left, remaining on South Lake Road. Continue 6.75 miles to the end of the road near South Lake. Backpackers must park in the overnight lot (when it is full, additional parking may be available 1.3 miles back down the road—a footpath connects to the trailhead). Dayhikers can park vehicles below the backpacker lot in spaces marked NO OVERNIGHT PARKING. Restrooms and water are available at the trailhead.

END: From Bishop, leave US 395, and turn west onto Line Drive, which is known as South Lake Road and Highway 168 outside of town. Proceed southwest 15 miles to a junction with Lake Sabrina Road, and continue ahead for 3 miles to the North Lake Road junction where you turn right. Follow single-lane, gravel road 1 mile to the day-use parking lot. Backpackers must travel another 0.6 mile to a right-hand turn onto a short spur leading to dual overnight parking lots directly west of North Lake.

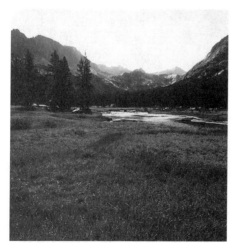

Lush meadowlands in Evolution Valley on the John Muir Trail

DESCRIPTION: As the first leg of the journey involves getting to the JMT, begin with a short, steep descent through lush vegetation, and then gently ascend above the east shore of South Lake through young aspens and lodgepole pines. Soon, break out into the open to fine views up the canyon, as a steeper climb ensues. Cross the wilderness boundary, and continue climbing to a Y-junction with the Treasure Lakes Trail (see Trip 116, page 418), 0.75 mile from the trailhead.

Veer left (southeast), and continue through light lodgepole forest to a plank-bridge crossing of a small, flower-lined creek. A moderate climb leads to an unmarked, faint junction, 1.4 miles from the trailhead, with the partly cross-country route to Marie Lakes. Solitude seekers can follow this route northeast to a marshy meadow and then steeply southeast to the lakes.

Just beyond the junction, come alongside and then cross another small stream. Short-legged switchbacks lead over granite outcrops and boulders to the north junction of the Chocolate Lakes Trail, 1.9 miles from the trailhead.

From the junction, an easy quarter-mile stroll leads to the north shore of aptly named Long Lake (10,753 feet). The elongated lake is bordered by green meadows, granite boulders, and scattered conifers. The crystal-blue surface is sprinkled with tiny islets and reflects the craggy images of Mt. Goode and Hurd Peak. Its fine scenery, proximity to a trailhead, and good fishing for rainbow, brook, and brown trout combine to make it a very popular destination. Overused campsites abound around the overused lakeshore, particularly on the knoll above the south end. The lake seems to go on forever, as you follow the trail along the east shore, occasionally right at the water's edge and other times a good distance away. Near the far end of the lake, 2.7 miles from the trailhead, you come to the south junction with the Chocolate Lakes Trail.

Beyond the junction, continue along the shore of Long Lake, cross the inlet from Ruwau Lake, and then begin to climb

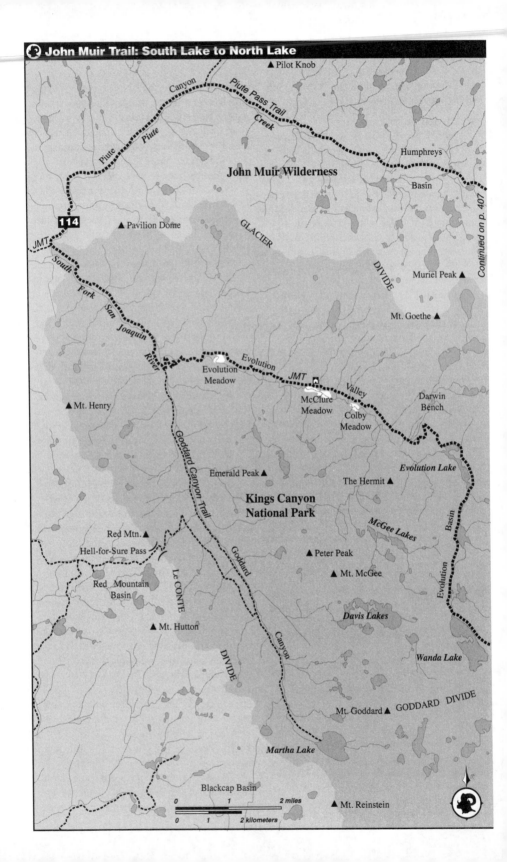

▲ Pilot Knob

Piute Pass Trail

Canyon

Creek

Piute

Piute

Piute

Humphreys

Basin

John Muir Wilderness

Continued on p. 407

114

▲ Pavilion Dome

GLACIER

DIVIDE

Muriel Peak ▲

JMT

South

Fork

San

Joaquin

River

Mt. Goethe ▲

Evolution

Evolution
Meadow

JMT

Valley

Darwin
Bench

▲ Mt. Henry

McClure
Meadow

Colby
Meadow

Goddard Canyon Trail

Emerald Peak ▲

Evolution Lake

The Hermit ▲

**Kings Canyon
National Park**

McGee Lakes

Red Mtn. ▲

Hell-for-Sure Pass

Goddard

▲ Peter Peak

Evolution

Basin

Le CONTE

Red Mountain
Basin

▲ Mt. McGee

Davis Lakes

▲ Mt. Hutton

Canyon

Wanda Lake

DIVIDE

Mt. Goddard ▲ GODDARD DIVIDE

Martha Lake

Blackcap Basin

0   1   2 miles

0   1   2 kilometers

▲ Mt. Reinstein

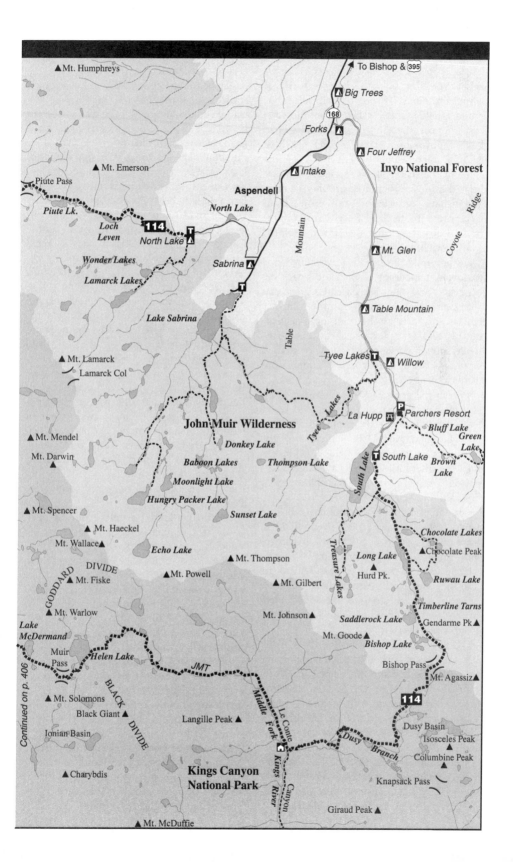

▲Mt. Humphreys

To Bishop & 395

🏕️ Big Trees

🏕️ 168

Forks 🏕️

🏕️ Four Jeffrey

▲ Mt. Emerson

🏕️ Intake

Inyo National Forest

Piute Pass

Aspendell

North Lake

Piute Lk.

Loch Leven

114 🅣

North Lake 🏕️

🏕️ Mt. Glen

Mountain

Coyote Ridge

Wonder Lakes

Sabrina 🏕️

Lamarck Lakes

🅣

🏕️ Table Mountain

Lake Sabrina

Table

▲ Mt. Lamarck

Lamarck Col

Tyee Lakes 🅣 🏕️ Willow

La Hupp 🅿️ 🏕️ Parchers Resort

Bluff Lake

John Muir Wilderness

Donkey Lake

Green Lake

▲ Mt. Mendel

Mt. Darwin ▲

Baboon Lakes   *Thompson Lake*

South Lake

🅣 *South Lake*

Brown Lake

Tyee Lakes

Moonlight Lake

Hungry Packer Lake

▲ Mt. Spencer

Sunset Lake

▲ Mt. Haeckel

Chocolate Lakes

Mt. Wallace▲

Echo Lake

▲Chocolate Peak

Treasure Lakes

Long Lake

DIVIDE

▲Mt. Powell

▲ Mt. Thompson

Hurd Pk.
▲

Ruwau Lake

GODDARD

▲ Mt. Fiske

▲Mt. Gilbert

Timberline Tarns

▲ Mt. Warlow

Mt. Johnson▲

Saddlerock Lake

Gendarme Pk ▲

Lake McDermand

Mt. Goode▲

Bishop Lake

Muir Pass

Helen Lake

JMT

Bishop Pass

114

Middle Fork

Le Conte

Mt. Agassiz▲

▲ Mt. Solomons

BLACK

Black Giant ▲

Langille Peak ▲

Dusy Basin

Ionian Basin

DIVIDE

Dusy Branch

Isosceles Peak

Columbine Peak
▲

Continued on p. 406

▲ Charybdis

Kings Canyon National Park

Canyon

Kings River

Knapsack Pass

Giraud Peak ▲

▲ Mt. McDuffie

again through a light to scattered forest of whitebark pines. Through small meadows, boulder fields, and patches of wildflowers, climb across the slope east of Spearhead Lake (approximately 10,730 feet), which is quite picturesque backdropped by the spine of the Inconsolable Range. There are limited campsites scattered around the lake, and fishing for rainbow and brook trout is reported to be fair. Easy cross-country travel leads west from the lake to isolated Margaret Lake.

A half-mile climb leads up a rocky slope to lovely Timberline Tarns, and sparkling waterfalls and tumbling cascades greet you along the way. Although most campers bypass this area, a handful of excellent, out-of-the-way campsites nearby are worthwhile spots for spending a night or two. A straightforward cross-country route from the east tarn leads north to Ruwau Lake.

From the tarns, a short climb leads up to island-dotted Saddlerock Lake (11,128 feet), 3.8 miles from the trailhead. Cradled in a glacier-scoured basin at the foot of the northeast buttress of towering Mt. Goode, the lake offers an austere haven for backpackers. Anglers can test their skill on rainbow and brook trout.

If you're planning on camping at Bishop Lake, follow an unmarked use trail from Saddlerock Lake over a low rise to irregularly shaped Bishop Lake (approximately 11,230 feet), as the Bishop Pass Trail skirts a hillside well to the east of the lake. There are good campsites on a low rise just north of the lake. Rainbow and brook trout also inhabit these waters.

Continuing on the Bishop Pass Trail, hike above timberline into the alpine zone on rocky tread composed of red metamorphosed rock. Soon the grade increases, where the winding trail passes through granite terrain on a climb of the dramatic cirque wall up to the pass. Through a seemingly endless sea of boulders and slabs, continue the laborious ascent, perhaps pausing occasionally to catch your breath while enjoying spectacular views of Mt. Goode and the spires of the Inconsolable Range.

Depending on the previous winter's snowpack, snow patches may cover the trail well into summer on the way to Bishop Pass (11,972 feet), 6 miles from the trailhead, where signs herald your arrival at the boundary of Kings Canyon National Park. The westward vista is quite striking, with the meadow-rimmed tarns of Dusy Basin directly below, backdropped nicely by Giraud and Columbine Peaks. To the southwest, beyond the deep chasm of Le Conte Canyon, the Black Divide casts a regal profile against the Sierra sky. Flanking the pass to the northeast, Mt. Agassiz beckons energetic climbers toward its summit.

After the taxing uphill climb, descend from the pass on sandy tread to some switchbacks, where a fairly defined use trail leads shortly to the top of a cliff, from where you have an excellent view of Dusy Basin and the surrounding peaks and ridges. Back on the main trail, continue the winding descent, encountering welcome patches of verdant meadow and an assortment of wildflowers, well watered through midseason by gurgling freshets. Along the descent, you will have plenty of fine views of Dusy Basin dramatically framed by the crags of the Palisades and Isosceles and Columbine Peaks.

Approximately 1.5 miles from the pass, a use trail branches left and leads to the uppermost tarn (approximately 11,350 feet) in the basin. You can follow this path to campsites around this tarn or continue to more secluded sites near Lake 11388 or Lake 11425. By continuing down the Bishop Pass Trail another 0.75 mile, you can access another use trail to campsites around the lower tarns.

Wherever you stay, Dusy Basin is an exquisitely beautiful area, with small pockets of luxuriant meadow and acres of sparkling granite bordering azure tarns and tiny, crystalline rivulets. The neighboring peaks create a splendid alpine backdrop, with rugged spires piercing the rarified air and precipitous faces and knife-edge ridges providing plenty of challenges for the hardiest mountaineer. The delicate alpine vegetation is colorfully vibrant and quite fragile—camp only in pockets of sandy soil devoid of plant life.

While traveling across the basin, follow the least noxious routes to damage the vegetation as little as possible. There are plenty of campsites throughout the basin, but campers seem to congregate in areas closest to the Bishop Pass Trail. Possibilities for seclusion increase at campsites around tarns farthest from the main trail. From a base camp, you could spend days exploring the more remote corners of the basin on dayhikes. Anglers may test their skill on golden and brook trout. Along with recreationists, photographers are also drawn to the incredible scenery in Dusy Basin; alpenglow on the west faces of the Palisades can create a dreamlike climax to a spectacular sunset, an ideal conclusion to a day in Dusy Basin.

Bound for Le Conte Canyon and a connection with the John Muir Trail (JMT), continue the scenic descent from Dusy Basin down the Bishop Pass Trail. Widely scattered whitebark pines grace the upper end of the basin and become slightly less scattered as the elevation drops. Interspersed between granite slabs and boulders are pockets of verdant meadow, clumps of willow and heather, and colorful wildflowers, including shooting star, penstemon, aster, and buttercup. Such vegetation greets you along the trail, which follows the winding Dusy Branch dancing toward the Middle Fork Kings River below in Le Conte Canyon. Just beyond Lake 10742, the trail reaches the lip of Dusy Basin, from where you gaze into the deep declivity of the canyon.

More switchbacks follow as the stiff descent continues, offering periodic views of the Dusy Branch spilling down a nearly vertical wall of granite. Gazing down the hillside below reveals an avalanche swath, where a large stand of trees was swept away in years past. The trail plunges down the slope to a lightly forested bench and a pair of crossings over the multibranched creek. Among the nearby trees are a number of excellent campsites along the creek.

Beyond the crossings, proceed down the canyon wall through light to scattered lodgepole pine forest, interrupted briefly by an open chaparral-covered slope offering a dramatic view of the canyon and towering Langille Peak. As the descent ends, the open vegetation gives way to a light covering of forest shading the floor of the canyon. Reach a signed junction with the JMT, 13 miles from the trailhead. Campsites are spread around the area on either side of the Le Conte Canyon Ranger Station.

From the Bishop Pass Trail junction, head northbound on the JMT on gently graded tread through light forest, passing numerous campsites on either side of the Le Conte Canyon Ranger Station and along the east bank of Middle Fork Kings River. The grade increases where the forest is left behind, the open terrain allowing impressive views of the towering profile of 12,018-foot Langille Peak looming over Le Conte Canyon. Until late summer, a prolific display of wildflowers lines the trail on the way to Little Pete Meadow, where the grade eases and the river mellows on a meandering course through the slightly sloping, grass-covered meadow. Sagebrush and lodgepole pines border the meadow and harbor a number of adequate campsites. Anglers should find fishing in the river for rainbow, brook, and golden trout to be good.

The climb resumes beyond the meadow through open terrain with fine views up the canyon of the now cascading river. After a couple of stream crossings, you drop into a lush wildflower garden intermixed with young aspens, pass through a drift fence, and then climb through scattered pines to Big Pete Meadow, 1.8 miles from the Bishop Pass junction. The mostly forested meadow harbors a number of campsites.

The JMT veers west, crosses some streams, and passes through an area extensively damaged by a previous avalanche, where massive Langille Peak continues to dominate the view. About a quarter mile beyond the meadow, the trail passes more campsites and closely follows the course of the river in and out of light forest cover. A moderate to moderately steep climb ensues between walls of granite, which can feel a bit like walking through an oven during hot and sunny afternoons. Above a talus slope, skirt a side canyon, and climb above granite slabs to a fine view of a waterfall on the turbulent Middle Fork. Follow the trail across a luxuriant, seep-watered hillside with a bounty of wildflowers to rocky switchbacks climbing above the fall and into a small basin filled with delightful tarns and verdant meadows. The grade eases momentarily on a stroll through this picturesque grotto, bordered by intermittent, mixed stands of mountain hemlocks and lodgepole, western white, and whitebark pines. After crossing a brook, a short climb leads to campsites nestled beneath a stand of trees near the trail.

More switchbacks lead up to views of a pond-filled basin, where there are primitive campsites scattered around the shorelines. After crossing the turbulent Middle Fork, wander around a tangle of rock humps and low ridges to a large tarn. Backpackers in need of overnight accommodations could set up camp on a rock shelf above the south shore or on a rise southwest of the tarn.

Amid diminishing whitebark pines, you leave the tarn behind and cross back over the nascent Middle Fork, follow the river for a bit, and then veer away before rejoining it farther up the slope. Climb past another unnamed tarn, and continue up the narrowing slot of the Middle Fork to the east shore of rockbound, sprawling, and majestic Helen Lake (11,617 feet), named for one of John Muir's daughters. With a little searching, you will find campsites scattered around this massive body of water, but the ground-hugging vegetation offers little protection from the elements. However, the stark beauty of the surroundings can be quite compelling.

Follow the southern edge of Helen Lake to where the trail weaves around some tarns to the base of the final slope leading up to the pass. From there, switchbacks zigzag up to Muir Pass (11,955 feet) along the Goddard Divide near the stone Muir Hut. Spread about before you is a fine view of the upper part of Evolution Basin, with gigantic Wanda Lake and the much smaller Lake McDermand the two prominent bodies of water visible.

MUIR HUT

The beehive-shaped stone Muir Hut was built by the Sierra Club in 1933 to honor the organization's most prestigious member, cofounder, and original president. The hut was also constructed to "offer protection and safety to storm-bound travelers." While it is available for temporary shelter, camping inside the hut and outside in the immediate vicinity is prohibited.

The descent from Muir Pass begins moderately and then eases to mild across the upper end of Evolution Basin. Less than a mile from the pass, you encounter lonely Lake McDermand (approximately 11,650 feet) and follow the west shore to the far end. A short drop in elevation leads to Wanda Lake, named for Muir's other daughter, where there are spartan campsites on the rise northeast of the lake, near the outlet, and on the far shore. Diminutive alpine vegetation in cracks and crannies attempts to soften the otherwise austere surroundings at Wanda Lake. However, the scenery is stunning, with glacier-clad Mt. Goddard rising sharply into the southwest sky, and Mts. Huxley, Spencer, Darwin, and Mendel filling the horizon to the north. From the outlet, a cross-country route travels over Davis Lake Pass to Davis Lake and onward into Goddard Canyon.

In the shadow of Mt. Huxley, continue a mild descent following the course of Evolution Creek, ford the creek, and then pass the next unnamed gem in the string of lakes. Soon, you drop into the depression holding beautiful Sapphire Lake (10,966 feet). Sapphire is perhaps the prettiest of the Evolution Lakes, the glacier-polished canyon sandwiched between towering summits on both sides of the trail. Campsites are even less prevalent here than at Wanda Lake. The trailless mini-basin to the east of the lake offers more remote campsites around smaller, 11,000-foot lakes and tarns sitting in scenic wonderland below a horse-shoe of soaring peaks, including Mounts Huxley, Warlow, Fiske, Wallace, Haeckel, and Spencer.

Proceeding through the deep cleft of the canyon, you drop down to Evolution Lake, the largest in the chain and perhaps the most hospitable for campers. Follow the trail around the east side of the lake, which is tucked into a long, narrow chasm at the north end of Evolution Basin and towered over by the hulks of Mt. Darwin and Mt. Mendel. Verdant strips of meadow soften the otherwise granite-laden bowl. Crest a low rise near the far end of the lake, and swing around to the north shore of a large cove to a small, slightly elevated peninsula, which has a number of scenic campsites amid very widely scattered whitebark pines. There are additional campsites around the northwest side along the outlet.

Before departing Evolution Lake, grab one more look at the scenic majesty of Evolution Basin, and then begin the descent toward Evolution Valley. Follow sandy tread past some tarns and over granite slabs to switchbacks heading down the north wall of the canyon. At the top of these switchbacks, cross-country routes depart the JMT and head toward crossings of Glacier Divide at

The Keyhole, Alpine Col, and Snow Tongue Pass and over the Sierra Crest via Lamarck Col. A thickening forest of lodgepole pines coincides with a drop in elevation, as you zigzag down toward the floor of Evolution Valley, with periodic gaps in the trees allowing views across the deep gorge. On the descent, a couple of flower-lined rivulets spill across the trail and, farther down, you first hear and then pass below a thundering waterfall on the creek draining the Darwin Bench area before reaching the valley floor.

Proceed down the valley on gently graded tread, passing through the shade from scattered stands of pines separated by small pocket meadows. Wandering past granite slabs and boulders, you reach Colby 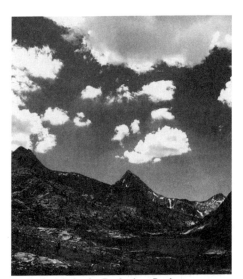 Meadow, first of the larger meadows in Evolution Valley. Good campsites beneath lodgepole pines around the edge of the meadow offer overnight accommodations, with pleasant views of the valley, winding creek, and surrounding peaks. Fishing in nearby Evolution Creek for golden trout is good.

Follow gently graded tread away from Colby Meadow and over a couple of side streams through light forest for 0.75 mile to the edge of McClure Meadow (approximately 9,620 feet), the largest of the meadows in Evolution Valley. The McGee Lakes cross-country route leaves the east end of the meadow, crosses Evolution Creek, and proceeds up McGee Creek. There are numerous campsites spread around the fringe of the meadow, some providing excellent views of Evolution Creek flowing sinuously through the verdant clearing. On a low rise north of the trail sits McClure Meadow Ranger Station, the summer home of a seasonal backcountry ranger. Beyond the cabin, gently graded trail continues toward the end of the meadow, where the creek starts to tumble again.

For the next couple of miles, you pass in and out of lodgepole pine forest and hop across a trio of tributaries draining the south side of Glacier Divide. Breaks in the forest allow occasional views of the canyon, including a major avalanche swath and a picturesque waterfall below Emerald Peak.

Evolution Lake in Evolution Basin

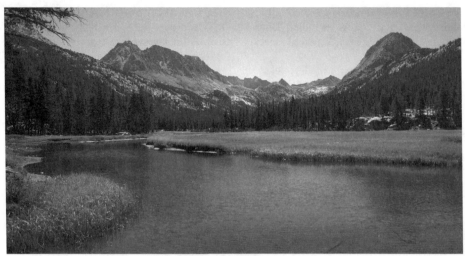

Evolution Creek coursing through McClure Meadow

Reach the fringe of Evolution Meadow (approximately 9,210 feet), and then skirt the north edge of the meadow under forest cover, passing a number of campsites along the way.

Nearing the west end of the meadow, at the crossing of a twin-channeled stream, the Packsaddle Pass and Lobe Pass cross-country routes head north toward Glacier Divide. Shortly beyond the meadow the trail curves south to reach a broad ford of Evolution Creek, 12.3 miles from Muir Pass. Except during the height of snowmelt, the ford is not particularly difficult, but it is usually deep enough to wet your lower legs.

Beyond the ford, gently graded trail leads along the south bank to where the lazy creek suddenly begins a raucous plunge, tumbling over slabs and careening around boulders, on the way toward a union with South Fork San Joaquin River below. The trail seemingly matches the creek's fall with a zigzagging descent down the exposed west-facing wall, with fine views of the canyon and the river along the way. Nearing the bottom of the canyon, reenter the welcome shade from a mixed forest of lodgepole pines, incense cedars, and aspens, and then stroll across the canyon floor to a wood bridge over the river and a junction with the Goddard Canyon Trail, 1.5 miles

from the ford. There are a number of well-used campsites spread around the junction on either side of the bridge.

Continuing northbound on the JMT, follow the river downstream through mixed forest, soon crossing and then briefly paralleling an unnamed tributary draining the area east of Mt. Henry. A mixed bag of vegetation greets you over the next mile, as the trail wanders in and out of scattered forest and across open, sagebrush- and currant-covered slopes with a fine assortment of drought-tolerant wildflowers, including lupine, paintbrush, penstemon, pennyroyal, cinquefoil, and Mariposa lily. A mile from the Goddard Canyon junction, just before crossing a bridge over the South Fork, reach a junction with a short spur on the left leading to pine-shaded campsites on a small flat above the south bank of the river.

Downstream from the bridge, the canyon narrows, powerfully propelling the river through a slim, rocky chasm. Proceed alongside this raging torrent until more placid waters return about a mile from the bridge. Just beyond a stream crossing is Aspen Meadow (approximately 8,235 feet), 2.3 miles from the Goddard Canyon junction, which turns out to be more of a grove than a typical meadow. The mainly aspen-covered flat is sprinkled with lesser amounts of pine and offers a few sheltered campsites.

Away from Aspen Meadow, proceed downstream alongside the South Fork through mostly open, rocky terrain, following the trail bending north around Muir Rock. Veer away from the river through widely scattered conifers to a lightly forested flat harboring a number of campsites. Just before a steel bridge spanning Piute Creek, a sign announces your departure from Kings Canyon National Park. Across the bridge is a junction with the Piute Pass Trail, 3.5 miles from the Goddard Canyon junction.

Leaving the JMT, turn right (north) and follow the Piute Pass Trail, initially close to tumbling Piute Creek. Farther on, the trail climbs steeply above the stream on poor tread across open, chaparral-covered slopes, which makes the stiff ascent feel unusually hot on a warm summer day. To add insult to injury, the trail occasionally loses and then regains precious elevation on the way up the canyon. The open terrain does allow for stunning views of the canyon and the highly fractured Pavilion Dome and other unnamed domes along the west end of Glacier Divide. Just beyond Turret Creek, the trail bends east, fords West Pinnacles Creek, and then climbs moderately steeply northeast beneath the welcome shade of a lodgepole pine forest. Nearing Hutchinson Meadow, you reach the Pine Creek Pass Trail junction, with several spacious campsites nearby, although horse packers have used most of them previously. Unless the stiff climb has tuckered you out, much better campsites await ahead in Humphreys Basin.

Away from the junction, the trail makes several fords of the braided creek draining French Canyon before resuming a moderate climb up Piute Creek canyon. Through midseason, a fine wildflower display accompanies the ascent through slowly thinning forest cover on the way to expansive Humphreys Basin. Once you reach the flower-sprinkled, sweeping basin, the options for campsites are virtually unlimited, provided you don't mind leaving the security of a maintained trail. Other than a 500-foot ban around Lower Golden Trout Lake, camping is allowed near any of the numerous lakes and tarns sprinkled across the basin. The distinctive summit of nearly 14,000-foot Mt. Humphreys above the east edge of the basin dominates the landscape. Extra layover days could be spent exploring the far reaches of the basin. Continuing up the trail, you pass a junction with a fairly well-defined old trail to Desolation Lake, followed by a faint use trail to Humphreys Lakes before climbing above Summit Lake on the way to 11,423-foot Piute Pass.

From the pass, head down North Fork Bishop Creek canyon, past Piute Lake, Loch Leven, and a handful of unnamed tarns and ponds. Beyond Loch Leven, the trail traverses the north wall of the canyon and then switchbacks below Piute Crags on a descent into thickening lodgepole pine forest. Cross the creek on a pair of log bridges and continue downstream to North Lake Campground and the end of single-track tread at the signed trailhead. From here, follow the campground access road out of the campground and over to the spur road leading to the overnight parking area above the northwest shore of North Lake.

Many options exist for further wanderings along this section of the JMT. Ionian Basin, south of Glacier Divide, is a knapsacker's paradise known for its stark, above timberline beauty, with convoluted terrain filled with austere lakes and surrounded by impressive peaks. The long distance from trailheads coupled with arduous terrain ensures that the region remains uncrowded. A number of classic High Sierra treks pass through the basin, including one from Helen Lake to Martha Lake in Goddard Canyon and two more difficult routes down Enchanted Gorge and Goddard Creek (south of Glacier Divide).

Black Giant Pass (approximately 12,200 feet, 0.5 mile west of Black Giant, Class 2) offers cross-country enthusiasts access to Ionian Basin from the JMT at the south end of Helen Lake. From the lake, climb just east of Lake 11939 to the broad saddle of

Black Giant Pass. Descend from the pass to Lake 11828, then head west past numerous tarns to Chasm Lake (11,011 feet). From there you have several choices, including a short return to the JMT that climbs northwest a half mile to Lake 11592 and then northeast over Solomons Pass (approximately 12,445 feet, 0.3 mile west-northwest of Mt. Solomons, Class 2) to Muir Pass. You could also head northwest from Lake 11592 to Wanda Pass (approximately 12,440 feet, 0.4 mile south of Wanda Lake, Class 2) and head around the west side of the lake to the JMT.

To continue toward Martha Lake and a connection to the Goddard Canyon Trail from Chasm Lake, climb around Peak 11078, and follow the south shore of Lake 11837 to a short climb up to a rocky saddle southwest of the lake. Proceed west to Lake 11818 and then around the south shore to the middle of the lake, where two peninsulas nearly touch. Boulder hop to the far side, and then climb northeast past the north shore of an unnamed tarn to Goddard Creek Pass (approximately 12,240 feet, 0.7 mile south of Mt. Goddard, Class 2). From there, descend rocky slopes to the east shore of Martha Lake. To return to the JMT, follow the outlet downstream, pick up the Goddard Canyon Trail, and head northwest.

To visit McGee Lakes, leave the JMT at the east end of McClure Meadow, and ford Evolution Creek. Head southeast through dense lodgepole pine forest toward McGee Creek canyon on traces of old trail, eventually drawing near the creek. Continue upstream to the lakes, where there are excellent campsites on the north shores of the two largest lakes. From the upper lake, head east past two small tarns to a distinct notch in the skyline ridge directly west of Sapphire Lake, and descend steeply but shortly to the lake. An alternate exit from McGee Lakes continues south from Lake 10821 past two tarns before arcing east past a third tarn to a gap above Lake 11293. From there, a short drop reconnects with the JMT in Evolution Basin on the west side of Lake 11293.

Two cross-country routes depart Evolution Meadow for trips over Glacier Divide. The first route climbs north and northeast 2.5 miles from the meadow to the Packsaddle Pass (approximately 12,400 feet, 2.7 miles east-southeast of Pavilion Dome, Class 2). Descend steeply for 300 feet, and then continue down easier terrain along a stream to Packsaddle Lake in Humphreys Basin. The second climbs north from the meadow along a stream toward Lake 11236 and ascends north then east for a half mile to Lobe Pass (approximately 12,320 feet, 2.2 miles east-northeast of Pavilion Dome, Class 2). Descend steep slopes, and then follow the inlet through a canyon to Lobe Lakes above Humphreys Basin.

Additional cross-country routes accessible from the JMT include Lamarck Col over the Sierra Crest (see Trip 121, page 431), and Alpine Col, The Keyhole, and Snow Tongue Pass over Glacier Divide.

[R] A wilderness permit is required for overnight stays. Bear canisters are required. Campfires are prohibited above 10,000 feet.

SOUTH LAKE TRAILHEAD

TRIP 115

Chocolate Lakes Loop

Ⓜ 🏊 **DH or BP**

DISTANCE: 7.2 miles, semiloop

ELEVATION: 9,845'/11,325',
+1,690'/-1,690'/±6,760'

SEASON: Early July to mid-October

USE: Moderate to heavy

MAPS: USGS's *Mt. Thompson* or Tom
Harrison Maps' *Bishop Pass
North Lake-South Lake Loop
Trail Map*

TRAIL LOG

0.75 Treasure Lakes Trail junction
1.9   Chocolate Lakes North Trail
      junction
2.3   Bull Lake
2.8   Middle Chocolate Lake
3.9   Ruwau Lake
4.5   Chocolate Lakes South Trail
      junction
7.2   South Lake Trailhead

INTRODUCTION: The relatively short
semiloop around aptly named Chocolate
Peak leads to a string of picturesque lakes.
Rewards include outstanding scenery and
a sense of relative seclusion away from the
steady stream of recreationists traveling the
heavily used Bishop Pass Trail. Unfortunately, backpackers wishing to spend a night
or two in the Chocolate Lakes basin must
compete for the same quota of wilderness
permits as the more popular trail.

However, the 7-mile distance is well
suited for a dayhike when you are unable
to secure a permit. Be forewarned that portions of the trail between the Chocolate
Lakes and Ruwau Lake are rough and indistinct in parts and indiscernible in others, but
the route-finding is fairly straightforward.
Anglers should find the fishing to be quite
decent.

DIRECTIONS TO TRAILHEAD: From Bishop,
leave US 395, and turn west onto Line
Drive, which is known as South Lake Road
and Highway 168 outside of town. Proceed
southwest 15 miles to a junction with Lake
Sabrina Road, and turn left, remaining on
South Lake Road. Continue 6.75 miles
to the end of the road near South Lake.
Backpackers must park in the overnight lot
(when it is full, additional parking may be
available 1.3 miles back down the road—a
footpath connects to the trailhead). Dayhikers can park vehicles below the backpacker lot in spaces marked NO OVERNIGHT
PARKING. Restrooms and water are available at the trailhead.

DESCRIPTION: Begin with a short, steep
descent through lush vegetation, and then
gently ascend above the east shore of South
Lake through young aspens and lodgepole
pines. Soon, break out into the open to fine
views up the canyon, as a steeper climb
ensues. Cross the wilderness boundary, and
continue climbing to a Y-junction with the
Treasure Lakes Trail (see Trip 116, page
418), 0.75 mile from the trailhead.

Veer left (southeast), and continue
through light lodgepole forest to a plank-
bridge crossing of a small, flower-lined creek.
A moderate climb leads to an unmarked,
faint junction, 1.4 miles from the trailhead,
with the partly cross-country route to Marie
Lakes. Solitude seekers can follow this route
northeast to a marshy meadow and then
steeply southeast to the lakes.

Just beyond the junction, come alongside and then cross another small stream.
Short-legged switchbacks lead over granite
outcrops and boulders to the north junction
of the Chocolate Lakes Trail, 1.9 miles from
the trailhead.

Turn left at the junction, cross a talus
slide, climb up a steep draw to a meadow,
and then immediately arrive at pretty Bull
Lake (approximately 10,775 feet). Its shoreline is blanketed with a light forest of
whitebark pines, wildflowers, and scattered
clumps of willow. There are plenty of campsites just off the trail. Anglers can ply the
waters for brook trout.

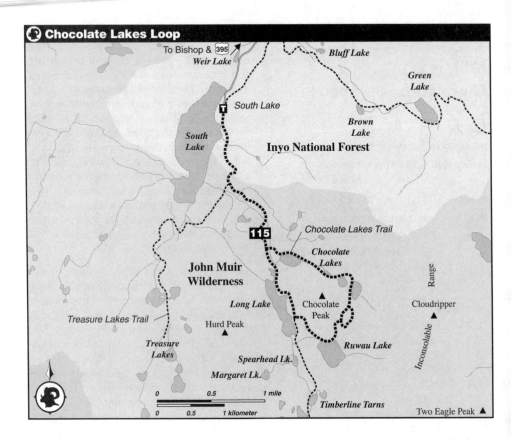

Chocolate Lakes Loop

Follow the trail around the north shore of the lake, cross the inlet, and then climb moderately steeply through a stunning display of wildflowers, including columbine, shooting star, and paintbrush. As the Inconsolable Range comes into view, climb into a rocky basin past a shallow, seemingly irregular pond, which actually turns out to be Lower Chocolate Lake (approximately 10,950 feet).

Above the lower lake, cross the creek again and climb up to Middle Chocolate Lake (approximately 11,060 feet), 2.8 miles from the trailhead. There are campsites scattered around the hillside above the north shore.

Continuing up the trail, you switchback up a hillside, cross a willow-lined creek, and ascend to Upper Chocolate Lake (approximately 11,075 feet), largest of the group. Surrounded by grasses, shrubs, and few trees, the lake sits at the base of a talus

slope, with fine views of the surrounding peaks and ridges. There are decent campsites spread around the lakeshore. Fishing is reportedly good at all three Chocolate Lakes for brook trout.

The trail continues to circumnavigate Chocolate Peak, as you climb moderately steeply away from the upper lake over rocky terrain. The *Mt. Thompson* quad indicates two trails leading out of Chocolate Lakes basin, over the ridgecrest, and down to Ruwau Lake. Both trails are unmaintained and a bit rough, with sections that virtually disappear for considerable distances. You have the option of heading straight toward the ridgecrest on a steep, tightly zigzagging climb or of following a route of longer-legged switchbacks up to the crest just southeast of a craggy knoll. The crest has fine views of the surrounding terrain.

Whichever uphill route you choose, avoid the temptation to descend the talus-filled gully on the far side of the crest, which deceptively appears to be the most direct line. The two routes merge at an undefined point and then follow faint tread down the hillside above and west of this gully. The trail becomes more defined farther down the slope, eventually arriving at the north shore of Ruwau Lake (11,044 feet), 3.9 miles from the trailhead.

Ruwau Lake is perhaps the most scenic of the Chocolate Lakes, sandwiched between Chocolate Peak and the Inconsolable Range and graced from all angles with views of craggy peaks and ridges. On warm afternoons, slabs on a tiny island near the north shore will entice sunbathers and swimmers willing to share the chilly waters with the resident rainbow trout. Whitebark pines shade campsites on a low hill above the north shore and around the outlet. Around the remaining shoreline, willow thickets and an assortment of wildflowers provide floral adornment. Although only a half mile away from the popular Bishop Pass Trail, the lake seems just far enough off the beaten path to provide a reasonable helping of solitude and serenity.

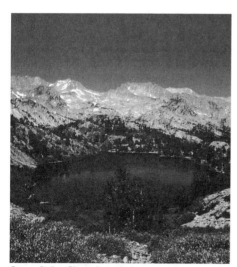

One of the Chocolate Lakes

To complete the loop section, follow the trail around the north shore toward the outlet. Through heather and scattered pines, you turn away from the lake and proceed northwest on a slight descent. After a brief climb, the trail descends in earnest on a steep, winding drop to Long Lake. At the bottom of a hill is a junction with the Bishop Pass Trail, 4.5 miles from the trailhead.

From the junction, turn right (north), and proceed on gently graded tread through scattered forest and wildflowers to a marshy pond. Soon, a part of aptly named Long Lake is visible to the left, along with a fine view of Mt. Goode rising to the southwest. A short climb over a low hump brings you alongside the picturesque lake for a while. Beyond the north shore, the descent increases, and the forest thickens on the way to the north junction of the Chocolate Lakes Trail at the close of the loop. From there, retrace your steps 1.9 miles to the South Lake Trailhead.

You can easily combine the Chocolate Lakes Loop with the Bishop Pass Trail for a number of extended journeys. An easy cross-country route from Ruwau Lake to Timberline Tarns provides a more direct route toward Bishop Pass than the trail down to Long Lake. Work your way around the west shore of Ruwau Lake and then up an obvious gully at the lake's south end via a use trail and intermittent boulder scrambles. From the top of the gully, you drop down toward Timberline Tarns, a stream crossing, and a connection with the Bishop Pass Trail.

A Class 2 route follows the southeast slope of Chocolate Peak up to fine views from the 11,682-foot summit. Cloudripper and Picture Puzzle Peak in the Inconsolable Range are Class 3 ascents.

A wilderness permit is required for overnight stays. Bear canisters are required. Campfires are prohibited.

TRIP 116

Treasure Lakes

Ⓜ ⁄ **DH or BP**

DISTANCE: 8 miles, out-and-back

ELEVATION: 9,845'/11,185',
+1,765'/-450'/±4,430'

SEASON: Early July to mid-October

USE: Moderate

MAPS: USGS's *Mt. Thompson* or Tom
Harrison Maps' *Bishop Pass
North Lake–South Lake Loop
Trail Map*

TRAIL LOG

0.75 Treasure Lakes Trail junction
2.8 Lake 10668
4.0 Lake 11175

INTRODUCTION: The Treasure Lakes Trail
leads away from the normal hubbub along
the Bishop Pass Trail to a group of relatively
secluded lakes in a granite basin near the
Sierra Crest. Over the short journey, you
pass through three distinct plant zones—
montane, subalpine, and alpine. The quite
scenic lakes offer campers serene settings
for pitching a tent and anglers excellent
fishing for golden trout. Some route-finding
and a bit of boulder hopping are necessary
to reach the upper lakes, but that should be
easy enough for all but beginning backpackers. Although the trail is open to equestrians, the absence of a path over rocky terrain
should dissuade the use of pack animals
above the first two lakes, increasing the
chances for an undisturbed visit for the
nonequine crowd. A straightforward cross-
country route offers an alternative to simply
retracing your steps back to the trailhead
(see options, page 420).

DIRECTIONS TO TRAILHEAD: From Bishop,
leave US 395, and turn west onto Line
Drive, which is known as South Lake Road

and Highway 168 outside of town. Proceed
southwest 15 miles to a junction with Lake
Sabrina Road, and turn left, remaining on
South Lake Road. Continue 6.75 miles
to the end of the road near South Lake.
Backpackers must park in the overnight lot
(when it is full, additional parking may be
available 1.3 miles back down the road—a
footpath connects to the trailhead). Dayhikers can park vehicles below the backpacker lot in spaces marked NO OVERNIGHT
PARKING. Restrooms and water are available at the trailhead.

DESCRIPTION: Begin with a short, steep
descent through lush vegetation, and then
gently ascend above the east shore of South
Lake through young aspens and lodgepole
pines. Soon, break out into the open to fine
views up the canyon, as a steeper climb
ensues. Cross the wilderness boundary, and
continue climbing to a Y-junction with the
Treasure Lakes Trail, 0.75 mile from the
trailhead.

Bear right (south) at the junction, and
head through scattered to light lodgepole
pine forest to easy crossings over two small
streams. The mild descent continues as
South Lake pops into view below and Mt.
Johnson, Mt. Gilbert, Mt. Thompson, and
Hurd Peak are revealed to the southwest.

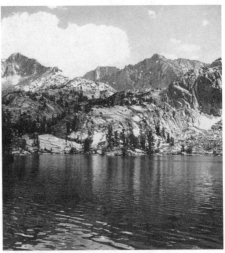

One of the Treasure Lakes

Soon, you follow an arcing descent to three crossings of South Fork Bishop Creek and a pair of tributaries, where willows, grasses, and wildflowers line the banks.

Now the real climbing begins, briefly interrupted by a short decline to a crossing of Treasure Creek. Beyond the creek, follow a winding, moderately steep climb beside granite boulders, over slabs, and through a mixed forest of lodgepole and whitebark pines. Work your way back to the creek, hop across, and then continue a winding climb through thinning forest. After passing a small pond, switchback up to Lake 10668, 2.8 miles from the trailhead.

The first and largest Treasure Lake is dotted with small rock islands and bordered by boggy turf along the north shore. Proceeding up gently graded trail above the east shore, you pass a number of exposed campsites nestled beneath clumps of pine.

A steep wall of rock on the opposite shore rises up to Peak 12047, providing a dramatic backdrop to the usually placid waters. Toward the south end, a use trail branches left past more campsites to the lake directly east of Lake 10668. Smaller and somewhat less scenic, this lake has a handful of campsites scattered around the shore.

Continuing south on the main trail, cross the stream connecting the first two lakes, and work your way alongside a creek coursing down a rock-filled gully. Clumps of willow and small patches of meadow sprinkled with monkeyflower soften the otherwise stark surroundings. Where the creek divides into two channels, follow the more gradual cleft to the right through large talus blocks. Farther up-canyon, Mt. Johnson and the long ridge connecting to Mt. Goode add to the rugged alpine atmosphere. Route-finding from here is

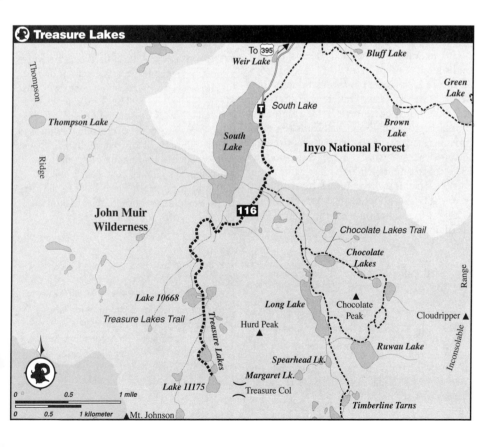

straightforward over rocky terrain on a traverse east over a low ridge to the left-hand fork, where a deep cirque west of Peak 12192 cradles a trio of lakes. Excellent campsites beneath whitebark pines near the northwest shore of the first lake will tempt overnighters. Anglers will find golden trout in all three lakes. Reach the last lake in the chain at 4 miles from the trailhead.

O Rather than retrace your steps, you can easily create a semiloop trip by following a straightforward cross-country route from Lake 11175. First, climb southeast up to a prominent saddle 550 feet above the lake. From there, descend northeast approximately 110 yards, and then angle over to a tiny creek. Follow this creek briefly, and then head directly toward Margaret Lake. Pick up a use trail near the lake's northwest shore, and head northeast to the south end of Long Lake. Ford South Fork Bishop Creek, and pass some campsites on the way to a connection with the Bishop Pass Trail.

A more difficult (Class 2) cross-country route, requiring an ice axe, heads up the right-hand canyon past the westernmost Treasure Lake and up a snow and ice chute to Treasure Col (approximately 12,000 feet, 0.3 mile north-northwest of Mt. Johnson). From there, steep, loose rock leads to easier travel along a stream to cliffs above Big Pete Meadow, where more route-finding is necessary to reach the John Muir Trail (JMT). The most direct return route follows the JMT southbound through Le Conte Canyon to a junction with the Bishop Pass Trail and over Bishop Pass to the South Lake Trailhead.

Mountaineers can ascend a Class 2 route from the uppermost Treasure Lake to the top of 12,871-foot Mt. Johnson. The southeast slope of Mt. Gilbert (13,106 feet) is Class 2 from Treasure Col, but an ice axe will likely be necessary to negotiate the steep chute on the northeast side of the col.

R A wilderness permit is required for overnight stays. Bear canisters are required. Campfires are prohibited.

SOUTH LAKE TRAILHEAD

TRIP 117

Tyee Lakes

M ✓ **DH** or **BP**

DISTANCE: 8 miles out-and-back

ELEVATION: 9,090'/11,600', +2,520'/negligible/±5,040'

SEASON: Mid-July to mid-October

USE: Light

MAPS: USGS's *Mt. Thompson* or Tom Harrison Maps' *Bishop Pass North Lake-South Lake Loop Trail Map*

TRAIL LOG

1.8 Cindy Lake
3.0 Clara Lake
4.0 Table Mountain View

INTRODUCTION: A little-used trail provides a short but steep route to a group of delightful lakes set in a high granite basin well east of the Sierra Crest. The 3-mile journey to the upper lake is well suited for either a day-hike, complete with a refreshing swim and a picnic lunch, or an overnight backpack. Anglers should find plenty of brook trout in all of the Tyee Lakes. The nearly mile-long, 600-foot climb from Clara Lake to the view from the plateau atop Table Mountain is certainly worth the extra effort.

TYEE LAKES

Somewhat inexplicably, the Tyee Lakes were named for a famed brand of salmon eggs. The origin of the various first names (Cindy, John, Jim, Ted, Clara, and Melissa) applied to the lakes is unknown.

DIRECTIONS TO TRAILHEAD: From Bishop, leave US 395, and turn west onto Line Drive, which is known as South Lake Road and Highway 168 outside of town. Proceed southwest 15 miles to a junction with Lake Sabrina Road, and turn left, remaining on South Lake Road. Continue 5 miles to the trailhead, which has parking along the gravel shoulder.

DESCRIPTION: Begin by crossing an impressive arched, wood bridge over South Fork Bishop Creek. Just beyond, follow a moderate, zigzagging climb up a sagebrush-covered hillside above the creek, through pockets of young aspens and lodgepole pines. The steady climb continues beyond a crossing of the Tyee Lakes outlet at 1.5 miles. The grade eases where you enter John Muir Wilderness, round a hillside, and reach Cindy Lake (approximately 10,300 feet), 1.8 miles from the trailhead.

There are a couple of fair campsites near the stream below the lake. A pleasant beach on the west shore invites sunbathers and swimmers, but marshy meadow, willows, and pockets of aspen border the rest of the lake, making access a tad difficult for anglers attempting to snag a brook trout.

Arc around the first lake, cross a trickling stream dribbling into the lake, and then resume the climb. A number of switchbacks lead steeply uphill to the second lake, John (approximately 10,595 feet). Surrounded by grasses, this lake is the smallest and shallowest in the chain. Across the outlet, a few pine-sheltered campsites occupy a hump of granite. Anglers will find brook trout here as well.

The trail leaves the west shore of John Lake and begins a moderately steep climb through whitebark pines over a granite bench. Switchbacks lead to a spot among dwarf pines and scattered boulders, offering

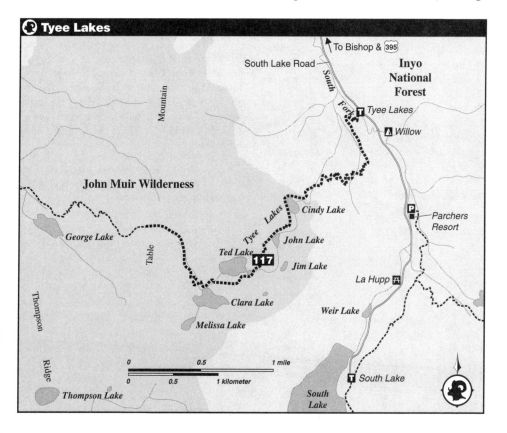

Tyee Lakes

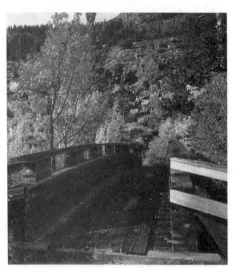

Bridge over South Fork Bishop Creek near the Tyee Lakes Trailhead

a bird's-eye view of John Lake and other lakes to the east of the trail (Jim is the largest of these). Then, a more moderate climb leads across Tyee Creek and past a small pond to the fourth lake, Ted (approximately 10,900 feet), one of the larger Tyee Lakes. Talus cascades down the hillside above the far shore. There are good campsites spread beneath whitebark pines.

Skirt the south side of the lake away from the shoreline, and then begin to climb moderately steeply up and over the talus-covered hillside to the narrow cleft of the stream connecting Ted Lake with its upstairs neighbor. Cross the stream, and climb up the cleft toward the next lake, Clara, 3 miles from the trailhead.

Clara (11,015 feet) is also one of the larger lakes in the chain, where rugged cliffs form a splendid backdrop and a few whitebark pines eke out a near-timberline existence. There are campsites above the northeast shore among the trees and in a sandy area near the northwest shore. Unlike in the lower lakes, anglers will find rainbow trout cohabitating with the characteristic brook trout at Clara. To reach the last Tyee Lake, Melissa (approximately 11,030 feet), head cross-country up the outlet from the Clara's southwest shore.

From Clara Lake, a 1-mile (each way) climb leads to a dramatic view from Table Mountain. Follow a winding course up the gorge of the delightful stream draining into the lake. Near the head of the drainage, the trail becomes a tad indistinct, but the route is obvious—simply head west toward the top of the plateau between Peaks 11684 and 11651, passing through a profusion of corn lilies along the way.

O With shuttle arrangements, you could continue from Clara Lake northwest over Table Mountain and past George Lake to the Lake Sabrina Trailhead. Along the way you will have excellent views from Table Mountain, and George Lake offers good campsites.

R A wilderness permit is required for overnight stays. Bear canisters are required. Campfires are prohibited.

TRIP 118

Sabrina Basin

Ⓜ ✒ **DH**, **BP**, or **BPx**

DISTANCE: 14 miles, out-and-back to
Hungry Packer Lake

ELEVATION: 9,080'/11,145',
+2,860'/-680'/±7,080'

SEASON: Mid-July to mid-October

USE: Moderate

MAPS: USGS's *Mt. Thompson* and
Mt. Darwin or Tom Harrison
Maps' *Bishop Pass North
Lake-South Lake Loop
Trail Map*

TRAIL LOG

1.3   George Lake Trail junction
3.0   Blue Lake
3.3   Donkey Lake Trail junction
4.7   Dingleberry Lake
5.5   Midnight Lake
7.0   Hungry Packer Lake

INTRODUCTION: The main quandary when
contemplating a trip to Sabrina Basin is
whether or not you have enough time to
visit all of the scenic lakes since they are
bountiful and there is nary a rotten apple
in the bunch. An array of options—well-
traveled trails, less-traveled use trails, and
cross-country routes—allow you to select
potential destinations compatible with a
wide range of skill levels. With so many
lakes to choose from, getting away from it
all should be a reasonable goal, especially if
you're willing to veer off the beaten path.

The lakes in the upper basin are particularly scenic, nestled in granite bowls, encircled by steep rock cliffs, and backdropped
by the towering Sierra Crest. Along the
way, delightful meadows, colorful wildflowers, picturesque waterfalls, and cascading
streams offer stunning visual treats. The
basin's mostly open nature provides strik-

ing panoramas throughout the journey.
Whether you are here for a day, a week, or
something in between, Sabrina Basin has
much to offer.

DIRECTIONS TO TRAILHEAD: From Bishop,
leave US 395, and turn west onto Line
Drive, which is known as South Lake Road
and Highway 168 outside of town. Proceed
southwest 15 miles to a junction with Lake
Sabrina Road, and continue ahead for 3
miles past the North Lake Road junction to
the parking area for the Lake Sabrina Trailhead. The actual trailhead is another half
mile up the road, just below the lake, where
there is a day-use parking lot. Overnight
users must park in the lot near the North
Lake Road junction.

DESCRIPTION: From the trailhead, follow
an old road through a cover of aspens until
it merges with single-track trail that leads
around a corner to a fine view up the canyon of Middle Fork Bishop Creek across
open sagebrush-covered slopes dotted with
junipers, Jeffrey pines, aspens, lodgepole
pines, mountain mahogany, and western
white pines. Immediately below is the blue
expanse of Lake Sabrina with the Middle
Fork cascading into a small cove at the far
end.

Farther up the canyon, the rugged Sierra
Crest is crowned by the 13,000-foot summits of Mt. Darwin, Mt. Haeckel, Mt.
Wallace, and Mt. Powell. Traverse across
a hillside, enter the John Muir Wilderness
near the lake's midpoint, and then climb
steadily up the slope to the far end of Lake
Sabrina. Reach a junction with the George
Lake Trail and a ford of its refreshing outlet, 1.3 miles from the trailhead.

Continuing ahead enter a light forest
of lodgepole pines, and climb moderately
via switchbacks up a hillside south of the
lake, crossing another stream on the way.
Sporadic openings in the forest allow splendid views back to Lake Sabrina and ahead
toward the Sierra Crest. More switchbacks,
interspersed with granite steps, lead up a
hillside through a rocky ravine, and past a
small pond, where the grade eases. Near the

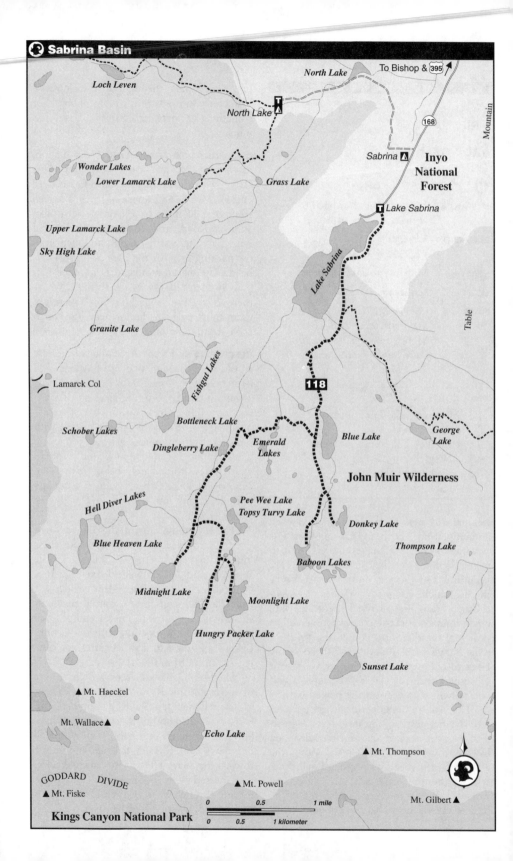

Loch Leven

North Lake

North Lake

To Bishop & 395

168

Sabrina

Inyo National Forest

Mountain

Wonder Lakes

Lower Lamarck Lake

Grass Lake

Lake Sabrina

Upper Lamarck Lake

Sky High Lake

Table

Granite Lake

Fishgut Lakes

Lamarck Col

118

Schober Lakes

Bottleneck Lake

Dingleberry Lake

Emerald Lakes

Blue Lake

George Lake

John Muir Wilderness

Hell Diver Lakes

Pee Wee Lake

Topsy Turvy Lake

Donkey Lake

Thompson Lake

Blue Heaven Lake

Midnight Lake

Baboon Lakes

Moonlight Lake

Hungry Packer Lake

Sunset Lake

▲ Mt. Haeckel

Mt. Wallace ▲

Echo Lake

▲ Mt. Thompson

GODDARD   DIVIDE

▲ Mt. Fiske

▲ Mt. Powell

Mt. Gilbert ▲

Kings Canyon National Park

0   0.5   1 mile

0   0.5   1 kilometer

pond, spy the north shore of Blue Lake, pass a couple of campsites, and then ford the outlet immediately below the lake, 3 miles from the trailhead.

Blue Lake (10,388 feet) is very photogenic, with an irregular shoreline bordered by weather-beaten lodgepole pines and granite benches, backdropped by the craggy, undulating crest of Thompson Ridge. There are plenty of campsites spread around the shore, but choose your site wisely since some are obviously too close to the water. Anglers can test their skill on brook and rainbow trout. Follow the trail around the west shore to a three-way junction with the Donkey Lake Trail near the midpoint, 3.3 miles from the trailhead.

SIDE TRIP TO BABOON AND DONKEY LAKES: From the three-way junction, head south through lodgepole pines and past granite slabs, well away from the shoreline of Blue Lake. Cross a seasonal stream, and continue climbing gently to an unmarked junction with a faint path heading south-southwest to Baboon Lakes. The trail disappears completely before reaching the lakes, but route-finding is straightforward along the outlet to the largest Baboon Lake (10,976 feet). Anglers can try their luck on rainbow trout at this lake and both rainbow and brook trout in the upper lakes. Adventurous cross-country types can extend the journey to Sunset Lake (11,464 feet) beneath the glacier-clad north face of Mt. Thompson.

To reach Donkey Lake, continue south a short distance from the unmarked junction mentioned above to a crossing of the creek draining Baboon Lakes. Proceed on faint tread around outcrops, past a small pool, and through a notch to Donkey Lake (approximately 10,590 feet), tucked into a narrow cleft at the base of Thompson Ridge. Anglers can expect decent fishing for brook trout. **END OF SIDE TRIP**

Turn right (northwest) from the junction to Baboon and Donkey Lakes, and proceed on gently graded trail over a low saddle, across a rocky slope, and then up

granite ledges to a grassy valley dotted with lodgepole pines. At 3.8 miles from the trailhead, cross the creek draining the small ponds known as Emerald Lakes, and curve around the marshy meadow adjacent to the lower lakes on the way to a junction with a faint use trail, which provides access to the larger lakes. The westernmost lake has fine campsites, and fishing there is reported to be good for brook and rainbow trout.

Remaining on the main trail, climb away from Emerald Lakes up granite steps and over slabs along the west side of a low ridge. Eventually, you wind down off the ridge to the southeast shore of Dingleberry Lake (10,489 feet), 4.7 miles from the trailhead. The lake is squeezed between cliffs and slabs of a low ridge on one side and the steep wall of Peak 13253's east ridge on the other. There are campsites at either end of the lake along the creek, but wet meadows on the south end create a haven for mosquitoes through midseason.

Beyond the south end of Dingleberry Lake, the foot and stock trails split for separate fords of Middle Fork Bishop Creek. After the ford, reconnect with the stock trail, and climb alongside a tributary to a picturesque meadow, where the serpentine stream winds lazily through grasses, willows, and wildflowers. Across the valley, a dazzling waterfall plunges from Topsy Turvy Lake. In the midst of the meadow, a faint use trail heads left toward campsites at Pee Wee and Topsy Turvy Lakes. At the head of the meadow, resume the climb over numerous low granite benches to the signed Midnight Lake Trail junction, 5.5 miles from the trailhead.

SIDE TRIP TO MIDNIGHT LAKE: Veer right at the junction, and after a short climb drop to a crossing of the stream draining Hell Diver Lakes. Gently graded trail leads away from the crossing, past a good-size tarn, and then across the outlet from Midnight Lake to a steeper climb over rock slabs. Eventually, the grades eases again, where you crest the lip of a basin and soon stroll over to the north shore of Midnight Lake (10,988 feet), 0.5 mile from the junction.

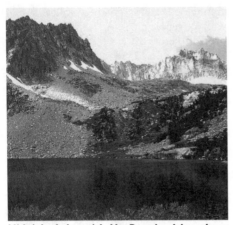

Midnight Lake, with Mt. Darwin rising above the far shore

This teardrop-shaped lake reposes in a granite bowl surrounded by talus slopes and steep, rugged cliffs, where snow patches cling to shady crevices and a waterfall cascades 300 feet into the lake. Reigning over the Sierra Crest, 13,831-foot Mt. Darwin looms in the background above the shimmering lake. Near timberline, widely scattered lodgepole pines hold on tenuously in the cracks of granite hummocks lining the outlet. The steep lakeshore inhibits camping, but you may find sites peppered along the outlet between the lake and the tarn downstream. Anglers fishing for the resident brook trout seem to fare quite well at Midnight Lake. **END OF SIDE TRIP**

From the Midnight Lake junction, turn southeast, and cross a pair of willow- and flower-lined streams. On a mild to moderate climb, arc around a spur ridge, and then head south through scattered whitebark pines to a sloping meadow filled with willow, heather, and an assortment of wildflowers, interspersed among sparkling granite slabs. A short climb leads to a stunningly picturesque basin brimming with crystalline streams and splendid cascades, backdropped by aptly named Picture Peak accenting the scene toward the head of the canyon. About 0.75 mile from the junction, reach an unmarked junction with a use trail to Moonlight Lake.

SIDE TRIP TO MOONLIGHT LAKE: Moonlight Lake (11,052 feet) is best approached via the use trail below (north of) Sailor Lake since a vast talus field inhibits easy access from the main trail to Hungry Packer Lake above. Follow the use trail to a ford of the outlet from Sailor Lake, cross the meadow below the lake, and then ascend Moonlight Lake's outlet to the rockbound lake's northwest shore. Campsites are limited to exposed spots along the outlet and the south end of a low rise above the west shore. In spite of the seemingly lifeless surroundings, the lake harbors a healthy population of brook trout. **END OF SIDE TRIP**

SAILOR LAKE

Sailor Lake was supposedly named for a patron of the Lake Sabrina Lodge, who was found asleep one day by packers, apparently recovering from the effects of too much to drink. Some older maps used the appellation "Drunken Sailor Lake," which seems a tad more colorful, but the shortened name is the accepted one.

From the use trail junction to Moonlight Lake, continue south on the main trail west of Sailor Lake (approximately 10,850 feet), which sits in an open, nearly treeless basin, bordered by sloping granite shelves and slabs and pockets of verdant meadow. There are a number of fine, although exposed, campsites scattered around the basin. Anglers can fish for both brook and rainbow trout in the lake and creek.

Proceed up the main trail, with the north face of Picture Peak dominating the scene, to the north shore of Hungry Packer Lake (11,071 feet), a narrow finger of water, 7 miles from the trailhead. From here, the view of the alpine peak across the lake's surface lives up to the billing, as Picture Peak towers above, with steep cliffs sweeping around the basin on either side. During snowmelt, thin ribbons of water plunge steeply down the cliffs, while throughout summer patches of snow cling to clefts in its north face. A granite peninsula on the lake's northwest shore is too close to the water for camping, but its slightly sloping slabs provide fine spots for afternoon sunbathing and chilly swimming. Rainbow trout will test the skill of anglers.

☒ With such a bounty of lakes, Sabrina Basin offers plenty of opportunities for further exploration, so much so that you could easily spend an entire week here. Cross-country routes extend the number of opportunities to more far-flung destinations, such as Fishgut and Hell Diver Lakes. Perhaps the most noteworthy route ascends the ridge east of Hungry Packer Lake to the boulder-strewn canyon above Moonlight Lake and then up to austere Echo Lake (11,602 feet), just north of the Sierra Crest below Clyde Spires.

From upper Sabrina Basin, experienced cross-country trekkers can choose from a number of strenuous, off-trail routes over the Sierra Crest to connect eventually with the John Muir Trail (JMT) in Evolution Basin. From the vicinity of Echo Lake, the Haeckel-Wallace Col (approximately 13,000 feet, 0.1 mile west-northwest of Mt. Wallace) and Wallace Col (approximately 12,960 feet, 0.2 mile south-southeast of Mt. Wallace) offer Class 2 routes over the crest. Echo Col (approximately 12,400 feet, 1 mile southeast of Mt. Wallace) is a more difficult Class 3 route. From the ridge between Hungry Packer and Midnight Lakes, Haeckel Col (approximately 12,680 feet, 0.3 mile northwest of Mt. Haeckel) also offers a Class 3 route over the crest. Haeckel-Wallace Col is usually the best option.

Nontechnical climbing routes from Sabrina Basin are few. The lone exception is a Class 2 route up the north slope of 13,377-foot Mt. Wallace. From a bench west of Echo Lake, head northwest into the cirque between Mt. Haeckel and Mt. Wallace, and then climb scree slopes to the top.

☒ A wilderness permit is required for overnight stays. Campfires are prohibited.

LAKE SABRINA TRAILHEAD

TRIP 119

George Lake

Ⓜ ↗ DH or BP

DISTANCE: 6.6 miles, out-and-back

ELEVATION: 9,080'/10,735', +2,025'/-170'/±4,390'

SEASON: Early July to mid-October

USE: Light

MAPS: USGS's *Mt. Thompson* or Tom Harrison Maps' *Bishop Pass North Lake-South Lake Loop Trail Map*

TRAIL LOG

1.3 George Lake Trail junction
3.3 George Lake

INTRODUCTION: Although George Lake is not the most picturesque lake accessible from the Lake Sabrina Trailhead, it is one of the least crowded, which is a bit of a mystery considering its relatively short distance from the trailhead. Anglers routinely make the journey to fish for brook and rainbow trout, but backpackers seem to bypass the lake in favor of more popular territory farther into Sabrina Basin. The delightful body of water makes a fine destination for either a dayhike or overnight backpack.

DIRECTIONS TO TRAILHEAD: From Bishop, leave US 395, and turn west onto Line Drive, which is known as South Lake Road and Highway 168 outside of town. Proceed southwest 15 miles to a junction with Lake Sabrina Road, and continue ahead for 3 miles past the North Lake Road junction to the parking area for the Lake Sabrina Trailhead. The actual trailhead is another half mile up the road, just below the lake, where there is a day-use parking lot. Overnight users must park in the lot near the North Lake Road junction.

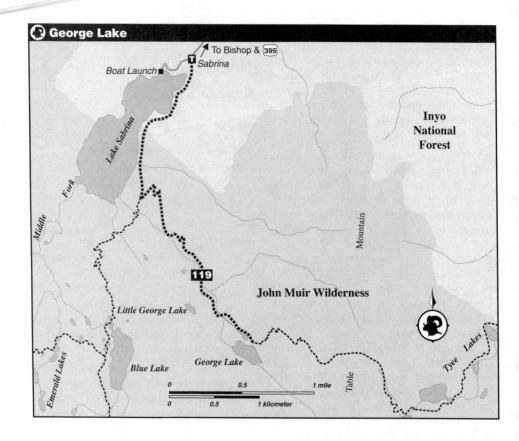

DESCRIPTION: From the trailhead, follow an old road through a cover of aspens until it merges with single-track trail that leads around a corner to a fine view up the canyon of Middle Fork Bishop Creek across open sagebrush-covered slopes dotted with junipers, Jeffrey pines, aspens, lodgepole pines, mountain mahogany, and western white pines. Immediately below is the blue expanse of Lake Sabrina with the Middle Fork cascading into a small cove at the far end.

Farther up the canyon, the rugged Sierra Crest is crowned by the 13,000-foot summits of Mt. Darwin, Mt. Haeckel, Mt. Wallace, and Mt. Powell. Traverse across a hillside, enter the John Muir Wilderness near the lake's midpoint, and then climb steadily up the slope to the far end of the lake. Reach a junction with the George Lake Trail and a ford of its refreshing outlet, 1.3 miles from the trailhead.

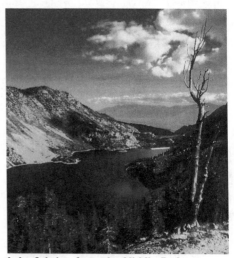

Lake Sabrina from the Middle Fork Lakes Trail

Turn left (northeast) at the junction, and follow moderately steep switchbacks up an exposed slope. About a half mile from the junction, scattered whitebark pines make an appearance. Farther on, cross George Creek a couple of times, and continue a winding climb until the grade eases beneath a thickening cover of forest near the lower end of a valley. Stroll up the valley, and cross the creek again near the head of a pleasant meadow, 2.5 miles from the trailhead. Proceed up the west bank for a quarter mile to where the trail veers left, crosses the creek once more, and then climbs above a willow-choked meadow, reaching the lake after another half mile.

There are fine campsites spread around the north shore of George Lake (10,716 feet). Once the anglers who frequent the area depart for the day, you'll likely enjoy a healthy dose of solitude.

Although the trail over Table Mountain is faint and even nonexistent in sections, the route is straightforward and offers fine views of the surrounding terrain. With shuttle arrangements, you could hike to the Tyee Lakes Trailhead instead of simply retracing your steps back to the Lake Sabrina Trailhead.

A wilderness permit is required for overnight stays.

NORTH LAKE TRAILHEAD

TRIP 120

Lamarck Lakes

M ⟋ **DH** or **BP**

DISTANCE: 6 miles, out-and-back

ELEVATION: 9,225'/10,920', +1,700'/-50'/±3,500'

SEASON: Early July to mid-October

USE: Moderate

MAPS: USGS's *Mt. Darwin* or Tom Harrison Maps' *Bishop Pass North Lake-South Lake Loop Trail Map*

TRAIL LOG

1.1   Grass Lake Trail junction
2.4   Lower Lamarck Lake
3.0   Upper Lamarck Lake

INTRODUCTION: The Lamarck Lakes Trail offers hikers and backpackers a short, but steep route to a pair of picturesque lakes amid rugged mountain scenery. While the distance is minimal, the elevation gain requires a fair amount of effort. Maintained tread dead-ends at the upper lake, but off-trail options extend to the lightly visited Wonder Lakes.

DIRECTIONS TO TRAILHEAD: From Bishop, leave US 395, and turn west onto Line Drive, which is known as South Lake Road and Highway 168 outside of town. Proceed southwest 15 miles to a junction with Lake Sabrina Road, and continue ahead for 3 miles to the North Lake Road junction, and turn right. Follow single-lane, gravel road 1 mile to the day-use parking lot. Backpackers must travel another 0.6 mile to a right-hand turn onto a short spur leading to dual overnight parking lots directly west of North Lake.

DESCRIPTION: From either the day-use or overnight parking lots, begin the journey

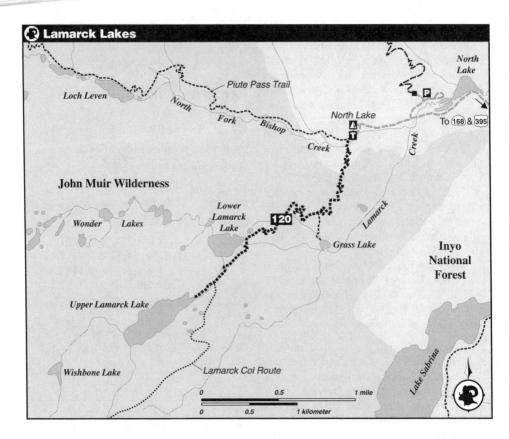

Lamarck Lakes

North Lake

Piute Pass Trail

Loch Leven

North Fork Bishop Creek

North Lake

To (168) & (395)

John Muir Wilderness

Lower Lamarck Lake

120

Wonder Lakes

Lamarck Creek

Grass Lake

Inyo National Forest

Upper Lamarck Lake

Wishbone Lake

Lamarck Col Route

Lake Sabrina

| 0 | | 0.5 | | 1 mile |
| 0 | | 0.5 | | 1 kilometer |

by hiking up the road toward North Lake Campground (1 mile from the day-use lot, 0.7 mile from the overnight lot). The trailhead is just beyond a sign at the entrance to the campground.

From the trailhead, follow single-track trail through aspens and pines through the campground to a junction near the far end. Bear left, cross a trio of willow-lined branches of North Fork Bishop Creek on wood-plank bridges, and then climb moderately steeply up a hillside via switchbacks, passing beneath aspen and lodgepole pine cover. Farther on, limber pines join the mixed forest near the approach to a signed junction, 1.1 miles from the junction. The trail straight ahead travels 0.2 mile to aptly named Grass Lake, which becomes less of a lake and more of a meadow as the season progresses.

Veering right at the junction, continue climbing through pine forest. Switchbacks resume where the trail becomes steep, rocky, and exposed near some cliffs, from where you have views of Grass and North Lakes. Eventually leaving the views behind, proceed through light forest, climbing another set of switchbacks. Pass above a small pond on the right, and then soon spy the lower lake through the trees. A short descent leads to a crossing of the outlet and then up to Lower Lamarck Lake (10,662 feet), 2.4 miles from the trailhead.

Lower Lamarck Lake is quite scenic, tucked beneath steep granite cliffs and backdropped by the triangular summit of Peak 12153. Clumps of limber pine shade a number of overused campsites near the outlet and slightly less-used sites above the northeast shore. Fishing for rainbow and brook trout should be fair.

From the lower lake, follow the trail through the rocky wash of Lamarck Creek. A series of short-legged switchbacks take you above and then down to a crossing of the creek. From there, continue upstream along the northwest bank through tiny meadows dotted with pines to where the creek exits Upper Lamarck Lake, 3 miles from the trailhead.

The stark surroundings of Upper Lamarck Lake, tucked into a narrow, steep-walled slot seem less hospitable than the lower lake. The only break in the cliffs and talus is found where some stunted pines cling desperately to the shallow soil on a rise above the southeast shore, where you may find campsites. Additional sites are also near some small tarns east of the lake. Upper Lamarck Lake harbors both brook and rainbow trout.

O Lower Lamarck Lake makes a fine base camp for off-trail forays to a string of neighboring lakes and tarns known as the Wonder Lakes. A trail follows the shoreline of the lower lake to the northwest side, where you must climb steeply to exit the lake's basin. A faint use trail, occasionally marked by cairns, follows the left bank of the outlet over rock slabs to the first lake.

Straightforward cross-country travel continues upstream to the higher lakes. The Wonder Lakes are bordered by meadows, scattered pockets of pines, and granite slabs and ramps. Steep cliffs and glacial moraines add a decidedly alpine feel to the area. Less developed campsites around the lower lakes will likely offer a higher degree of solitude than those around Lamarck Lakes. Anglers will find small brook trout in the lower lakes.

R A wilderness permit is required for overnight stays. Campfires are prohibited.

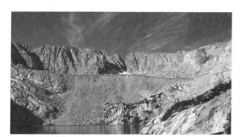

Austere Upper Lamarck Lake

NORTH LAKE TRAILHEAD

TRIP 121

Evolution Basin via Lamarck Col

Ⓜ ✒ DH or BP

DISTANCE: 21 miles, out-and-back

ELEVATION: 9,225'/12,920'/10,852', +4,510'/-1,600'/±12,220'

SEASON: Late July to late October

USE: Light

MAPS: USGS's *Mt. Darwin* or Tom Harrison Maps' *Bishop Pass North Lake-South Lake Loop Trail Map*

TRAIL LOG

1.1	Grass Lake Trail junction
2.4	Lower Lamarck Lake
5.5	Lamarck Col
7.2	Lake 11592
8.0	Darwin Bench
9.6	John Muir Trail
10.5	Evolution Lake

INTRODUCTION: A classic glacier-scoured canyon rimmed by jagged peaks and graced by a string of crystalline lakes makes Evolution Basin one of the premier destinations in the High Sierra. The lengthy distance from a trailhead necessary to reach the basin is perhaps the only reason this incredibly scenic area is not completely overrun by adoring devotees. By maintained trail, the closest trailheads are at South Lake, 23 miles away, and North Lake, 30 miles away. However, armed with a spirit of adventure and the requisite navigational skills, backpackers fluent in off-trail travel can shorten the distance to a mere 10.5 miles by accepting the challenge of this route over 12,920-foot Lamarck Col.

Only a small portion of this route can truly be considered cross-country. Beyond the maintained Lamarck Lakes Trail a

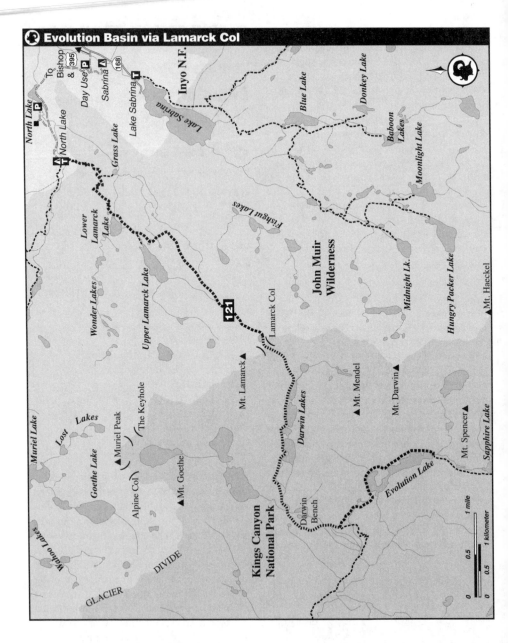

Evolution Basin via Lamarck Col

well-defined use trail leads all the way to a permanent snowfield just below the col. Negotiating the snowfield and the talus-filled, 1,000-foot descent on the far side of the col is the most difficult stretch. Depending on conditions, the moderate-angle snow slope may require an ice axe. Below the col, clambering over boulders and ankle-twisting talus can be quite tedious. Once you reach Darwin Lakes, you can follow a use trail from there to verdant, pond-dotted Darwin Bench and then all the way down the north wall of the canyon, with a view across it of The Hermit, to connect to the John Muir Trail (JMT) just below beautiful Evolution Basin.

The route to Lamarck Col is physically demanding, gaining more than 3,600 feet in 5.5 miles. Additionally, at nearly 13,000 feet, the altitude presents dual concerns about proper acclimatization and the potential for afternoon lightning storms. All but very strong parties should opt to camp the first night at one of the Lamarck Lakes instead of climbing over the col in one day. Descending poor footing below the col when you are fatigued is not a smart idea. Although it is not as technically challenging as many cross-country routes over the Sierra Crest, the Lamarck Col route should not be taken lightly.

While Evolution Basin may be the ultimate goal of this trip, there are additional highlights to consider along the way, as well as optional destinations beyond. The austere setting of Darwin Lakes and Darwin Canyon is quite scenic in its own right and offers a degree of solitude rare for this section of the High Sierra. Above the lakes, the towering cliffs of the Sierra Crest and Mt. Mendel and Mt. Darwin, with ice-filled couloirs and clinging pocket glaciers, create an alpine ambiance as dramatic as any in the range. Darwin Bench, although only a mere 400 vertical feet below the lakes, experiences enough of an altitude difference to create a completely different subalpine environment, composed of delightful tarns, bordered by sparkling slabs of granite and pockets of lovely, wildflower-covered meadows.

DIRECTIONS TO TRAILHEAD: From Bishop, leave US 395, and turn west onto Line Drive, which is known as South Lake Road and Highway 168 outside of town. Proceed southwest 15 miles to a junction with Lake Sabrina Road. Continue ahead for 3 miles to the North Lake Road junction, and turn right. Follow single-lane, gravel road 1 mile to the day-use parking lot. Backpackers must travel another 0.6 mile to a right-hand turn onto a short spur leading to dual overnight parking lots directly west of North Lake.

DESCRIPTION: From either the day-use or overnight parking lots, begin the journey by hiking up the road toward North Lake Campground (1 mile from the day-use lot, 0.7 mile from the overnight lot). The trailhead is just beyond a sign at the entrance to the campground.

From the trailhead, follow single-track trail through aspens and pines through the campground to junction near the far end. Bear left, cross a trio of willow-lined

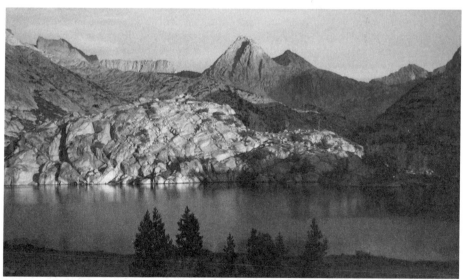

Sunset at Evolution Lake

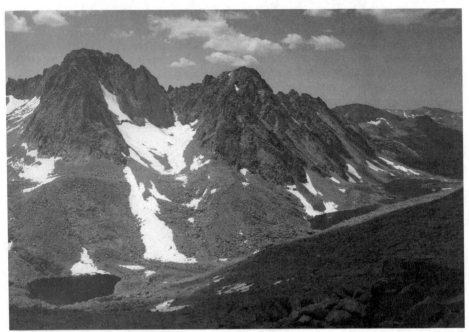

Darwin Lakes from Lamarck Col

branches of North Fork Bishop Creek on wood-plank bridges, and then climb moderately steeply up a hillside via switchbacks, passing beneath aspen and lodgepole pine cover. Limber pines join the mixed forest, where you approach a signed junction, 1.1 miles from the junction. The trail straight ahead travels 0.2 mile to aptly named Grass Lake, which becomes less of a lake and more of a meadow as the season progresses.

Veering right at the junction, continue climbing through pine forest. Switchbacks resume where the trail becomes steep, rocky, and exposed near some cliffs, from where you have views of Grass and North Lakes. Eventually leaving the views behind, proceed through light forest, climbing another set of switchbacks. Pass above a small pond on the right, and then soon spy the lower lake through the trees. A short descent leads to a crossing of the outlet and then up to Lower Lamarck Lake (10,662 feet), 2.4 miles from the trailhead.

Lower Lamarck Lake is quite scenic, tucked beneath steep granite cliffs and backdropped by the triangular summit of

Peak 12153. Clumps of limber pine shade a number of overused campsites near the outlet and slightly less-used sites above the northeast shore. Fishing for rainbow and brook trout should be fair.

From the lower lake, follow the trail through the rocky wash of Lamarck Creek. A series of short-legged switchbacks take you above and then down to a crossing of the creek. From there, continue upstream along the northwest bank through tiny meadows dotted with pines. Keep your eyes peeled for a use trail on the left, which departs the main trail several hundred yards before reaching Upper Lamarck Lake.

Cross the creek, and make a short climb up the rise to the southeast. Continue up the use trail past campsites and a small pond to a sloping meadow bisected by a gurgling stream. With the aid of cairns, make a winding ascent beside boulders and rocks up a steep hillside to the crest of a ridge, from where there are good views of Grass Lake, Lamarck Lakes, North Lake, Lake Sabrina, Owens Valley, and the White Mountains beyond.

The grade eases as you follow the route around the left side of a ridge through widely scattered pines to a lushly vegetated hillside, well watered by seasonal seeps. Leaving this oasis behind, zigzag more steeply up an arid hillside to an ascending traverse. Farther on, more climbing is necessary to surmount another hill, after which the trail heads into a sloping valley angling up toward the Sierra Crest. Proceed up the vale toward the perennial snowfield with a small tarn at the base just below the col. Carefully cross the snowfield and continue over some rock to Lamarck Col (12,920 feet), 5.5 miles from the trailhead. This lofty aerie offers a stunning view of Mt. Mendel, Mt. Darwin, and the Darwin Glacier, as well as the Darwin Lakes below backdropped by the deep cleft of Evolution Creek.

Aside from the brief crossing of the snowfield on the east side of the col, you should be able to follow discernible tread all the way to the col in an average season. However, the descent to Darwin Lakes is another matter. You'll probably have to pick your way down the boulder- and talus-filled slope without aid of a maintained trail. Although it can be tedious while carrying a full backpack, the route to the lakes is clear. The going becomes easier once you reach Lake 11623 (the middle lake), where a faint path runs along the north shore. There are a few decent campsites near the shore of the next lake, Lake 11592, 7.2 miles from the trailhead.

Past the lakes, continue following the faint tread of the use trail along the stream draining Darwin Canyon to beautiful, tarn-dotted Darwin Bench (approximately 11,225 feet), 8 miles from the trailhead. After the time-consuming descent of the barren, rock-filled terrain above the lakes, this area seems to be an even more verdant oasis. Little-used campsites scattered around the bench offer beautiful vistas across Evolution Valley.

Leaving Darwin Bench, swing south on a 0.75-mile traverse across a series of granite benches toward the JMT. Your goal is to meet the famed trail near the top of the switchbacks coming up from Evolution Valley at approximately 10,700 feet. From there, Evolution Lake is a mile-long stroll southeast on the well-trod trail. There are good campsites near the small peninsula on the northwest shore and by the outlet.

O Multiday options abound once you reach Evolution Basin, including a variety of loops to North Lake for those who don't want to simply backtrack to the trailhead. The most straightforward alternative is to head northbound on the JMT through Evolution Valley to a junction with the Piute Pass Trail, then up through Piute Canyon and Humphreys Basin before cresting the range at Piute Pass and then dropping to North Lake.

Experienced cross-country travelers have even more to choose from. More technically challenging routes over Glacier Divide at The Keyhole (approximately 12,520 feet, Class 3), Alpine Col (approximately 12,320 feet, Class 2), or Snow Tongue Pass (approximately 12,200 feet, Class 2–3) access Humphreys Basin and a connection with the Piute Pass Trail back to the North Lake Trailhead.

Nontechnical mountaineers have a pair of ascents to consider. From Lamarck Col, Lamarck Peak is a straightforward Class 2 climb. The south slope of 13,264-foot Mt. Goethe is an easy Class 1 ascent from the isthmus between Lakes 11540 and 11546 from the basin just northwest of Darwin Canyon.

R A wilderness permit is required for overnight stays. Campfires are prohibited.

TRIP 122

Piute Pass Trail to Humphreys Basin and Piute Canyon

MS / **DH, BP**, or **BPx**

DISTANCE: 14 miles, out-and-back to Humphreys Basin

34 miles, out-and-back to the John Muir Trail

ELEVATION: 9,225'/11,423'/10,800', +2,175'/-450'/±5,250'

9,225'/11,423'/8,075', +2,600'/-3,800'/±12,800'

SEASON: Mid-July to late October

USE: Moderate

MAPS: USGS's *Mt. Darwin, Mt. Tom, Mt. Hilgard,* and *Mt. Henry* or Tom Harrison Maps' *Bishop Pass North Lake-South Lake Loop Trail Map*

TRAIL LOG

2.2	Loch Leven
3.3	Piute Lake
4.6	Piute Pass
7.1	Lower Golden Trout Lake
11.9	Hutchinson Meadow and Pine Creek Pass Trail junction
17.0	John Muir Trail

INTRODUCTION: Just north of the Glacier Divide, which forms the north boundary of Kings Canyon National Park, is a large, lake-dotted alpine basin rivaling any in the High Sierra for sweeping beauty. You will spend most of the effort required to reach such mountain splendor on a moderate, 4.6-mile climb along a well-maintained trail to 11,423-foot Piute Pass. A gentle descent from there propels you toward a bountiful assortment of pristine lakes and tarns sprinkled across the wide expanse of Hum-

phreys Basin. Since the Piute Pass Trail is the only maintained path through the basin, reaching most of the lakes requires following use trails or traveling cross-country. A base camp in Humphreys Basin may well be an off-trail enthusiast's nirvana, with straightforward travel over open terrain to a plethora of picturesque lakes. Piercing the skyline above the basin is a fine assortment of high peaks, culminating in 13,986-foot Mt. Humphreys, guardian of the basin, whose airy summit is a feather in any mountaineer's cap since the least difficult route to the top is rated Class 4.

Backpackers blessed with more time can continue from Humphreys Basin down Piute Canyon to a connection with the John Muir Trail (JMT). From there, you have many options for extended trips, including a fairly popular route southbound to the Bishop Pass Trail and then a climb over Bishop Pass to the South Lake Trailhead (which requires a short shuttle between trailheads).

With elevations around 11,000 feet, Humphreys Basin requires proper acclimatization, especially for hikers residing near sea level. Spending the night before your trip at one of the many Forest Service campgrounds in the area would be a great help to the process. Additionally, the open terrain at this altitude is no place to be during a lightning storm.

DIRECTIONS TO TRAILHEAD: From Bishop, leave US 395, and turn west onto Line Drive, which is known as South Lake Road and Highway 168 outside of town. Proceed southwest 15 miles to a junction with Lake Sabrina Road. Continue ahead for 3 miles to the North Lake Road junction, and turn right. Follow single-lane, gravel road 1 mile to the day-use parking lot. Backpackers must travel another 0.6 mile to a right-hand turn onto a short spur leading to dual overnight parking lots directly west of North Lake.

DESCRIPTION: From either the day-use or overnight parking lots, begin the journey by hiking up the road toward North Lake Campground (1 mile from the day-use lot, 0.7 mile from the overnight lot).

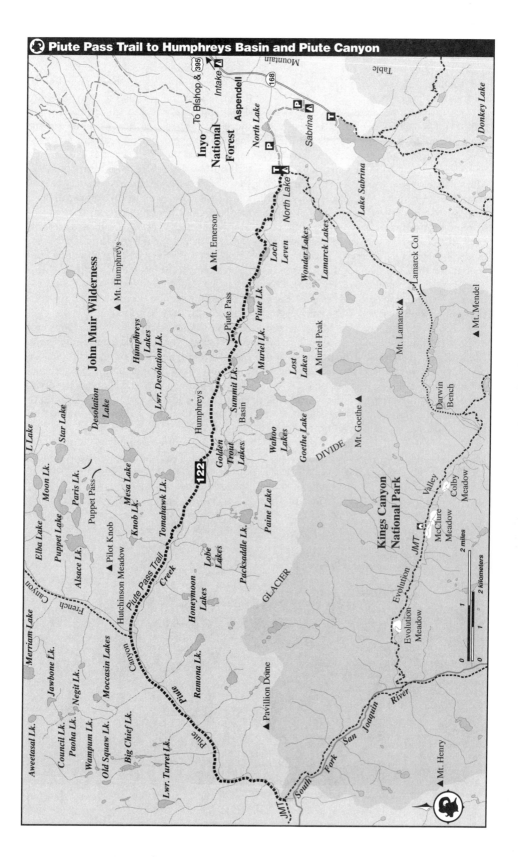

The trailhead is just beyond a sign at the entrance to the campground.

From the trailhead, follow single-track trail through aspens and pines through the campground to junction near the far end. Veer right at the junction, and follow the Piute Pass Trail, soon passing into John Muir Wilderness. Climb gently through aspen groves, stands of lodgepole pines, and meadow patches dotted with seasonal wildflowers. Beyond a pair of crossings of North Fork Bishop Creek, the grade increases to moderate, where a series of switchbacks lead above the canyon floor, followed by a long, gently ascending traverse. Fine views include a waterfall on the North Fork plunging steeply out of the basin above, Peak 12691 on the left, and Mt. Emerson and the multihued Piute Crags on the right. Rock steps and more switchbacks take you up the narrowing canyon through diminishing lodgepole pines and limber pines.

At 2.2 miles, surmount a headwall, and reach the shore of Loch Leven (10,700 feet), which has picnic spots and overused, exposed campsites scattered around its shore. You may find more solitude around rockbound Emerson Lake (11,219 feet), accessible via a 0.3-mile cross-country route from Loch Leven's southeast shore. Anglers may find the fishing for brook and rainbow trout to be fair at Piute Lake.

From Piute Lake, head northwest toward timberline, climbing over granite slabs and passing through meadowlands sliced by refreshing brooks and dotted with tiny ponds. A final traverse leads to 11,423-foot Piute Pass, 4.6 miles from the trailhead, from where you have stunning views both near and far. Immediately below and to the west is the wide expanse of scenic, lake-dotted Humphreys Basin, towered over to the southwest by the rugged crest of Glacier Divide, including Muriel Peak and Mt. Goethe. To the north, the dramatic and impressive profile of Mt. Humphreys tops out just below 14,000 feet. To the west, distinctive Pilot Knob rises above the deep cleft of the South Fork San Joaquin River.

If decision-making is not your long suit, you'll surely be troubled in Humphreys Basin, where myriad lakes tempt you in every direction. A modicum of navigational skill will allow you to travel across the open basin to a wide variety of destinations. If you are willing to leave the security of maintained trail, you have ample opportunities for bountiful amounts of solitude and exploration. Enjoying the numerous ponds, tarns, and lakes could consume several splendid days.

If Muriel Lake is your goal, find a use trail heading southwest from just below Piute Pass. Otherwise, follow a winding

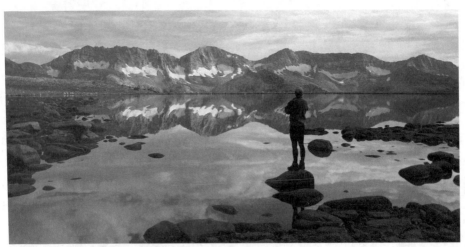

Mesa Lake and the Glacier Divide

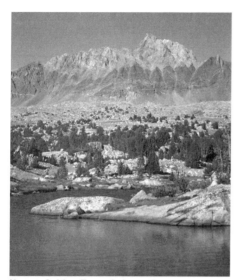

Upper Golden Trout Lake and Mt. Humphreys

descent down the Piute Pass Trail, passing hummocks of granite and tiny brooks coursing through verdant meadows on the way around Summit Lake (11,225 feet), where anglers may see brook trout gliding through pale blue waters. The trail passes well above the level of the lake and then continues on gently descending tread through the basin. Approximately 1.5 miles from the pass, reach a junction with use trails branching both north and southwest. The more heavily used path heading southwest travels nearly a mile to the popular Golden Trout Lakes, where camping is prohibited within 500 feet of Lower Golden Trout Lake (10,786 feet). The north-trending path leads up to large, aptly named Desolation Lake (11,375 feet), which provides a fine base camp for short jaunts to smaller, neighboring lakes.

The Piute Pass Trail is a gateway to some of Kings Canyon's most impressive scenery. By continuing westward from Humphreys Basin, you descend through increasingly dense lodgepole pine forest to subalpine gardens lining Piute Creek, where a wide array of wildflowers splash color across the green meadowlands through midseason. At 11.9 miles, you cross the braided creek draining French Canyon and reach fine

campsites in Hutchinson Meadow (9,438 feet) near a junction with the Pine Creek Pass Trail heading north. From the meadow, you have picturesque views of Pilot Knob and the surrounding peaks and ridges. Anglers may find the fishing for rainbow and golden trout good in both Piute and French Canyons.

Away from Hutchinson Meadow, descend gently through lodgepole pine forest to a ford of East Pinnacles Creek. Beyond the ford, the rate of descent increases on an oftentimes rocky, sometimes winding trail down the canyon toward South Fork San Joaquin River below. Follow plunging Piute Creek to an easy ford of West Pinnacles Creek, across a pair of bridged crossings over gullies. The trail bends south and soon crosses braided Turret Creek. Eventually, the lodgepole forest gives way to chaparral, granting fine views of Pavilion Dome to the east. Continue the rocky descent along Piute Creek to a junction with the JMT, 17 miles from the North Lake Trailhead. There are plenty of good campsites near the junction.

Possibilities for additional wanderings in Humphreys Basin are too numerous to adequately detail. The basin is a cross-country enthusiast's delight. Generally, the terrain south of the trail below Glacier Divide offers steep-walled cirques filled with talus. North of the trail, the terrain is more rolling and open. Technically challenging routes over Glacier Divide include The Keyhole (approximately 12,520 feet, Class 3), Alpine Col (approximately 12,320 feet, Class 2), and Snow Tongue Pass (approximately 12,200 feet, Class 2–3). Puppet Pass (Class 2) offers a relatively easy route from Desolation Lake to a handful of lakes on a bench above French Canyon. You can take a fine loop trip by descending from the bench into French Canyon and then heading down the Piute Creek Pass Trail back to the Piute Pass Trail.

A wilderness permit is required for overnight stays. Camping within 500 feet of Lower Golden Trout Lake is prohibited. Campfires are also prohibited.

Appendices

Highest Peaks and Largest Giant Sequoias in Sequoia and Kings Canyon National Parks

\multicolumn{7}{c}{Highest Peaks in the Sierra Nevada}
Rank in CA	Rank in Sierra	Name	Feet	Meters	USGS 7.5-minute quad
I	I	Mt. Whitney	14,484	4,418	*Mount Whitney*
2	2	Mt. Williamson	14,375	4,382	*Mt. Williamson*
4	3	North Palisade	14,242	4,334	*North Palisade*
6	4	Mt. Sill	14,153	4,314	*North Palisade*
7	5	Mt. Russell	14,086	4,293	*Mt. Whitney*
8	6	Split Mountain	14,058	4,293	*Split Mountain*
9	7	Middle Palisade	14,040	4,279	*Split Mountain*
10	8	Mt. Langley	14,028	4,275	*Mt. Langley*
11	9	Mt. Tyndall	14,018	4,273	*Mt. Williamson*
12	10	Mt. Muir	14,009	4,270	*Mount Whitney*
13	11	Thunderbolt Peak	14,003	4,268	*North Palisade*

Note: Although several points in the Sierra are higher than some of the mountains listed above, they are not considered peaks. Among these subpeaks are Keeler Needle (14,272 feet), Starlight Peak (14,220 feet), West Horn of Mt. Williamson (14,160 feet), East Horn of Mt. Williamson (14,125 feet), and Polemonium Peak (14,000 feet). Mount Shasta (14,162 feet), in the Cascade range in far northern California, is the fifth largest peak in California.

Largest Giant Sequoias in Sequoia and Kings Canyon National Parks

Rank in CA	Rank in SEKI	Name	Volume (cubic feet)	Height (feet)	Circumference (feet)	Location
1	1	General Sherman	52,508	274.9	102.6	Giant Forest
2	2	Washington	47,950	254.7	101.1	Giant Forest
3	3	General Grant	46,608	268.1	107.6	Grant Grove
4	4	President	45,148	240.9	93.0	Giant Forest
5	5	Lincoln	44,471	255.8	98.3	Giant Forest
8	6	Boole Tree	42,472	268.8	113.0	Converse Basin
9	7	Franklin	41,280	223.8	94.8	Giant Forest
10	8	King Arthur	40,656	270.3	104.2	Garfield Grove
11	9	Monroe	40,104	247.8	91.3	Giant Forest
12	10	Robert E. Lee	40,102	254.7	88.3	Grant Grove
13	11	John Adams	38,956	250.6	83.3	Giant Forest
14	12	Ishi Giant	38,156	248.1	105.1	Kennedy Grove
15	13	Unnamed	37,295	243.8	93.0	Giant Forest
17	14	Unnamed	36,292	239.4	75.5	Giant Forest
18	15	Unnamed	36,228	281.5	95.1	Giant Forest
21	16	Pershing	35,855	246.0	91.2	Giant Forest
22	17	Diamond	35,292	286.0	95.3	Atwell Grove
24	18	Roosevelt	35,013	260.0	80.0	Redwood Mountain
26	19	(AD)	34,706	242.4	99.0	Atwell Grove
27	20	Hart	34,407	277.9	75.3	Redwood Mountain
29	21	Chief Sequoyah	33,608	228.2	90.4	Giant Forest

APPENDIX II
Contact Information

General	
Campground reservations (NPS and USFS)	877-444-6777 www.recreation.gov
CalTrans (road conditions)	800-427-7623 www.dot.ca.gov/
United States Geological Survey (USGS)	888-275-8747 www.usgs.gov/

Inyo National Forest	
Information	760-873-2400 www.fs.usda.gov/inyo
Eastern Sierra Inter Agency Visitor Center	760-876-6222
Mt. Whitney Ranger District	760-876-6200
White Mountain Ranger District	760-873-2500
Wilderness Permit Office	760-873-2485 (information) 760-873-2483 (reservations) 760-873-2484 (fax)

Sequoia and Kings Canyon National Parks	
Information	559-565-9700 (phone) 559-565-3730 (fax) www.nps.gov/seki/
Wilderness Office	559-565-3766 (phone) 559-565-4239 (fax)
Sequoia Natural History Association	559-565-3759 (phone) 559-565-3728 (fax) www.sequoiahistory.org

Giant Sequoia National Monument	
Information	559-781-4744 www.fs.fed.us/r5/sequoia/gsnm.html
High Sierra Ranger District	559-855-5355
Hume Lake Ranger District	559-338-2251

Lodging

Delaware North Park Services (Wuksachi)   888-252-5757
www.nps.gov/seki/planyourvisit/lodging

Kings Canyon Park Services   866-522-6966
(John Muir Lodge, Grant Grove Cabins,   www.nps.gov/seki/planyourvisit/lodging
and Cedar Grove Lodge)

Kings Canyon Lodge   559-335-2405

Montecito Sequoia Lodge   800-227-9900,
www.montecitosequoialodge.com

Silver City Resort   559-561-3223
www.silvercityresort.com

Stony Creek Lodge   866-522-6966
www.sequoia-kingscanyon.com/
stonycreeklodge

Suggested Reading

Arnot, Phil. *High Sierra: John Muir's Range of Light*. San Carlos, CA: Wide World Publishing/Tetra, 1996.

Backpacking California. Berkeley, CA: Wilderness Press, 2008.

Blehm, Eric. *The Last Season*. New York City: Harper Collins, 2008.

Browning, Peter, ed. *Splendid Mountains: Early Explorations in the Sierra Nevada*. Lafayette, CA: Great West Books, 2007.

Cutter, Ralph. *Sierra Trout Guide*. Portland, OR: Frank Amato Publications, 1991.

Dilslayer, Larry M., and William C. Tweed. *Challenge of the Big Trees*. Three Rivers, CA: Sequoia Natural History Association, 1991.

Farquhar, Francis P. *History of the Sierra Nevada*. 2nd edition. Berkeley, CA: UC Press, 2007.

Horn, Elizabeth L. *Sierra Nevada Wildflowers*. Missoula, MT: Mountain Press Publishing Company, 1998.

Jackson, Louise A. *Beulah: A Biography of the Mineral King Valley of California*. Tucson, AZ: Westernlore Press, 1988.

Johnston, Verna R. *Sierra Nevada: The Naturalist's Companion*. Berkeley, CA: UC Press, 2000.

Krist, John. *50 Best Hikes in Yosemite and Sequoia/Kings Canyon*. Berkeley, CA: Wilderness Press, 1993.

Moore, James G. *Exploring the Highest Sierra*. Stanford, CA: Stanford UP, 2000.

Morey, Kathy. *Hot Showers, Soft Beds, and Dayhikes in the Sierra Nevada*. 3rd edition. Berkeley, CA: Wilderness Press, 2008.

———, Mike White, et al. *Sierra South: Backcountry Trips in California's Sierra Nevada*. Berkeley, CA: Wilderness Press, 2006.

Petrides, George A., and Olivia Petrides. *Trees of the California Sierra Nevada*. Mechanicsburg, PA: Stackpole Books, 2005.

Roper, Steve. *The Climber's Guide to the High Sierra*. San Francisco, CA: Sierra Club Books, 1995.

———. *The Sierra High Route: Traversing Timberline Country*. 2nd edition. Seattle, WA: The Mountaineers Books, 1997.

Secor, R. J. *The High Sierra: Peaks, Passes, and Trails*. 3rd edition. Seattle, WA: The Mountaineers Books, 2009.

Smith, Genny, ed. *Sierra East: Edge of the Great Basin*. Berkeley, CA: UC Press, 2000.

Sorensen, Steve. *Day Hiking Sequoia.* Three Rivers, CA: Fuyu Press, 1996.

Stone, Robert. *Day Hikes in Sequoia and Kings Canyon.* Red Lodge, MT: Day Hike Books, Inc., 2001.

Strong, Douglas H. *From Pioneers to Preservationists, A Brief History of Sequoia and Kings Canyon National Parks.* Three Rivers, CA: Sequoia Natural History Association, 2000.

Tweed, William. *Beneath the Giants: A Guide to the Moro Rock-Crescent Meadow Road of Sequoia National Park.* Three Rivers, CA: Sequoia Natural History Association, 1986.

———. *Kaweah Remembered.* Three Rivers, CA: Sequoia Natural History Association, 1986.

Weeden, Norman F. *A Sierra Nevada Flora.* 4th edition. Berkeley, CA: Wilderness Press, 1996.

Wenk, Elizabeth, with Kathy Morey. *John Muir Trail: The Essential Guide to Hiking America's Most Famous Trail.* Berkeley, CA: Wilderness Press, 2010.

Index

About the Author

Mike White was raised in the suburbs of Portland, Oregon, in the shadow of Mt. Hood (whenever the Pacific Northwest skies cleared enough to allow such things as shadows). As a teenager, Mike began hiking, backpacking, and climbing in the Cascades of Oregon and Washington and then honed his outdoor skills while attending Seattle Pacific University. After he acquired a B.A. in political science, Mike and his new wife, Robin, relocated to the high desert of Reno, Nevada, from where he discovered the joys of exploring the Sierra Nevada. After leaving his last "real" job, he began a full-time writing career. He is the author or coauthor of seventeen outdoor guides, including award-winning books *Top Trails Lake Tahoe* and *50 Classic Hikes in Nevada*. He also has contributed to *Sunset* and *Backpacker* magazines and the *Reno Gazette Journal* newspaper. A former community college instructor, Mike is also a popular featured speaker for outdoor groups.

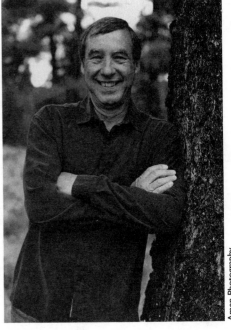

Amen Photography